Optical Mapping of Cardiac Excitation and Arrhythmias

Edited by

David S. Rosenbaum, MD

Director, Heart and Vascular Research Center
Associate Professor of Medicine,
Biomedical Engineering, and
Physiology and Biophysics
MetroHealth Campus
Case Western Reserve University
Cleveland, Ohio

and

José Jalife, MD

Professor and Chairman of Pharmacology
Professor of Medicine and Pediatrics
SUNY Upstate Medical University
Syracuse, New York

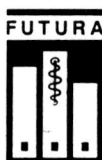

FUTURA

Futura Publishing Company, Inc.
Armonk, NY

Library of Congress Cataloging-in-Publication Data

Optical mapping of cardiac excitation and arrhythmias / edited by David S. Rosenbaum and José Jalife.
    p. ; cm.
  Includes bibliographical references and index.
  ISBN 0-87993-481-6 (alk. paper)
  1. Arrhythmia—Imaging. 2. Electroluminescent devices. 3. Electrophysiology. 4. Heart—Contraction. 5. Fluorescence microscopy. 6. Video microscopy. I. Rosenbaum, David S. II. Jalife, José.
  [DNLM: 1. Arrhythmia—diagnosis. 2. Diagnostic Imaging. 3. Electric Countershock. 4. Microscopy, Fluorescence. 5. Microscopy, Video. WG 330 062 2001]
  RC685.A65 O65 2001
  616.1′2807547—dc21

                                                                00-054355

Published by
Futura Publishing Company
135 Bedford Road
Armonk, New York 10504
www.futuraco.com

LC#: 00-054355
ISBN#: 0-87993-481-6

Printed in the United States of America on acid-free paper.

Dedication and Acknowledgments

The editors are extremely grateful to Paloma Jalife and Anita, Ben, and Elliot Rosenbaum for their unwavering love and support. We are also grateful to Rose Viskovic for her tireless assistance in the preparation of this book. We thank the research trainees, past and present, of the Heart and Vascular Research Center at Case Western Reserve University and the Heart Group of the Department of Pharmacology at SUNY Syracuse for their inspiration and friendship. Finally, we gratefully acknowledge the support of Guidant and Medtronic in our scientific endeavors.

This book is dedicated to the memory of Benjamin C. Rosenbaum (DSR's father), who showed all around him how to achieve excellence with grace, charitableness, and humor.

Foreword

The concept of mapping rhythmic activation of the heart is nearly 100 years old. From the first time that Mayer[1] watched rhythmic muscular contraction around the ring of a jellyfish in 1906, to Mines'[2] description and mapping of reentry in the turtle heart, to the first systematic mapping of sinus rhythm and then atrial flutter by Lewis et al.,[3] the importance of activation mapping to understand the mechanisms and locations of arrhythmias has continued to evolve. Barker et al.[4] were the first to map the human heart. During most of the middle two thirds of the 20th century, the discussions about mapping related primarily to describing unipolar versus bipolar signals and relating them to local activation as well as to determining the effects of pathologic abnormalities in myocardium on these recordings.[5] The first mapping was performed primarily using single probes moved to different positions in the heart. Durrer and his group in Amsterdam[6] had developed computerized mapping of the epicardium of the human heart. Computerized mapping was first used in the Wolf-Parkinson-White syndrome, and eventually led to the surgical cure of this arrhythmia. In 1970, Durrer et al.[7] also used computerized mapping of the entire human heart in Langendorff preparations. The ability to record activation from several hundred sites simultaneously has expanded our knowledge of atrial and ventricular arrhythmias in experimental preparations and, to a lesser extent, in humans.

The technical problems associated with amplifications, gains, sampling rates, signal-to-noise ratio, and the inability to see signals during high-voltage shocks, led to the development and use of voltage-sensitive dyes as a means to map not only activation, but recovery. Voltage-sensitive dyes, when excited, provide an optical signal that mimics an action potential and thus allows one to see both the activation and recovery processes at the same time in any region under view. This allows one to precisely evaluate the propagation of a wave of excitation and to measure its wavelength visually. This was a great step above multisite acquisition mapping with extracellular electrograms, by which only activation times can be obtained. The refractory periods can never be simultaneously measured with current standard extracellular mapping techniques. Heterogeneity of refractoriness and activation times can only be simultaneously assessed using these optical techniques. The ability to accurately evaluate simultaneously both the activation and recovery properties of a tissue allows one to determine the exact mechanism of initiation, maintenance, and termination of reentrant arrhythmias, and to assess the roles of curvature and anisotropy of the propagation of activation wave front.

Optical mapping techniques use discrete photodiodes and a planar detector array and imaging devices such as charged-coupled device video cameras with the heart being illuminated and either continuously or spatially scanned. This permits very high spatial resolution. Laser scanning has also been used to evaluate intact hearts, although the spatial resolution is less. The basis for all these techniques is the use of voltage-sensitive dyes that bind to or interact with cell membranes. These dyes can transduce changes in membrane voltage into optical signals that are linearly related to those voltage changes during both depolarization and repolarization. While the voltage changes mimic the time course of an action potential, these are not identical to action potentials, since no absolute level of membrane potential is recorded. The technique is also limited by contraction artifacts (deflections), which require, in many cases, a calcium-free environment, paralysis of the muscle, or calcium blockers in order to allow assessment of the repolarization components. Optical mapping also does not provide intramural data and hence is not as useful as some extracellular electrograms, which can provide information about interactions of wavefronts. The major advantages of optical mapping systems are their insensitivity to artifacts from high-voltage shocks allowing for the study of defibrillation of both the atrium and the ventricle, the ability to assess propagation in very small cells or sheets of cells which are not amenable to standard microelectrode techniques, and the ability to see impulse propagation and heterogeneity of recovery at the same time. These advantages have led to widespread and growing use of voltage-sensitive dyes in experimental cardiac electrophysiology research.

This text is the only resource for the basic science investigators as well as clinical electrophysiologists who are interested in the application of optical mapping techniques to cardiac electrophysiology. The book is divided into four sections, all of which are written by leaders in the field. The first section discusses the basic principles of optical mapping from a historical perspective and a mechanistic view. The second section discusses the use of optical mapping in the study of propagation and repolarization of the cardiac impulse. This section not only covers normal propagation in homogeneous cardiac tissue, but also discusses intercellular coupling and structural discontinuities associated with the influence of tissue anisotropy on the propagation to and through the atrioventricular junction. The third section of the text deals with cardiac arrhythmias and the role of optical mapping in studying these arrhythmias. Specifically discussed are the role of the concept of the cardiac wavelength in the mechanism of initiation and perpetuation of reentrant arrhythmias, optical mapping of ischemic substrates of ventricular tachyarrhythmias and video imaging of cardiac fibrillation, and the role of spiral waves in mechanisms of arrhythmias, and finally studies in transgenic mice with cardiomyopathy in which the proarrhythmic substrate is explored. The final section is on cardiac defibrillation. As noted earlier, optical mapping provides a unique opportunity to study the mechanism of defibrillation of cardiac tissue, since these dyes are insensitive to high-voltage shocks. This section includes the most up-to-date information regarding the mechanism of defibrillation. Each of the last three sections is followed by a discussion by a clinical investigative electrophysiologist to evaluate the application of optical mapping in current and future research.

In sum, this book is a unique addition to any library on electrophysiology. It bridges the gap between basic science and clinical electrophysiology. The ability to bridge cellular and clinical electrophysiology with optical mapping techniques will surely lead to a better understanding of arrhythmogenesis, of the mechanism of action of antiarrhythmic agents, and of the mechanism of defibrillation, all of which will ultimately lead to better care of our patients. Drs. Rosenbaum and Jalife should be immensely proud of this text, which will serve as a resource for all those interested in new methods to enhance our understanding of cardiac electrophysiology.

MARK E. JOSEPHSON, MD
Professor of Medicine
Harvard Medical School
Boston, MA

References

1. Mayer AG. *Rhythmical Pulsation in Scyphomedusae.* Washington, DC: Carnegie Institution of Washington, Publication 47. 1906:1–62.
2. Mines GR. On dynamic equilibrium in the heart. *J Physiol* 1913;46:349–382.
3. Lewis T, Feil S, Stroud WD. II. The nature of auricular flutter. *Heart* 1920;7:131–346.
4. Barker PS, Mcleod AG, Alexander J. The excitatory process observed in the exposed human heart. *Am Heart J* 1930;5:720–742.
5. Durrer D, Formijne P, Van Dam RTN, et al. The electrogram in normal and some abnormal condition. *Am Heart J* 1961;61:303–314.
6. Durrer D, Roos JP. Epicardial exultation of the ventricles in a patient with Wolf-Parkinson-White Syndrome (type B). *Circulation* 1967;35:15–21.
7. Durrer D, Van Dam RT, Frend GE, et al. Total excitation of the isolated human heart. *Circulation* 1970;41:899–912.

Contributors

William T. Baxter, PhD Research Scientist, Wadsworth Laboratories, Albany, NY

Yuanna Cheng, MD Research Associate, Department of Cardiology, The Cleveland Clinic Foundation, Cleveland, OH

Bum-Rak Choi Departments of Cell Biology and Physiology, University of Pittsburgh, Pittsburgh, PA

Jorge M. Davidenko, MD Research Associate Professor, Department of Pharmacology, SUNY Health Science Center, Syracuse, NY

Stephen M. Dillon, PhD University of Pennsylvania Health System, Division of Cardiovascular Medicine, Philadelphia, PA

Igor R. Efimov, PhD Elmer L. Lindseth Associate Professor of Biomedical Engineering, Case Western Reserve University, Cleveland, OH

Vladimir G. Fast, PhD Research Assistant Professor, Department of Biomedical Engineering, University of Alabama at Birmingham, Birmingham, AL

Steven D. Girouard, PhD Research Associate, Department of Biomedical Engineering, MetroHealth Campus, Case Western Reserve University, Cleveland, OH

Richard A. Gray, PhD Assistant Professor, Biomedical Engineering, Cardiac Rhythm Management Laboratory, University of Alabama at Birmingham, Birmingham, AL

José Jalife, MD Professor and Chairman of Pharmacology, Professor of Medicine and Pediatrics, SUNY Upstate Medical University, Syracuse, NY

André G. Kléber, MD Professor of Physiology, Department of Physiology, University of Bern, Bern, Switzerland

Stephen B. Knisley, PhD Associate Professor, Department of Biomedical Engineering of the School of Medicine, The University of North Carolina at Chapel Hill, Chapel Hill, NC

Jan P. Kucera, MD Research Fellow, Department of Physiology, University of Bern, Bern, Switzerland

Kevin F. Kwaku, MD, PhD   Cardiology Fellow, Beth Israel Deaconess Medical Center, Cardiovascular Division, Harvard Medical School, Boston, MA

Kenneth R. Laurita, PhD   Assistant Professor of Medicine and Biomedical Engineering, MetroHealth Campus, Case Western Reserve University, Cleveland, OH

L. Joshua Leon, PhD   Associate Professor, Department of Electrical and Computer Engineering, University of Calgary, Calgary, Alberta, Canada

Shien-Fong Lin, PhD   Research Assistant Professor of Physics, Living State Physics Group, Department of Physics and Astronomy, Vanderbilt University, Nashville, TN

Leslie M. Loew, PhD   Professor of Physiology, Director, Center for Biomedical Imaging Technology, University of Connecticut Health Center, Farmington, CT

Imad Libbus, MS   Research Associate, Department of Biomedical Engineering, MetroHealth Campus, Case Western Reserve University, Cleveland, OH

Todor N. Mazgalev, PhD   Director, Basic Cardiac Electrophysiology Laboratories, Department of Cardiology, The Cleveland Clinic Foundation, Cleveland, OH

Gregory E. Morley, PhD   Research Assistant Professor, Department of Pharmacology, SUNY Upstate Medical University, Syracuse, NY

Douglas L. Packer, MD   Professor of Medicine, Mayo Graduate School, Mayo Foundation, Rochester, MN

Joseph M. Pastore, PhD   Research Associate, Department of Biomedical Engineering, MetroHealth Campus, Case Western Reserve University, Cleveland, OH

Patricia A. Penkoske, MD   Clinical Professor of Surgery, Department of Surgery, St. Louis University Hospital, St. Louis, MO

Stephan Rohr, MD   Associate Professor, Department of Physiology, University of Bern, Bern, Switzerland

David S. Rosenbaum, MD   Director, Heart and Vascular Research Center, Associate Professor of Medicine, Biomedical Engineering, and Physiology and Biophysics, MetroHealth Campus, Case Western Reserve University, Cleveland, OH

Guy Salama, PhD   Professor of Cell Biology and Physiology, Department of Cell Biology and Physiology, University of Pittsburgh School of Medicine, Pittsburgh, PA

Faramarz Samie, PhD   Fellow, Department of Pharmacology, SUNY Upstate Medical University, Syracuse, NY

Leslie Tung, PhD   Associate Professor of Biomedical Engineering, Department of Biomedical Engineering, The Johns Hopkins University, Baltimore, MD

Dhjananjay Vaidya, PhD   Postdoctoral Research Associate, Department of Pharmacology, SUNY Upstate Medical University, Syracuse, NY

Karen L. Vikstrom, PhD   Assistant Professor, Department of Pharmacology, SUNY Upstate Medical University, Syracuse, NY

Albert L. Waldo, MD   The Walter H. Pritchard Professor of Cardiology, Professor of Medicine, and Professor of Biomedical Engineering, Case Western Reserve University; Director, Clinical Cardiac Electrophysiology Program, University Hospitals of Cleveland, Cleveland, OH

John P. Wikswo, Jr., PhD   A.B. Learned Professor of Living State Physics, Professor of Physics, Living State Physics Group, Department of Physics and Astronomy, Vanderbilt University, Nashville, TN

Herbert Windisch, PhD   Professor, Institut für Medizinische Physik und Biophysik, Karl-Franzens-Universität, Graz, Austria

Francis X. Witkowski, MD, FRCP(c)   Professor, Department of Medicine, University of Alberta School of Medicine, Edmonton, Alberta, Canada

Douglas P. Zipes, MD   Distinguished Professor of Medicine, Pharmacology, and Toxicology, Director of the Krannert Institute of Cardiology and of the Division of Cardiology, Indiana University School of Medicine, Indianapolis, IN

Contents

Section III. Cardiac Arrhythmias

Section IV. Cardiac Defibrillation

Glossary

Absorption: The loss in total light intensity as incident light is directed onto biological media, caused by absorption of light energy by the media. Absorption is dependent on depth of light penetration, the physical characteristics of the tissue, and the wavelength of the incident light.

AC coupling: A technique used to subtract slow, time-dependent variations from a signal.

Acousto-optic deflector: A device that relies on the interaction between a laser beam and ultrasound waves to cause an angular deflection of the laser beam. In optical mapping, this is most often used to excite fluorescence sequentially and rapidly from very small spots on the surface of the heart. By tracking the position of the laser at every point of time, it is possible to map optical action potentials from multiple sites on the heart's surface with a single detector.

Autofluorescence: The fluorescence that tissues emit in the absence of a fluorescent probe; i.e., fluorescence that is intrinsic to the tissue. For example, in the heart autofluorescence of NADH in response to excitation with ultraviolet light can be used to map metabolic activity at multiple sites on the heart.

Beam splitter: A partially opaque mirror that reflects one portion of incident light and transmits the other portion. Often used to direct images to two detectors simultaneously.

Charged coupled device (CCD): The detector used in video cameras; a light-sensitive device that uses metal-oxide semiconductor capacitors to transduce incident photons to electrical potential charges. These charges, which accumulate during image acquisition, are shifted sequentially to neighboring capacitors and eventually shifted off the array where they are read off by an analog-to-digital converter. The amount of charge is related to the intensity of the image at each pixel.

Chromophore: That part of a dye molecule which is responsible for its fluorescent properties, and which reacts to excitation light. Also referred to as a chromophoric group, fluorophore, or fluorophoric group.

Cold mirror: A semitransparent mirror that permits infrared radiation to be transmitted while reflecting the visible portion of light. Used to remove excessive heat (infrared) from an excitation light source.

Dichroic mirror: A beam splitter that has high transmittance to a specific range of wavelengths and high reflectance to other wavelengths. Dichroic mirrors can be manufactured as high-pass, low-pass, or band-pass filters. Its primary use is to allow one to direct excitation and emission light through the same light path for epi-illuminating a preparation.

Emission: Process, analogous to fluorescence, in which light is emitted by a dye molecule upon return (following excitation) to its ground state.

Emission filter: An optical filter through which fluorescent light emitted by a fluorescent probe (e.g., voltage-sensitive dye) is passed for the purpose of isolating fluoresced light emitted by the probe (i.e., the signal of interest) from reflected light emitted from the excitation light source (i.e., noise). In voltage-sensitive dye mapping, these are usually long-pass optical filters.

Emission spectrum: Measured with a spectrofluorometer, indicates the intensity of light fluoresced or emitted by a fluorescent dye molecule (measured during excitation with light of one constant wavelength) as a function of wavelength of the fluoresced light. The emission spectrum of a dye can be used to select the dyes and emission filters used in optical mapping because every dye fluoresces light over a distinct range of wavelengths.

Epi-illumination: A type of fluorescent excitation that uses the same lens to both focus the excitation light onto, and collect emitted light from, the preparation.

Excitation: Process required to elicit fluorescence from voltage-sensitive dyes by exciting a dye molecule to a higher energy state. Usually light having a specific wavelength is used to excite fluorescence from a dye molecule since certain wavelengths of light excite more fluorescence than do others.

Excitation filter: An optical filter through which light emitted by a source used to excite fluorescence (e.g., tungsten-halogen lamp) is passed for the purpose of exposing the dye molecule to selected wavelengths of light that are optimal for exciting fluorescence of that particular dye. In voltage-sensitive dye mapping, these are usually band-pass interference filters.

Excitation spectrum: Measured with a spectrofluorometer, indicates the intensity of light emitted by a fluorescent dye molecule (measuring emission of light at one constant wavelength), as a function of wavelength of excitation light used to excite fluorescence. The excitation spectrum of a dye can be used to select the dyes and excitation filters used in optical mapping because certain wavelengths of light will maximally excite fluorescence from a particular dye.

Fluorescence: The emission of a photon from an excitable molecule during the transition from excited state (provoked by excitation light) to a ground state. The energy (i.e., wavelength or color) of the emitted photon is dictated by the change in molecular energy when passing from the excited to the ground state, less the energy lost in the process.

Fluorescent probe: A molecule or substance that exhibits fluorescence in response to changes in the local environment (e.g., voltage, ion concentration, etc.).

Focal length: The distance from the center of a lens to the point at which light rays passing through the lens converge. This is related to the magnifying power of a lens.

Frame rate: The number of images that are acquired as a function of time. For a CCD video camera, it is analogous to sampling rate.

Gain: The amount of signal amplification applied before digitization. High gain makes the image brighter but also increases noise.

Integration time: A fixed period over which charge is collected in a single element (pixel) of a CCD video detector. The intensity or amplitude of the signal diminishes as integration time is reduced. Long integration times can cause blurring artifacts (temporal blurring).

Interference filter: An optical filter used to pass light within a range of wavelengths. Most often used as excitation filters in voltage-sensitive dye mapping.

Isosbestic point: The wavelength at which the intensity of the fluorescence spectra is not sensitive to the parameter being measured (e.g., voltage).

Laser (Light Amplification by Stimulated Emission of Radiation): A light source that produces a highly monochromatic, collimated (parallel), and phase-coherent output.

Motion artifact (MA): A distortion of the fluorescence signal due to contraction of the heart.

Numerical aperture (NA): An index of the light collection efficiency of a lens. The higher the numerical aperture, the more light that is passed through the lens.

Objective lens: The lens of a microscope that is closest to the preparation.

Offset: With regard to CCD video cameras, also called the black level, is an additive shift to the signal that determines what brightness level will appear as black in the resulting image. It is useful to be able to manipulate the gain and offset; some cameras have nonadjustable factory-preset levels.

Patterned growth technique: A technique applied to tissue culture monolayers that permits cell growth to occur in a prespecified 2-dimensional pattern.

Photobleaching: An irreversible photochemical oxidation reaction that causes fluorescence of dye molecules to attenuate with exposure to excitation light over time.

Photodetector: A light-sensitive element that is capable of transducing light energy into electrical energy.

Photodiode array (PDA): A photodetector that consists of multiple silicon devices, each of which converts light energy to electrical current. A PDA has a fast response time, and the amplitude of the current is dependent on the wavelength of the incident light and the spectral response of the photodiode.

Photodynamic effect: Also called phototoxicity. It is irreversible injury to a myocyte stained with fluorescent dye upon exposure to excitation light. This is thought to be free-radical–mediated cell death. Intact heart preparations are relatively resistant to this effect.

Photomultiplier tube: A light detector that transduces and amplifies incident photons to electrons.

Phototoxicity: See photodynamic effect.

Pixel: A single element within a 2-dimensional photodetector array.

Pixel binning: Combining neighboring pixels to yield a super-pixel. Often used with CCD video cameras to increase frame rate at the expense of spatial resolution.

Potentiometric dye: Also known as voltage-sensitive dye. It is a fluorescent probe whose fluorescence intensity is proportional to transmembrane potential.

Quantum efficiency: See quantum yield.

Quantum yield: Also known as emission efficiency of a dye molecule. It is the ratio of emitted energy to absorbed energy, and is an important factor determining the strength of signal one can record with a fluorescent probe.

Quenching: Refers to decreasing fluorescence intensity. This is due to changes in dye absorption or emission characteristics with time or dilution (i.e., washout).

Sampling rate: The rate (usually expressed in samples/s or Hertz) at which an analog signal representing an action potential is converted to a digitally sampled data point. If the signal is generated by a photodiode array, the total time required to acquire a sample from all photodiode pixels is usually the frame rate. If the signal is acquired by a CCD video camera, all pixels are sampled simultaneously, so the sampling rate equals the frame rate.

Saturation: With regard to CCD video cameras, the point at which the pixel elements cannot convert any more photons. It is sometimes called well size (how deep the well or bucket is) and measured in units of charge.

Scattering: Excitation light that is incident to a dye molecule that is not absorbed by the molecule (i.e., not used toward exciting fluorescence), but is scattered into the tissue.

Sensitivity: With regard to CCD video cameras, indicates the lowest detectable light level. It may be expressed as the amount of voltage generated per unit of light intensity or, alternatively, as the least amount of light that will generate an image either at or just above the noise floor. Thus, camera makers express sensitivity in a variety of units, both photometric and electronic: lux, footcandles, $A/W/cm^2$, or $coulomb/J/cm^2$. Comparison of cameras is made even more difficult by the fact that manufacturers may report sensitivity without specifying whether the gain was off (i.e., equal to 1) or at maximum value.

Signal-to-noise (S/N) ratio: The ratio of the magnitude of a fluorescent signal to baseline noise.

Spatial resolution: The smallest distance between two adjacent recording sites from which distinct and independent fluorescent signal can be resolved. Usually given by distance between recording pixels of the detector and the extent to which recorded image is magnified onto the detector; i.e., higher magnification gives greater spatial resolution.

Spectrofluorometer: An instrument used to measure excitation and emission spectra of a dye molecule.

Stokes' shift: The difference in wavelength of light used to excite fluorescence from a dye molecule, from wavelength of light actually fluoresced or emitted by the molecule. Typically, between the process of excitation and emission there is a shift toward longer wavelengths. In optical mapping, the Stokes' shift is exploited for the purpose of distinguishing excitation light from fluoresced light.

Tandem lens: An arrangement of two photographic lenses placed face to face and focused at infinity. The heart preparation is placed at the focal plane of the first lens, while the image is formed at the focal plane of the second lens. Optical magnification is determined by the ratio of focal lengths of the two lenses. Tandem lens systems are used to optimize light throughput and, therefore, signal intensity.

Temporal resolution: Elapsed time between two samples. Inverse of sampling rate.

Transillumination: A technique of optical recording that uses an objective lens to collect light emitted from one side of the specimen as a result of excitation through a condenser on the opposite side of the specimen. Also known as transmitted illumination.

Vignetting: Fading of an image at its periphery. This artifact is often associated with use of sequential lenses as in tandem lens optics.

Wavelength: Light can be considered as a periodic sinusoidal wave having a distance over which the wave completes one cycle or period. This distance (usually expressed in nanometers) is referred to as wavelength. The wavelength determines important properties of light such as its color and the depth to which incident light will be reflected, absorbed, and penetrated into tissue. Wavelength of light is inversely related to its frequency.

Section I

Basic Principles

Introduction:

Optical Mapping of Cardiac Excitation and Arrhythmias:

A Primer

David S. Rosenbaum

The chapters of this textbook contain detailed and authoritative discussions of the principles and applications of the powerful technique of optical cardiac mapping. The book is divided into four major sections: I. Basic Principles; II. Microscopic Propagation; III. Cardiac Arrhythmias; and IV. Cardiac Defibrillation, with the latter three covering the major applications of optical mapping to date. Before delving into applications, however, it is essential to understand the basic principles underlying the technique of voltage-sensitive dye recordings in the heart. At first, this may seem a bit intimidating to some life scientists or clinicians, because understanding the principles of optical mapping calls upon knowledge from multiple disciplines of science including physical chemistry (e.g., molecular mechanisms of dye fluorescence), optics (e.g., cameras, lasers, and fiberoptics used to generate and record optical signals), solid state physics (e.g., optical detectors), data acquisition (e.g., high-speed multichannel action potential recordings), computer science (e.g., analysis software), and, of course, physiology. In many instances, nomenclature can be a greater barrier to understanding than the basic concepts, which are, in fact, reasonably straightforward. Therefore, a glossary of technical terms is included in this textbook.

The aim of this first section of the textbook is to convey the principles and concepts that underlie optical mapping in a manner that can be useful for experts in this field as well as interested scientists, students, and clinicians who many never perform an optical mapping experiment. To this end, this brief introduction is intended to serve as a primer on the basic principles for those without substantial prior knowledge or training in optical mapping techniques.

An optical mapping system consists of three major components: 1) the heart preparation, which is stained with a voltage-sensitive dye; 2) a system of optics, which filters the fluoresced light emanating from the preparation and focuses it onto a photodetector; and 3) a photodetector, which measures the fluoresced light. The components of a commonly used system are shown schematically in Figure 1.

Voltage-Sensitive Dyes

Voltage-sensitive dyes are molecules that bind to the cell membrane with high affinity (Fig. 2). Dye can be delivered to cardiac cells within the

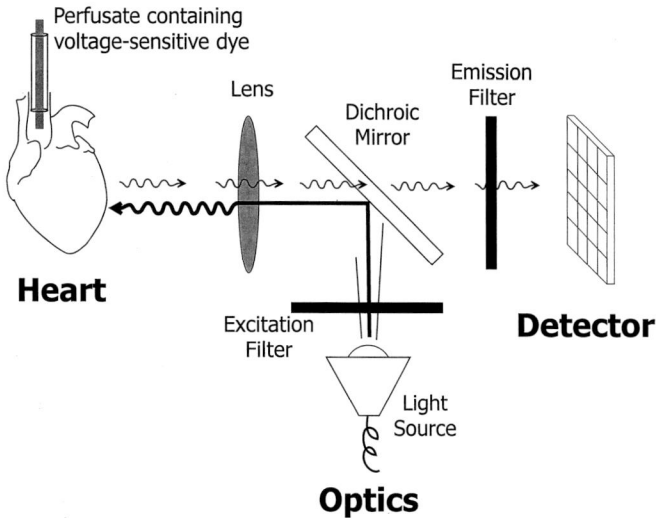

Figure 1. Typical optical mapping system consisting of three major components: 1) the heart preparation; 2) a system of optics; and 3) a detector. An excitation filter is used to pass selected wavelengths of light from the light source to a dichroic mirror, which semiselectively reflects light of this wavelength and directs it toward the preparation. In response to excitation light, voltage-sensitive dye molecules bound to the heart cells fluoresce light in proportion to the membrane potential of the cell to which they are bound. Light emitted from the dye has a longer wavelength, and therefore passes through (it is not reflected) the dichroic mirror, undergoes a final stage of filtering, and is focused onto the detector.

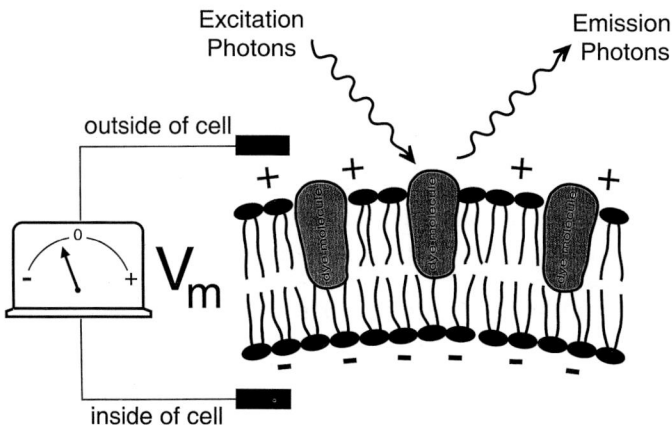

Figure 2. Schematic representation of voltage-sensitive dye molecules bound to cardiac cell membrane. After being struck by excitation photons from a light source, dye molecules emit photons (i.e., fluorescence). The intensity of fluorescence varies, and is directly proportional to transmembrane potential (V_m). Therefore, dye molecules transduce the voltage signal, V_m, into light. This light signal is later transduced back to an electrical signal by a photodetector (not shown).

intact heart, to isolated myocardial tissues or cells, or to cardiac cells grown in tissue culture via coronary perfusion or superfusion. While bound to the membrane of cardiac cells, the dye molecules fluoresce light in direct proportion to transmembrane voltage. Therefore, voltage-sensitive dyes function as highly localized transducers of membrane potential, transforming a change of membrane potential into a change in fluorescence intensity. Herein lies a major advantage of optical mapping. One is only required to measure light noninvasively (i.e., from the cells viewpoint), obviating the need for impaling cells with electrodes which, in turn, minimizes risk of cellular injury and permits essentially unlimited spatial resolution between recording sites.

The process of fluorescence requires two basic steps: 1) excitation: membrane-bound dye molecules must be excited by light (i.e., photons) of a specific wavelength into a higher energy state, and 2) emission: as the molecule returns from its excited state to its ground state, it emits a photon of longer wavelength than the initially absorbed photon. Although voltage-sensitive dyes can be divided into two classes, distributive and electrochromic dyes (according to their response to membrane potential), for all practical purposes only electrochromic dyes are used exclusively for cardiac optical mapping because of their very rapid time response. For instance, excitation and emission of electrochromic dyes require approximately 10^{-12} and 10^{-6} ms, respectively. Therefore, the total process of voltage-sensitive fluorescence (i.e., $10^{-12} + 10^{-6}$ ms) is several orders of magnitude faster than the most rapid change in membrane potential (i.e., rapid upstroke of the action potential is about 10^0 ms). Consequently, these dyes can faithfully track the time course of any electrical change occurring across the cell membrane.

So how do voltage-sensitive dyes work? For any given constant excitation light intensity and wavelength, light is emitted by voltage-sensitive dyes over a range of wavelengths that can be represented by emission spectra as shown in Figure 3. The key property of voltage-sensitive dyes is that they display an emission spectrum that is voltage-dependent. A depolarization of transmembrane potential during the rapid upstroke of the action potential (Fig. 3) causes the fluorescence emission spectrum to shift to the right. One can use a filter to selectively record only those wavelengths that are longer than the cut-off wavelength of the filter (Fig. 3, vertical line). The shift in the emission spectra changes the magnitude of fluoresced light that is passed by this filter and is measured by a light detector (Fig. 3, shaded region). Since the area of the shaded region (i.e., amount of light passed) is proportional to relative membrane potential, the light detector actually measures relative membrane potential. It is important to emphasize that the precise shape of any emission spectra does not correspond to any absolute voltage; hence, only relative potential change is detected. However, it is very well established that the timing and shape of the optically recorded action potentials follows that of the action potential recorded with a microelectrode with considerable accuracy. Therefore, voltage-sensitive dyes provide a means of determining the timing of cellular depolarization and repolarization, in addition to revealing important details on action potential shape. Of course, a major advantage of optical mapping over microelectrode techniques is that one can acquire such information on cel-

Voltage-Dependent Changes In Dye Emission Spectra

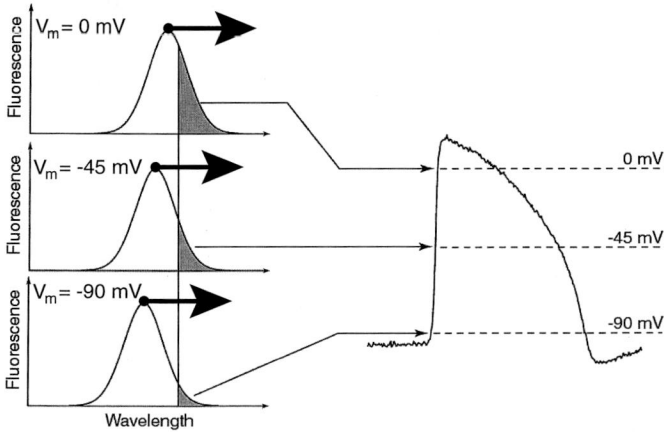

Figure 3. Schematic representation of the principle of voltage-sensitive fluorescence. Emission spectra for voltage-sensitive dye molecule changes with membrane potential, V_m. As the cell depolarizes from its resting voltage ($V_m = -90$ mV) toward less negative potentials (-45 mV and 0 mV, respectively), the emission spectrum of the dye shifts progressively to the right (arrows). An emission filter placed in front of the light detector (see Fig. 1) excludes light emitted from the dye below a specific wavelength, as depicted by the vertical line that passes through each spectrum. Therefore, the amount of light that strikes the photodetector is the shaded area under each spectrum. This is the principle by which voltage-sensitive dyes convert membrane potential into light intensity. Note that for many voltage-sensitive dyes, fluorescence intensity can actually decrease as voltage increases, resulting in an inverted action potential trace. In either case, the same principles underlie voltage-sensitive fluorescence.

lular activity simultaneously from hundreds of sites on the heart. This allows one to examine cell-to-cell interactions and cellular activity within propagating arrhythmias in a manner that is not possible with conventional techniques.

Optics

As mentioned above, voltage-sensitive dye must be excited by light to induce fluorescence (Fig. 2) . The most common excitation light sources are tungsten-halogen lamps, mercury arc lamps, and argon ion lasers. Each has its own limitations and advantages. Optical mapping requires collection of emitted light having relatively low intensity. Therefore, light collection efficiency must be maximized to allow elements of the action potential to be distinguished from background noise. When a lens is used to magnify and focus an image onto a photodetector, the amount of light collected is inversely proportional to the square of the magnification. Maximizing light collection efficiency is particularly important at high magnifications, when the source of fluorescence is reduced (i.e., relatively few cells contribute to the optical signal).

The source of each optical action potential is derived from a minute spot of tissue that can be composed of as few as one to as many as hundreds of cardiac cells, depending on the extent of optical magnification used. Therefore, an optically recorded potential often represents the average potential from a small aggregate of neighboring cells. The greater the magnification, the smaller the spot of tissue from which the optical potential is derived, the more closely the optical action potential will correspond to a single cell recording.

High-quality images can be acquired with a microscope or with photographic lenses. Fluorescence microscopes are commercially available with objective lens magnifications ranging from 4× to 100×, allowing for mapping of very small preparations (1 to 5 mm). Because high magnifications are used, light collection efficiency must be optimized, which is why microscope objectives are designed with high numerical apertures (NAs). Photographic lenses are better suited for magnifications under 10×, permitting one to map action potentials from larger preparations (5 to 50 mm). A simple photographic lens system is shown schematically in Figure 1. The preparation is placed at a specific distance from the focal plane of the lens. The photodetector is placed on the other side of the lens at the position at which the image is formed. The photographic camera lens system has the advantage of being simple and sufficient for many applications.

Not all optical mapping systems require lenses to collect the fluoresced light. For example, optical fibers have been successfully used to focus voltage-sensitive fluorescence onto a photodetector. Alternatively, laser scanning systems have been used to record optical maps from cardiac tissue. Because only a small region of the tissue is excited at one time, all the fluoresced light can be collected with a single photodetector without the use of a collector lens. As the laser scans the preparation, a 2-dimensional map of the tissue can be obtained.

Photodetectors

Voltage-sensitive fluorescence emitted by the preparation is measured with a photodetector. The most widely used photodetectors in optical mapping are photodiode arrays and charged coupled device (CCD) video cameras. Both devices are capable of obtaining 2-dimensional maps, but each has its own advantages and disadvantages.

A photodiode array contains up to several hundred individual photodiodes, each of which is a semiconductor light sensor. When a photon of fluoresced light strikes the photodiode, the energy is converted into a current. A change in membrane potential causes fluorescence intensity to change such that more photons strike the detector; this in turn causes the photodetector to produce more current. The current output from each photodetector must be passed through a current-to-voltage converter so that a voltage signal having amplitude that is proportionate to membrane potential can be transferred to a data acquisition computer. A major advantage of a photodiode array is that it generates photocurrent in response to membrane potential changes continuously, allowing one to digitally sample the action potential at very rapid rates (i.e., high sampling rate) without compromising the fidelity of the recorded action potential. Therefore, these detectors are very useful for measuring details in the time course and mor-

phology of the action potential. They are limited by the number of photodetectors on the array (typically 256 or less).

A CCD video camera is also a semiconductor device that has been seg-
mented into an array of light-sensitive recording pixels. In contrast to a
photodiode array, a CCD camera can contain hundreds of thousands of
pixels, permitting greater spatial resolution between recording sites. When
a photon strikes a CCD detector, it releases an electron, which is stored
within the recording pixel. Electrons accumulated and stored within each
pixel since the previous frame are read off at regular time intervals (i.e.,
the frame rate). Limitations of CCD cameras include the relatively slow
frame rates associated with video cameras, and the fact that any attempt to
increase frame rate comes at the expense of signal fidelity.

The principles summarized above are covered in detail in this section
of the book. It is appropriate that we start with a chapter by Dr. Guy
Salama, who was the first to have applied these principles to optical mapping of the heart.

Chapter 1

Optical Mapping:
Background and Historical Perspective

Guy Salama

Introduction

In biological systems, the potential across the cellular membrane plays an important role in maintaining normal function and, in excitable cells, serves as a signaling mechanism for cell-to-cell communication and as a trigger for normal organ function. Most of what we know regarding membrane potential changes in multicellular preparations comes from potentials measured by impaling cells with glass pipette microelectrodes. In many experimental conditions, the difficulties in maintaining the microelectrode tip in the intracellular space and the damage to the cells limit the use of the method. Moreover, microelectrode techniques are not applicable to small cells (<3 μm in diameter) and subcellular organelles, nor are they practical in situations in which the simultaneous monitoring of membrane potential from multiple sites is required. A great deal has been learned regarding the cardiac action potential in heart muscle from studies with intracellular microelectrode recordings in which the method can be applied to isolated cells and papillary muscles. However, in intact hearts, the forceful contractions of the muscle make it difficult to maintain stable intracellular microelectrode impalements or to track voltage changes in an electrical syncytium by recording from multiple sites. For these and other reasons, attempts were made in the late 1960s to develop new techniques to monitor membrane potential. The aim of this chapter is to focus on the development of this field of research from a historical perspective and to provide technical background of the method as it relates to cardiac electrophysiology. Areas in which the method has made an important scientific impact, as well as future exciting directions, are highlighted. Later chapters in this book elaborate on exciting applications to cardiac electrophysiology, provide further details on techniques, and describe new findings. Readers are referred to an earlier review that dis-

These studies were supported over the years by the Western Pennsylvania American Heart Association, the National American Heart Association, and currently by NIH grant HL57929.

From Rosenbaum DS, Jalife J (eds): *Optical Mapping of Cardiac Excitation and Arrhythmias.* ©Futura Publishing Co., Inc., Armonk, NY, 2001.

cussed in greater details optical measurements of membrane potential in heart, the screening of dyes, photodynamic damage, linearity of the voltage-dependent optical response, voltage-clamp experiments, spectral studies, and techniques used to map electrical activity in heart.[1]

Early Studies

Initial attempts to measure voltage-dependent optical signals in biological systems were based on intrinsic signals recorded in the absence of exogenously added dye or probe. Changes in light scattering or birefringence measured from various types of nerve cells and frog skeletal fibers appeared to mimic the time course of their action potential.[2–5] However, the signal-to-noise (S/N) ratio of such signals was too poor to be of practical value, and extensive time averaging (10^4 sweeps) was required to resolve these signals. In the search for voltage-dependent optical signals with greater S/N ratio, various classes of dyes were tested as possible probes of transmembrane potential. Axons were stained with dyes such as aniline-8-naphthalene sulfonate (ANS) or 2-p-toluidinonaphthalene-6-sulfonate (TNS), and dye fluorescence during electrical stimulation was correlated with changes in membrane potential or current.[6–8] Some reports suggested that the *extrinsic* fluorescence (i.e., emission from exogenously added dye) from ANS or TNS was related to changes in membrane conductance,[7,9] and others that it reflected the time course of the membrane potential.[10–12] *Extrinsic* optical signals improved the S/N ratio by a factor of approximately 10 compared with intrinsic signals, but were still impractical for most physiological investigations. Nevertheless, these studies changed the direction of investigations from intrinsic to extrinsic optical signals and more than 300 hundred dyes were screened by Cohen and his colleagues.[13] Many of the dyes responded to potential changes through changes in absorption and/or fluorescence (>50%) and several changed up to 0.1% of the resting intensity during an action potential, with S/N ratio ≥10:1 in a single sweep.[13] The most promising signals were obtained from the absorption and fluorescence changes of Merocyanine 540 (M-540), which were found to mimic the time course of giant axon action potentials with high fidelity.[14] However, the practical value of the method was still in doubt because of severe phototoxic damage that limited the recording time to a few seconds.

Dyes were also screened (approximately 100) in amphibian and mammalian heart muscles for possible voltage-dependent optical responses. Investigators followed spectral changes during membrane depolarization induced by high extracellular potassium.[1,15] Of the dyes tested, a class called Merocyanine dyes demonstrated for the first time that optical recordings of membrane potential could prove to be useful in physiological investigations.[16]

Screening for Possible Potentiometric Probes in Heart

To function satisfactorily as a probe of membrane potential, a dye must exhibit several essential properties: 1) it must bind or interact with the plasma membrane to act as a sensor of membrane potential; 2) it should exhibit large fluorescence and/or absorption changes that vary (preferably linearly) with changes in membrane potential; 3) its optical responses must be specifically related to potential changes and not to ion concentration, transmembrane currents, or membrane conductance; 4) staining of the heart with the dye should not result in pharmacological or toxic effects to the preparation; 5) the dye should be optically stable in its local environment and not prone to photobleaching on exposure to intense light. Dyes were screened in two types of preparations; Langendorff-perfused hearts or sheets of atrial and ventricular tissue stretched on a ring.[15]

Staining Procedures

Concentrated dye solutions were typically prepared in ethanol or dimethyl sulfoxide (DMSO) and were kept in the dark to avoid photobleaching. Heart muscles were bathed in Ringer's solution containing 1 to 1000 μmol/L of dye for 10 to 30 minutes, then washed in dye-free solutions. Muscles stained by superfusion in dye solution required long periods of dye exposure since the penetration of the dye depends on its diffusion in the tissue. When examined under the light microscope, the muscles were found to be superficially stained (<100 μm) and had consistently smaller voltage-dependent optical responses. To improve the delivery of dye and the homogeneity of staining deep in the myocardium, the dye was delivered through the coronary perfusate in Langendorff-perfused hearts.[1,16,17] The "health" of the preparation was continuously monitored by measuring electrical activity with surface electrograms, as well as aortic and ventricular pressures before, during, and after the washout of dye. Staining the heart through the coronary perfusate offered several important advantages. The tissue stains uniformly and deeply, and 10 to 20 times lower dye concentrations were needed to obtain optical responses with 5 to 20 times greater S/N ratio. A perfused ventricular sheet preparation was developed to measure absorption and fluorescence spectra across the myocardial wall (± dye) and to measure electrical activity at different resting lengths of the muscle.[18] Sheets of heart muscle were stretched, sutured to a stainless steel ring, and electrically stimulated. The force of contraction was measured with a strain gauge mounted on the ring. The preparation was ideal for measurements of intrinsic absorption and fluorescence and for comparison of the spectral characteristics of the dye in solution versus dye bound to the myocardium. In most experiments, the heart was stained in the Langendorff mode then sheets of muscle were dissected and sutured to the ring for spectral measurements.

The dyes tested in heart muscle fell into one of five categories.[1] 1) Some dyes simply did not bind to the muscle regardless of the staining procedure. 2) Other dyes bound to heart muscle but only after a depolarization with high extracellular K$^+$, and were taken up by the cells with toxic consequences. 3) Acridine dyes seemed to exhibit voltage-dependent responses but they also induced large positive inotropic effects in rat and frog ventricular muscle. The addition of β-antagonists reversed the positive inotropic effects but was associated with a loss of membrane-bound dye. Higher concentrations of Acridine Orange (>5×10^{-6} M) were toxic and resulted in a state of contracture. 4) Membrane permeable cyanine dyes were ineffective at less than 5 μmol/L and tended to be toxic at higher concentrations (up to 60 μmol/L), particularly when added to the coronary perfusate. The toxic effects were in part due to the poor solubility of cyanine dyes in Ringer's solution and to the precipitation of dye crystals in the coronary vessels. Cyanine dyes were not toxic to heart muscle bathed in dye solutions, but the staining was negligible and no convincing voltage-dependent signals were detected. 5) Merocyanine, oxonol, styryl, and pyridinium compounds exhibited voltage-dependent responses in heart muscle. All these dyes bind to heart muscle and did not readily wash out after several hours of perfusion in dye-free solution. An important feature of these dyes is their hydrophobic structure, which accounts for tight binding to the cellular membrane and a localized negatively charged group (SO_3^-) that prevents its diffusion inside cells. As a result, these dyes are trapped on the membrane where large electrical field changes occur and exhibit "fast" voltage-dependent responses. As of now, all probes of membrane potential in heart have these molecular features (a hydrophobic moiety and a localized charged group), bind tightly to the sarcolemma (i.e., a feature of "fast" response dyes), and can be successfully used to measure cardiac action potentials.

Merocyanine Dyes

Polar Merocyanine dyes are highly solvatochromic (peak excitation and/or emission shift as a function of the solvent's polarity) since they exhibit wavelength shifts of 270 nm or more in their maximum absorption by being transferred from a polar to a nonpolar solvent.[19,20] In general, the molecular structure of Merocyanine dyes is that of an uncharged chromophore, but charged molecules can be synthesized by covalently attaching a sulfonate group on their hydrocarbon ring, as in M-540 (also called Merocyanine I). The charge remains localized rather than delocalized over the entire chromophore and this property reduces the membrane permeability of the dye so that the dye does not diffuse in healthy cells. Besides M-540, two weakly fluorescent dyes, Merocyanine-Rhodanine and Merocyanine-Oxazolone, should be mentioned because of their high sensitivity to membrane potential changes, their lack of phototoxic effects, and their potentiometric responses at long wavelengths (>700 nm). When bound to heart muscle, these "absorption" dyes fluoresce weakly but exhibit large changes in absorption during potential changes. A disadvantage is that muscle contractions produce larger optical artifacts in the absorption than fluorescence mode. However, they offer advantages of low toxicity (see "Photodynamic Effect"), greater S/N ratio, and signal from cells deeper in the tissue because of their longer wavelengths.

Characteristics of Voltage-Dependent Optical Signals

The first measurements of optical action potentials were obtained with M-540. Although more sensitive dyes with less phototoxicity have replaced M-540, the same general principles apply to all "fast" dyes. When bound to heart muscle, M-540 has two absorption peaks at 540 and 570 nm, and fluoresces at 585 nm when excited at either 540 or 570 nm. Electrical stimulation of the muscle results in absorption decreases (0.1% to 1%) and increases (0.01% to 0.5%) at 540 and 570 nm, respectively. With either 540- or 570-nm excitation, electrical stimulation produces a 1.3% increase in fluorescence quantum yield. Figure 1A illustrates a basic instrument to measure a light signal from a 1-mm light spot focused on a sheet of frog ventricular muscle. Electrical stimulation of the unstained preparation produces a change in light scattering ($\Delta I/I$) due to the muscle contraction (Fig. 1B, top left). After the muscle is stained with M-540, electrical stimulation results in a rapid voltage-dependent optical response, which is coincident with the stimulus and is superimposed on the slower motion artifact (MA) (Fig. 1B, top right). After the muscle is bathed in a zero Ca^{2+} solution, contractions are suppressed and the voltage-dependent fluorescence response ($\Delta F/F$) has the time course of the cardiac action potential (Fig. 1B, bottom).

The voltage-dependent optical response provides a detailed measurement of the shape and kinetics of the cardiac action potential but no "direct" information on the actual value of transmembrane potential. Attempts to develop an internal calibration of membrane potential using "fast" dyes have thus far failed because of the nature and origins of these responses. The baseline fluorescence is due to dye bound to the tissue (e.g., as deduced from the staining procedure) and depends on the optical apparatus (i.e., cross-talk between excitation and emission filters). The dye can 1) bind to the extracellular matrix; 2) bind to the membrane of cardiomyocytes; 3) bind to the surrounding endothelial cells; and 4) be internalized in the cytosol. The absorption and/or fluorescence spectra of the chromophore depend on the local environment such that only dye molecules associated with the excitable membrane of cardiomyocytes will transduce potential changes to an optical response. The fractional absorption (or reflectance, $\Delta R/R$) and/or fluorescence ($\Delta F/F$) change per action potential will depend on the "sensitivity" of the dye to voltage, the fraction of dye molecules bound to excitable membranes, and the sum of potential changes from all cells (healthy and sick) seen by the detector. In principle, $\Delta F/F$ (and/or $\Delta R/R$) recorded during an action potential can be related to the depolarization of cardiac cells (i.e., approximately 100 mV). However, the situation is more complex because the baseline fluorescence tends to drift. This was documented for M-540 but applies to all dyes albeit with different time courses. In hearts stained with M-540, the fluorescence baseline increases, reaches a maximum (approximately 10 min), then gradually decreases. The most likely explanation[1] is that a combination of dye washout and photobleaching is responsible for these patterns of baseline drift. With an initially high concentration of dye bound to the tissue, the fluorescence would be self-quenched. During exposure to light, the washout and photo decomposition of the dye would produce a decrease in fluorescence quenching resulting in an increase in baseline fluorescence and an increase in optical action potential amplitude. The fluorescence intensity and the amplitude of action potential would reach a maximum value then decrease slowly with further loss of dye. For these reasons, the fluorescence baseline does not strictly depend on the absolute

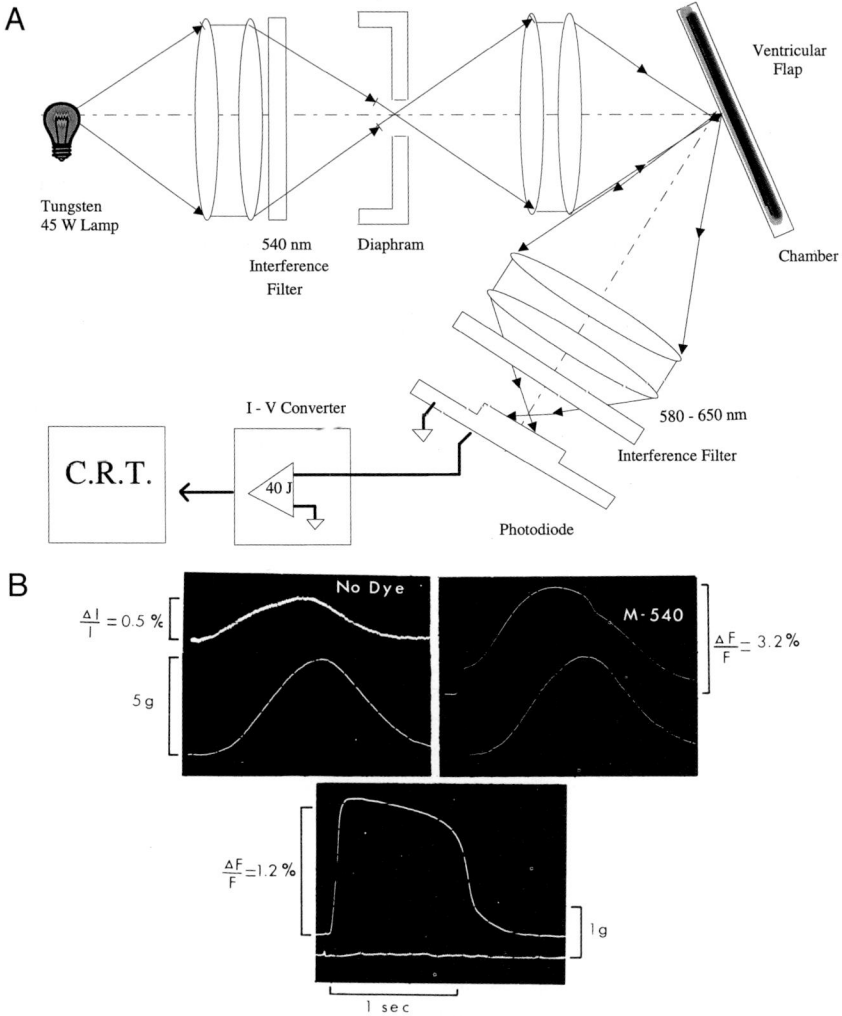

Figure 1. Optical recording of an action potential from a voltage-sensitive dye. **A.** Schema of a simple apparatus to measure optical action potentials. Light from a tungsten-halogen lamp is collimated, passed through a 540 ± 20 nm interference filter and a diaphragm, and is refocused (1-mm-diameter beam) on the surface of a perfused sheet of ventricular muscle. Fluorescence and scattered light from the surface of the muscle is collected with a camera lens (Nikon f1:1.4), passed through a 580- to 650-nm filter, focused on a photodiode, and read from the voltage output or a current-to-voltage converter. **B.** Fluorescence and force measurements from a sheet of ventricular muscle. *Top left:* In the absence of dye, changes in light scattering (i.e., motion artifact [MA]) follow the time course of developed force from a frog ventricular sheet. *Top right:* After the tissue is stained with Merocyanine 540 and washed with dye-free and Ca^{2+}-free solution, electrical stimulation elicits a rapid increase in the fluorescence of dye bound to the tissue followed by a slower recovery and decrease in signal coincident with the MA. *Bottom:* After washing with Ca^{2+}-free solution, contractions are abolished and the fluorescence signal has the shape and time course of the action potential. Force is measured by suturing the ventricular sheet to an annealed stainless steel ring (a 3-mm cut on the ring produces a stiff spring) on which a transducer is mounted. Adapted from reference 16.

resting membrane potential, and the fractional fluorescence change per action potential is proportional to a change in membrane potential, $\Delta F/F \propto \Delta V_m$ but the coefficient proportionality is variable. Even though the dyes can interact at many sites, the percent $\Delta R/R$ and/or $\Delta F/F$ is remarkably reproducible from heart to heart and from one species to another as long as the heart is "healthy" and the staining procedure is not altered.[1] Thus, as originally demonstrated for M-540, "fast" dyes like the most widely used pyridinium dye, di-4-ANEPPS, measure the kinetics of action potentials but the voltage values must be deduced from simultaneous recordings of action potentials by optical and microelectrode techniques.[21]

Linearity of Voltage-Dependent Optical Responses

Optical signals from potentiometric dyes clearly have the shape and time course of action potential recorded with microelectrodes. However, there are noticeable differences: the upstroke velocity and, more infrequently, the rate of repolarization of optical signals are slower than those recorded with electrodes. The slower kinetics of optical action potentials can be attributed to the propagation of action potential and the asynchronous firing of action potential in the patch of tissue viewed by the detector. The high fidelity of optical and microelectrode traces shows that fast dyes monitor potential and not membrane current or conductance changes. Nevertheless, the potential dependence of the signals could be coincidental (i.e., valid under some conditions but not others) and/or nonlinear. In all cases tested thus far, optical signals recorded under a variety of ionic (e.g., changes in extracellular Ca^{2+}, K^+, or Na^+, addition of Cd^{2+} or Ni^{2+}) and pharmacological (e.g., Ca^{2+} channel blockers and β adrenergic agonists) interventions monitored the same changes detected with microelectrodes. Optical action potentials recorded from different regions of the heart recorded the expected shape and time course of action potentials from sinoatrial nodal, atrial, and ventricular cells.[1,15,16] The sucrose gap technique was adapted for optical recordings during voltage-clamp steps of test nodes, cylindrical muscle strips (0.6 mm in diameter $\times$ 0.8 mm in length). For Merocyanine dyes, optical responses varied linearly with potential changes in hyperpolarizing and depolarizing voltage-clamp steps.[1,17] An important feature of these probes is that their voltage-dependent responses follow direct current (DC) changes in membrane potential and show no signs of alternating current coupling step changes in potential, even for long (200 to 300 ms) voltage-clamp steps. This feature is particularly important in heart, where the precise time course of the action potential plateau is required to analyze action potential durations (APDs).

Kinetics of Voltage-Dependent Optical Responses

The ability of potentiometric probes to track rapid voltage changes was investigated by two methods: by using the sucrose gap technique[17] and by using a laser's narrow beam (90 to 200 μm in diameter) to excite one or more cells and compare the upstroke velocity of optical and intracellular microelectrode.[22] The sucrose gap apparatus makes it possible to hold all cells in the "test node" at the same membrane potential and to synchronously depolarize the node to a set command potential. Sucrose gap experiments showed that the rise times of optical upstrokes were similar to those recorded with intracellular electrodes, within the resolution of the voltage-clamp (10 to 100 μs).[1,15,17] Figure 2 illustrates simultaneous action potential recordings with optical and microelectrode techniques from the test node of a muscle strip in a sucrose gap apparatus. Examples are shown using M-540 (top panels) or Merocyanine-Oxazolone (NK 2367, bottom panels). The left panels compare the two measurements at slow sweep speeds and show the excellent fidelity of both optical probes to microelectrode recordings. Optical signals can thus be calibrated from absolute potential measurements, and the rise times of optical signals are in excellent agreement with those obtained with microelectrodes. Another approach that has been used to analyze the response characteristics of optical probes is to compare upstroke velocity from a single cell intracellular microelectrode with an optical recording using narrow laser excitation

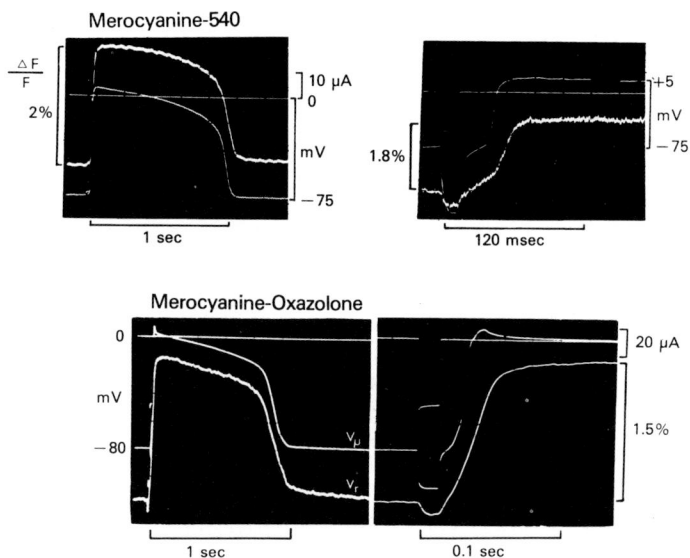

Figure 2. Comparison of action potentials recorded optically and with an intracellular microelectrode. A ventricular muscle strip is placed in sucrose gap voltage-clamp apparatus and stained with Merocyanine 540 (*top panels*) or Merocyanine-Oxazolone (*bottom panels*) and equilibrated in 50-μmol/L Ca^{2+} to suppress contractions. *Left:* Action potentials are recorded at a slow sweep speed optically, and when a microelectrode (V_μ) was impaled in one of the cells excited with the 1-mm-diameter incident beam, the action potentials recorded optically and with a microelectrode were in excellent agreement. *Right:* Action potentials recorded at fast sweep speeds show that under voltage-clamp conditions the rise times of optical and microelectrode action potentials upstrokes are comparable. Note that hyperpolarizing stimulus impulses produces an artifactual hyperpolarization on the microelectrodes that does not appear on the optical traces (*left panels*). The optical action potentials sense the local potential changes (i.e., within a molecular distance of the dye) and do not detect the stimulus-induced potential across the series resistance between the reference electrode and the cell.

beams.[22] In rat ventricular myocardium, the rise time of optical action potentials measured with a laser excitation was slower than, equal to, or faster than that recorded with an intracellular microelectrode, depending on the diameter of the excitation beam. With a large-diameter excitation beam (>130 μm), optical responses are the sum of action potential from several cells and were slower than microelectrode recordings, because the cells fire out of phase. With a 130-μm-diameter beam, the two signals were identical whereas with a 90-μm-diameter beam, optical upstrokes were faster than those of the electrode, most likely because of current leaks caused by the intracellular microelectrode.[22]

The possible interplay between the dye and pharmacological agents and the linearity of voltage-dependent responses has been primarily investigated for Merocyanine dyes but not for other fast dyes such as styryl, oxonol, and pyridinium dyes. For the latter dyes, the linearity of their voltage-dependent responses has been deduced from the high fidelity of optical action potentials to microelectrode recordings, which can be an adequate confirmation of linearity, particularly for long APDs (>300 ms).

Mechanism of Potentiometric Response

Several mechanisms have been suggested to explain the potentiometric response of fast dyes in heart.[1] Of all the potentiometric dyes, those in the Merocyanine class were the most extensively studied in axons and in heart muscle. These dyes were chosen because they are highly solvatochromic, that is, they also exhibit spectral changes as a function of their local environment. The solvent properties of Merocyanine dyes made them excellent candidates as potentiometric probes because changes in membrane potential alter the local environment. In theory then, such an "electrochromic" dye would exhibit wavelength shifts in peak fluorescence emission and/or absorption due to a change in membrane potential. Voltage-dependent spectral changes or "action spectra" were measured with a linear array spectrograph, to scan spectra at high speeds during various phases of the cardiac action potential. The instrument recorded a spectrum from 200 to 800 nm in 20 ms, and high-speed spectral analysis of M-540 revealed that the peak fluorescence and absorption of the dye changed with membrane depolarization with no wavelength shifts, with an accuracy of ±1 nm.[1,15,17] In the absence of an electrochromic effect, other mechanisms were proposed: 1) the local potential changes can shift dye molecules partially in or out the membrane or can alter the dielectric around the dye to produce spectral changes; 2) dye molecules in the membrane undergo dimer-to-monomer transitions as a function of membrane depolarization; and 3) the transition dipole moment vector of the chromophore interacts with the local electrical field vector such that changes in electrical field produce a rotation of the chromophore in the plane of the membrane. High-speed spectral changes measured as a function of membrane potential suggested that a membrane depolarization elicited a decrease in absorption at 540 nm and an increase at 570 nm which is consistent with a rotation of M-540 dye molecules from perpendicular to parallel to the plane of the membrane.[1,15] Few studies have focused on the mechanism responsible for the potentiometric response of fast dyes, and most were carried out in artificial membranes or squid giant axons using spectral analysis and polarized light to track the orientation of the chromophore (e.g., dipole moment) in the membrane. In the absence of definitive proof regarding the mechanism, the design of new probes remains largely empirical. The goal would be to obtain probes with greater sensitivity and "self-calibration" of membrane potential without requiring intracellular electrodes. "Self-calibration" can be achieved in theory with dyes that exhibit large electrochromic shifts. For instance, imagine a dye that has a peak fluorescence emission that varies systematically as a function of transmembrane potential. The dye, for example, fluoresces with a sharp maximum at 600 nm when the potential is -100 mV, 650 nm at -50 mV, 700 nm at 0 mV, etc. Then a calibration curve can be generated from a plot of peak fluorescence versus potential. A measurement of the peak emission wavelength automatically calibrates the membrane potential. At this time, the dye with the most desirable features for cardiac electrophysiology is di-4-ANEPPS [1-(3-sulfonatopropyl)-4-[β-[2-(di-n-butylamino)-6-naththyl]vinyl]pyridinium betaine].[21] As confirmed in numerous studies, it exhibits large fractional fluorescence changes during an action potential (8% to 15%) with low toxicity and photobleaching, and its signal amplitude and kinetics are stable for 2 to 4 hours without restaining the preparation.[21] The pyridinium class of dyes (di-5-ASP and di-4-ANEPPS) was developed based on a theoretical model of an electrochromic mechanism produced by a voltage-dependent intramolecular charge-shift.[23,24] In oxidized cholesterol vesicles and in HeLa cells, di-4-ANEPPS was used to measure and calibrate the membrane potential. In these preparations, di-4-ANEPPS exhibits a large electrochromic shift, and ratiometric fluorescence measurements ($\lambda_{emission} = 610$ nm) using two excitation wavelengths (F_{440}/F_{505}) was found to be linearly related to membrane potential.[25] In heart, there are no reports of ratiometric calibration of potential with pyridinium dyes and no evidence of a sufficiently large electrochromic shift to be of practical value for a calibration procedure.

Photodynamic Effect

Early studies described a phenomenon called "photodynamic effect" produced by exposing neurons to a chromophore and an intense excitation beam, resulting in increased membrane permeability, membrane depolarization, decreased inward sodium current (I_{Na+}), and eventual loss of excitability.[26] Photodynamic damage to biological membranes caused by electromagnetic radiation is enhanced by light intensity, oxygen, and the presence of certain chromophores. A mechanism that is consistent with the available data is that the excitation of the chromophore by intense light, in the presence of oxygen, generates oxygen free radicals which in turn cause lipid peroxidation and denature proteins. The severity of photodynamic damage was highly dependent on the potentiometric dye. For instance while M-540 produced severe photodynamic damage to axons causing complete loss of neuronal excitability in seconds,[13,14] other dyes from the same chemical class (i.e., Merocyanine-Rhodanine and Merocyanine-

Oxazolone) caused little photodynamic damage. In whole heart or large preparations, the photodynamic damage caused by M-540 was negligible, but in smaller papillary or muscle strips, damage was considerably more severe.[16,17] Phototoxicity seen in muscle strips had the hallmarks of photodynamic damage reported by earlier investigators. It was exacerbated by dissolved oxygen in the perfusate, by high light intensity, and by dye concentration. The greater protective effects in heart compared with axons and by large compared with small preparations was consistent with increased protection by the presence of oxygen free radical scavengers.[1,15,17] The results imply that preparations with a "healthy" metabolic state can better neutralize free radicals (produced by the excitation of the dye) by reducing these oxidants with intrinsic reducing agents (i.e., reduced glutathione [GSH]). In some cases, the addition of exogenous free radical scavengers can be protective against photodynamic effects and this approach may be valuable in studies when the metabolic state of the preparation is compromised. For instance, ischemia and hypoxia enhance oxidative stress and alter Ca^{2+} transport by the sarcoplasmic reticulum (SR).[27] Such metabolic deficits are associated with a lower ratio of reduced to oxidized glutathione (GSH/GSSG) and reduced protection against photodynamic damage, but the oxygen content is also reduced which decreases free radical production and the potential for photodynamic damage.[28] Potentiometric dyes like di-4-ANEPPS produce no detectable photodynamic damage in healthy, perfused, intact heart preparations and thus give an incorrect impression that these dyes simply do not cause photodynamic damage. As shown in Figure 3, optical action potentials recorded from a guinea pig heart stained with di-4-ANEPPS were stable for

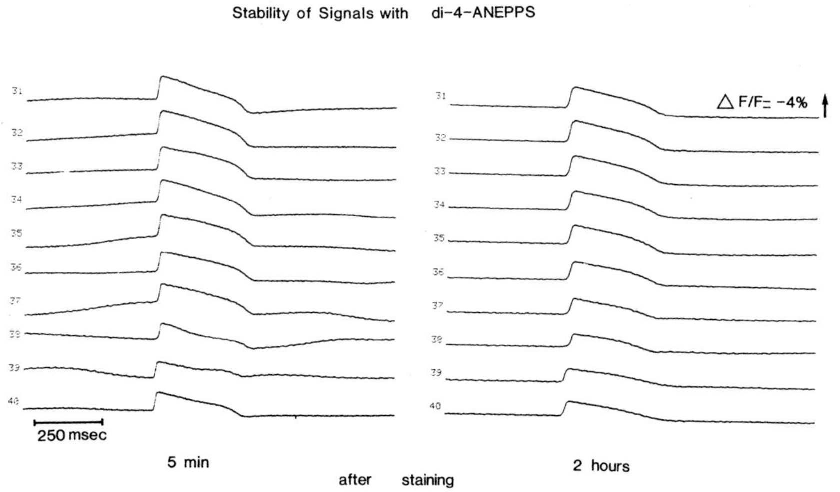

Stability of Signals with   di-4-ANEPPS

Figure 3. Lack of photodynamic damage by di-4-ANEPPS in perfused hearts. A guinea pig heart was perfused and stained with di-4-ANEPPS (10 μmol/L) and action potentials were recorded every 5 minutes. At the end of 2 hours, the S/N ratio and the shape and time course of action potential recordings remained stable with long plateau phases indicative of a "healthy" preparation.

2 hours with no detectable toxicity. However, when working with single cardiac cells or cultures myocytes in monolayers, the light intensity is typically increased to improve the S/N ratio, and in these conditions the same dye exhibits photodynamic effects.[29,30]

Dealing with MAs

Once an action potential could be measured using optical probes, it became particularly attractive to apply the technique to simultaneously record action potentials from multiple sites and thereby map patterns of cardiac activation (depolarization) and recovery (repolarization). Several approaches were developed to optically map or scan the surface of heart muscle: 1) photodiode arrays (PDAs)[31,32]; 2) laser scan or flying spot technique[33]; and 3) video[34] and charged coupled device (CCD) cameras.[35] A major technical difficulty faced by all the mapping techniques was the vigorous muscle contractions, which produce large MA that are superimposed on the voltage-dependent signals. MA is a more severe problem in intact perfused hearts than in muscle strips or in sheets of tissue because the latter can be stretched to reduce gross movement of the tissue. Several methods have been used to abate MA; each approach has advantages and disadvantages and its suitability is dependent on the question being addressed.

Mechanical Stabilization by the Chamber

To map activation and repolarization from "working" or Langendorff-perfused hearts,[32,36,37] a chamber was designed to abate MA by providing mechanical stabilization while maintaining physiological conditions (i.e., normal levels of extracellular Ca^{2+}). The aortic cannula was passed through two Delrin platforms and locked in a desired position by compressing an O-ring between the two platforms. The front of the chamber, a cylindrical frame with a glass window, was attached to the platform by dovetails and the window was adjusted to make contact with the epicardium. The aortic cannula could be rotated to select the region of the heart viewed by the optical apparatus or displaced "up and down" to adjust the vertical position of the heart to the center of the window. The front part of the chamber was displaced until the glass made gentle contact with the epicardium and then was locked in place to prevent excess pressure between the glass and the heart. A second cylindrical frame or "rear part" slid as a piston inside the "front part" of the chamber to make a watertight seal (Fig. 4). The coronary effluent filled the chamber, bathed the heart, then drained out through an overflow port located on top of the chamber. Temperature was set at a chosen value and regulated to within 1°C with a thermistor placed near the base of the ventricle and with a feedback control system of a heat-exchange coil. Temperature gradients within the chamber were prevented by opening a valve at the bottom of the chamber to better mix the perfusate in the chamber. The pressure applied to heart by the chamber is designed to reduce MA on the front window while allowing the muscle to contract against the back part or the piston. A potential criticism of this approach is that the chamber applies excess pres-

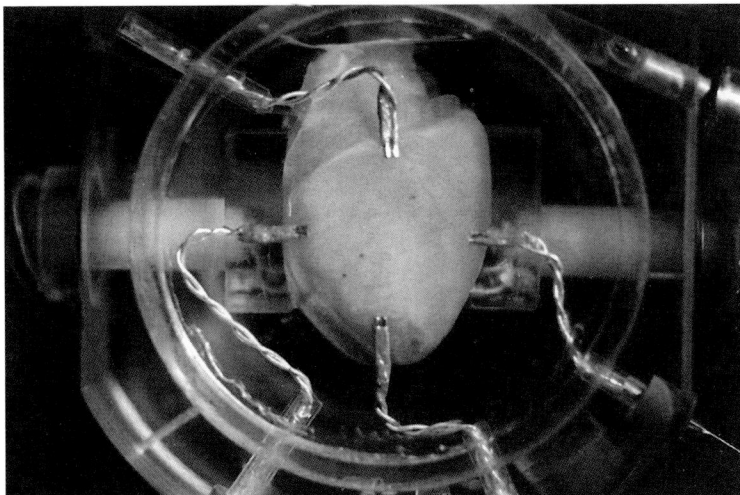

Figure 4. Photograph of a guinea pig heart in a chamber to reduce motion artifacts. The left ventricle faces the optical axis and is viewed by a photodiode array. Side pads on the anterior and posterior edges of the left ventricle contain bipolar electrodes for electrogram recordings and four $Ag^+/AgCl$ bipolar electrodes are placed around the field of view to stimulate the heart from different sites.

sure to the heart and its coronary vessels and reduces coronary flow, resulting in regional ischemia. Other concerns include the possibility of spatial heterogeneities of pressure and temperature across the myocardium, which could produce erroneous heterogeneities of action potentials. Numerous studies have shown that these concerns are not severe: 1) Guinea pig hearts were placed in the chamber and an action potential was recorded from the center of the epicardium at the first site to make contact with the glass window, with no pressure on the heart. The distance between the front and rear part of the chamber was then systematically decreased to compress the heart in 0.5-mm steps. After the heart was compressed by 2.0 to 2.5 mm, which raised diastolic pressure by 10 to 15 cm H_2O, MA were effectively abated but there were no changes in APD or amplitude. Further squeezing in the range of 5 to 6 mm (approximately 15-mm-diameter heart) was needed to reduce APD; this was tantamount to applying greater than 60 cm H_2O. 2) A "roving" thermistor was placed between the epicardium and the glass window and temperature was uniform through the epicardium to within 1°C, with or without exposing the heart to the excitation beam. 3) APDs were measured for several hours from hearts placed in the chamber but signs of ischemia could not be detected. As shown in Figure 3, optical action potential recordings were stable for 2 hours without signs of regional ischemia; i.e., decreases in APDs, triangulation of the plateau phase, and decreases in conduction velocity. 4) Maps of APDs measured from hearts in the chamber were compared with those measured from isolated, perfused ventricular sheets in the absence of a stabilizing chamber. Activation and repolarization maps were similar when recorded from the left and right epicardium of Langendorff and isolated sheet preparations, respectively.[18] 5) Displacement of the myocardium "in and out" of the field of view of a photodiode during a contraction would also preclude accurate measurements of APDs. Using a similar stabilizing chamber, Girouard et al.[38] inserted minutia pins on the myocardium at the corners of a 1×1-cm field of view to track the displacement of the tissue during contractions. In a freely beating heart, the displacement was 440±14 μm and was markedly reduced to 135±5 μm by the chamber.[38] Still, it is necessary to use stabilizing chambers cautiously. In all experiments, coronary flow rate and diastolic and systolic pressures are continuously monitored once the chamber is placed, to ensure that it does not alter cardiac function.

Diacetyl Monoxime

The membrane permeant oxime, diacetyl monoxime (DAM) or 2, 3-butane-dione monoxime, was shown to inhibit force development in a variety of muscles at 5 to 20 mmol/L in a reversible manner.[39,40] DAM uncouples excitation from contraction in cardiac muscle primarily by inhibiting myosin ATPase activity and cross-bridge formation. For this reason it has been an attractive approach to abolish force and MA in studies based on optical mapping techniques. However, it is now apparent that DAM influences other cellular systems involved in the regulation of myocardial contraction and electrical activity and thereby alters the substrate being studied. In rabbit and guinea pig ventricular myocytes, DAM inhibited the inward and delayed rectifier currents and reduced L-type Ca^{2+} currents, resulting in a decrease in APD and refractory periods.[41,42] DAM at low concentrations (1 to 5 mmol/L) had no effect on intracellular Ca^{2+} transients (Cai) but inhibited Cai at higher DAM concentrations (5 to 30 mmol/L). This effect of DAM does not involve a decrease in the Ca^{2-} affinity of troponin C but is due to a stimulation of Ca^{2+} release from the SR resulting in a decrease in Ca^{2+} load in the SR and of subsequent Cai transients.[42] A most serious pharmacological effect of DAM may be a rapid, dose-dependent blockade of gap junction conductance in rat ventricular myocytes,[43] which in principle reduces conduction velocity in heart muscle. Most studies report the pharmacological effects of DAM in superfused cardiac muscles and find that these effects are reversible upon washout. However, we found that when delivered through the coronary perfusate (in guinea pig and rabbit hearts), DAM (at 10 to 15 mmol/L for >45 min) can cause a loss of electrical excitability, in a time- and dose-dependent manner. In dog hearts, DAM changes the shape and time course of the "spike and dome" action potential on the epicardium (data not shown), most likely by inhibiting the transient outward K^+ current, I_{to}. The rate dependence and nonuniform distribution of I_{to} contributes to the temporal and spatial heterogeneities of APDs (i.e., differences in APD between the epicardial, endocardial, and M cells), which in turn have been invoked to explain the induction of arrhythmias.[44] In the rabbit atrioventricular (AV) node, DAM (10 to 15 mmol/L for more than 30 min) first prolonged AV delays, produced Wenckebach effects, then produced complete AV block. These time-dependent effects could be reversed if DAM was washed within 30 minutes but became irreversible once AV block occurred.[45] Thus, DAM must be used judiciously, particularly when delivered through the coronary perfusate. Most "side effects" of DAM are concentration-dependent and therefore can be minimized as required by experimental needs.

Ca^{2+} Channel Blockers

Another approach to abate MA is to perfuse hearts with an inhibitor of L-type Ca^{2+} channels, verapamil, which alters APDs and may have antiarrhythmic effects, and interferes with mechanoelectrical feedback. In some cases such as investigations of the effects of defibrillation shocks on myocardial depolarization, verapamil offers a suitable approach to abate MA.

Optical Mapping Techniques

Three optical mapping techniques have been used to map action potentials in heart: PDAs, laser scans, and CCD cameras. The advantages and disadvantages of these methods have been discussed in previous review articles.[1,46] Several aspects of the optical apparatus must be considered to maximize the quality of the signals (e.g., the S/N ratio of optical action potentials) that can be obtained in heart, including the light source, (e.g., noise characteristics, homogeneity of the excitation beam, intensity), the collection of light from the surface of the tissue under observation, and the detection of voltage-dependent absorption and/or fluorescence changes.

Light Sources

Three kinds of light sources have been used to measure optical action potentials in heart muscle: tungsten-halogen filament lamps, mercury/xenon arc lamps, and laser emission.

Filament Lamps. Tungsten-halogen lamps provide the most stable light source but have low intensity per unit area compared with arc lamps and laser emission. We have found that "projection" lamps consisting of a filament at the focal point of a parabolic mirror yield particularly stable excitation light and high intensity in the visible range and are commercially available at a variety of wattage outputs. It is not difficult to drive these lamps with a low ripple DC power supply, but switching DC supplies should be avoided. Only filament lamps have sufficiently low noise characteristics to measure action potential through absorption changes of the dye.[17,46] Light from the lamp is passed through a diaphragm placed at the focal plane of the focusing mirror, collected with a condensing lens, and is focused on the surface of the heart. These lamps are turned on during actual recordings (0.5 to 4 min) and are then turned off to avoid excessive heat to the lamp bases and electrodes. Once ignited, the lamps reach a stable running temperature in seconds, for data acquisition.

Arc Lamps. Xenon (75, 100, 250, and 300 W) arc lamps, lamp housings, and power supplies are available from several companies, with noise that is in the range of 1 part in 10^4 or 10 times greater than that for filament lamps. Arc lamps provide a fine illumination spot with 2 to 3 times greater intensity than the equivalent filament lamp, and are particularly advantageous when examining small fields of view (1- to 3-mm-diameter spots). For large fields of view (i.e., $\geq 1 \times 1$ cm), arc lamps have not been shown to significantly improve the S/N ratio. Two major disadvantages are the low-frequency light noise caused by oscillations or "arc wander" between the cathode and anode and the damage to electronic boards and components during the ignition of the arc lamp. The criterion for whether or not to use an arc lamp depends on the amplitude of the optical action potential with respect to dark noise and shot noise. If the dark noise of the detector is dominant, as is often the case for fluorescence measurements from single cells, then the S/N ratio will improve linearly with intensity, and if the shot noise is dominant, it will improve as the square root of intensity.[46] As a general rule, filament lamps provide sufficient intensity to measure action potentials from tissues and the extra intensity from an arc lamp improves the S/N ratio slightly at the expense of increased photobleaching and/or photodynamic damage. Nevertheless, the extra intensity of arc lamps is most useful for studies on cardiomyocytes because the area of excitable membrane and levels of membrane-bound dye limit the S/N ratio.

Laser Excitation. Lasers provide high-intensity monochromatic light spots, a requirement for the acousto-optic deflectors used in the laser or "flying spot" scanning technique.[33] Tungsten-halogen filament lamps are the most stable light sources, with light output fluctuations of 1 part in 10^5, whereas laser light is 10 to 50 times more noisy because of amplitude fluctuations (2 parts in 10^5) and laser speckle.[47] The pure monochromatic light of lasers does not often match the peak excitation wavelength of the dye molecule. Instead, the laser's wavelength excites a minor vibronic state of the dye and for dyes with broad excitation spectra, laser light is less effective at raising dye molecules to an excited fluorescent state. The higher noise and pure wavelength of laser light sources may be partly compensated by their high intensity per unit area, particularly for narrow excitation beams (<1 mm in diameter).

Detectors

Many factors must be considered when choosing an imaging system, including quantum efficiency of the sensor and, most importantly, the requirement for spatial and temporal resolution. Increases in either temporal or spatial resolution reduce the S/N ratio because in a shot noise limited measurement, the S/N ratio is proportional to the number of measured photons.

Photodiode Arrays. The PDA technique was first introduced to simultaneously record electrical activity from multiple sites in invertebrate ganglia,[48] processes of a cultured neuron,[49] and cardiac muscle.[31,32] Figure 5 shows a typical PDA apparatus. Light from tungsten-halogen lamps is collected, projected, passed through appropriate interference filters, and focused on the surface of a perfused heart in its chamber. The fluorescence or reflectance from the surface of the heart is collected with a camera lens mounted on bellows, passed through a cut-off or interference filter, and focused on the surface of a PDA by a second lens. The magnification (M) of the image of the heart falling on the array depends on several parameters:

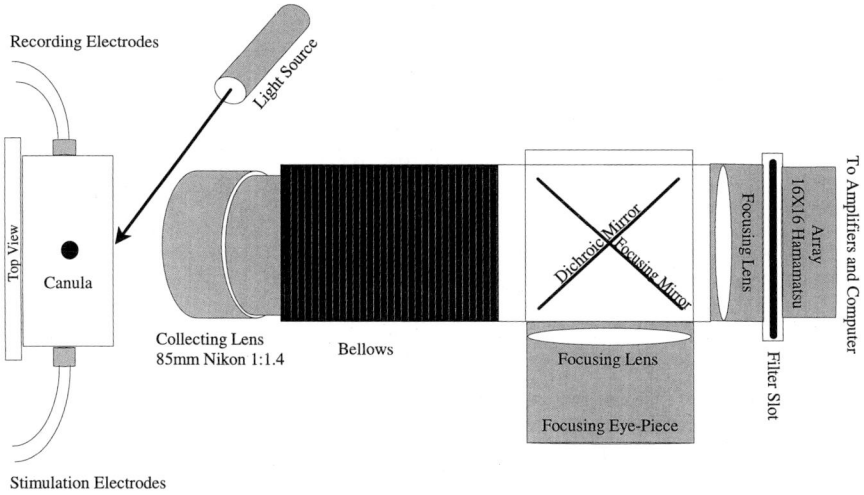

Figure 5. Top view of optical apparatus. The heart is placed in the chamber shown in Fig. 4 and is illuminated by the beam of a tungsten-halogen lamp. Fluorescent light from the dye bound to the heart is collected with a camera lens, passed though a dichroic mirror to transmit light greater than 610 nm to a 16×16 element photodiode array and to reflect light less than 610 nm to a focusing screen, another array, or a charged coupled device camera (not shown). The 256 channels of signals from the diodes are processed in parallel circuits, amplified, filtered, digitized, and stored in computer memory (see text).

the focal lengths (f1 and f2) of the collecting and focusing lenses, respectively; the "object" distance between the heart and the collecting lens; the distance between the two lenses; and the "image" distance between the focusing lens and the array. These distances are variable such that magnifications from 6× to −4× can be obtained with commercially available lenses for 35-mm cameras (e.g. Nikon 50-mm, f1:1.2, f1:1.4, or f1:1.8 and 85-mm f1:1.4 [Nikon Corp., Torrance, CA]). The focusing lens is a 40-mm-diameter, double convex lens with 100-mm focal length (Edmund Scientific, Barrington, NJ). The first mapping system was designed with a 12×12 matrix of photodiodes (Centronic Ltd., Craydon, UK, model MD 144, or MD 100–5PV for a 10×10 element array). Every diode detects light from a different region of the image that corresponds to light levels from a specific site on the heart. Arrays were provided with gold leaf wires as output lines to read the photocurrents from individual diodes. Analog circuits, the interface, and the computer hardware and software were built in-house. Details of the first interface and computer algorithms appeared in a previous review.[1] A major advantage of PDA systems is the high temporal resolution achieved by the parallel readout of the diodes. Another advantage is the high spatial resolution achieved by the large number of diodes that can be used to resolve the spread of electrical activity in myocardium. Disadvantages of these systems have included the need to design and construct most of the components and to develop software for data acquisition and analysis. The task of building a new system has been markedly simplified over the last few years, particularly with respect to the interface and the computer hardware and software. An array with increased spatial resolution became available from Centronic with 464 pixels (MD-464),[50] but this array has not been used in cardiac studies because of concerns regarding reliability (up to 10% of the diodes fail) and difficulties of building an interface with 464 parallel channels of data. A 16×16 array is now available from Hamamatsu Photonics Corp. (Bridgewater, NJ) with several choices of feedback resistors for the current-to-voltage converters on first-stage amplifiers. Other silicon diode imaging systems have been developed for neuroscience applications. Some are noteworthy because of increased spatial resolution, with as many as 1020 diodes, and a combination of parallel and serial readouts of the diode elements is used to achieve high sampling rates.[46]

Laser Scan. The advantages and disadvantages of the laser scan technique were previously discussed.[1,33,51] Of note has been the combination of laser excitation (argon ion laser, Innova 70-4, Coherent Inc., Palo Alto, CA) with 256 bifurcated light guides and 256 photodiodes aligned in a matrix to record electrical activity from in vivo (open-chest) dog heart.[51] The high intensity (1 W) of the laser is shared by a matrix of 16×16 fiberoptic probes spaced on 3-mm centers which form a recording plaque with a total recording area of 45×45 mm, on the heart. Each fiberoptic probe consists of six return fibers to collect fluorescence that surround a central fiber used to deliver the laser excitation. The fluorescence from the six return fibers on each fiberoptic probe is measured by an individual photodiode and the 256 diodes are read at 2000 frames per second (fps) through a parallel interface.[51] Laser light is noisier than conventional light sources and a laser stabilization system was devised to reduce the noise caused by a factor of 10 to improve the S/N ratio of optical action potential recordings.[51]

Vacuum Photocathode and CCD Cameras. The low quantum efficiency of vacuum photocathodes (0.15 compared with 0.9 for photodiodes) is a disadvantage but may be preferable when the signals can be time-averaged to improve the S/N ratio. In studies of the response properties of the monkey striate cortex, neuronal activity measured with a voltage-sensitive dye required particularly high spatial resolution.[34] Images of the monkey visual cortex were focused on a Newvicon television camera (model 5300, Cohu Inc., San Diego, CA) using an objective with 0.1 to 0.1 numeral aperture. The video signal was fed to an image processor (Imaging Technology Inc., Woburn, MA), which consisted of a digitizer with a flash 8-bit analog-to-digital (A/D) converter, four frame buffers, and an arithmetic unit processor. Video images taken under different conditions of visual stimulation were accumulated in separate frame buffers for subsequent manipulation by the arithmetic processor. The limited dynamic range of the A/D converters (256 gray levels) and the small fractional fluorescence changes (approximately 0.1%) during electrical activity required additional circuitry for the following reasons: 1) to flatten the signal so that all parts of the image had roughly equal values; 2) to boost the small signal gain, which contains most of the voltage-dependent information; and 3) to eliminate DC bias (reduce the apparent white level). This circuitry put radiant changes greater than 0.01% within the range of the flash A/D converter. It also introduced and amplified noise, which was removed through averaging.[34] Tests with the calibrated emission of a light-emitting diode (LED) indicate that a photocathode video camera detects radiant changes greater than 0.01% if they persist long enough (approximately seconds) to be time averaged.

CCD cameras have greater quantum efficiency than do photocathodes, but the dynamic range is still limited by the accuracy of the A/D conversion and saturation at light levels obtained from cardiac tissue. A dynamic range of 10^3 is not easily achieved.[46] CCD cameras have been used extensively to map activation[35,52,53] and fibrillation.[54,55] With CCD cameras, the standard frame rate (30 Hz or 33.3 fps) can be speeded up at the expense of spatial resolution. The standard video rate can be accelerated twofold to 16.7 ms/frame by using noninterlaced video, reducing the number of vertical lines from 480 to 240 video lines.[56] It can be further speeded up by using an external reset feature, decreasing the number of usable horizontal lines; at 4.2, 8.3, and 16.7 ms/frame there are 60, 120, and 240 usable horizontal lines, respectively.[56] In the absence of spatial filtering, the S/N ratio of a CCD pixel is too low to detect an optical action potential in a single sweep. With a spatial Gaussian filter of 2.5 to 3 pixels, an S/N ratio of 1.6 can be achieved at a frame rate of 4.2 ms/frame.[56] The improved spatial resolution comes at the cost of poor temporal resolution and S/N ratio, which can blur measurements of conduction velocity particularly for fast velocities or when action potentials propagate in 4 to 8 ms across the heart.[32,57] Refinements of digital cameras will most likely improve the dynamic range, accuracy, and frame rate. A camera made by PixelVision, Inc. (Tigard, OR) with 80×80 elements, large pixels (18 μm), 14-bit accuracy, and 1500 fps promises a turn-key interface with improved spatial and temporal resolution.

Optics

Numerical Aperture (NA). The need to maximize the collection of fluorescent photons and the S/N ratio dominates the choice of optical components. The number of photons collected by an objective lens during the formation of an image is proportional to $(NA)^2$. In epi-illumination, both the excitation and the emission pass through the objective and the intensity is proportional to the fourth power of the NA.[47] Thus, objectives with high NA are of critical importance to maximize the S/N ratio. For mapping the surface of guinea pig, rabbit, or other mammalian hearts of similar dimensions, the magnification of the image of the heart was in the range of 0.6× to 4×. For low magnifications, conventional microscope objectives have low NA, and we therefore took advantage of high-NA camera lenses to image the heart on the array.[52] A direct comparison of camera versus microscope lenses, at 4× magnification, showed that the fluorescence intensity detected with the camera lens was 100× greater than that detected with a microscope objective.[46]

Energy Transfer Function. The intensity of the light reaching the image plane depends on the light-collecting efficiency of the lens; this is largely but not strictly determined by the magnification and NA. The intensity depends primarily on the *"energy transfer function"* which is sometimes available from the manufacturer. Alternatively, the energy transfer function can be determined by systematically displacing an LED in the object x-y plane of the lens and recording the energy distribution reaching the detector in the image plane. The goal is to compare several "fast" lenses (i.e., camera lenses that can capture images after brief exposure of the film) to maximize the intensity of the image and the S/N ratio of the signals.

Spatial Resolution and Depth of Field. The depth of focus of a lens can be measured by focusing an object then displacing it along the optical or z-axis until it appears blurred. This subjective measurement can be quantified by focusing the light from an LED on a diode on the array and defocusing the image of the LED (moving along the z-axis) until the intensity decreases by 50% while it increases in the neighboring diodes. In heart muscle, the optical action potential detected by each diode will represent the sum of signals from a volume of cells (V) equal to the area of tissue (A) viewed by the diode times twice the depth of field (DF), $V = A \times 2DF$. The DF of the apparatus depends on the NA of the collecting lens, the emission wavelength (λ_{ex}), and the magnification (M), and can be calculated from an empirical equation[58] DF $(in\ \mu m) = 1000\ \mu m/[(7\ NA \times M) + \lambda_{ex}\ (\mu m)/2\ (NA)^2]$.

Application of Voltage-Sensitive Dyes and Future Directions

Optical mapping is still a relatively new technique, but it is coming into its own as a powerful tool to address fundamental questions in cardiac electrophysiology. The method offers important advantages, which are being increasingly appreciated and used to investigate areas that could not be satisfactorily addressed by conventional methods. As shown in the succeeding chapters, it offers new insights into many important basic science and clinical problems. For instance, the voltage-sensitive dye response is impervious to shock artifacts and can be used to examine in detail the depolarization of the myocardium close to and far from the shock electrodes. The high spatial and temporal resolution that can be achieved allows us, for the first time, to visualize action potential wave fronts within a single cell, in patterned cultured cells with complex organization, in heart muscle as it curls around obstacles and forms vortices with or without an anatomical obstacle, and during fibrillation. The spatial resolution offers the opportunity to map impulse propagation across the AV node and address fundamental questions regarding the mechanisms of AV node delay, facilitation, and Wenckebach phenomena. Several investigators are involved in mapping the small hearts of mice to take advantage of molecularly engineered hearts with specific ion channel modifications. In some cases, optical methods have produced controversy, but again it is still the most potent approach to resolve it, and the potential development of depth-resolved images for 3-dimensional mapping will guarantee the method a long and bright future.

Acknowledgments I am indebted to William Hughes and Scott MacPherson, staff of the Departmental Machine Shop, for their skill and professionalism, and to Jim VonHedemann and Greg Szekeres, staff of the Electronic Shop, for their continuous help and ability to solve instrumentation problems. Thanks are due to my graduate student, Mr. Bum-Rak Choi, for his collaboration and proof reading the manuscript, and to Alexander R. Terrill, for helping with some of the figures.

References

1. Salama G. Optical measurements of transmembrane potential in heart. In Loew L (ed): *Probes of Membrane Potential.* Boca Raton: Uniscience Press; 1988:137–199.
2. Cohen LB, Keynes RD, Hille B. Light scattering and birefringence changes during nerve activity. *Nature* 1968;218:438–441.
3. Cohen LB, Hille B, Keynes RD. Light scattering and birefringence changes during activity in the electric organ of *Electrophorus electricus. J Physiol (Lond)* 1969;203:489–509.
4. Cohen LB, Hille B, Keynes RD. Changes in axon fluorescence during an action potential. *J Physiol (Lond)* 1971;211:495–515.
5. Tasaki I, Watanabe R, Sandlin R, Carnay L. Changes in fluorescence, turbidity, and birefringence associated with nerve excitation. *Proc Natl Acad Sci U S A* 1968;61:883–888.
6. Conti F, Tasaki I. Changes in extrinsic fluorescence in squid axons during voltage-clamp. *Science* 1970;169:1332–1324.
7. Conti F, Tasaki I, Wanke E. Fluorescence signals in ANS-stained squid giant axons during voltage-clamp. *Biophysik* 1971;8:58–70.
8. Conti F, Wanke E. Changes produced by electrical stimulation in the extrinsic ANS fluorescence of nerve membranes. *EU Biophys Congress* 1971;1:199.
9. Conti F. Fluorescent probes in nerve membranes. *Annu Rev Biophys Bioeng* 1975;4:287–310.
10. Davila HV, Cohen LB, Salzberg BM, et al. Changes in ANS and TNS fluorescence in giant axons from Loligo. *J Membr Biol* 1974;15:29–46.
11. Tasaki I, Carnay L, Watanabe A. Transient changes in extrinsic fluorescence of nerve produced by electrical stimulation. *Proc Natl Acad Sci U S A* 1969;64:1362–1368.
12. Tasaki I, Carnay L, Sandlin R. Fluorescence changes during conduction in nerves stained with Acridine Orange. *Science* 1969;163:683–685.
13. Cohen LB, Salzberg BM, Davila HV, et al. Changes in axon fluorescence during activity: Molecular probes of membrane potential. *J Membr Biol* 1974;19:1–36.
14. Davila HV, Salzberg BM, Cohen LB, et al. A large change in axon fluorescence that provides a promising method for measuring membrane potential. *Nat New Biol* 1973;241:159–160.
15. Salama G. *Merocyanine Dyes as Optical Probes of Membrane Potential.* [PhD thesis] University of Pennsylvania. Ann Arbor: University Microfilms International; 1978.
16. Salama G, Morad M. Merocyanine 540 as an optical probe of transmembrane electrical activity in the hearts. *Science* 1976;191:485–487.
17. Morad M, Salama G. Merocyanine dyes as optical probes of membrane potential in heart. *J Physiol (Lond)* 1979;292:267–295.
18. Kanai A, Salama G. Optical mapping reveals that repolarization spreads anisotropically and is guided by fiber orientation in guinea pig hearts. *Circ Res* 1995;77:784–802.
19. Brooker LGS, Keyes GH, Spague RH, et al. Color and constitution. X. Absorption of the Merocyanines. *J Am Chem Soc* 1951;73:5332.
20. Brooker LGS, Craig AC, Heseltine DW, et al. Color and constitution. XIII. Merocyanines as solvent property indicators. *J Am Chem Soc* 1965;87(11):2443–2450.
21. Loew L, Cohen LB, Dix J, et al. A naphthyl analog of the aminostyryl pyridinium class of potentiometric membrane dyes shows consistent sensitivity in

a variety of tissue, cell and model membrane preparations. *J Membr Biol* 1992;130:1–10.

22. Windish H, Muller W, Tritthart H. Fluorescence monitoring of rapid changes in membrane potential in heart muscle. *Biophys J* 1985;48:877–884.

23. Loew LM, Scully S, Simpson L, Waggoner AS. Evidence for a charge-shift electrochromic mechanism in a probe of membrane potential. *Nature* 1979; 281:497–499.

24. Loew LM, Bonneville GW, Surrow J. Charge shift optical probes of membrane potential. *Biochemistry* 1978;17:4065–4071.

25. Montana V, Farkas DL, Loew LM. Dual-wavelength ratiometric fluorescence measurements of membrane potential. *Biochemistry* 1989;28:4536–4539.

26. Arvanitaki A, Chalazonitis N. Excitation and inhibitory process initiated by light and infrared radiation in single excitable nerve cells (giant ganglion cells of Aplysia). In Florey E (ed): *Nervous Inhibition*. New York: Pergamon Press; 1961:194.

27. Kagan KE, Ritov VB, Gorbunov NV, et al. Oxidative stress and Ca^{2+} transport in skeletal and cardiac sarcoplasmic reticulum. In Reznick A (ed): *Oxidative Stress in Skeletal Muscle*. Basel, Switzerland: Birkhäuser Verlag; 1998:181–199.

28. Salama G, Kanai A, Huang DT, et al. Hypoxia and hypothermia enhance spatial heterogeneities of repolarization in guinea pig hearts: Analysis of spatial correlation of optically recorded action potential durations. *J Cardiovasc Electrophysiol* 1998;9:164–183.

29. Rhor S, Salzberg BM. Multiple site optical recordings of transmembrane voltage in patterned growth heart cell cultures: Assessing electrical behavior with microsecond resolution on a cellular and subcellular scale. *Biophys J* 1994;67:1301–1315.

30. Schaffer P, Ahammer H, Muller W, et al. Di4-ANEPPS causes photodynamic damage to isolated cardiomyocytes. *Eur J Physiol* 1994;426:548–551.

31. Salama G, Sanger T, Cohen LB. Optical recordings of action potential propagation in intact heart. *Biol Bull* 1981;61:316.

32. Salama G, Lombardi R, Elson J. Maps of optical action potentials and NADH fluorescence in intact working hearts. *Am J Physiol* 1987;252(2 Pt. 2):H384–H394.

33. Dillon SM, Morad MA. A new laser scanning system for measuring action potential propagation in heart. *Science* 1981;214:453–456.

34. Blasdel G, Salama G. Voltage-sensitive dyes reveal a modular organization in monkey striate cortex. *Nature* 1986;321:579–585.

35. Davidenko JM, Pertsov AV, Salomonz R, et al. Stationary and drifting spiral waves of excitation in isolated cardiac muscle. *Nature* 1992;355:349–351.

36. Salama G, Rosenbaum D, Kanai A, et al. Data analysis techniques for measuring spatial inhomogeneity in repolarization using optical transmembrane potentials. *Proc Ann Int Conf IEEE Eng Med Biol Soc* 1989;11:222–223.

37. Efimov IR, Ermentrout B, Huang DT, Salama G. Activation and repolarization patterns are governed by different structural characteristics of ventricular myocardium: Experimental study with voltage-sensitive dyes and numerical simulations. *J Cardiovasc Electrophysiol* 1996;7:512–530.

38. Girouard SD, Laurita KR, Rosenbaum DS. Unique properties of cardiac action potentials recorded with voltage sensitive dyes. *J Cardiovasc Electrophysiol* 1996;7:1024–1038.

39. Wiggins JR, Reiser J, Fitzpatrick DF, Bergey JL. Inotropic actions of diacetyl monoxime in cat ventricular muscle. *J Pharmacol Exp Ther* 1980;212:217–224.

40. Li T, Sperelakis N, Teneick RE, Solaro RJ. Effects of diacetyl monoxime on cardiac excitation-contraction coupling. *J Pharmacol Exp Ther* 1985;232:688–695.

41. Liu Y, Cabo C, Salomonz R, et al. Effects of diacetyl monoxime on the electrical properties of sheep and guinea pig ventricular muscle. *Cardiovasc Res* 1993;27:1991–1997.

42. Gwathmey JK, Hajjar RJ, Solaro RJ. Contractile deactivation and uncoupling of crossbridges. Effects of 2,3-butanedione monoxime on mammalian myocardium. *Circ Res* 1991;69:1280–1292.
43. Verrechia F, Hervé JC. Reversible blockade of gap junctional communication by 2,3-butanedione monoxime in rat cardiac myocytes. *Am J Physiol* 1997;272:C875–C885.
44. Antzelevitch C, Sicouri S. Clinical relevance of cardiac arrhythmias generated by afterdepolarizations. Role of M cells in the generation of U waves, triggered activity and torsade de pointes. *J Am Coll Cardiol* 1994;23:259–277.
45. Choi B-R, Salama G. Optical mapping of the rabbit atrio-ventricular node reveals discontinuities of propagation from atrial to nodal cells. *Am J Physiol* 1998;43(3):H829–H845.
46. Wu JY, Lam YW, Falk CX, et al. Voltage-sensitive dyes for monitoring multi-neuronal activity in the intact CNS. *J Histochem* 1998;30:169–187.
47. Cohen LB, Lesher S. Optical monitoring of membrane potential: Method of multisites optical measurements. In DeWeer P, Salzberg BM (eds): *Optical Methods in Cell Physiology*. New York: Wiley-Interscience; 1986:72.
48. Grinvald A, Cohen LB, Lesher S, Boyle MB. Simultaneous optical monitoring of activity of many neurons in invertebrate ganglia using a 124-element photodiode array. *J Neurophysiol* 1981;45(5):829–840.
49. Grinvald A, Ross WN, Farber I. Simultaneous optical measurements of electrical activity from multiple sites on processes of cultured neurons. *Proc Natl Acad Sci U S A* 1981;78:3245–3249.
50. Senseman DM. High-speed optical imaging of afferent flow through rat olfactory bulb slices: Voltage-sensitive dye signals reveal periglomerular cell activity. *J Neurosci* 1996;16:313–324.
51. Hill B, Courtney K. Design of multi-point laser scanned optical monitor of cardiac action potential propagation: Application to microentry in guinea pig atrium. *Ann Biomed Eng* 1987;15:567–577.
52. Cabo C, Pertsov AM, Baxter WT, et al. Wave-front curvature as a cause of slow conduction and block in isolated cardiac muscle. *Circ Res* 1994;75:1014–1028.
53. Pertsov AM, Davidenko JM, Salomonz R, et al. Spiral waves of excitation underlie reentrant activity in isolated cardiac muscle. *Circ Res* 1993;72:631–650.
54. Gray RA, Pertsov AM, Jalife J. Spatial and temporal organization during cardiac fibrillation. *Nature* 1998;392:75–78.
55. Witkowski FX, Leon JL, Penkoske PA, et al. Spatiotemporal evolution of ventricular fibrillation. *Nature* 1998;392:78–82.
56. Baxter WT, Davidenko JM, Loew LM, et al. Technical features of a CCD camera system to record cardiac fluorescence data. *Ann Biomed Eng* 1997;25(4):713–725.
57. Salama G, Efimov RI, Kanai A. Subthreshold stimulation of the Purkinje system interrupts ventricular tachycardia as monitored with voltage-sensitive dyes and imaging techniques. *Circ Res* 1994;74(3):1–16.
58. Piller H. *Microscope Photometry*. New York: Springer-Verlag; 1977:16.

Chapter 2

Mechanisms and Principles of Voltage-Sensitive Fluorescence

Leslie M. Loew

Introduction

Potentiometric dyes are designed to either assay average membrane potentials in cell population measurements with a spectrofluorometer or determine spatial patterns of voltage distribution associated with tissues, individual cells, or organelles. The latter types of applications are the primary interest of this laboratory and have directed our dye chemistry development. Several important general purpose dyes have emerged from this effort, including di-5-ASP,[1] di-4-ANEPPS,[2,3] di-8-ANEPPS,[4,5] TMRM, and TMRE.[6] Such dyes have been of great utility to neuroscientists interested in mapping patterns of electrical activity in complex neuronal preparations, with numerous examples spanning the last two decades.[7-9] In addition, the dyes have been used to map the spatial[4,10,11] and temporal[12,13] patterns of electrical activity along single cell membranes and have measured potentials in fine processes and at synapses.[14] We have even been able to measure the membrane potentials across the inner membranes of individual mitochondria within a single living cell.[15] All of these experiments could not be accomplished with conventional electrical measurements using microelectrode or patch-clamp techniques.

The availability of optical methods has had an especially important impact on the study of patterns of electrical activity in cardiac tissue. Guy Salama was one of the pioneers of this technology and, with W. Müller and H. Windisch, also introduced the use of di-4-ANEPPS to the study of cardiac electrophysiology.[3,16-18] The technology was then significantly advanced when it was demonstrated that video cameras could produce high spatial and temporal resolution records of spiral waves in isolated cardiac muscle with this fluorescent dye.[19,20] Di-4-ANEPPS now is the probe of choice for a number of laboratories that are studying complex patterns of activity in heart, as exemplified by many of the chapters in this volume.

The purpose of this chapter is to describe the physical and chemical

I would like to acknowledge the consistent support of the NIH through grant no. GM35063.

From Rosenbaum DS, Jalife J (eds): *Optical Mapping of Cardiac Excitation and Arrhythmias*. ©Futura Publishing Co., Inc., Armonk, NY, 2001.

properties of potentiometric dyes so that they may be rationally chosen and applied to problems in cardiac physiology. Emphasis is placed on describing the known mechanisms for the response of dyes to membrane potential changes. The solubility of the dyes and their mode of binding to membranes is also discussed as this relates to their utility in preparations of different thickness. Finally, some new ideas for optical mapping based on recent developments in microscopy are presented.

Mechanisms of Spectral Sensitivity to Membrane Potential

There are many factors that contribute to deciding on a choice of dye for a given preparation and experimental objective. A primary aim of this chapter is to provide background information about the dye chemistries that is sufficient to assure that these choices have a rational basis. In this section we concentrate on the central issue of the mechanisms by which dyes can display spectral changes in response to changes in membrane potential. Figure 1 summarizes three broad categories of dye responses to membrane potential and Figure 2 details a fourth mechanism, electrochromism, which is the putative source of the sensitivity of many styryl dyes like di-4-ANEPPS. Table 1 lists examples of some commonly used dyes representing all of the major mechanisms and classes of chromophores. These mechanisms are now discussed and the general classes of dyes that use them identified.

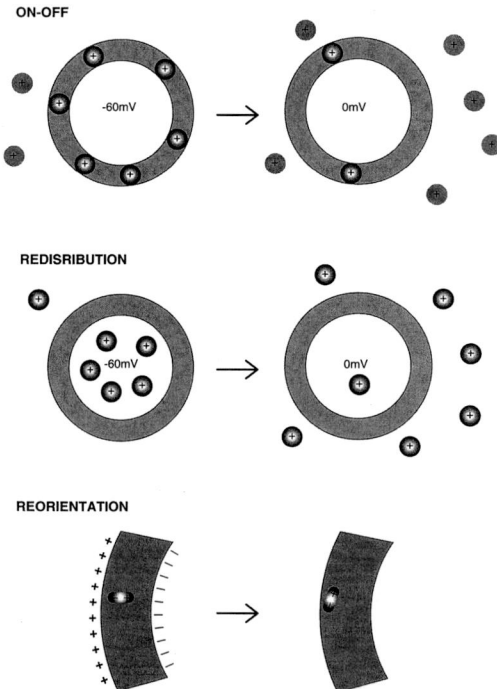

Figure 1. Common mechanisms for the spectral sensitivity of dyes to membrane potential. *Left:* The state of the dyes when the membrane is polarized. *Right:* The effect of depolarization. The gray ring represents the cell membrane for the ON-OFF and REDISTRIBUTION mechanisms while only a portion of the membrane is represented as a gray arc for the REORIENTATION mechanism. The bright objects represent fluorescent dye molecules, while the dull gray objects represent poorly fluorescent dye molecules. Detailed explanations of each mechanism are given in the text.

Figure 2. Electrochromic mechanism for dye response to membrane potential. *Top:* The key characteristics of an electrochromic probe are illustrated for di-4-ANEPPS. The chromophore portion of the molecule undergoes a charge shift upon excitation from the ground state to the excited state because of the reorganization of the electronic structure. Also critical is that the molecule contains appended polar groups and nonpolar hydrocarbon chains arranged in such a way as to orient the rod-shaped chromophore parallel to the intramembrane electrical field. This orientation is shown at the *bottom,* where the chromophore is represented as a hatched rectangle embedded in a shaded membrane. The field produced inside a polarized membrane lowers the energy difference between the ground and excited states and therefore shifts the dye spectra to higher wavelengths (cf. Fig. 3).

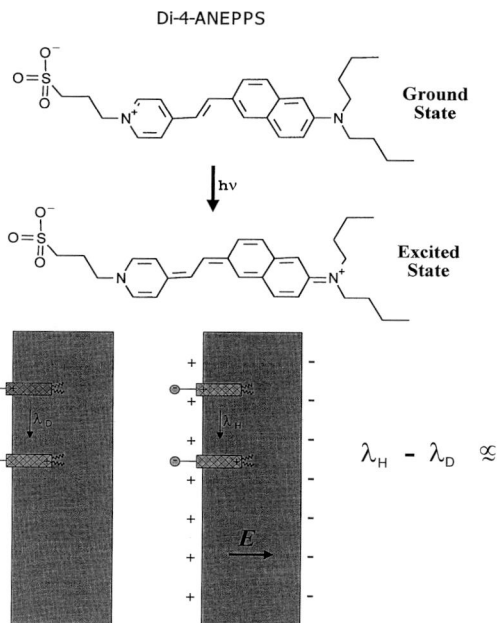

The ON-OFF mechanism is common to many cyanine and oxonol dyes.[21–23] The cyanines are positive dyes and the oxonols are negatively charged. Figure 1 depicts only the case for a positive dye. In its simplest form, a positively charged dye will have a greater binding constant to a polarized than to a depolarized membrane; the opposite holds for negative dyes. Most dyes exhibit significant fluorescence enhancements when associated with a hydrophobic and viscous environment. Therefore, the fluorescence of cyanine dyes that obey a pure ON-OFF mechanism goes down upon depolarization while that of oxonols goes up.

An understanding of the details of the physical-chemical interactions involved in the ON-OFF mechanism can help in the design of applications. The concentrations of dye and membrane must be adjusted so that there will be a close balance between the concentration of aqueous and membrane-bound forms; only under this condition of balance can a change in potential effect a large change in the relative populations of the two forms. Of course, the optimal concentration of dye should also provide a large fluorescence signal while minimizing any deleterious photodynamic or pharmacological effects. The key point is that one cannot simply increase the concentration of dye to obtain a large signal-to-noise (S/N) ratio, as the sensitivity to potential is also dependent on dye concentration. Clearly, the optimal concentrations can vary tremendously from preparation to preparation and from dye to dye.

To be useful for measuring electrical activity in cardiac preparations, the dyes must respond to changes in potential with time constants on the order of 0.01 seconds. For the ON-OFF mechanism, which requires a significant molecular translocation from a membrane to an aqueous environ-

Table 1
Properties of Selected Potentiometric Dyes

Name	Chromophore	Description	ABS (nm)	EM (nm)	Structure
M-540	Merocyanine	One of the original and most thoroughly studied potentiometric dyes. First heart dye. Reorientation mechanism. t: ms	555	578	
TMRE	Rhodamine	Rhodamine redistribution dye for single cell and mitochondrial potential measurements. t: s - min	548	597	
Di-S-C3(5)	Cyanine	Very sensitive dye for cell suspensions. Can give 10-fold intensity changes by a redistribution/self-quench mechanism. t: s - min	550	568	
Rhodamine-123	Rhodamine	Redistribution dye for mitochondrial staining. t: min	505	534	
DiBaC4(3)	Oxonol	Anionic on:off indicator. Also called "Bis-oxonol"; t:ms-s	493	516	
Di-4-ANEPPS	Naphthyl Styryl	Versatile fast styryl dye. Most common heart dye. Electrochromic mechanism. Dual wavelength ratio is an option. t: <μs	502	723	
RH155	Oxonol	Good choice for absorbance measurements. No fluorescence signals. t: ms	638		
RH795	Styryl	Good styryl dye for penetration into cortex; t: ms	530	712	

ment, such rapid speeds are often not attained. There is evidence of a variant ON-OFF mechanism for many of the dyes in which the movement occurs from the membrane to a near-membrane aqueous binding site; such a mechanism would be expected to be faster.[24] Another factor that influences the speed of the response is the kinetic barrier for movement of the dye through the membrane-aqueous interface. The size of this barrier depends on the degree of charge delocalization within the dye chromophore and the size of the dye molecule. In general, the more highly delocalized the charge and the larger the molecule holding the charge, the more readily does the dye move from the aqueous to the lipid phase. The polar headgroups of the lipid molecules produce a dipole potential[25] that also affects the barrier to movement of ions from the aqueous to the membrane phases. Because this electrostatic potential rises steeply for the first several angstroms into the membrane, anions can penetrate the membrane much faster than cations can. Therefore, all other factors being equal, oxonols generally can achieve more rapid responses to potential changes than can cyanines by the ON-OFF mechanism. The "bisoxonol" dyes, e.g., diBaC$_4$(3) in Table 1, are among the more sensitive ON-OFF dyes.

The REDISTRIBUTION mechanism is shown in its simplest form in the center of Figure 1. A fluorescent membrane-permeant cation distributes between the extracellular medium and the cytosol according to the Nernst equation:

$$\Delta V = -60\log\left(\frac{[dye]_{in}}{[dye]_{out}}\right) mV \qquad (1)$$

This mechanism is the basis for microscope-based methods where the ratio of fluorescence from inside and outside a cell is directly related to the membrane potential.[26,27] Cationic rhodamine dyes, such as TMRE (Table 1), are frequently employed for such measurements. However, this simple mechanism would not produce a fluorescence change when a population of cells or a multicellular region of an organ is being sampled by the measuring optics, as would be the case for optical mapping of cardiac activity. This is because the fluorescence of the individual dye molecules does not change, and therefore the redistribution depicted in Figure 1 will not cause a change in fluorescence measured from the averaged population of dye molecules in a large multicellular region of a preparation.

However, a more complex form of the REDISTRIBUTION mechanism can produce a change in total fluorescence signal with a change in membrane voltage. This combines the Nernstian redistribution shown in Figure 1 with a concentration-dependent aggregation of the dye molecules. Cyanine dyes are especially prone to this phenomenon.[21,24,28,29] Dye aggregates are usually nonfluorescent or can have highly red-shifted fluorescence spectra. If the optical system is set up with filters corresponding to the optimal wavelengths for the fluorescent monomeric dye, fluorescence changes of as much as a factor of 100 can be realized for a voltage change of 60 mV. This is because the dye aggregate is not membrane permeant; aggregation, by mass action, therefore pulls monomer across a polarized membrane at levels beyond what would be predicted by the Nernst equation.[30]

Unfortunately, dyes using the REDISTRIBUTION mechanism are invariably too slow to be useful for following cardiac action potentials. This is because of the need to have dyes re-equilibrate completely between two aqueous compartments separated by a membrane barrier following a potential change. The fastest REDISTRIBUTION kinetics are on second time scales and some dyes can take minutes to fully equilibrate. Still, it may be possible to detect incomplete changes in dye distribution at a time scale corresponding to cardiac action potentials. But the primary reason for the inclusion of this mechanism, in addition to historical completeness, is that the high sensitivity could be useful in designing experiments in which the aim is to follow potential on a slow time scale, such as variations in average or resting potential. Also, many dyes can respond to membrane potential via a composite of several mechanisms. So to properly interpret dye signals, it is helpful to have a comprehensive understanding of all known mechanisms. Indeed, di-S-C$_3$(5) (Table 1) can behave with either a REDISTRIBUTION or an ON-OFF mechanism, depending on the concentrations of dye and membrane, but in most applications it uses a combination of REDISTRIBUTION and aggregation to produce huge potential-dependent fluorescence changes.

In contrast, the molecular motion in the REORIENTATION mechanism, shown at the bottom of Figure 1, is relatively modest and therefore typically displays submillisecond kinetics. It is therefore well suited to faithfully monitoring cardiac action potentials. On the other hand, the magnitude of the fluorescence change with potential is small compared with the other mechanisms. As in the ON-OFF mechanism, the sensitivity to potential depends on the existence of a delicate free energy balance between two or more states of the dye; in the present case, however, the states correspond to different orientations of the dye within the membrane. A change in the intramembrane electrical field can then shift the balance via an electrostatic interaction with the dye dipole moment. For the pure REORIENTATION mechanism, the fluorescence change arises from the intrinsic optical anisotropy of the preparation and would not, for example, be seen in a homogenous cell suspension. The basic principle that is at work here is that the transition moment of a dye must be aligned with the oscillating electrical field of the incident light; the latter is perpendicular to the direction of propagation of the light wave. Therefore, dye molecules oriented parallel to the incident light beam, as on the lower left of Figure 1, will be very poorly excited. Upon reorientation after depolarization (bottom right), the geometry is appropriate for absorption of a photon and detection of the fluorescence emission with the epifluorescence optical path common to most microscopes. The heart is appropriately anisotropic and this is the putative mechanism for the first dye applied to optical mapping of cardiac activity, Merocyanine 540.[16,31]

As for the other mechanisms, there are important variations of the REORIENTATION mechanism that have been described. At high concentrations of dye, dimerization or aggregation of dye monomers can occur in the membrane, with a preference for molecules that can associate with each other in an antiparallel manner. Such an antiparallel arrangement will only be possible for dyes that are not aligned by the intramembrane electrical field, as is shown on the bottom right of Figure 1. Whereas the simple REORIENTATION mechanism has a potential-dependent relative fluorescence change that is independent of dye concentration, the coupling of the mechanism to a fluorescence change due to aggregation imparts a strong concentration dependence. Merocyanine 540, one of the first dyes used to monitor action potentials (Table 1), can produce potential-dependent responses with or without an aggregation step, depending on its surface density on the cell membrane. Another mechanistic variant combines a change in orientation with a change in the nature of membrane environment surrounding the dye that could cause a change in the dye excitation or emission spectrum. This is similar to the variant of the ON-OFF mechanism in which the dye moves from a binding site associated with the aqueous interface to a binding site in the hydrophobic core of the membrane with a concomitant increase in fluorescence.

Indeed, it should again be stressed that the depiction of the mechanisms in Figure 1 is idealized and that dye responses to membrane potential are commonly composed of complex combinations of these and other processes. As noted, the sensitivity of a dye using these motion-based mechanisms depends on both kinetic and thermodynamic factors that will vary according to the nature of the biological preparation and the concentrations of both dye and membrane. Another hallmark of these motion-based mechanisms is that they depend on the interaction of the potential with the charge(s) on the dye molecule; so a change in the magnitude, distribution, or sign of the charge(s) on the dye molecule will invariably alter the nature of the potential-dependent response.

If a large redistribution of charge within a nonsymmetric chromophore accompanies photoexcitation, the intramembrane electrical field can change the spectrum of the dye without involvement of any molecular motion. This is the basis of the ELECTROCHROMISM mechanism depicted in Figure 2. The charge shift that accompanies excitation is illustrated at the top of Figure 2 for di-4-ANEPPS. In the ground state, the chromophore has its positive charge localized near the pyridinium end on the left. In the excited state, the positive charge is localized near the aniline moiety on the right. Another way of thinking about this is that, upon excitation, the negative electron cloud shifts from a density on the aniline side to the pyridinium side of the chromophore. By appending a hydrophilic sulfonate group and lipophilic hydrocarbon chains to opposite ends, binding of the molecule to the membrane is engineered in such a way that the chromophore aligns itself along the lipid molecules (Fig. 2, bottom). Such an alignment assures that the excitation-induced electronic charge shift will be parallel to the direction of the intramembrane electrical field. In a polarized membrane, this coupling of the electrical field with the chromophore charge distribution will decrease the energy difference between the ground and excited states resulting in a red shift of both the excitation and emission spectra. When the membrane is depolarized, the spectra are blue shifted. Therefore, as illustrated in Figure 3, when fluorescence is monitored with filters that select the high wavelength range of excitation and emission, a decrease in signal would ac-

Figure 3. Voltage-dependent spectral shift for an electrochromic dye. Depolarization produces a decrease in fluorescence at the red wing of the spectrum and an increase when fluorescence is monitored on the blue wing of the spectrum. For an ideal electrochromic mechanism, the spectrum will only shift and not change shape or amplitude. In practice, this ideal behavior is rarely observed.

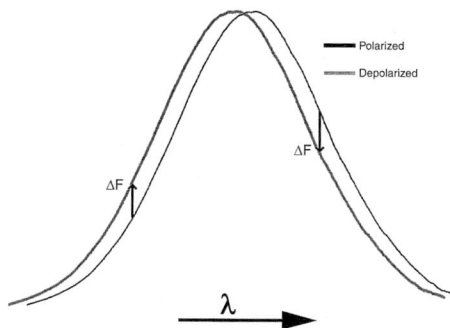

company an action potential; if wavelengths are chosen to the blue of the excitation and emission maxima, an increase in fluorescence would be anticipated. In fact, it is best to choose wavelengths at a steep portion of the spectrum to maximize the change. If the relative fluorescence change, $\Delta F/F$, is being measured, it is also best to choose a wavelength near the wings of the spectrum so that the denominator is minimized. Somewhat counterintuitively, but as can be appreciated from Figure 3, the wavelength of maximum fluorescence should be avoided because that is where F is large while ΔF is minimal. Dual wavelength schemes have also been developed to maximize the signal and normalize away nonpotentiometric contributions to the fluorescence.[5,32]

The electrochromic mechanism was originally attractive because it lends itself well to the design of new molecular probes via molecular orbital theory.[33,34] In a survey of common dye chromophores, it was found that the p-aminostyryl-pyridinium chromophore produced large charge shifts upon photoexcitation.[33] In addition, the structure of the chromophore lent itself to the incorporation of appended organic chains that would properly align it in the membrane. It was predicted that this mechanism would be more robust and universal than other mechanisms because it depends on the fundamental photophysics of the chromophore rather than a delicate balance between different chemical states of the dye. Also, because electrochromism does not involve any molecular motion, a fast response to voltage changes is guaranteed. The naphthylstyryl chromophore that is incorporated into di-4-ANEPPS has the same properties[2] and has been found to be a stable and reliable probe in many preparations including heart.[3]

However, it is generally not possible to transfer a calibration of the electrochromic dye response from one preparation to another—the dyes must be independently calibrated against voltage change under the specific conditions of a given experimental protocol. An obvious reason is that the precise characteristics of the optical configuration, particularly the choice of wavelength ranges for emission and excitation, will affect the size of the response. But the characteristics of the cells or tissue that are being studied can also affect the fractional change in fluorescence following an action potential. This is because the relative change in the optical signal with voltage depends on the size of the background signal from stained nonexcitable cells and can also be contaminated with responses due to other collateral mechanisms[35] (indeed, other styryl dyes, e.g., RH795 [Table 1], may have a minor contribution from electrochromism to a potential-dependent fluorescence response depending on the preparation and wavelengths). Further, the electrochromic response requires that the dye only stain one leaflet of the lipid bilayer (Fig. 2). Therefore, as the dye becomes internalized and its density becomes equalized on the extracellular and cytoplasmic surfaces of the plasma membrane, the voltage-dependent signal will diminish. The rate of this process depends on the cell that is being stained and also on the sidechains of the dye. Di-8-ANEPPS was developed to retard this internalization process.[4,5] Thus, while the electrochromic dyes have been broadly applicable and give reliable responses in many different preparations and experimental configurations, care is required especially when the goal is quantitative information on the amplitudes of voltage changes. More details on the factors involved in the choice of an electrochromic dye are given in the next section of this chapter.

Experimental Design: Choice of Dyes

There are many issues that must be considered in the choice of dye for a given experiment. Obviously, a large sensitivity to potential is always advantageous. Also important are low rates of photobleaching and minimal toxicity, pharmacological, or photodynamic effects. These can vary not only from dye to dye but also from preparation to preparation and are often exacerbated in well-oxygenated environments. Generally, the styryl dyes are relatively stable and benign, but high exciting light levels and long exposures to the excitation are not possible even with these dyes. As mentioned above, the relative fluorescence change can depend on how well the dye is confined to the excitable membrane in a complex tissue or organ, as staining of nonexcitable cells will produce a large background signal. In the choice of excitation and emission wavelength, there can be a tradeoff between relative fluorescence change and S/N ratio. The latter is often limited by total fluorescence signal, which is maximal at the peak of the spectral bands; the relative fluorescence change is often maximal at the wings of the spectrum (Fig. 3). The solubility properties of the dyes will determine their persistence in experiments of long duration and their ability to penetrate deeply into tissue. Studying the structures and characteristics of a series of styryl dyes can provide an appreciation of these factors.

Table 2 lists a selection of dyes, all containing the same chromophore as di-4-ANEPPS. These dyes were tailored to meet the very different requirements of a variety of cell and tissue preparations and experimental goals. The electrochromic mechanism permits this kind of molecular engineering without sacrificing the intrinsic ability of the chromophore to respond to membrane potential. In other words, changing the lipophilicity and charge does not produce an a priori change in the dye sensitivity, as it would for the mechanisms depicted in Figure 1. On the other hand, such changes can improve the binding, penetration, persistence, or solubility properties of the dyes as might be required for a particular application, and thus indirectly improve the voltage-dependent optical signal. Each dye is discussed to show how modification of the base structure of di-4-ANEPPS produces a desired change in molecular properties.

JPW-1063 replaces the negatively charged propylsulfonate in di-4-ANEPPS with a positively charged ethyltrimethylammonium group. This produces a divalent cation probe as opposed to the neutral internal salt structure of the "ANEPPS" dyes. Interestingly, this drastic change in the charge does not significantly affect the voltage sensitivity in model membranes—consistent with the electrochromic mechanism. However, the added positive charge does improve the aqueous solubility of the dye and permits it to penetrate more deeply into thick tissue. It is important to be aware, however, that the double positive charge would be expected to per-

Table 2

Naphthylstyryl Dyes Engineered for Various Applications

Name	Chromophore	Description	ABS (nm)	EM (nm)	Structure
JPW-1063	Naphthylstyryl	Doubly cationic relative of di-4-ANEPPS. Higher solubility gives better penetration into thick tissue. In cardiac studies, has given better signals from hearts taken from large animals.	540	695	
JPW-1113	Naphthylstyryl	More soluble analog of di-4-ANEPPS. Good tissue penetration for brain slices.	498	717	
JPW-1114	Napththylstyryl	Highly water soluble. Best potentiometric dye for microinjection. Also good tissue penetration when applied externally, but may wash out quickly.	529	725	
Di-8-ANEPPS	Naphthylstyryl	More slowly internalized than di-4-ANEPPS. Relatively insoluble in water and therefore requires Pluronic F127 to stain.	500	705	
JPW-2045	Napththylstyryl	Potentiometric dye for neuronal tracing and long-term studies. Highly persistent over the many hours required for retrograde transport.	513	717	
JPW-2066	Naphthylstyryl	Di-linoleyl-ANEPPS is oil soluble. An oil solution may be microinjected to stain the endoplasmic reticulum or other selective staining.	497	707	

turb the surface potential of cell membranes and could therefore affect the electrophysiological properties of the system.

Another way of improving the water solubility of the probes is to shorten the alkyl chains on the amino nitrogen, as in JPW-1113. This dye penetrates thick tissue but, because of the lowered hydrophobicity, does not bind as strongly to membrane as does di-4-ANEPPS. Its persistence can therefore be problematic, but it will give signals if the experiment is of short duration and does not require constant superfusion.

The dye JPW-1114 was designed for microinjection studies. It is highly soluble and can be loaded into a microinjection pipette at concentration of approximately 10 mg/mL. Because this divalent cation is held inside a microinjected cell by the resting potential, long-term experiments can be performed. For example, it has been used to study a single cell in an intact invertebrate ganglion after many hours of incubation.[36]

Interestingly, long-term experiments with dyes applied to the outside require highly insoluble dyes with longer alkyl chains. This is the principle behind the design of di-8-ANEPPS. The major factors that limit the duration of an experiment is dye washout and dye internalization. Longer alkyl chains solve both of these problems. However, the low solubility of compounds like di-8-ANEPPS requires that they be applied to the preparation via a vehicle like Pluronic F127, a high molecular weight nonionic detergent. For the same reason, the utility of this dye is limited to the staining of surface layers of tissue.

JPW-2045 has both a double positive charge and long alkyl chains. It is sufficiently persistent for long-term experiments. It has been used in a chick spinal cord preparation in which the ends of the cells were stained by direct application of the dye. After several hours of dye retrograde transport, recordings can be obtained from opposite ends of the neurons.[37,38] The positive charges probably lead to dye internalization and entrapment over this long period, assuring that only those cells that have been initially exposed to the dye will show remote signals.

The long unsaturated hydrocarbon chains in JPW-2066 make this dye soluble in nonpolar organic solvents. It can be dissolved in soybean oil and applied to a cell as a microdroplet. The dye is slowly transferred from the oil to the cell membrane and diffuses throughout the cell surface. Alternatively, the oil solution can be microinjected to stain intracellular organelles. Such a technique was originally developed to stain the endoplasmic reticulum with a nonpotentiometric fluorescent dye.[39]

New Approaches to Potentiometric Dye Measurements

Until very recently only this laboratory and that of Amiram Grinvald had been actively working on new potentiometric dye design and synthesis. In 1995, the laboratory of Roger Tsien joined the effort.[40,41] These investigators developed a scheme based on the change in fluorescence resonance energy transfer when an anionic acceptor dye undergoes potential dependent redistribution across a membrane and thereby changes its proximity to a donor that is fixed to the outer membrane surface. The sensitivity is high and the signals are sufficiently rapid to accurately track action potentials. However, large dye concentrations are required to achieve sufficient energy transfer efficiencies, risking dye toxic and photodynamic effects; also, the application of this dye-pair technology is cumbersome, especially for complex multicellular preparations. Still, this approach has great promise, especially if both the donor and acceptor chromophores can be engineered into the same molecule. Another exciting new scheme incorporates green fluorescent protein into the shaker potassium channel.[42] This construct can be expressed in cells and shows a 5% fluorescence change per 100-mV change in potential. This approaches the sensitivity of the existing organic dyes. However, the time course does not reflect a response of the chromophore to the fast conformational change associated with the gating charges within the protein—it is much slower. The slow response permits integration of the signal for better S/N ratios but precludes the monitoring of electrical spikes in neuronal preparations. The general concept of introducing fluorescent protein segments into gated channels could produce improved constructs with greater sensitivity and speed.

Dual wavelength ratiometric measurements with existing naphthylstyryl dyes[4,32,43] can have several advantages at the expense of somewhat more complex instrumentation. The approach is based on the shift in spectrum shown in Figure 3, and the measurement of fluorescence from opposite wings of the spectral band, and calculating their ratio. Since the potentiometric signal is opposite at these two wavelengths, the sensitivity of the ratio is approximately double that realized with single wavelength measurement. Another advantage is that the ratio is independent of the level of dye binding in different regions of the preparation or of photobleaching over time. It can therefore provide a much cleaner spatiotemporal map of the distribution of membrane potential than single wavelength measurements.

Nonlinear optics may offer new opportunities for optical mapping of cardiac activity. One nonlinear optical effect that has been applied to microscopy is 2-photon excitation of fluorescence.[44] In this technique, two near infrared photons combine to excite a visible light electronic transition in a chromophore. This excited state can then produce ordinary fluorescence. Because this is a low-probability transition and depends on the square of the incident light intensity, very high power laser pulses are required and the effect only takes place at the focal point where the light is most highly concentrated. The major advantages of this approach are minimal photobleaching, deep penetration into thick tissue, and the ability to produce 3-dimensional reconstructions. A similar but newer approach is second harmonic generation, in which two near infrared photons interact with the dye to produce a single photon with half the wavelength. This effect, also called frequency doubling, has been shown to be highly voltage-dependent.[45–47] A detailed description of these methods is beyond the scope of this chapter, but it is important for the optical mapping community to be aware of these technologies. Indeed, the second edition of this text may see inclusion of a separate chapter on these approaches.

Acknowledgments   I would like to thank all those coworkers who have contributed to the work in this lab over the years. In particular, Larry Cohen has been an excellent colleague and collaborator since the beginning.

References

1. Loew LM, Scully S, Simpson L, et al. Evidence for a charge-shift electrochromic mechanism in a probe of membrane potential. *Nature* 1979;281:497–499.
2. Fluhler E, Burnham VG, Loew LM. Spectra, membrane binding and potentiometric responses of new charge shift probes. *Biochemistry* 1985;24:5749–5755.
3. Loew LM, Cohen LB, Dix J, et al. A naphthyl analog of the aminostyryl pyridinium class of potentiometric membrane dyes shows consistent sensitivity in a variety of tissue, cell, and model membrane preparations. *J Membr Biol* 1992;130:1–10.
4. Bedlack RS, Wei M-D, Loew LM. Localized membrane depolarizations and localized intracellular calcium influx during electric field-guided neurite growth. *Neuron* 1992;9:393–403.
5. Loew LM. Voltage sensitive dyes and imaging neuronal activity. *Neuroprotocols* 1994;5:72–79.
6. Ehrenberg B, Montana V, Wei M-D, et al. Membrane potential can be determined in individual cells from the Nernstian distribution of cationic dyes. *Biophys J* 1988;53:785–794.

7. Grinvald A, Cohen LB, Lesher S, et al. Simultaneous optical monitoring of activity of many neurons. *J Neurophysiol* 1981;45:829–840.
8. Kauer JS, Senseman DM, Cohen LB. Odor-elicited activity monitored simultaneously from 124 regions of the salamander olfactory bulb using a voltage-sensitive dye. *Brain Res* 1987;418:255–261.
9. Wu J-Y, Cohen LB, Falk CX. Neuronal activity during different behaviors in aplysia: A distributed organization? *Science* 1994;263:820–822.
10. Gross D, Loew LM, Webb WW. Spatially resolved optical measurement of membrane potential. *Biophys J* 1985;47:270.
11. Bedlack RS, Wei M-D, Fox SH, et al. Distinct electric potentials in soma and neurite membranes. *Neuron* 1994;13:1187–1193.
12. Shrager P, Rubinstein CT. Optical measurement of conduction in single demyelinated axons. *J Gen Physiol* 1990;95:867–890.
13. Antic S, Zecevic D. Optical signals from neurons with internally applied voltage-sensitive dyes. *J Neurosci* 1995;15:1392–1405.
14. Salzberg BM. Optical recording of voltage changes in nerve terminals and in fine neuronal processes. *Ann Rev Physiol* 1989;51:507–526.
15. Loew LM, Tuft RA, Carrington W, et al. Imaging in 5 dimensions: Time dependent membrane potentials in individual mitochondria. *Biophys J* 1993;65:2396–2407.
16. Morad M, Salama G. Optical probes of membrane potential in heart muscle. *J Physiol* 1979;292:267–295.
17. Müller W, Windisch H, Tritthart HA. Fast optical monitoring of microscopic excitation patterns in cardiac muscle. *Biophys J* 1989;56:623–629.
18. Rosenbaum DS, Kaplan DT, Kanai A, et al. Repolarization inhomogeneities in ventricular myocardium change dynamically with abrupt cycle length shortening. *Circulation* 1991;84:1333–1345.
19. Davidenko JM, Pertsov AV, Salomonsz R, et al. Stationary and drifting spiral waves of excitation in isolated cardiac muscle. *Nature* 1992;355:349–351.
20. Pertsov AM, Davidenko JM, Salomonsz R, et al. Spiral waves of excitation underlie reentrant activity in isolated cardiac muscle. *Circ Res* 1993;72:631–650.
21. Sims PJ, Waggoner AS, Wang C-H, et al. Studies on the mechanism by which cyanine dyes measure membrane potential in red blood cells and phosphotidylcholine. *Biochemistry* 1974;13:3315–3330.
22. Smith JC, Frank SJ, Bashford CL, et al. Kinetics of the association of potential-sensitive dyes with model and energy-transducing membranes: Implications for fast probe response times. *J Membr Biol* 1980;54:127–139.
23. George EB, Nyirjesy P, Basson M, et al. Impermeant potential sensitive oxonol dyes: I. Evidence for an "On-Off" mechanism. *J Membr Biol* 1988;103:245–253.
24. Waggoner AS, Wang CH, Tolles RL. Mechanism of potential-dependent light absorption changes of lipid bilayer membranes in the presence of cyanine and oxonol dyes. *J Membr Biol* 1977;33:109–140.
25. Flewelling RF, Hubbell WL. The membrane dipole potential in a total membrane potential model. Applications to hydrophobic ion interactions with membranes. *Biophys J* 1986;49:541–552.
26. Loew LM: Confocal microscopy of potentiometric fluorescent dyes. In Matsumoto B (ed): *Cell Biological Applications of Confocal Microscopy. Methods in Cell Biology.* Orlando: Academic Press; 1993:194–209.
27. Loew LM. Measuring membrane potential in single cells with confocal microscopy. In Celis JE (ed): *Cell Biology: A Laboratory Handbook.* Vol. 3. San Diego: Academic Press; 1998:375–379.
28. Emerson ES, Conlin MA, Rosenoff AE, et al. The geometrical structure and absorption spectrum of a cyanine dye aggregate. *J Phys Chem* 1967;71:2396–2403.
29. Reers M, Smith TW, Chen LB. J-Aggregate formation of a carbocyanine as a

quantitative fluorescent indicator of membrane potential. *Biochemistry* 1991;30:4480–4486.

30. Loew LM, Rosenberg I, Bridge M, et al. Diffusion potential cascade. Convenient detection of transferable membrane pores. *Biochemistry* 1983;22:837–844.

31. Dragsten PR, Webb WW. Mechanism of the membrane potential sensitivity of the fluorescent membrane probe Merocyanine 540. *Biochemistry* 1978; 17:5228–5240.

32. Montana V, Farkas DL, Loew LM. Dual wavelength ratiometric fluorescence measurements of membrane potential. *Biochemistry* 1989;28:4536–4539.

33. Loew LM, Bonneville GW, Surow J. Charge shift optical probes of membrane potential. Theory. *Biochemistry* 1978;17:4065–4071.

34. Loew LM, Simpson L. Charge shift probes of membrane potential. A probable electrochromic mechanism for ASP probes on a hemispherical lipid bilayer. *Biophys J* 1981;34:353–365.

35. Loew LM, Cohen LB, Salzberg BM, et al. Charge shift probes of membrane potential. Characterization. *Biophys J* 1985;47:71–77.

36. Zecevic D. Multiple spike-initiation zones in single neurons revealed by voltage-sensitive dyes. *Nature* 1996;381:322–325.

37. Wenner P, Tsau Y, Cohen LB, et al. Voltage-sensitive dye recording using retrogradely transported dye in the chicken spinal cord: Staining and signal characteristics. *J Neurosci Methods* 1996;170:111–120.

38. Tsau Y, Wenner P, O'Donovan MJ, et al. Dye screening and signal-to-noise ratio for retrogradely transported voltage-sensitive dyes. *J Neurosci Methods* 1996;170:121–129.

39. Terasaki M, Jaffe LA. Organization of the sea urchin egg endoplasmic reticulum and its reorganization at fertilization. *J Cell Biol* 1991;114:929–940.

40. Gonzalez JE, Tsien RY. Voltage sensing by fluorescence resonance energy transfer in single cells. *Biophys J* 1995;69:1272–1280.

41. Gonzalez JE, Tsien RY. Improved indicators of membrane potential that use fluorescence resonance energy transfer. *Chem Biol* 1997;4:269–277.

42. Siegel MS, Isacoff EYIN: A genetically encoded optical probe of membrane voltage. *Neuron* 1997;19:735–741.

43. Zhang J, Davidson RM, Wei M, et al. Membrane electrical properties by combined patch clamp and fluorescence ratio imaging in single neurons. *Biophys J* 1998;74:48–53.

44. Denk W, Strickler JH, Webb WW. Two-photon laser scanning fluorescence microscopy. *Science* 1990;248:73–76.

45. Bouevitch O, Lewis A, Pinevsky I, et al. Probing membrane potential with nonlinear optics. *Biophys J* 1993;65:672–679.

46. Ben-Oren I, Peleg G, Lewis A, et al. Infrared nonlinear optical measurements of membrane potential in photoreceptor cells. *Biophys J* 1996;71:1616–1620.

47. Campagnola PJ, Wei M-D, Lewis A, Loew LM. High resolution optical imaging of live cells by second harmonic generation. *Biophys J* 1999;77:3341–3349.

Chapter 3

Optical Properties of Cardiac Tissue

William T. Baxter

Optical mapping with potentiometric dyes is a valuable technique for monitoring electrical activity in heart tissue. It has been successfully applied in a variety of tissue preparations, to study normal propagation as well as cardiac arrhythmias.[1–4] In bulk tissue, this approach almost always uses epi-illumination, in which the light source and photodetector are aimed at the same surface. The signal contributing to the resulting optical action potentials has been estimated to come from a thin layer of cells at the heart surface[2,3]; this is advantageous because it assures that action potentials measured from the heart surface are not contaminated by signals originating in deeper layers of myocardium. However, the ventricles of the heart may be many millimeters thick, thus the 3-dimensional propagation of electrical waves in cardiac tissue must be inferred from surface recordings. It is possible to obtain some information about what is occurring in the thickness of the ventricles using transillumination, in which the light source and detector are on opposite sides of the preparation. If excitation light irradiates a preparation perfused with a voltage-sensitive dye, the fluorescence escaping from layers deep inside thick ventricular tissue can be detected, yielding identifiable action potentials.[5] This approach has been used to record intramural activity in thick ventricles.[6,7] The precise interpretation of such signals remains problematic due to the complex optical characteristics of tissue. This chapter reviews the optical properties of cardiac tissues that come into play when transillumination is used in optical mapping studies. More general reviews of light transport in biological media may be found in references 8 through 10.

Transillumination

In the mid 19th century, testicular cancer was diagnosed by holding a lamp behind the testes and noting the shadows cast by tumors. For over 150 years, detection of internal lesions by shining light through tissues has been used to study pathology in the skull, teeth, scrotum, and female breast.[11] Transillumination of the breast, formerly called diaphanography

From Rosenbaum DS, Jalife J (eds): *Optical Mapping of Cardiac Excitation and Arrhythmias.* ©Futura Publishing Co., Inc., Armonk, NY, 2001.

and now often referred to as optical mammography, was first described in 1929 by Cutler et al.,[12] who placed a lamp with white light against the breast and found that shadows were cast by tumors and blood vessels by virtue of their excessive absorption of light. This approach could not be used to detect small lesions, and required so much light as to cause heating of the skin. The technique acquired various improvements throughout the years. Cooling of the light source permitted higher power and thus deeper penetration of light.[13] Filtering of the light to use the longer more useful wavelengths (630 nm and 800 nm) also allowed deeper penetration with less scattering.[14] Using laser collimated transillumination in a scanning mode, Jarry et al.[15] obtained high spatial resolution for metal objects inserted deep into tissues (kidneys, thoracic wall; maximum width 1.5 cm). Sensitivity was further increased by capturing images on color infrared film. Interest in transillumination stemmed mainly from the fact that it used safer, nonionizing radiation compared with x-ray radiography. However, a review of breast imaging techniques concluded that while diaphanography could provide some additional information in certain cases, it could not compete with x-ray mammography.[16]

The major problem with transillumination is the decrease in lateral spatial resolution due to light scattering, the predominant attenuation process in tissue.[17] Excited fluorophores act as isotropic point sources of emission photons,[10,18] scattering light in all directions, laterally within the myocardium, as well as toward the photodetector. This induces significant blurring during image formation, with deeper layers having greater blurring. However, development of corrective methods has brought renewed interest to optical imaging of tissues, including transillumination of the breast.[19,20] The spatial resolution of transillumination may be improved by approaches such as coaxial collimation and time-of-flight imaging, which distinguish scattered versus nonscattered photons based on their angle of exit or their time of arrival at the photodetector.[21–23] Chang et al.[24] showed that image reconstruction methods could be used for imaging of fluorescence in highly scattering media. Arridge and Hebden[25] published a general survey of reconstruction methods for overcoming the effects of scattering in optical imaging.

For optical mapping studies using transillumination, a major goal is the estimation of the relative contributions from different depths to the total recorded fluorescence. In other words, where is the emitted light coming from? This question may be divided into two parts: 1) Given a slab of tissue irradiated by light, what is the amount of excitation light reaching a point at depth z? 2) How much of the fluoresced light at depth z escapes from the tissue and is thus available to reach the detector? Answering these questions requires a description of the interaction of light with biological tissue. The medical uses of light have included imaging,[13,17] photoradiation therapy,[26] and surgical lasers for diagnosis and ablation.[8] Development of these applications has focused efforts on understanding the distribution of light within tissues that is produced by external light sources. Estimation of light distribution within a medium requires knowledge of the optical properties of the medium, as well as a model of how light propagates in that medium. If tissues were homogeneous media that only absorbed light, light distribution could be simply described by exponential decay according to the Lambert-Beer law of absorption.[27] But biological tissues are highly scattering, and this introduces great complexity in the estimation of light distribution.

Absorption

Figure 1 schematically illustrates a collimated beam incident on a slab of tissue. Once light enters the medium, photons may be absorbed, scattered, or transmitted. Absorption by a fluorophore may result in the emission of another photon, which is then subjected to more scattering. The amount of light at a given point z within the tissue is called the fluence rate, $\phi(z)$, in W/m^2, defined as amount of light incident on that point from all directions.[9] Propagation of light in tissue is governed by scattering and absorption, and calculation of the fluence rate requires knowledge of these properties.

A tissue's ability to absorb light is characterized by its absorption coefficient μ_a (mm^{-1}). According to the Lambert-Beer law, light decreases exponentially as it passes through a medium of width L: $I = I_o \exp(-\mu_a L)$, where I_o is the incident light, and I is the transmitted light emerging from the medium. Biological tissues have very high absorption in the ultraviolet and infrared regions. At wavelengths shorter than 300 nm, most light is absorbed by water, proteins, and nucleic acids. Water is also the primary absorber above 1200 nm. Between the absorption-dominant wavelength bands in the infrared and ultraviolet, there is a "window" where scattering events predominate over absorption. The ratio of scattering to absorption is expressed by a quantity called the albedo (see below). Absorption still occurs at the visible wavelengths, primarily by hemoglobin, flavins, cytochromes, and carotenoids, resulting in great variability in light absorption in tissues at different wavelengths.[8,28,29]

In absorption, the incident light actually "disappears"; the photon is converted to some other form of energy, usually heat, or, in the case of fluorophores (such as voltage-sensitive dyes), it raises the molecule to an excited state. For fluorescence to take place the photon must first be absorbed.

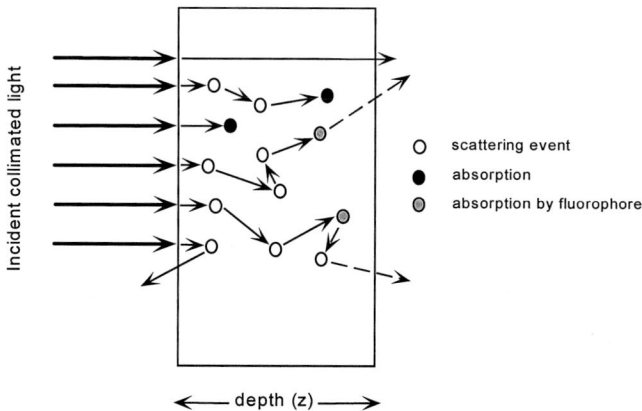

Figure 1. Events occurring during the interaction of light with matter.

For a photon to be absorbed by a molecule, its energy must match the energy difference of the allowable excited states of the electron bond in the molecule. Once the molecule is raised to an excited energy state by absorption of a photon, it may de-excite by a variety of competitive pathways. The energy of a fluoresced photon will always be less than the absorbed photon due to loss of energy in the absorption and de-excitation process.[27]

Scattering

Light passing through a medium is also attenuated by scattering, in which case it is not actually lost, but it does not reach the detector because it is scattered away in different directions. In Figure 1, some of the incident photons are scattered back into the air, some are scattered toward absorbing molecules, many change direction multiple times. The major part of light reflected from tissue is caused by scattered photons escaping from the inside. The zigzag path of multiply scattered photons keeps them within the material for longer periods, increasing their probability of being absorbed. All photons that penetrate deeper than a few tenths of a millimeter have been subjected to multiple scattering and thus may reach a molecule from any direction. Thus, if scattering is high, it can act as a diffusing process. Scattering therefore increases reflection, enhances absorption, and results in an isotropic distribution of light in regions distal to the surface.[17,26]

Scattering is principally an elastic mechanism in which the photon retains its energy but changes direction. Absorption is a competing mechanism, and is a quantum effect in which all of the photon's energy is given up. There are multiple forms of scattering[30]: Rayleigh scattering occurs when a photon interacts with objects whose size is less than the wavelength (atoms, molecules). It is isotropic, that is, the photon will take off in any new direction with equal probability. Rayleigh scattering is inversely proportional to the fourth power of the wavelength; therefore, short wavelengths experience the greatest scattering, which is why the sky is blue. For interaction with objects roughly the size of the wavelength (organelles and small cells), scattering is still inversely proportional to wavelength, thus favoring the more energetic short-wavelength photons. But it is not isotropic, instead being somewhat forward directed. Mie scattering is operational for objects that are very large compared to the wavelength (cell and tissue boundaries, gross structures); this scattering is highly forward directed and is essentially wavelength-independent. All three types of scatter occur significantly in biological tissues.[31]

Interdependence of Scattering and Absorption

When light traverses tissue, it undergoes both absorption and scattering. If scattering were negligible, light would obey the simple absorption law, with the attenuation rate fixed by the medium's absorption coefficient. However, scattering in tissues is appreciable: light is attenuated exponentially, with scattering coefficient μ_s. Therefore, the amount of light reaching a point within the medium is attenuated by both absorption and scattering, and may be expressed as $\phi(z) = I_o \exp(-[\mu_a + \mu_s] z)$, where $\phi(z)$ is the fluence rate of collimated light at position z. The absorption and scattering coefficients may be combined into a total attenuation coefficient $\mu_t = \mu_a + \mu_s$. The penetration depth δ (mm) of the collimated beam is the depth at which the light has been reduced to 37% (i.e., $1/e$ of the original magnitude), and is defined as the reciprocal of the total attenuation coefficient: $\delta = 1/\mu_t$. The penetration depth and absorption and scattering coefficients are all wavelength-dependent. The absorption and scattering coefficients, μ_a and μ_s (in mm^{-1}), and their inverse values, $1/\mu_a$ and $1/\mu_s$ (in mm), may also be thought of as probabilities, representing the mean free path before absorption occurs, or between scattering events, respectively.[10,32]

Because scattering has been found to be highly anisotropic in tissue,[32,33] the probability of a photon's new direction must be incorporated into calculations of the fluence rate. $S(\theta)$ is the angular scattering phase function, i.e., the probability, per unit solid angle, of scattering into angle θ.[32] The directionality of scattering is usually represented by the anisotropy factor g, the mean cosine of the angular phase function. For isotropic scattering, $g = 0$; for totally forward scattering, $g = 1$. The phase function may be measured, e.g., by irradiating a thin specimen with a collimated beam and rotating the detector around the specimen in a 180° arc.[32,33] For biological tissues, it has been found that the angular distribution is highly forward peaked. In most tissues g ranges from 0.64 to 0.97, with muscle usually above 0.9.[9] In models of light propagation (see below), anisotropy must be taken into account either by explicit angular scattering cross-sections (in Monte Carlo and exact methods) or implicitly by a modified diffusion coefficient (in diffusion theory). The "reduced" scattering coefficient μ'_s is obtained from the scattering coefficient and the anisotropy: $\mu'_s = \mu_s(1-g)$. Similarly, this gives a reduced total attenuation coefficient: $\mu'_t = \mu_a + \mu'_s$. The degree to which either scattering or absorption predominates in a medium is quantified by the albedo, $a = \mu'_s/(\mu_a + \mu'_s)$, which approaches 1 for a totally scattering medium, and 0 for a completely absorbing medium. At 630 nm, the wavelength most frequently used in laser studies, muscle tissue has small mean free paths (<0.1 mm), high albedo (>0.99), and significant forward scattering ($g \geq 0.9$).[32]

The parameters μ_a, μ_s, μ_t, and their reduced forms are considered "microscopic" properties of tissues.[32] They are distinguished from macroscopic properties, the values actually measured in bulk tissues, denoted by the effective attenuation coefficient, μ_{eff} (mm^{-1}), and its reciprocal, the effective penetration depth, $\delta_{eff} = 1/\mu_{eff}$. The microscopic properties are important for theoretical analysis, including computer simulations, but experiments in tissues typically measure macroscopic properties and then attempt to infer the former from the latter. The relationship between the fundamental microscopic properties and the measured quantities is complex. But far from the boundaries, in the case where scattering is much greater than absorption, scattering acts as a diffusion process, and diffusion theory predicts $\mu_{eff} = \sqrt{3\mu_a(\mu_a + \mu'_s)}$.[10,17,34]

Measurement of Optical Properties

In many soft tissues, optical albedo is high (i.e., scattering predominates over absorption), scattering is highly forward peaked, and the mean free path between photon interactions is small, making it difficult to measure the absorption and scattering coefficients.[32,35] Tissue properties are typically classified into microscopic properties (absorption and scattering coefficients, and the scattering phase function) versus macroscopic properties (the effective attenuation coefficient, total diffuse reflectance, and total diffuse transmittance). Measurement techniques can be separated into direct versus indirect methods. Direct methods use tissue samples that are thin enough (<100 μ) so that multiple photon scattering is negligible, i.e., only a single scattering event is assumed.[36] Because measurements are made from optically thin samples, direct methods do not require any propagation model. Direct methods tend to be technically difficult, with subtle variations in tissue sample preparation leading to inconsistent results. Indirect methods are simpler, since the tissues do not have to be optically thin. However, indirect methods require some model of light propagation. They are based on in vivo or in vitro measurements of macroscopic optical properties from bulk tissue, from which the microscopic coefficients are deduced by applying a light propagation model. Indirect techniques include 1) external methods, with the light detectors outside the tissue volume, such as the integrating spheres technique[33]; 2) internal methods, such as insertion of optical fibers through the tissue[37]; and 3) perturbation methods, in which measurements are made after the addition of a substance with known optical characteristics.[38] The measured optical properties of biological tissues vary considerably depending on the wavelength, the type of tissue, the species, and the geometry of the preparation and irradiation. However, even within the same tissue, the literature contains tremendous variations in estimated values for the optical coefficients (see below).

Models of Light Propagation in Tissue

Scattering of light in turbid media (i.e., media in which scattering predominates) has been studied in applications using optics in the atmosphere, in the ocean, in biological media, and in interstellar space.[31] The existing theoretical models are still not satisfactory for explaining many data. In turbid material, light is scattered and absorbed due to inhomogeneities and to the absorption characteristics of the medium. The two main mathematical descriptions of light propagation and scattering are analytical theory and transport theory. In analytical theory, Maxwell's equations governing electromagnetism consider the statistical nature of the medium and the statistical moments of the wave. In principle, this is the most fundamental approach, but exact solutions of Maxwell's equations governing the propagation of electromagnetic waves are not practical, because light passing through biological tissues encounters numerous heterogeneities and multiple scattering events.

Transport theory deals directly with the transport of power through turbid media. The development of transport theory is heuristic, and all proposed models have been numerical or approximate analytical solutions of the neutral particle transport equation. That is, the wave properties of light are ignored and propagation is described in terms of discrete photons, which may be scattered conservatively (without energy loss) or may be absorbed.[39] The transport of neutral particles such as neutrons or photons may be calculated by the Monte Carlo method or by solution of the linear Boltzmann equation. The Boltzmann equation is used in reactor physics and applied to x-ray or gamma photons to compute, for example, cases of radiation shielding. Photon transport is expressed in terms of energy fluence rate (also called space irradiance). Photons are treated as neutral particles that are transported in tissue, as neutrons propagate in a reactor. In 1976, Duderstadt and Hamilton[40] explained how to derive the classic Boltzmann transport equation for an arbitrary volume.

Except for a few extremely simple cases, the Boltzmann equation cannot be solved analytically. Therefore, the transport equation is usually solved numerically, using computer programs developed for neutron and gamma ray transport calculations. These are usually the Monte Carlo or the discrete ordinates techniques. The method of discrete ordinates amounts to a numerical solution of a discrete version of the Boltzmann equation.[40,41] Approximate analytic solutions to the transport equation include diffusion theory[17,31] and the Kubelka-Munk method.[34,42]

Diffusion Theory

Diffusion theory provides a simple though approximate approach to solving the Boltzmann equation.[43] It is only valid for highly scattering conditions. The integro-differential transport equation may be simplified to a partial differential equation, the diffusion equation of neutron physics, which is then solved by standard techniques.[39] Only in infinite planar geometry is the $1/e$ penetration depth equal to the diffusion length. Diffusion theory tends to break down near boundaries, localized sources, and strong absorbers.[44] Therefore, diffusion theory may be used when absorption is small compared to scattering; scattering is nearly isotropic, and regions near the source, boundaries, and strong absorbers are not included. The diffusion equation is solved subject to boundary and surface source conditions. The diffusion length D (in mm) is a function of the absorption and scattering coefficients and the mean cosine of the angle of scattering: $D = 1/(3[\mu_a + \mu_s(1 - g)])$. The $1/e$ effective penetration depth for light is $\delta = \sqrt{D/\mu_a}$.[10,17]

The Kubelka-Munk method is an even more approximate and limited method for estimation of the energy fluence rate in tissue.[42] It is a 2-flux model (inward and outward flux), which describes the diffuse reflectance, R, and transmittance, T, for light incident on a tissue slab in terms of the absorption and scattering coefficients. Under certain conditions, it is equivalent to diffusion theory.[39]

Monte Carlo Model of Light Distribution

The term "Monte Carlo" refers to the technique of formulating a deterministic problem in terms of random elements, then solving it by large-scale sampling. It has come to describe any simulation problem that uses random numbers. In Monte Carlo simulations, individual photon histories are generated to calculate macroscopic parameters or space irradiance distributions for arbitrary geometries. It is thus the preferred technique for 3-

dimensional geometry problems. Monte Carlo programs for light transport essentially simulate a random walk of a photon. The distance from the source or last collision is randomly selected from an exponential distribution, characterized by the mean free path or inverse of μ_t, the total attenuation. The new coordinates are calculated by trigonometry. The weight of the photon is multiplied by the ratio of the scattering-to-total attenuation coefficient. At the end of the random walk tracking, the loss in weight at each collision is tallied to compute the absorption. A new direction is randomly selected from the scattering phase function, and the process continues until the weighted photon escapes or its weight reaches a cut-off. Then a new source photon is launched. It is a computationally expensive process; tracking may be stopped after a small number of collisions, which may underestimate the energy fluence rate.[43,45]

However, given enough computer time, Monte Carlo simulations are generally considered the gold standard of light distribution in tissue,[10,44] with which the other approximate methods are compared to assess their validity.[39] Both Monte Carlo techniques and solution of the transport equation require knowledge of the absorption coefficient μ_a, the scattering coefficient μ_s, and the scattering phase function $S(\theta)$. These are difficult to calculate from inhomogeneous tissue. As described above, the measurement of optical properties of biological tissues has itself been an area of intense research.

Most of the above models have been developed in efforts to model light distributions for dosimetry planning in laser coagulation treatments. Another application of light uses fluorescence for diagnosis.[46,47] In this approach, the observed fluorescence spectrum is dependent on the fluence rate distribution of excitation light and the fraction of emitted fluorescence emerging from the tissue, termed the "escape function."[18] Several studies of fluorescence have used simple analytic expressions describing light transport derived from Monte Carlo simulations. Jacques[48] summarized analytic expressions for several simple tissue and irradiation geometries using a "standard" set of tissue optical properties. This approach was extended to more general light sources in reference 10. Girouard et al.[3] estimated the penetration of excitation light into guinea pig hearts and the resulting emitted fluorescence from the epi-illuminated surface using exponential decay based on the transmission properties of their preparations. Gardner et al.[18] used similar expressions for excitation light and emitted fluorescence with an additional corrective factor in the estimation of excitation fluence rate to account for boundary perturbations (see below). They validated their analytic expressions by comparing them with Monte Carlo simulations and tissue phantoms over a large range of diffuse reflectance values. These expressions were used by Baxter[7] in transilluminated cardiac tissue to estimate the relative contributions of internal layers to the total recorded fluorescence.

Wavelength Sensitivity of Tissues

Biological tissues exhibit characteristic spectral sensitivity: longer wavelengths have a higher transmittance, i.e., are able to penetrate more deeply, while shorter wavelengths are quickly attenuated.[3,49,50] Tissue spectra typically show a large increase in transmission around 600 nm. This has implications for many voltage-sensitive fluorescent dyes, such as di-4-ANEPPS, in that the short wavelength excitation light is unable to penetrate very deeply, but once a fluorophore is excited, the longer wavelength fluoresced light is more likely to escape from the tissue. Superimposed on the overall shape of the spectrum are specific minima, corresponding to absorption by various substances such as hemoglobin and lipid. The transmissivity of muscle lies approximately midway between relatively transparent tissues such as gray matter and more opaque tissues such as liver. However, even heart and skeletal muscle may be distinguished by differences in their spectra. The transmittance of skeletal muscle is relatively flat in the 700- to 1000-nm range, while cardiac muscle often shows a more gradual increase above 600 nm.[51]

Exponential Decay of Light

For a given wavelength, the attenuation of light within tissues exhibits two general features: exponential decay of light deep within the preparation, and a small decrease in light just below the illuminated surface.[7] The exponential decrease of light in biological media is well-known and results from the interaction of the absorption and scattering characteristics. The subsurface decrease in light results from the loss of scattered photons combined with the reflective and refractive properties of the irradiated tissue surface.

The effective penetration depth δ_{eff} characterizes the $1/e$ attenuation of light in tissue for a given wavelength.[10,34,50] Measurements of δ_{eff} for muscle at specific wavelengths vary greatly in the literature. Wilson et al.,[50] positioning optical fibers at different depths in rabbit muscle, calculated penetration depths around 2 and 3 mm for 514- and 630-nm light, respectively. Girouard et al.[3] used transmission spectra of guinea pig ventricle to calculate decay constants of 0.289 and 0.434 mm for 540 and 640 nm, the excitation and emission wavelengths of di-4-ANEPPS. This dye was also used in isolated sheep ventricles, where penetration depths of 0.8 mm and 1.3 mm were obtained for the excitation and emission bands.[7] In a review of methods for measuring optical properties, Wilson[35] pointed out that the development of accurate measurement techniques is itself an active field of research. He also noted that in the exhaustive list of optical properties published by Cheong et al.,[34] and updated in the appendix to his chapter,[35] there were significant inconsistencies in the published data. The variance across different laboratories is even greater than the variance across tissue types, most probably due to variations in experimental technique and methods of tissue preparation.

Reflection and Refraction

Light interacts with the surface of the medium in the form of reflection and refraction. When light passes from one medium to another, reflected light bounces back into first medium, and refracted light passes into second medium. In general, the greater the angle of incidence, the more light is reflected. Light reflected from tissue includes both this normal type of reflection (called specular reflection) and diffuse reflection. The latter consists of photons that enter the tissue and are scattered back out across the illuminated surface. Diffuse reflectance depends on the scattering and absorption properties of the tissue.[35] Refraction depends on the angle of incidence and nature of the two media. According to Snell's law, if light moves into a medium with a greater refractive index, it bends toward the normal. The greater the angle of incidence, the greater the angle of refraction.[27] For simplicity, most models assume a broad beam of collimated incident light (i.e., all rays are parallel). The significance in reflection and refraction lies in the perturbations in light they effect at the tissue boundary. Baxter[7] observed a pronounced boundary effect in profiles of light attenuation in the form of a peak beneath the surface. It was hypothesized that this effect played a role in causing the bulk of the transilluminated signal to originate from subsurface layers. This subsurface peak of light distribution in highly scattering media with slab geometry has been observed in analytical solutions to the light transport equation[52] and in simulations based on diffusion theory[43,44] and Monte Carlo models,[10,18] as well as empirically in phantoms and muscle tissue.[18,53] It has been explained as resulting from the loss of scattered photons from tissue near the surface.[26,43]

The boundary also interacts with escaping light (diffuse reflectance) in the form of a refractive mismatch. Calculations for diffuse reflectance have been published[10,18] for refractive mismatches of 1.38 (n_{tissue}/n_{air}) and 1.33 (n_{water}/n_{air}), where n_x is the index of refraction for medium x. It has been shown that as the refractive mismatch approaches 1 (index matching), the fluence profile exhibits a well-defined maximum within the medium.[44,52] Tissue preparations immersed in saline bath solutions probably have a refractive mismatch closer to 1 ($n_{tissue}/n_{water} = 1.38/1.33$), further adding to the prominence of the subsurface peak. For isolated hearts suspended in air, fewer photons leak out of the surface, probably due to the increased total internal reflection just under the surface, which traps photons within the tissue.

Summary

Proper use of cardiac optical mapping requires understanding the properties of light transmission through tissue. This is influenced by many factors, including the wavelengths used, the irradiation geometry, the type of the tissue and its surrounding environment, specimen preparation and thickness, the presence of blood, and nonuniformities within the tissue. The optical properties of biological media include the fundamental microscopic properties of absorption and scattering, as well as macroscopic quantities such as reflectance and effective penetration depth. There is some gap between these two, as the former are required in theoretical descriptions while the latter represent what can be easily obtained empirically. The relationship between these two can only be easily described under extremely simplified conditions such as infinite planar geometry far from any boundaries. The interaction of light and matter has been described by various models of light transport through tissue. There is interdependence between these models and the optical properties: most techniques for measuring optical properties require a model of light propagation, while the models themselves require knowledge of the optical properties of the medium. If the geometry of irradiation and the medium are simple enough, simple analytical expressions have been found to provide accurate descriptions of fluorescence excitation and emission, which depend only on the measured effective penetration depths.

References

1. Salama G, Kanai A, Efimov IR. Subthreshold stimulation of Purkinje fibers interrupts ventricular tachycardia in intact hearts. Experimental study with voltage-sensitive dyes and imaging techniques. *Circ Res* 1994;74:604–619.
2. Knisley SB. Transmembrane voltage changes during unipolar stimulation of rabbit ventricle. *Circ Res* 1995;77:1229–1239.
3. Girouard SD, Laurita KR, Rosenbaum DS. Unique properties of cardiac action potentials recorded with voltage-sensitive dyes. *J Cardiovasc Electrophysiol* 1996;7:1024–1038.
4. Dillon SM, Kerner TE, Hoffman J, et al. A system for in-vivo cardiac optical mapping. *IEEE Eng Med Biol Mag* 1998;17:95–108.
5. Pertsov AM, Baxter WT, Cabo C, et al. Transillumination of the myocardial wall allows optical recording of 3-dimensional electrical activity. *Circulation* 1994;90:I-411.
6. Baxter WT, Pertsov AM, Berenfeld O, et al. Demonstration of three dimensional reentry in isolated sheep right ventricle. *Pacing Clin Electrophysiol* 1997;20:1080.
7. Baxter WT, Mironov SF, Zaitsev AV, et al. Visualizing excitation waves inside cardiac muscle. *Biophys J* 2001;80:516–530.
8. van Gemert MJ, Welch AJ, Jacques SL, et al. Light distribution, optical properties, and cardiovascular tissues. In Abela GS, Norwell MA (eds): *Lasers in Cardiovascular Medicine and Surgery: Fundamentals and Techniques.* New York: Kluwer Academic Publishers; 1990:93–110.
9. Welch AJ, van Gemert MJ, Star WM, Wilson BC. Definitions and overview of tissue optics. In Welch AJ, van Gemert MJ (eds): *Optical-Thermal Response of Laser-Irradiated Tissue.* New York: Plenum Press; 1995:15–46.
10. Jacques SL. Light distributions from point, line and plane sources for photochemical reactions and fluorescence in turbid biological tissues. *Photochem Photobiol* 1998;67:23–32.
11. Bright R. *Reports of Medical Cases Selected with a View of Illustrating the Symptoms and Cure of Diseases by a Reference to Morbid Anatomy.* London: Longman, Rees, Orme, Brown, Green, Highley; 1831:431–435.
12. Cutler M. Transillumination as an aid to diagnosis of breast lesions. *Surg Gynecol Obstet* 1929;48:721–729.
13. Key H, Jackson PC, Wells PN. New approaches to transillumination imaging. *J Biomed Eng* 1988;10:113–118.
14. Gros C, Quenneville Y, Hummel Y. [Breast diaphanology]. *Journal de Radiologie, d Electrologie, et de Medecine Nucleaire* 1972;53:297–306.
15. Jarry G, Ghesquiere S, Maarek JM, et al. Imaging mammalian tissues and organs using laser collimated transillumination. *J Biomed Eng* 1984;6:70–74.
16. Sabel M, Aichinger H. Recent developments in breast imaging. *Phys Med Biol* 1996;41:315–368.
17. Profio AE, Navarro GA, Sartorius OW. Scientific basis of breast diaphanography. *Med Phys* 1989;16:60–65.
18. Gardner CM, Jacques SL, Welch AJ. Light transport in tissue: Accurate ex-

pressions for one-dimensional fluence rate and escape function based upon Monte Carlo simulation. *Lasers Surg Med* 1996;18:129–138.

19. Müller G, Chance B, Alfano R (eds): *Medical Optical Tomography: Functional Imaging and Monitoring.* Bellingham, WA: SPIE Press; 1993.

20. Alfano RR. Advances in optical biopsy and optical mammography. *Ann N Y Acad Sci.* Vol. 838; 1998.

21. Hebden JC, Kruger RA. Transillumination imaging performance: Spatial resolution simulation studies. *Med Phys* 1990;17(1):40–47.

22. Berg R, Andersson-Engels S, Svanberg S. Time-resolved transillumination imaging. In Müller G, Chance B, Alfano R (eds): *Medical Optical Tomography: Functional Imaging and Monitoring.* Bellingham, WA: SPIE Press; 1993:397–424.

23. Gandjbakhche AH, Nossal R, Bonner RF. Resolution limits for optical transillumination of abnormalities deeply embedded in tissues. *Med Phys* 1994;21(2):185–191.

24. Chang J, Graber HL, Barbour RL. Imaging of fluorescence in highly scattering media. *IEEE Trans Biomed Eng* 1997;44(9):810–822.

25. Arridge SR, Hebden JC. Optical imaging in medicine: II. Modeling and reconstruction. *Phys Med Biol* 1997;42:841–853.

26. Svaasand LO. Optical dosimetry for direct and interstitial photoradiation therapy of malignant tumors. *Prog Clin Biol Res* 1984;170:91–114.

27. Jenkins FA, White HE. *Fundamentals of Optics.* 3rd ed. New York: McGraw-Hill; 1957.

28. Weisskopf VF. How light interacts with matter. *Sci Am* 1968;219:60–71.

29. Johnson CC, Guy AW. Nonionizing electromagnetic wave effects in biological materials and systems. *Proc IEEE* 1972;60:692–721.

30. van de Hulst HC. *Multiple Light Scattering: Tables, Formulas, and Applications.* New York: Academic Press; 1980.

31. Ishimaru A. *Wave Propagation and Scattering in Random Media.* New York: Academic Press; 1978.

32. Wilson BC, Patterson MS, Flock ST. Indirect versus direct techniques for the measurement of the optical properties of tissues. *Photochem Photobiol* 1987;46:601–608.

33. Wilksch PA, Jacka F, Blake AJ. Studies of light propagation through tissue. *Prog Clin Biol Res* 1984;170:149–161.

34. Cheong WF, Prahl SA, Welch AJ. A review of the optical properties of biological tissues. *IEEE J Quantum Electron* 1990;26:2166–2185.

35. Wilson BC. Measurement of tissue optical properties: Methods and theories. In Welch AJ, van Gemert MJ (eds): *Optical-Thermal Response of Laser-Irradiated Tissue.* New York: Plenum Press; 1995:233–274.

36. Flock ST, Wilson BC, Patterson MS. Total attenuation coefficients and scattering phase functions of tissues and phantom materials at 633 nm. *Med Phys* 1987;14:835–841.

37. Wilson BC, Jeeves WP, Lowe DM, Adam G. Light propagation in animal tissues in the wavelength range 375–825 nanometers. *Prog Clin Biol Res* 1984; 170:115–132.

38. Wilson BC, Patterson MS, Burns DM. The effect of photosensitizer concentration in tissue on the penetration depth of photoactivating light. *Laser Med Sci* 1986;1:235–244.

39. Wilson BC, Patterson MS. The physics of photodynamic therapy. *Phys Med Biol* 1986;31:327–360.

40. Duderstadt JJ, Hamilton LJ. *Nuclear Reactor Analysis.* New York: Wiley; 1976:103–144.

41. Profio AE, Doiron DR. Dosimetry considerations in phototherapy. *Med Phys* 1981;8:190–196.

42. Kubelka P. New contributions to the optics of intensely light-scattering mate-

rials. *J Opt Soc Am* 1948;38:448–457.

43. Profio AE, Doiron DR. Transport of light in tissue in photodynamic therapy. *Photochem Photobiol* 1987;46:591–599.

44. Flock ST, Patterson MS, Wilson BC, Wyman DR. Monte Carlo modeling of light propagation in highly scattering tissue—I: Model predictions and comparison with diffusion theory. *IEEE Trans Biomed Eng* 1989;36:1162–1168.

45. Jacques SL, Wang L. Monte Carlo modeling of light transport in tissues. In Welch AJ, van Gemert MJ (eds): *Optical-Thermal Response of Laser-Irradiated Tissue*. New York: Plenum Press; 1995:73–100.

46. Andersson-Engels S, Johansson J, Svanberg K, Svanberg S. Fluorescence imaging and point measurements of tissue: Applications to the demarcation of malignant tumors and atherosclerotic lesions from normal tissue. *Photochem Photobiol* 1991;53:807–814.

47. Ramanujam N, Mitchell MF, Mahadevan A, et al. In vivo diagnosis of cervical intraepithelial neoplasia using 337-nm-excited laser-induced fluorescence. *Proc Natl Acad Sci U S A* 1994;91:10193-10197.

48. Jacques SL. Summarizing Monte Carlo simulations by simple analytic expressions to describe photon transport in tissues. *Proceedings of Photon Transport in Highly Scattering Tissue* 1994;September:2–10.

49. Preuss LE, Bolin FP, Cain BW. A comment on spectral transmittance in mammalian skeletal muscle. *Photochem Photobiol* 1983;37:113–116.

50. Wilson BC, Jeeves WP, Lowe DM. In vivo and post mortem measurements of the attenuation spectra of light in mammalian tissues. *Photochem Photobiol* 1985;42:153–162.

51. Bolin FP, Preuss LE, Cain BW. A comparison of spectral transmittance for several mammalian tissues: Effects at PRT frequencies. *Prog Clin Biol Res* 1984;170:211–225.

52. Star WM, Marijnissen JP, van Gemert MJ. Light dosimetry in optical phantoms and in tissues: I. Multiple flux and transport theory. *Phys Med Biol* 1988; 33:437–454.

53. Marynissen JPA, Star WM. Phantom measurements for light dosimetry using isotropic and small aperture detectors. *Prog Clin Biol Res* 1984;170:133–148.

Chapter 4

Optics and Detectors Used in Optical Mapping

Kenneth R. Laurita and Imad Libbus

In 1906, Mayer described reentrant excitation from visualization of pulsatile waves in the jellyfish.[1] Since then, our understanding of the fundamental mechanisms of arrhythmias has relied on the development of new experimental techniques to measure the electrical activity of the heart. Following the emergence of high-speed digital computers, it became technologically feasible to measure cardiac extracellular potentials simultaneously from hundreds of recording sites in the experimental and clinical laboratory.[2] Multichannel extracellular mapping techniques provided some of the first detailed images of impulse propagation in the intact heart during complex ventricular[3] and atrial arrhythmias.[4] Similarly, advances in micropipette patch-clamp techniques have taught us a great deal about cardiac electrophysiology at the level of the single cell and ion channel.[5]

As detailed in previous chapters, recent developments in fluorescent probes and imaging techniques have made it possible to measure action potentials from hundreds of sites at the level of the single cell or whole heart. Undoubtedly, optical mapping will continue to provide a basic understanding of the cellular mechanisms of arrhythmias and will play an important role in bridging the gap between macroscopic activation of the heart and ion channel electrophysiology. Although both convey electrical activity of the heart, it is important to emphasize that there are fundamental differences between conventional electrical and optical recording modalities. It will be evident that linking electrophysiological measurements to a system of optics imposes several unique characteristics to optically recorded action potentials that must be considered when interpreting these signals. This chapter focuses on some of the unique properties of optical action potentials and the special techniques used to measure them.

Source of Optical Action Potentials

The source of optical action potentials originates from dye molecules bound to the cell membrane from within a specific tissue area and depth. Thus, the optical action potential signal arises from a volume of cells that

From Rosenbaum DS, Jalife J (eds): *Optical Mapping of Cardiac Excitation and Arrhythmias.* ©Futura Publishing Co., Inc., Armonk, NY, 2001.

depends on optical magnification. This property gives the optical action potential several unique characteristics.[6] This issue is complicated by the fact that optical magnification also defines spatial resolution. Figure 1A demonstrates the effect of optical magnification on spatial resolution (i.e., distance between neighboring recording pixels, r in inset). Assuming a 1.5-mm center-to-center distance between photodiode elements, a spatial resolution of 1.5 to 0.15 mm can be achieved with an optical magnification range of 1× to 10×. Compared with spatial resolution, the recording area (Fig. 1B) and number of cells per recording area (Fig. 1C) decrease more rapidly with increasing optical magnification. Therefore, as spatial resolution increases (i.e., as r decreases) with optical magnification, the source of the optical action potential and, thus, the measured action potential amplitude decrease rapidly. Assuming that noise inherent to the detector and electronics is independent of optical magnification, signal-to-noise (S/N) ratio will decrease with increasing optical magnification. Figure 2 demon-

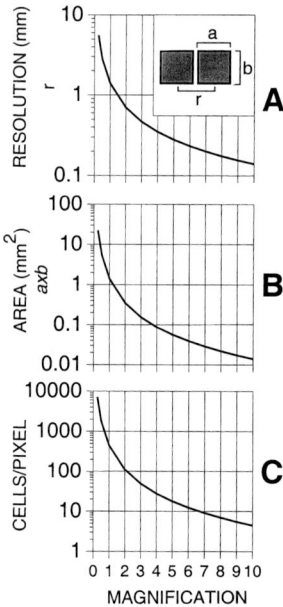

Figure 1. Influence of optical magnification on spatial resolution (A), pixel area (B), and cells per recording pixel (C). Calculations are based on a 2-dimensional recording pixel (i.e., ignoring depth of each pixel) having equal height and width (inset, a & b) and interpixel separation, r. A. Spatial resolution, r, varies as the inverse of magnification. B. Surface area of tissue imaged onto each photo element (pixel area = a×b). C. Estimated number of cells that contribute to the signal focused onto any individual photodetector. Reprinted from reference 6.

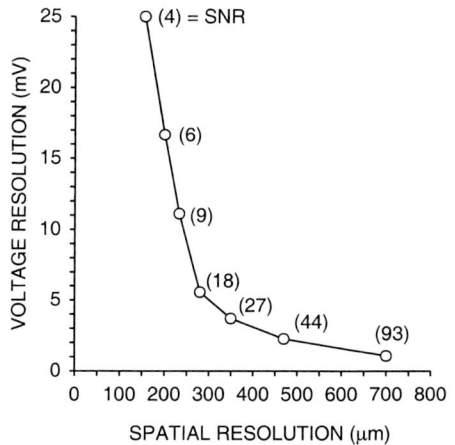

Figure 2. Voltage resolution and signal-to-noise ratio (SNR) plotted as a function of spatial resolution. As spatial resolution increases (i.e., pixel area decreases) voltage resolution and signal fidelity fall rapidly because fewer cells are contributing to the optical action potential signal while system noise and illumination intensity remain constant. Reprinted from reference 6.

strates this characteristic of optical action potentials. Shown is a graph of voltage resolution and S/N ratio calculated from optical action potentials measured at different spatial resolutions (i.e., interpixel separation). As interpixel separation is decreased, S/N ratio and voltage resolution deteriorate rapidly. Therefore, improvement of spatial resolution always occurs at a cost of lower S/N ratio. When high magnifications are required, additional measures such as maximizing light collection efficiency become increasingly important.

An optical action potential represents a multicellular spatial average of transmembrane potential from cells within a volume of tissue. Thus, as magnification decreases, more cells contribute to the optical action potential. At very low magnifications, a decrease in the rate of rise (i.e., prolongation) of the optical action potential upstroke may occur due to spatial averaging. Figure 3 shows the rise time of the optical action potential upstroke at a relatively low magnification ($1\times$), corresponding to a recording area of 1.5 mm $\times$ 1.5 mm per photodiode element. Compared with transmembrane potential recorded from a single cell within the same region using a glass microelectrode, the upstroke (i.e., rise time) of the optical action potential is slowed (Fig. 3, inset). However, when optical magnification is increased, the upstroke of the optical action potential approaches that measured from a single cell. These data are shown more quantitatively in the graph where rise time of the action potential, recorded optically (open circles) and with a microelectrode (shaded bar),

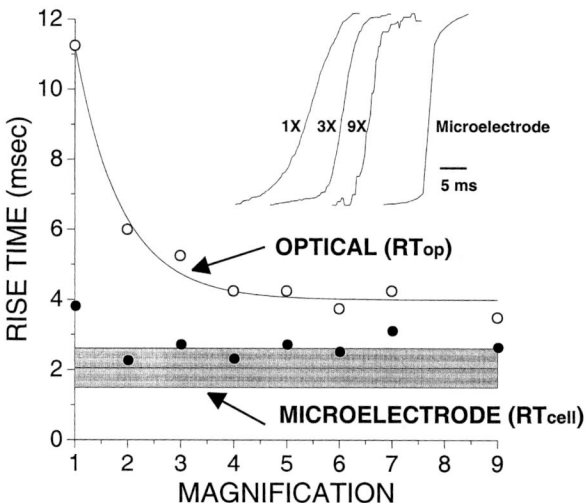

Figure 3. Rise time of optical action potentials (RT_{op}) measured as a function of optical magnification (open circles). For comparison, the mean ($\pm$ SD) rise time measured from single cells with glass microelectrodes is shown by the shaded bar. Single cell rise times (RT_{cell}, filled circles) calculated from optically recorded action potentials (open circles), conduction velocity (θ), and spatial resolution (r) using $RT_{cel} = RT_{op} - r/\theta$ closely correspond to rise times measured with microelectrodes. The inset demonstrates the effect of increasing optical magnification on phase 0 rise time of optical action potentials. Reprinted from reference 6.

were calculated as a function of optical magnification. Assuming uniform conduction velocity and planar wave front propagation, rise time prolongation can be corrected.[7] Shown in Figure 3 (graph) are corrected rise times (closed circles) calculated for each data point (open circles). The corrected rise times closely match rise times measured with the microelectrode. It is also possible that during slow impulse propagation the upstroke of the optical action potential may become artificially prolonged at normal magnifications. Prolongation of the optical action potential upstroke under these circumstances may not necessarily imply upstroke prolongation of transmembrane potential. If upstroke prolongation due to slow conduction is a concern, either higher magnification or a correction calculation can be used to better approximate the actual transmembrane potential upstroke.[7]

Because light can penetrate into cardiac tissue, the source of the optical action potential also includes a contribution from deeper tissue layers (see chapter 3 for detailed discussion). Excitation light must first penetrate to deeper layers and then fluoresced light originating from deeper layers must exit from the surface of the heart. To determine the contribution of deeper layers, the light transmission properties of ventricular myocardium were previously characterized.[6] The decay of light into and out of the myocardium can be modeled as a product of two exponentials:

$$I_{fl} = \gamma \int_0^D I_0 \left[e^{-x/\delta_{fl}} \right] \left[e^{-x/\delta_{ex}} \right] dx \qquad (1)$$

where, I_{fl} is the total fluorescence signal from the surface of the heart with thickness D, I_0 is the excitation light intensity at the surface of the heart, γ is the quantum yield of the dye (0.3 for di-4-ANEPPS), and δ_{ex} (0.289 mm) and δ_{fl} (0.434 mm) are the wavelength-dependent decay constants calculated from the transmission spectrum of guinea pig ventricle. Figure 4 shows the percent of fluoresced light originating from each 100-μm layer. Approximately 95% of the signal detected from the epicardial surface originates from a depth of less than 500 μm, with the majority coming from the first 100 μm. These results are in agreement with those reported previously.[8] Therefore, under these circumstances the source of optical signals is essentially a 2-dimensional layer of cells.

Light Collection

Optical mapping requires the collection of fluorescent light at relatively low intensities. Light collection should be maximized to allow elements of the action potential such as repolarization to be distinguished from background noise. When a lens is used to magnify and focus the image onto a photodetector, the amount of light collected is directly proportional to the square of the numerical aperture (NA) (i.e., an index of light gathering power) of the lens and inversely proportional to the square of the magnification.[9] Maximizing light collection efficiency is especially important at high magnifications, when the source of fluorescence is reduced.

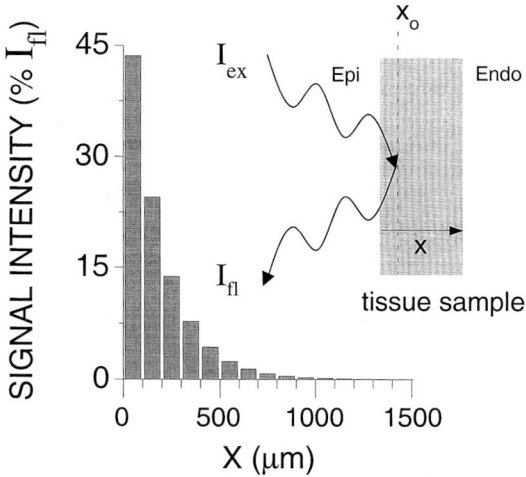

Figure 4. For an action potential generated by a cell located at a depth x_O below the epicardial surface to influence an optically recorded action potential recorded from the epicardial surface, excitation light (I_{ex}, 540 nm) must penetrate the tissue to excite voltage-sensitive dye bound to the cell. In turn, fluoresced light emitted by the dye (I_{fl}, >610 nm) must escape out of the tissue to the epicardial surface. Because excitation and fluoresced light intensity decay exponentially with depth, the contribution of subepicardial cells to the epicardial action potential falls as the product of these two exponential processes. Signal intensity is expressed as a percent of the total signal detected from the surface. Individual bars sum the contribution from each 100 μ of depth. Reprinted from reference 6.

Moreover, improving light collection efficiency maximizes signal fidelity without the adverse effects associated with intense excitation light, such as photobleaching.

High-quality images can be acquired with either microscope or photography lenses. Fluorescence microscopes are commercially available with objective lens magnifications ranging from 4× to 100×, allowing for the mapping of preparations smaller than 4 mm². Because high magnifications are used, high light collection efficiency is required. Therefore, microscope objectives are designed with high NAs, ranging from 0.5 to 1.3. In fluorescence microscopy, the preparation is epi-illuminated, meaning that the objective lens also acts as the condenser. As a result, epi-illumination efficiently and evenly illuminates the preparation.[9] Microscope objectives have been optimized for observing small preparations at short working distances (i.e., distance from lens to preparation); however, the advantages of microscope objectives are not maintained at lower magnifiations.

Photographic Lenses

Photographic lenses are better suited for magnifications less than 10×, where they have NAs ranging from 0.25 to 0.4. The working distance varies depending on the lens configuration and is on the order of 30 mm, much longer than the working distance of a microscope objective. The simplest way to use photographic lenses is to image a preparation with a single lens (Fig. 5A). The preparation (solid arrow) is placed at a specific distance (i.e., X_o) from the focal plane of the lens. Magnification can be calculated as a function of the focal length (i.e., f) and the distance between the object and the focal plane,[10]

$$M = \frac{f}{x_o} \tag{2}$$

A photodetector is placed at the position where the image is formed (dashed arrow) on the other side of the lens as determined by,[10]

$$x_i = \frac{f^2}{x_o} \tag{3}$$

The tandem lens configuration is a variation of the single lens design, and consists of two lenses aligned along an optical axis and separated by a distance, d (Fig. 5B). To implement the tandem lens configuration, two camera lenses are focused at infinity and are placed face to face.[11,12] The preparation is placed at the focal plane of the first lens (f_1), and the image is formed at the focal plane of the second lens (f_2). Magnification can be calculated as the ratio of the focal lengths of the two lenses,[10]

$$M = \frac{f_2}{f_1} \tag{4}$$

It should be noted that the magnification is not dependent on the separation of the two lenses. Changing magnification is simply a matter of

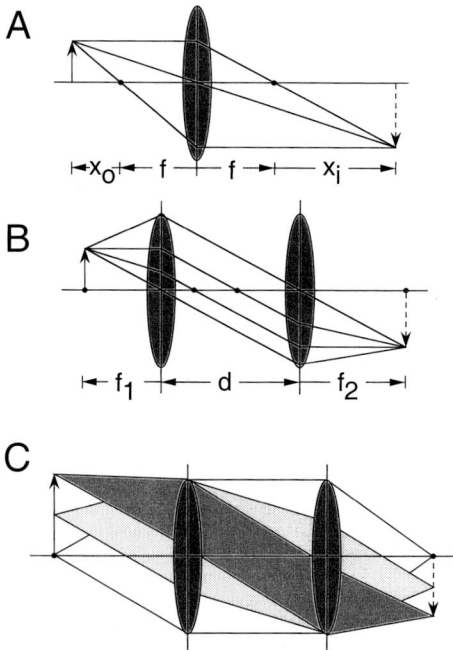

Figure 5. A. Single lens configuration. The object (i.e., preparation) is placed at a specific distance (x_o) from the focal plane (f) of the lens. The image is formed on the other side of the lens, at a specific distance (x_i) from the focal point. The single lens design can be implemented with a standard photographic lens. **B.** Tandem lens configuration. Two lenses are aligned along an optical axis and separated by a distance (d). The object is placed at the focal plane of the first lens (f_1), and the image is formed at the focal plane of the second lens (f_2). The magnification is equal to the ratio of the focal lengths (M = f_2/f_1). The tandem lens design can be implemented with two photographic lenses, focused at infinity and placed face to face. As a point on the object moves further away from the axis, the cone of rays that reach the image plane becomes narrower as indicated by the darker shades of gray (**C**). The edges of the lenses act as effective aperture stops, blocking a portion of the cone of light from reaching the image plane. As the distance between the lenses (d) increases, light originating from object points off axis becomes narrower, and the effect of vignetting increases.

changing one of the two lenses so that the ratio of the focal lengths of the two lenses yields the desired magnification. In addition, working distance is determined by the focal length of the first lens (typically 30 mm) and, unlike the single lens design, is independent of magnification.

Vignetting

As indicated in Figure 5B, in the tandem lens configuration the light between the two lenses that originates from any single point within the object is collimated. However, with the exception of light originating from the center of the image, light is not parallel to the optical axis. As a point on the object moves away from the optical axis, the cone of light rays originating from that point that reaches the image plane becomes narrower as indicated by the decreasing area of regions shaded in darker gray (panel C). Even if there is no other aperture limiting the light, the finite diameter of the lenses acts as effective aperture stops, blocking a portion of the light from reaching the image plane.[10,13] The result is a fading out of the image at the periphery, known as vignetting, which occurs regardless of detector size. Because the object (i.e., preparation) in a tandem lens configuration is close to the lens, the loss of light at the periphery of the image can be abrupt. As the distance between the two lenses increases, the cone of light reaching the second lens narrows, and the effect of vignetting increases. The effect of lens separation on vignetting (Fig. 6) was measured by increasing the distance between lenses starting from the minimum separation that could be

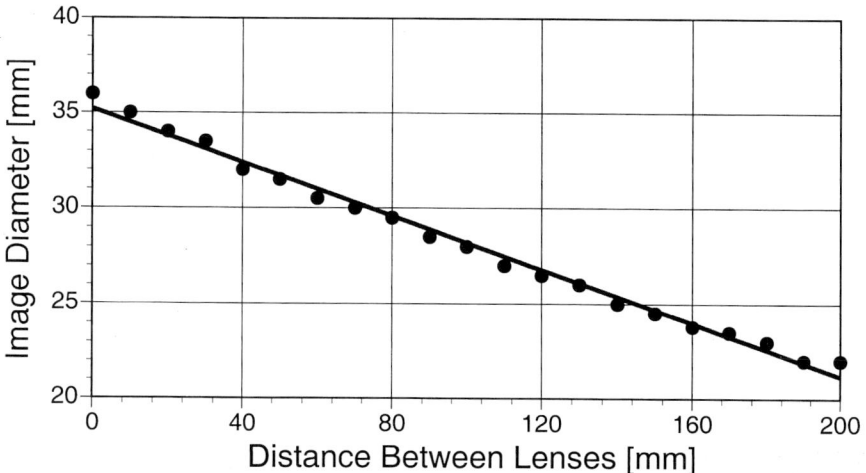

Figure 6. Effect of lens separation on image diameter in tandem lens configuration. Two camera lenses with focal lengths of 85 mm were placed in a tandem lens configuration, yielding a magnification of 1×. The distance between the lenses was increased in increments of 10 mm, beginning at the point of least possible lens separation (0 mm). For each distance tested, a grid was placed at the focal plane of the first lens (f_1) and imaged onto an oversized screen placed at the focal plane of the second lens (f_2). Image diameter was defined as the diameter of the grid that was visible on the screen. For this lens combination, the maximum image diameter is 35 mm.

obtained (0 mm.) At each distance, a grid was placed at the focal plane of the first lens (f_1) and imaged onto an oversized screen placed at the focal plane of the second lens (f_2). Image diameter was defined as the diameter of the grid that was visible on the screen. For the lens combination tested (85 mm/f1.4, 85 mm/f1.8), the maximum image that could be obtained occurred at the minimum separation and was approximately 35 mm in diameter. As the distance between the lenses increased, the image diameter decreased linearly. With use of this lens configuration and an 18 mm × 18 mm photodiode array (PDA) detector (i.e., a screen of limited size), vignetting was not a problem at separations less than 140 mm.

In addition to lens separation, NA also affects the degree of vignetting. Since NA is inversely proportional to focal length, it is difficult to change magnification without also changing the NA. To quantify the effect of different lens combinations with different apertures on vignetting, lenses with focal lengths ranging from 24 mm to 180 mm were placed in the tandem lens configurations, yielding magnifications ranging from 0.13× to 7.5×. The distance between the two lenses was fixed at 100 mm for each lens combination, and the amount of vignetting was measured using a test grid as described above. Figure 7 shows the relationship between magnification and image diameter for a variety of lens combinations. Each curve is labeled with the focal length of the second lens (i.e., lens closer to image), and points within each curve represent different first lens (i.e., lens

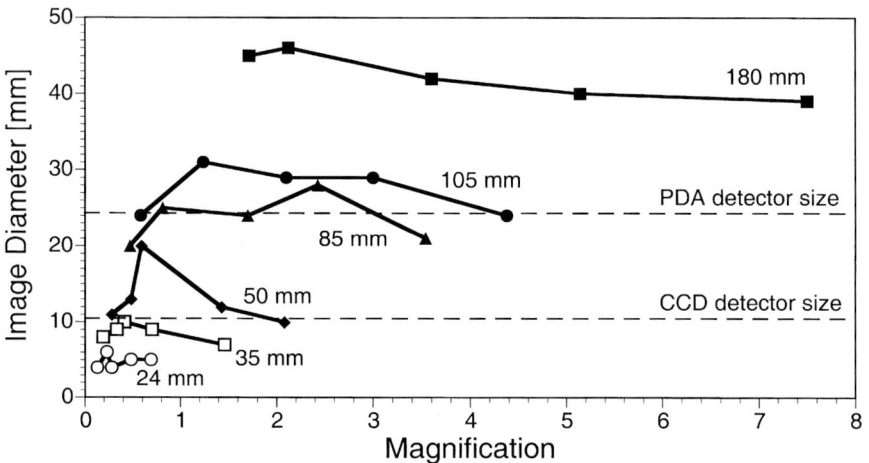

Figure 7. Effect of tandem lens combinations on image magnification and diameter. Camera lenses with focal lengths ranging from 24 mm to 180 mm were placed in the tandem lens configuration, yielding magnifications ranging from 0.13× to 7.5×. The lens focal lengths and NAs were: 24 mm/f2.0, 35 mm/f1.4, 50 mm/f1.8, 85 mm/f1.4, 105 mm/f1.8, and 180 mm/f2.8. For each lens combination tested, the distance between the lenses was fixed at 100 mm. A grid was placed at the focal plane of the first lens and imaged onto an oversized screen placed at the focal plane of the second lens. Image diameter was defined as the diameter of the grid that was visible on the screen. Each plot is labeled with the focal length of the second lens, which has a disproportionate effect on image diameter. Dashed lines indicate the size of a typical photodiode array (PDA) detector and charge-coupled device (CCD) detector.

closer to object) focal lengths. It is evident that different lens combinations produce different image diameters independent of magnification. The differences are due to the focal length and NA of the lenses used to obtain the desired magnification. Moreover, the second lens has a disproportionately large effect on image diameter compared with the first lens. Dashed lines indicate the size of a typical PDA detector and charged coupled device (CCD) detector. Depending on the detector used, lens combinations should be selected that produce the desired magnification and an image diameter greater than the detector size; otherwise, the periphery of the object will be clipped by the vignetting artifact.

Light Collection Efficiency

Previously, Ratzlaff and Grinvald[12] acquired fluorescence images with a tandem lens macroscopic that were 100 times brighter than those obtained with a commercial microscope. However, a comparison between the light collection efficiency of the single and tandem lens configuration had not previously been made. To quantitatively compare light collection efficiency of the single and tandem lens configurations, each system of optics was used to focus the light from a light-emitting diode (LED) onto a photodetector. Magnifications ranging from 0.8× to 2.1× were tested. As shown in Figure 8, the signal-to-noise ratio of recordings made with the tandem lens configuration was significantly greater than the signal-to-noise ratio of recordings made with the single lens configuration ($P <$ 0.001). At all magnifications, there was at least a threefold improvement in image quality ($P = 0.03$) and at some magnifications (e.g., 1.24×), the improvement was as high as fivefold. As expected, signal-to-noise ratio was also dependent on magnification as well as on the NAs of the lenses. As magnification increased, a smaller area of the LED (i.e., small source) was recorded by each photodiode. As a result, the signal amplitude and, therefore, the signal-to-noise ratio decreased with increasing magnification. For the single lens configuration, there was a linear relationship between magnification and signal-to-noise ratio (Fig. 8A, squares). For the tandem lens configuration, different magnifications were obtained with different lens combinations, resulting in a nonlinear relationship between magnification and signal-to-noise ratio (panel A, circles). However, the signal-to-noise ratio generally decreased with increasing in magnification for both the single and tandem lens configurations. The improvement in signal-to-noise ratio associated with the tandem lens configuration is obvious from actual optical action potentials recorded with each configuration at the same magnification using the same lenses (Fig. 8B).

Tandem Lens System Design

Improved light collection efficiency is not the only advantage of the tandem lens configuration. As Figure 5B illustrates, the light between the two lenses that originates from the same point is collimated. By placing a dichroic mirror (or beam splitter) between the lenses, collimated light can be diverted to a third lens, where it can be focused onto a second detector.

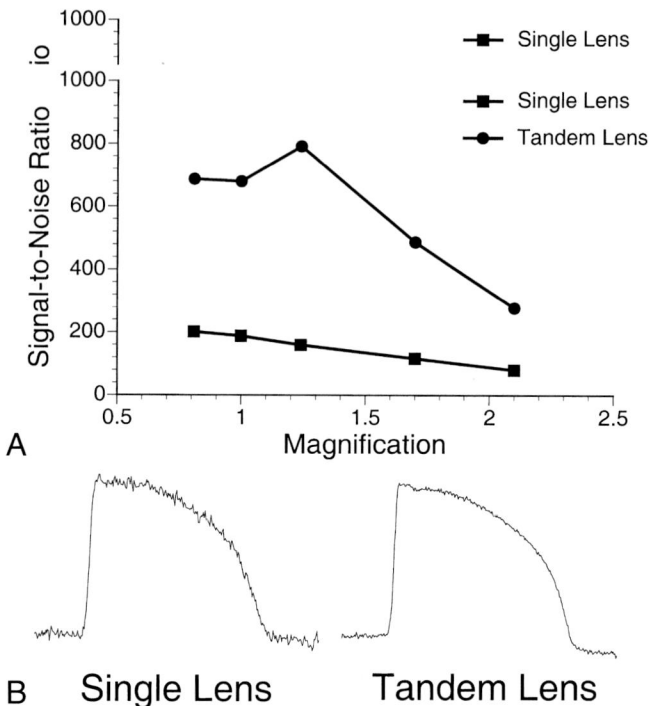

Figure 8. Relationship between signal-to-noise ratio and magnification for tandem and single lens configurations. Tandem and single lens optics were used to focus the light from a square light-emitting diode onto a photodiode array at magnifications ranging from 0.8× to 2.1× (**A**). Signal-to-noise ratio was defined as the signal amplitude divided by the standard deviation of the noise, and the values from the center pixels were averaged to obtain the signal-to-noise ratio at each magnification. At each magnification, the signal-to-noise ratio of recordings made with the tandem lens configuration are significantly greater than the signal-to-noise ratio of recordings made with the single lens ($P > 0.001$). **B.** Representative optical action potentials acquired using single and tandem lens configurations, illustrating the improvement in signal quality of the tandem lens configuration. Both recordings were made at a magnification of 1.0×. The single lens recording was made with an 85-mm/f1.4 lens, and the tandem lens recording was made with two 85-mm lenses, f1.4 and f1.8.

Figure 9 shows a tandem lens system that uses this principle to epi-illuminate the preparation and simultaneously image fluorescence with two detectors.[12] Excitation light provided by a light source is focused (lenses 4 and 1) onto the preparation through a dichroic mirror. Fluoresced light emitted by the preparation passes through the tandem lens (lenses 1 and 2, and mirror 1) and is focused onto a photodetector (detector 1). Simultaneously, a fraction of the light is diverted by a second dichroic mirror or beam splitter (mirror 2) onto a second detector (detector 2). Lenses 1 and 3 serve as the tandem lenses for detector 2. Although the two tandem lens configurations share a common first lens, the magnification of the image formed on each detector can be independently modified by changing the appropriate second lens.[12] In this configuration, two detectors can be used to image voltage simultaneously from the same preparation by using a 50/50 beam splitter. The beam splitter splits light evenly at all wave-

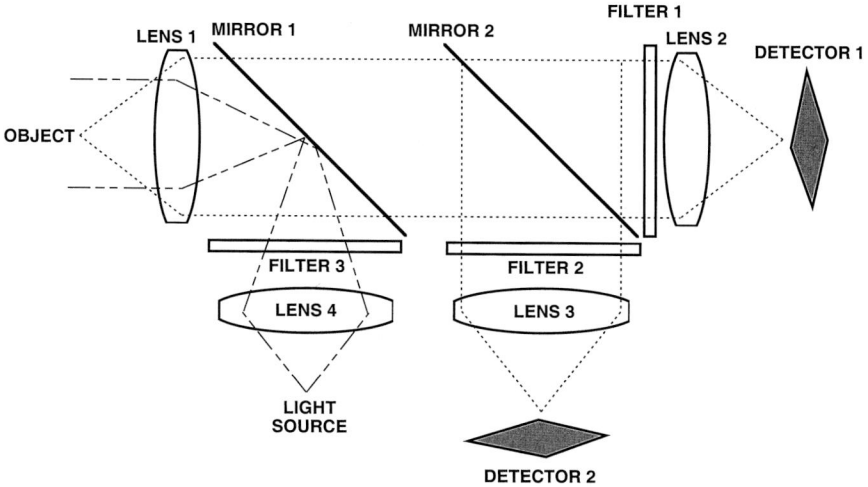

Figure 9. Schematic diagram of a tandem lens configuration that allows the object to be epi-illuminated and imaged simultaneously with two photodetectors. Excitation from a light source is filtered and reflected by the first dichroic mirror (mirror 1) onto the preparation (i.e., object). Fluoresced light collected by lens 1 passes through mirror 1 and a portion through the second dichroic mirror (mirror 2) and focused by a second lens (lens 2) onto a photodetector (detector 1). The remaining fluoresced light is diverted by mirror 2, collected by a third lens (lens 3), and focused onto a second photodetector (detector 2). All optical filters (filter 1, filter 2, and filter 3) are chosen to isolate excitation and emission wavelengths of interest.[12]

lengths, so that fluorescent light emitted by the preparation is split between the two detectors. As a result, each detector records an image of the preparation that is approximately half the intensity of the original image. Alternatively, a dichroic mirror can be used as the second mirror to selectively pass fluoresced light above a particular wavelength to detector 1 and reflect light at wavelengths below to detector 2. If the preparation is stained with a second fluorophore, a judicious selection of dichroic mirrors can allow the first detector to map voltage while the second detector maps, for example, NADH[14] or intracellular calcium (see Future Directions).

Detectors

Fluoresced light collected from a preparation must be focused onto a detector so that light intensity can be converted into an electrical signal. The CCD video camera and PDA are detectors with high sensitivity in the visible light range and are commonly used in optical mapping systems. Photomultiplier tubes are also used in laser scanning optical mapping systems,[15] but these are not discussed in this chapter. Photodiode and CCD arrays are similar in the way that they transduce light energy into electrical energy. When photons of sufficient energy strike a detector material, electron-hole pairs are created (i.e., the photoelectric effect). These photo-generated charge carriers can be either instantaneously converted to current flow or collected over a finite period. Photodiode and CCD arrays are also similar in that both detector types are typically configured as 2-dimensional arrays. PDAs typically consist of several hundred individual photodiodes with a total area of approximately 3 cm². CCD arrays contain several hundred thousand elements and are typically smaller in total detector area compared with PDAs. Beyond these similarities, both detectors have unique properties that must be considered.

Photodiode Arrays

PDAs for optical mapping applications are configured to instantaneously convert photoexcited charge carriers to current flow (i.e., photocurrent). The magnitude of photocurrent is directly proportional to the light intensity falling on a single photodiode element, and is converted to a voltage using a current-to-voltage preamplifier. Each photodiode is connected to its own preamplifier, where a feedback resistance (1 to 500 MΩ) determines the current-to-voltage gain. In most configurations, feedback resistance also influences the frequency response of the preamplifier. Therefore, a higher feedback resistance increases gain but may also attenuate high-frequency components of the optical action potential. At low optical magnifications this is not a concern because the optical action potential is larger in amplitude and a smaller gain is required. Furthermore, the optical action potential contains less high-frequency components at low magnification (Fig. 3). At high magnification the optical action potential signal is smaller in amplitude and, thus, requires a larger gain (i.e., larger feedback resistance). However, at higher magnifications the upstroke of the action potential contains higher frequency components that could, in theory, be attenuated by a larger feedback resistance. Therefore, when high magnifications are required, the feedback resistance must be chosen cautiously. It may be possible, for example, to increase overall gain by adding signal amplification to subsequent stages rather than the preamplifier stage.

Following current-to-voltage conversion, additional signal conditioning such as alternating current (AC) coupling (i.e., offset removal), antialiasing filtering, and gain can be added. It is important to note that the first stage of amplification is typically not AC coupled and can pass large direct current offsets. Therefore, a high gain in combination with large background fluorescence can saturate the first stage electronics independent of any offset removal in subsequent stages. Finally, because the current from each photodiode is converted and amplified in parallel, standard multichannel analog to digital conversion techniques can be used to achieve very high sampling rates (more than 4000 Hz per channel).

CCD Arrays

CCD detectors differ from photodiodes in that photoexcited charge carriers are collected within a single element (i.e., pixel) over a finite period (i.e., integration time). The quantity of charge collected is linearly proportional to the incident light intensity and integration time. The longer the integration time, the more charge will be collected and, thus, the larger the signal amplitude will be. However, too much light or too long of an integration time can saturate the charge capacity of a pixel. In addition, long integration times can cause blurring artifact due to the integration of fluoresced light over time.[16] Once integration is complete, the charge collected in each pixel is simultaneously moved in the same direction to a neighboring pixel, which acts as a temporary storage location. This process is repeated until all pixels are read out one at a time. This process of moving or coupling charge is, in fact, where the CCD (i.e., charge-coupled device) array gets its name. Finally, the magnitude of charge from each pixel is sequentially converted to an analog video signal and then passed to a frame grabber that digitizes and stores each successive frame. Standard image processing software can be used to subtract background fluorescence and enhance contrast.

In general, the time required to simultaneously collect an image and then read out each individual pixel determines the sampling or frame rate. Given that a CCD array contains several hundred thousand pixels and that each pixel is read out sequentially, readout time is a major factor that limits the sampling rate of CCD systems. In some configurations (e.g., CCDs that support frame transfer) it is possible to read out one image while simultaneously collecting the next, and thus increase sampling rate. It is also possible to significantly increase sampling rate by reducing the number of pixels read out by combining adjacent pixels into super pixels (i.e., binning) during readout. Because the surface area of a single CCD element (pixel) is small compared with a photodiode element, binning has the added benefit of increasing the effective pixel area and, thus, signal amplitude relative to readout noise. However, CCDs in general have a lower dynamic range than photodiode detectors, which limits the signal-to-noise ratio that can be achieved. A low dynamic range makes it difficult to capture large background fluorescence while providing adequate voltage resolution for the action potential. This is important because the total fluorescence measured consists mostly (90%) of background fluorescence. Nevertheless, recent improvements in CCD technology have dramatically increased the dynamic range and, thus, the signal-to-noise ratio that can be achieved.

Temporal and Spatial Sampling Requirements

Theoretically, the frequency content of an optical action potential determines the minimum temporal sampling rate required to accurately reconstruct the action potential from digital samples. Because optical action potentials represent an average of several cells, the frequency content of an action potential recorded from a microelectrode is expected to be higher and, thus, can be used to approximate the upper limit of sampling rate required for an optical action potential. Floating microelectrode recordings from the epicardial surface of the intact guinea pig ventricle indicate that approximately 90% of the total energy of the action potential is contained below 150 Hz.[6] Sampling theory requires that temporal sampling rate be at least 2 times greater than the highest frequency component in order to correctly reconstruct the original signal; otherwise, unwanted distortion (i.e., aliasing) may be introduced. Therefore, optical action potential recordings are typically made at 3 to 5 times the highest frequency component (i.e., 450 to 750 Hz). Certain tissue preparations (e.g., Purkinje fibers) may contain action potentials with higher frequency components and, thus, may require higher sampling rates.

As in the time domain, the spatial complexity (i.e., frequency) of propagating wave fronts dictates the spatial required resolution. For example, greater spatial resolution is required to accurately depict the complex wave fronts that occur during fibrillation and microreentry,[17] or to investigate the discrete nature of propagation at the cellular level.[18] However, it is often difficult to know, a priori, the spatial complexity of wave fronts and, thus, to place an upper and lower limit on the required spatial resolution. Independent of wave front complexity, when CCD or photodiode detectors are used with spatial resolutions greater than 1 mm, many cells contribute to the optical action potential, and this can result in significant blurring of the action potential upstroke (Fig. 3). Therefore, a spatial resolution larger than 1 mm is not recommended. It is important to note that, independent of spatial resolution, an insufficient temporal sampling rate makes it impossible to accurately depict wave front propagation, in time and space. Despite the difficulties associated with determining the necessary spatial resolution, one of the advantages of optical mapping is that spatial resolution can be changed as easily as changing the lens of a camera.

The choice of photodetector can limit, in some cases, the temporal and spatial resolutions that can be achieved. A typical CCD detector has several orders of magnitude more recording sites than does a PDA. Practically, however, the effective number of recording sites is much less, due to the spatial averaging and pixel binning that are typically required to raise signal-to-noise ratio and sampling rate to an acceptable level. Nevertheless, the effective number of recording sites for a CCD detector is greater than that of a PDA and, therefore, CCD detectors are more appropriated for mapping larger areas at low magnification so that spatial resolutions of approximately 1 mm or less can be maintained. On the other hand, the low signal-to-noise ratio and temporal sampling rate characteristic of CCD detectors make them inappropriate for high magnifications when the source of fluorescence signal is small and the frequency content of the optical action potential approaches that measured from a single cell. Photodiode detectors, on the other hand, contain fewer elements and are therefore unable to meet the minimum spatial sampling requirements when mapping larger preparations. However, the high sampling rates and signal-to-noise ratio that can be achieved with PDAs make them ideal for higher optical magnification when temporal resolution and signal fidelity are critical.

Future Directions

Motion Reduction

One of the most frustrating problems associated with optical mapping is motion artifact (MA) due to contraction of the heart. MA arises from changes in the reflectance properties of the tissue as the heart contracts, and from changes in the source of fluorescence associated with the movement of the tissue underneath one recording element.[19] Shown in Figure 10A is an example of MA present on an optical action potential. Typically, the upstroke of the action potential is unaffected by MA. In contrast, the plateau and repolarization phase of the action potential can become distorted, making it difficult to determine the timing of repolarization unless appropriate measures are taken. Current approaches to minimizing MA include administering pharmacological agents that inhibit mechanical contraction,[20–22] reducing extracellular calcium concentration, and mechanically constraining movement of the heart within the mapping field. None of these techniques are ideal. Pharmacological suppression of contraction using compounds such as 2,3 butanedione monoxime or verapamil, or reduced extracellular calcium concentration, can lead to unwanted electrophysiological side effects[23,24] (Fig. 10B, thin action potential). In contrast, mechanically constraining motion of the heart does not significantly alter the electrophysiology.[6] However, MA cannot always be completely eliminated. We have found that by mechanically constraining the heart, it is possible to attain detailed analysis of activation and repolarization[25] without the side effects associated with pharmacological agents. These approaches have been very successful; however, in smaller preparations in which high magnification is required (e.g., intact mouse heart), MA can be significant. New approaches using ratiometric imaging[19] may better suppress MA.

Intracellular Calcium and Transmembrane Potential Imaging

One of the advantages of optical mapping is that measurements are not limited to transmembrane potential. Fluorescent probes of intracellular calcium[26] have been used extensively to measure calcium transients and

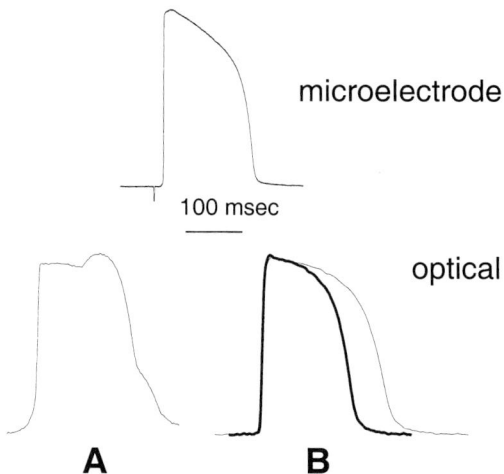

Figure 10. Ventricular action potential recorded with microelectrode techniques is compared with optical action potentials recorded with voltage-sensitive dye. **A.** Optical action potential recorded from unrestrained freely contracting heart. **B.** Action potentials recorded with voltage-sensitive dye using two methods of motion reduction; the bold action potential was recorded using mechanical stabilization of the heart with a Langendorff chamber and a moveable piston, the thin action potential was recorded during low calcium perfusion without mechanical stabilization. Both motion reduction techniques effectively eliminate motion artifacts. However, low calcium perfusion significantly prolonged action potential duration. Reprinted from reference 6.

intracellular calcium at the level of the intact heart[27–29] and single cell.[30] Because the peak excitation and emission wavelengths of fluorescent indicators vary from ultraviolet to near infrared, it is possible to measure more than one parameter in the same heart by measuring fluorescence intensity at separate wavelengths. To do so, one must select dyes that fluoresce light at different wavelengths (i.e., dyes with minimal overlap of emission spectra).[31–34] Such is the case with di-4-ANEPPS and indo-1, which are used for measuring transmembrane potential and intracellular calcium, respectively. We have previously shown that minimal spectral overlap exists between the emission spectra of di-4-ANEPPS and indo-1.[31] It is possible to measure action potentials and calcium transients simultaneously by using a dichroic mirror to direct fluorescence from each dye to separate detector arrays. As mentioned above, the tandem lens system, which simplifies the integration of a dichroic mirror and multiple detectors, is ideally suited for this procedure. Figure 11 shows an action potential and calcium transient measured from the same site in the intact guinea pig heart (panel A) and simultaneously recorded contour maps of activation time and the time of calcium transient onset (panel B) recorded simultaneously. As expected, a rapid increase in intracellular calcium follows the upstroke of the action potential by several milliseconds, while the decline of intracellular calcium is much slower, extending beyond the re-

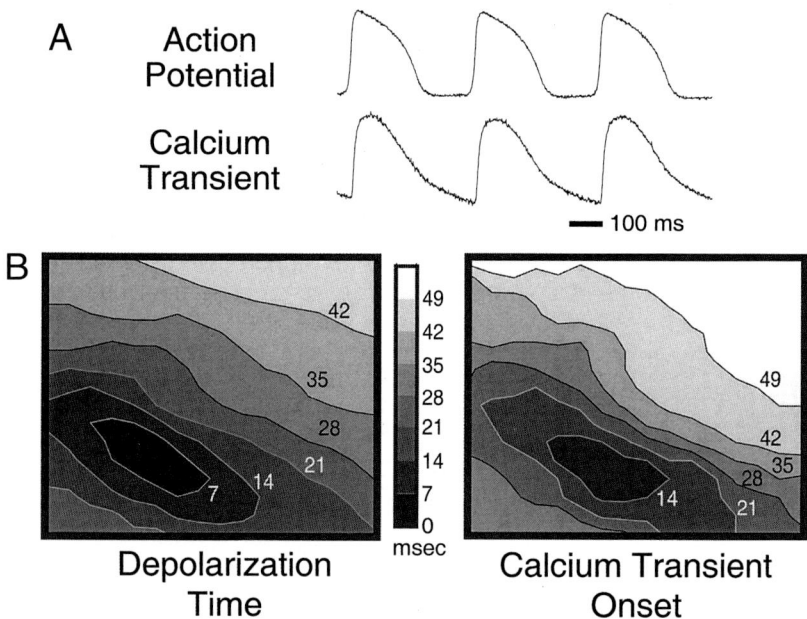

Figure 11. One of 256 ventricular action potentials and calcium transients recorded from an intact heart perfused with di-4-ANEPPS and indo-1 (**A**). Action potential and calcium transient recordings were made simultaneously with use of a dichroic mirror (550-nm cut-off) to redirect fluoresced light from each dye to separate detector arrays. **B.** Simultaneously recorded contour maps of activation time and calcium transient onset calculated from action potentials and calcium transients, respectively.

polarization phase of the action potential. Under normal conditions, this holds true throughout the entire mapping field (panel B). Using such techniques it is has been possible to investigate abnormalities of repolarization associated with intracellular calcium handling, such as the cellular mechanisms of T wave alternans,[35] and to examine the relationship between action potentials and calcium transients during reentrant excitation.[36]

References

1. Mines GR. On dynamic equilibrium in the heart. *J Physiol* (*Lond*) 1913; 46:349–383.
2. Ideker RE, Smith WM, Wallace AG, et al. A computerized method for the rapid display of ventricular activation during the intraoperative study of arrhythmias. *Circulation* 1979;59(3):449–458.
3. Klein GJ, Ideker RE, Smith WM, et al. Epicardial mapping of the onset of ventricular tachycardia initiated by programmed stimulation in the canine heart with chronic infarction. *Circulation* 1979;60:1375–1384.
4. Boineau JP, Mooney CR, Hudson RD, et al. Observations on re-entrant excitation pathways and refractory period distributions in spontaneous and experimental atrial flutter in the dog. In Kulbertus HE (ed): *Re-entrant Arrhythmias: Mechanisms and Treatment.* Baltimore; University Park Press, 1976:72–98.
5. Neher E, Sakmann B. Single-channel currents recorded from membrane of denervated frog muscle fibres. *Nature* 1976;260:799–802.
6. Girouard SD, Laurita KR, Rosenbaum DS. Unique properties of cardiac action potentials recorded with voltage-sensitive dyes. *J Cardiovasc Electrophysiol* 1996;7:1024–1038.
7. Girouard SD, Pastore JM, Laurita KR, et al. Optical mapping in a new guinea pig model of ventricular tachycardia reveals mechanisms for multiple wavelengths in a single reentrant circuit. *Circulation* 1996;93:603–613.
8. Knisley SB. Transmembrane voltage changes during unipolar stimulation of rabbit ventricle. *Circ Res* 1995;77:1229–1239.
9. Taylor DL, Salmon ED. Basic fluorescence microscopy. *Methods Cell Biol* 1989;29:207–237.
10. Hecht E. *Optics.* Reading, MA: Addison-Wesley Publishing Co.; 1987.
11. Lefkowitz L. *The Manual of Close-Up Photography.* Garden City, NY: American Photographic Book Publishing Co., Inc.; 1979.
12. Ratzlaff EH, Grinvald A. A tandem-lens epifluorescence macroscope: Hundredfold brightness advantage for wide-field imaging. *J Neurosci Methods* 1991;36:127–137.
13. Jenkins FA, White HE. *Fundamentals of Optics.* New York: McGraw Hill; 1976.
14. Salama G, Lombardi R, Elson J. Maps of optical action potentials and NADH fluorescence in intact working hearts. *Am J Physiol* 1987;252:H384–H394.
15. Dillon SM, Morad MA. A new laser scanning system for measuring action potential propagation in the heart. *Science* 1981;214:453–456.
16. Baxter WT, Davidenko JM, Loew LM, et al. Technical features of a CCD video camera system to record cardiac fluorescence data. *Ann Biomed Eng* 1997;25:713–725.
17. Spach MS, Josephson ME. Initiating reentry: The role of nonuniform anisotropy in small circuits. *J Cardiovasc Electrophysiol* 1994;5:182–209.
18. Windisch H, Ahammer H, Schaffer P, et al. Optical monitoring of excitation patterns in single cardiomyocytes. *IEEE EMBS* 1990;12:1641–1650.
19. Brandes R, Figueredo VM, Camacho SA, et al. Suppression of motion artifacts in fluorescence spectroscopy of perfused hearts. *Am J Physiol* 1992;263:H972–H980.

20. Pertsov AM, Davidenko JM, Salomonsz R, et al. Spiral waves of excitation underlie reentrant activity in isolated cardiac muscle. *Circ Res* 1993;72:631–650.
21. Dillon S. Synchronized repolarization after defibrillation shocks. *Circulation* 1992;85:1865–1878.
22. Wu J, Biermann M, Rubart M, Zipes DP. Cytochalasin D as excitation-contraction uncoupler for optically mapping action potentials in wedges of ventricular myocardium [see comments]. *J Cardiovasc Electrophysiol* 1998;9:1336–1347.
23. Liu Y, Cabo C, Salomonsz R, et al. Effects of diacetyl monoxime on the electrical properties of sheep and guinea pig ventricular muscle. *Cardiovasc Res* 1993;27:1991–1997.
24. Hirata Y, Kodama I, Iwamura N, et al. Effects of verapamil on canine Purkinje fibers and ventricular muscle fibers with particular reference to the alternation of action potential duration after a sudden increase in driving rate. *Cardiovasc Res* 1979;13:1–8.
25. Girouard S, Laurita K, Rosenbaum DS. Optical mapping can resolve propagation and recovery in the intact beating heart. *Pacing Clin Electrophysiol* 1993;16:II104. Abstract.
26. Grynkiewicz G, Poenie M, Tsien RY. A new generation of Ca^{2+} indicators with greatly improved fluorescence properties. *J Biol Chem* 1985;260:3440–3450.
27. Mohabir R, Clusin TW, Lee HC. Intracellular calcium alternans and the genesis of ischemic ventricular fibrillation. In Zipes DP, Jalife J (eds): *Cardiac Electrophysiology: From Cell to Bedside.* Philadelphia: W.B. Saunders Co.; 1990:448–456.
28. Brandes R, Figueredo V, Camacho S, et al. Quantitation of cytosolic $[Ca^{2+}]$ in whole perfused rat hearts using Indo-1 fluorometry. *Biophys J* 1993;65:1973–1982.
29. Knisley SB. Mapping intracellular calcium in rabbit hearts with fluo3. *Proc 17th Annu Int Conf IEEE Eng Med Biol Soc* 1995. Abstract.
30. Blinks JR, Wier WG, Hess P, Prendergast FG. Measurement of Ca^{2+} concentrations in living cells. *Prog Biophys Mol Biol* 1982;40:1–114.
31. Laurita KR, Singal A. Mapping action potentials and calcium transients simultaneously from the intact heart. *Am J Physiol* In Press.
32. Bum-Rak C, Salama G. Spatio-temporal relationship between action potentials and Ca^{2+} transient in anterior region of guinea pig hearts. *Pacing Clin Electrophysiol* 1999;22:702. Abstract.
33. Fast VG, Ideker RE. Simultaneous optical mapping of transmembrane potential and intracellular calcium in myocyte cultures. *J Cardiovasc Electrophysiol* 2000;11:547–556.
34. Johnson PL, Smith W, Baynham TC, Knisley SB. Errors caused by combination of di-4 ANEPPS and fluo3/4 for simultaneous measurements of transmembrane potentials and intracellular calcium. *Ann Biomed Eng* 1999;27:563–571.
35. Laurita KR, Singal A, Pastore JM, Rosenbaum DS. Spatial heterogeneity of calcium transients may explain action potential dispersion during T-wave alternans. *Circulation* 1998;98(17):I187. Abstract.
36. Laurita KR, Singal A, Pastore JM, Rosenbaum DS. High-resolution optical mapping of intracellular calcium and transmembrane potential during reentry. *Pacing Clin Electrophysiol* 1999;22:II702.

Chapter 5

Optimization of Temporal Filtering for Optical Transmembrane Potential Signals

Francis X. Witkowski, Patricia A. Penkoske, and L. Joshua Leon

Introduction

Despite decades of study, our understanding of clinically important cardiac rhythm disturbances, such as ventricular and atrial fibrillation, is incomplete. A recent journal issue[1] highlights the state of the art in this understanding for ventricular fibrillation (VF). The measurement of cardiac transmembrane potential changes with voltage-sensitive dyes is in increasing experimental use and will, we believe, provide major new insights into these important clinical problems. On a broader scale, the entire arena of fluorescent probes has recently erupted, with such advances as the linking of the green fluorescent protein gene to other genes.[2] This enabling development, which produces a fluorescent product without the need for exogenous substrates or cofactors, has proven to be a catalyst for a revolution in molecular biology that allows the process of gene expression and protein localization to be followed optically in living cells.

Two basic approaches have been used to record optical signals from voltage-sensitive dyes: silicon photodiodes and imaging devices such as charged coupled device (CCD) video cameras, with the heart being illuminated and either continuously or spatially scanned. The largest commercially available silicon photodiode array is 16×16 (256 pixels—picture elements). The advantage of silicon photodiode detectors is their rapid response time, good (80%) quantum efficiency, and relatively low

Regretfully, Dr. Witkowski passed away shortly after he completed this chapter. We would therefore like to dedicate this chapter to the memory of Frank Witkowski, who, in addition to being a prolific contributor to our field, was a cherished friend and colleague. He will be missed.

The authors gratefully acknowledge support from MRC grants (FXW, PAP, LJL) and the Alberta Heritage Foundation for Medical Research (FXW).

From Rosenbaum DS, Jalife J (eds): *Optical Mapping of Cardiac Excitation and Arrhythmias.* ©Futura Publishing Co., Inc., Armonk, NY, 2001.

dark current (the amount of signal present even though no light is present). The quantum efficiency dictates how many electrons per second (current) will be generated for a given photon per second level of irradiation over the surface area of the device. Using voltage-sensitive dyes in the intact heart, it is possible to achieve signal-to-noise (S/N) ratios in excess of 30. The largest (one of a kind) fiberoptic bundle-oriented photodiode-based system was reported by Hamamatsu Photonics Research Lab and contained 2500 pixels (50 × 50), with 2500 discrete photodiodes with 12-bit analog-to-digital (A/D) conversion on each pixel.[3] Unfortunately, the temporal resolution desired to characterize the electrophysiological events of interest at the whole heart level is on the order of 1 ms, which corresponds to a frame rate of 1000 frames/s.

The state of the art in scanned laser illumination imaging has recently been described by Bove and Dillon,[4] who reported the details of a system capable of 100x100 scanned points at a frame rate of 200 frames per second with 600 frames of continuous storage capacity. Detection of the very small fluorescent alterations associated with voltage-sensitive dyes using large multiplexed arrays such as CCD cameras at high sampling rates has proved challenging. The use of CCD cameras to visualize cardiac electrophysiology was pioneered by Jalife and colleagues.[5-7] Their initial recordings had a temporal resolution of 16.7 ms dictated by a frame rate of 60 frames per second, 8-bit A/D dynamic range, and continuous recording capability of 2 seconds, and had a reported S/N ratio of approximately 1 before processing.[6] Until recently, the state of the art in high-frame-rate (one of a kind) nonimage-intensified CCD cameras was represented by the 540-frame-per-second, 12-bit, thinned and back-illuminated (improves quantum efficiency), low-read-noise (6.5 e$^-$ root mean square [rms]) system developed by the group (headed by the late F.S. Fay) at the University of Massachusetts in Worcester.[7]

We recently described the details of our approach to the design of an image-intensified fiberoptically coupled CCD camera system constructed from commercially available components that provided 128 × 128 pixels of spatial resolution, 12-bit A/D conversion, and a frame rate of 838 frames per second.[8] Preliminary results using this system to investigate VF have already presented some interesting observations.[9] We were able to show that in isolated perfused dog hearts, high spatial and temporal resolution optical transmembrane potential mapping could readily detect transiently erupting rotors during the early phase of VF. This activity was characterized by a relatively high spatiotemporal cross-correlation. During this early fibrillatory interval, frequent wave front collisions and wavebreak generation[5] were also dominant features. Interestingly, this spatiotemporal pattern was found to undergo an evolution to a less highly spatially correlated mechanism devoid of the epicardial manifestations of rotors, despite continued myocardial perfusion.[9]

The fundamental parameters that ultimately limit CCD performance are 1) read noise; 2) charge-transfer efficiency; 3) quantum efficiency; and 4) charge-collection efficiency.[10] The use of CCD arrays for imaging voltage-sensitive dyes in cardiac muscle has been limited by the level of signal to noise. This usually requires significant averaging to improve the S/N ratio. Voltage-sensitive dyes (such as di-4-ANEPPS, RH-421, RH-237, or WW781, all commercially available from Molecular Probes Inc., Eugene, OR) act as molecular transducers, converting the transmembrane potential into optical signals. When the dye senses the transmembrane potential alterations, the magnitude of the emitted fluorescence changes when it is stimulated by an appropriate stable source of photons. This fluorescent change can be an increase (e.g., WW781 excited at 632 nm) or a decrease (e.g., di-4-ANEPPS excited at 500 nm). The magnitude of this small fluorescence change that corresponds to the transmembrane potential alteration resides on a baseline fluorescence level, and is approximately 2% to 10% of the baseline level. The response time for the fast dyes presently in use is rapid, and their response is linear with respect to transmembrane potential. The ideal potentiometric probe would have little or no tendency to harm the preparation as the result of pharmacological or phototoxic side effects. The molecular mechanism of photodynamic damage is believed secondary to the generation of free radicals[11] and can lead to rapid death of the cell/tissue being studied if photon irradiance is not limited.[12] Indeed long-term optical recordings have been reported with illumination levels less than 100 mW/cm² for durations measured in hours, with essentially no deterioration in the optical signals recorded with a silicon photodiode.[13] Both laser (bandwidths of <1 nm) and broader sources (up to 80 nm full width at half maximum) have been successfully used for optical excitation.

We present in this chapter some of our observations on how the noisy signals as presented by CCD cameras might be optimally processed. In the real experimental world, all we have available is a noisy version of the biological signal of interest. We used modeling data of spiral wave reentry to provide a noise-free gold standard against which two signal processing approaches could be compared for their ability to recover the signal of interest from varying degrees of noise degradation. Boxcar averaging with averaging windows of variable length is compared with median filtering with windows of variable length.

Mathematical Model of Spiral Wave Reentry

The rectangular sheet model is a single layer of parallel and uniformly spaced identical excitable cables, transversely interconnected by a regular resistive network in the form of a brickwall pattern (Fig. 1). Each resistor, R_n, may be viewed as an average representation of a local transverse junction resistance between adjacent myocardial strands. The center-to-center intercable spacing is fixed at 166 μm, and the inter-resistor spacing (Δ) is 200 (Δ) is 200 μm.

The cable (radius = 5 μm) has an intracellular resistivity (r_i) of 400 Ω-cm. It is described by the well-known cable equation in which the membrane potential (V) varies with time (t) and distance (x). Its resting length constant is 598.6 μm, and its steady-state conduction velocity is 50 cm/s. The excitable membrane is represented by a modified Beeler-Reuter model,[14,15] with $C_m = 1$ μF/cm² as the membrane capacitance and $I_{ion} = I_{Na} + I_{Si} + I_K$ as the total membrane ionic current. The sodium current is $I_{Na} = g_{Na}m^3$ hj $(V - E_{Na})$, where g_{Na} is the maximum conductance, m the ac-

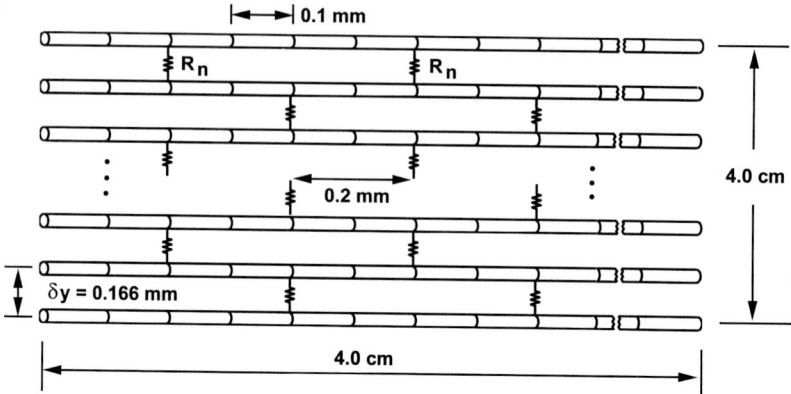

Figure 1. Diagram of the single layer model used to simulate 2-dimensional reentrant cardiac excitation. Preparation shows the arrangement of cables into fibers, with transverse regularly spaced resistive network (R_n) in the form of a brickwall pattern. Center-to-center intercable spacing is fixed at 166 μm, and the inter-resistor spacing is 200 μm as shown. See text for further details of model.

tivation variable, h and j the inactivation variables, and E_{Na} the reversal potential. The secondary inward current is $I_{si} = g_{si}df(V-E_{si})$, where g_{si} is the maximum conductance, d the activation variable, f the inactivation variable, and E_{si} the reversal potential. As in our previous studies of 2-dimensional reentry,[16,17] we divided the time constants of I_{si} by K = 4 in order to reduce the action potential duration and lessen the requirements on the overall sheet size. The total potassium current, $I_K = I_{x1} + I_{K1}$, includes a delayed component (I_{x1}) with an activation variable x1, and a time-independent component I_{K1}.[17]

Because of the parallel-cable arrangement of the sheet, the longitudinal flat wave conduction velocity (θ_L) is equal to that of an isolated cable. Current flow in the transverse direction is governed by R_n, r_i, and Δ. The transverse flat wave conduction velocity (θ_T) was varied by changing R_n, keeping r_i and Δ constant. The sheet anisotropy ratio (AR) is defined as AR = θ_L/θ_T. The sheet parameters are as follows: length = 4.0 cm, width = 4.0 cm, R_n = 1.0 MΩ, θ_L = 50 cm/s, θ_T = 29 cm/s, and AR = 1.6.

On a given cable of the sheet, the resting length constant of 598 μm and δx of 100 μm allow us to calculate a longitudinal discretization factor of 100/598.6 = 0.167. The cable is then equivalent to a uniform network in which equal segments (membrane area of 3.14×10^{-5} cm²) are joined by resistors of 5.2 MΩ. The spatial accuracy is sufficient to avoid significant numerical errors while keeping the computation time within reasonable limits.[18] For transverse plane wave propagation, the sheet can be assimilated to a discontinuous cable[15] with periodically varying radius and junction resistance.

Numerical solutions were obtained using a previously described computing technique.[15] Propagation on any given cable of the sheet is taken to be governed by the standard cable equation, and at each time instant its potential distribution is first calculated assuming that the cables are completely isolated from one another. Then a perturbation is added to account for current flow between adjacent cables. Programs were written in FOR-TRAN and run on a Silicon Graphics 12-processor Challenge computer.

Results and Discussion

With use of the modeling approach outlined above, reentry was initiated by a variation of the cross-shock protocol, first postulated in theory by Winfree.[19] A transverse plane wave was first generated by a conditioning stimulus S1 (1 ms in duration, 1.5 × diastolic threshold) applied along the upper longitudinal edge of the sheet, followed by a premature stimulus S_2 (1 ms in duration, 1.5 × diastolic threshold) applied uniformly over one quarter of the sheet surface (Fig. 2). The time interval between S_1 and

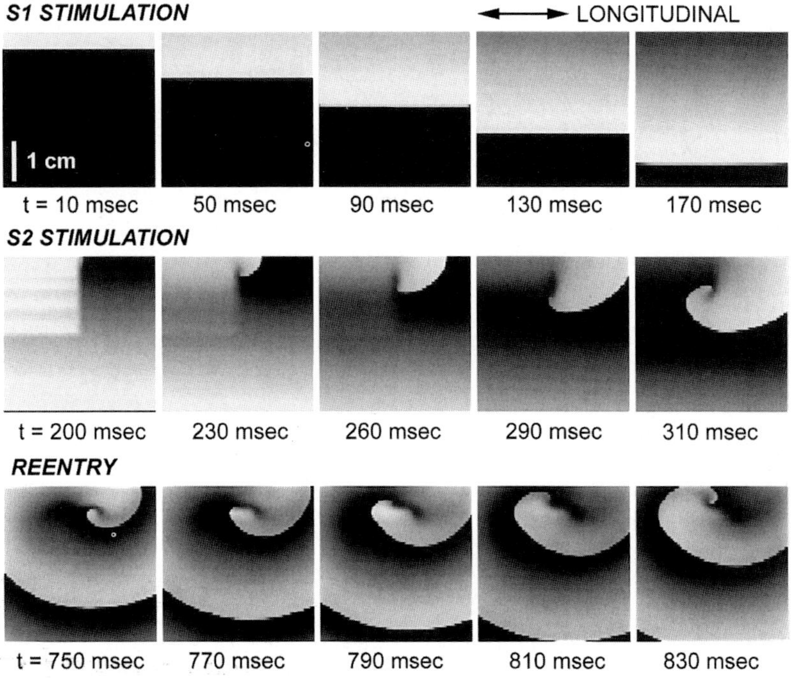

Figure 2. Map of the spatial distribution of simulated transmembrane potentials using the model described in Fig. 1. Image resolution is 128 × 128 pixels. Black encodes for fully repolarized potentials and white indicates fully depolarized transmembrane potentials. Selected frames at varying interframe intervals were chosen to convey the signals of interest. The beginning of the simulation occurred at time = 0 ms, and times are measured relative to that reference. The top five frames (S1 stimulation) depict the initial downwardly propagating wave front of activation that was launched to propagate in the transverse fiber direction with a linear wave front morphology. The middle five frames (S2 stimulation) indicate that the left upper quadrant of the model was stimulated beyond threshold during the inhomogeneous repolarization that succeeded the S1 activation wave front and resulted in the initiation of a reentrant activation wave front. The bottom five frames (Reentry) depict 80 ms of the spiral wave reentry after a few cycles had elapsed. These five frames will form the basis for comparison for Fig. 5.

S_2 was chosen such that some excitability recovery existed near the upper longitudinal edge of the sheet.

The time series of the transmembrane potential from a single site of the sheet after the induction of stable reentrant spiral wave activity was initiated was then normalized to a peak-to-peak value of 1 and a mean value of 0 (Fig. 3). This noise-free signal would be used as the gold standard for all subsequent data analysis procedures. Randomly generated noise with a Gaussian distribution and a mean value of 0 and a standard deviation of 1 (Fig. 3) was then added to the noise-free normalized transmembrane potential data in varying amounts to simulate the range of S/N values reported in the literature for optical transmembrane potential recordings (Fig. 4). We define S/N as the peak-to-peak noise-free signal (in our case this has been normalized to a value of 1.0) divided by the rms value of the noise. The rms value is very nearly equal to the standard deviation for large values of data points. The statistic used to calculate the error in the noisy signal is the sum of the squared differences between each

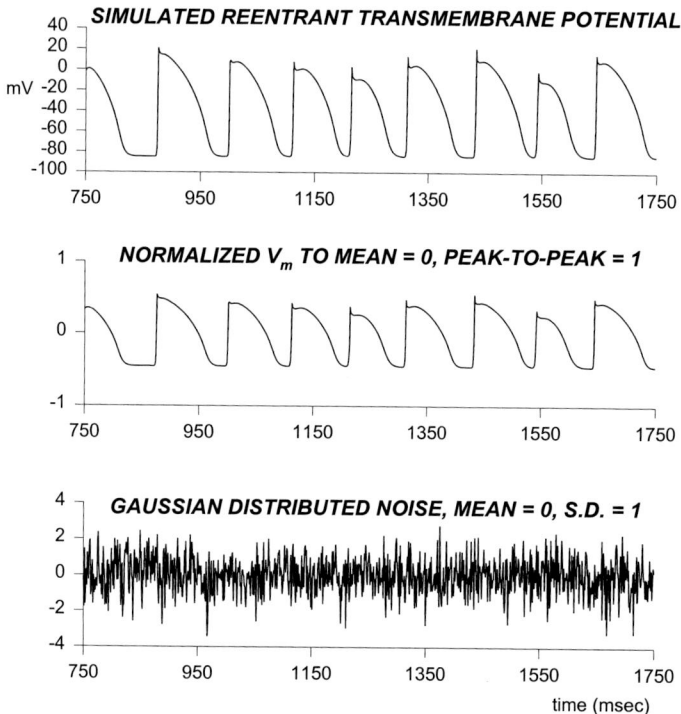

Figure 3. One second (1-ms temporal resolution) of a transmembrane potential time series (*top panel*) from a single site of the 128 × 128 pixels of simulated anisotropic tissue after spiral wave reentry was initiated demonstrating the expected irregular timing associated with meandering reentrant spiral waves. The middle panel is the same noise-free time series as just described but depicted with amplitude adjusted to yield a peak-to-peak value of 1 and a 0 mean value. The bottom panel is the white noise that will be added in varying amounts to achieve the desired signal-to-noise (S/N) ratios for our subsequent analyses. Our definition of S/N is the peak-to-peak value of the signal of interest divided by the root mean squared value of the noise.

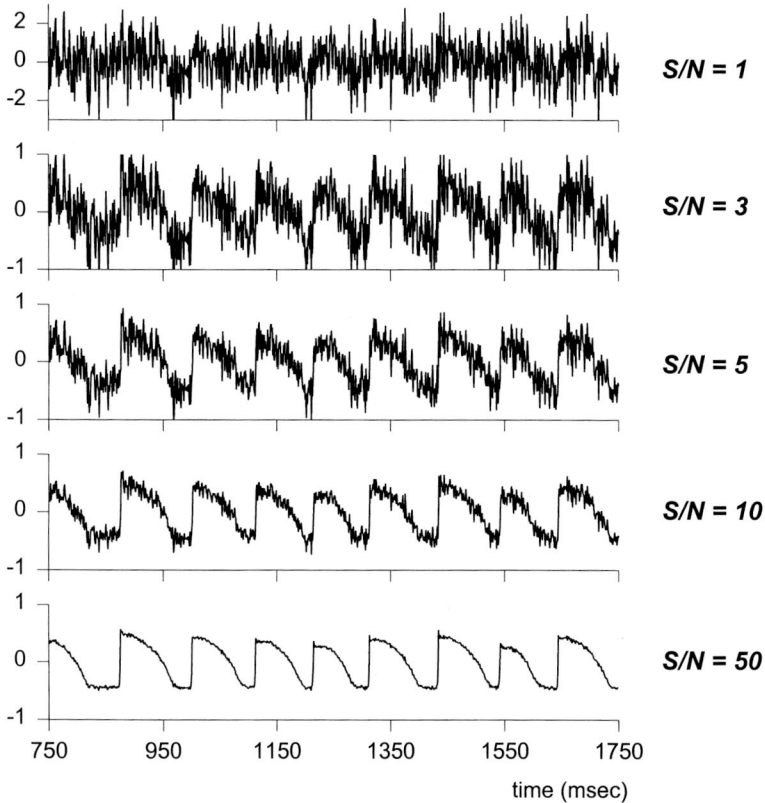

Figure 4. The noise-free time series of action potentials from Fig. 3 with varying amounts of additive white noise to achieve the five different signal-to-noise (S/N) ratios depicted. Note at the S/N = 1 that the y-axis has a different scale than the remainder of the time series. It is virtually impossible to visualize the original transmembrane potential waveform at an S/N = 1 when only the time series from a single site is available for inspection.

of the data points in the noise-free signal and the signal for comparison. The division by the number of data points, which would then be the mean squared error, was eliminated to provide error values greater than unity. The sum squared error for the noise-free signal is obviously 0. Data points from 800 to 1700 in the time series were used in the error calculations to avoid the boundary effects of the filtering schemes used.

An attempt to "see" the action potential waveforms shown in Figure 4 at an S/N = 1 readily demonstrates the difficulty presented by such low levels of signal. It has been stated in the neurophysiological literature that indeed an S/N ratio must be approximately equal to 3 (or larger) to observe a spike reliably in a single optical record.[13] Of interest, when the spatial information content from the entire 128 × 128 simulation sites is included, a hint of the spiral wave can still be seen even at S/N = 1 (Fig. 5).

The effect of boxcar averaging at three different S/N ratios is shown in Figures 6 through 8. Boxcar averaging simply replaces the value at a time

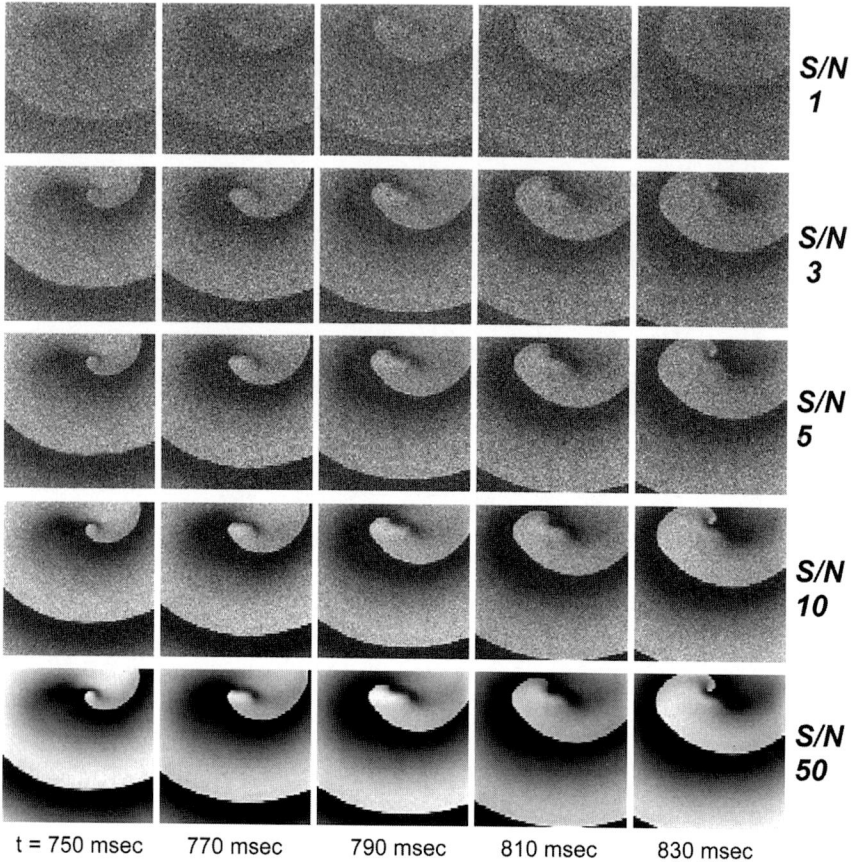

Figure 5. The same five panels of reentrant simulated activation as shown in Fig.2 with varying amounts of signal degradation. The signal-to-noise (S/N) ratios given refer to the values at each of the pixels. All pixels were assigned identical values of S/N. Note that with the additional information content presented by the 16,384 pixels of information (128 × 128), at the S/N = 1 the reentrant spiral wave is barely discernible when these five frames are viewed sequentially.

with the ensemble average over a time range that includes the point of interest. We have used boxcar lengths that symmetrically encompass the point of interest, and hence the minimal boxcar length is 3. The reduction in the squared error term as a function of boxcar averaging is presented as a percentage to allow comparison between quite disparate S/N ratios. The minimal error boxcar averaging for the S/N = 3 signal was found at a boxcar length of 15 (Fig. 6). The progressive lengthening of the boxcar resulted in further attenuation of the fast rise time components of the filtered signal, and resulted in a smoother signal but one that deviated further from the noise-free baseline. Interestingly, the boxcar length at which this minimum occurred was a function of the amount of noise present. For an S/N = 5 (Fig. 7), the minimum now was found at a boxcar length of 9. Interestingly, for the worst case scenario of S/N = 1 (Fig. 8), the error was found

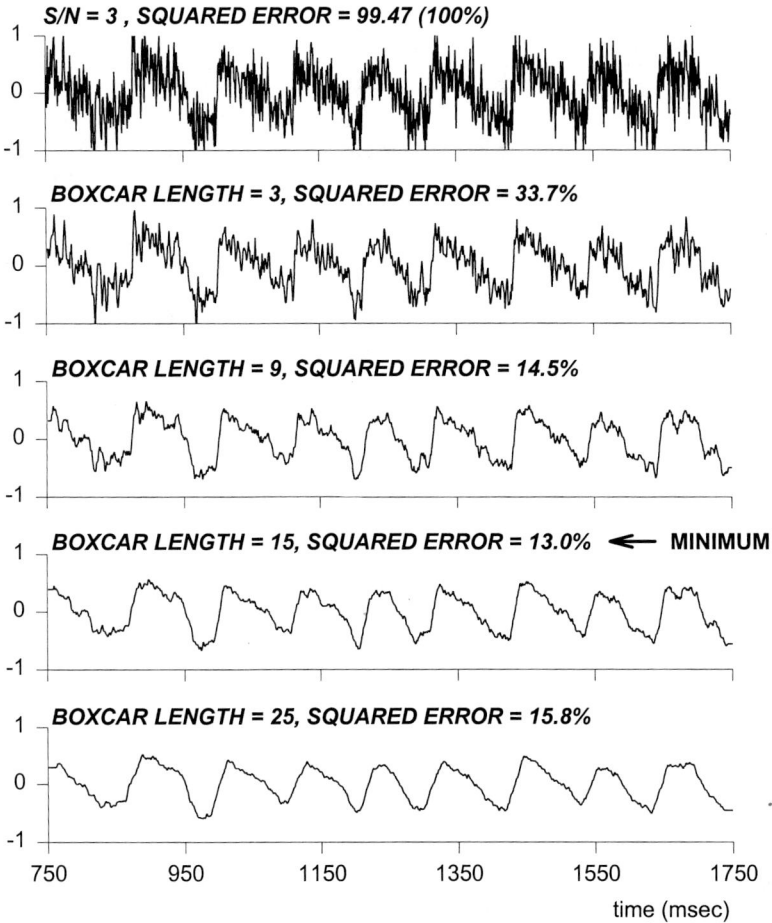

Figure 6. Effect of varying lengths of boxcar averaging on the cumulative squared error for the time series degraded with additive noise to a signal-to-noise (S/N) ratio of 3. The noise-free signal is identical to the one provided in Fig. 3. The overall value of the error for this noisy signal was 99.47, which was considered the 100% mark against which the effects of filtering were expressed as a percentage. Note that at a boxcar length of 15, a minimal squared error was obtained.

to monotonically decrease with no obvious minimal value observed. A summary for all boxcar lengths for four different S/N ratios is given in Figure 9, and clearly demonstrates that a minimal degree of smoothing is highly desirable if one has the luxury of dealing with S/N ratios in excess of 10. For experimentally derived signals, however, we do not have the luxury of knowing the S/N at each pixel of a CCD imaging a heart stained with a voltage-sensitive chromophore. Additionally, the S/N may vary from site to site in the same preparation due to inhomogeneities of dye loading, illumination levels, etc.

Median filtering does not shift edges for signals such as are depicted in Figure 3 which consist of vertical transitions to plateau levels that are

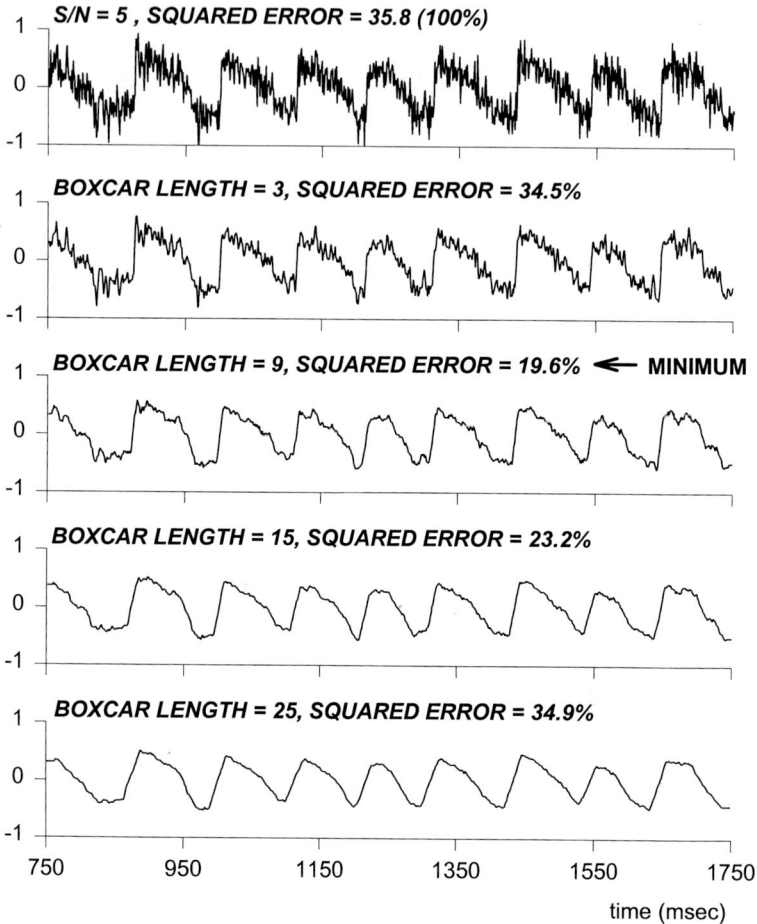

Figure 7. Waveforms similar to those in Fig. 6 with the initial signal for processing degraded to a signal-to-noise (S/N) ratio of 5. Note that the overall value of the computed error is now less than that found in Fig. 6 at S/N = 3, but now the minimal error was obtained at a slightly different boxcar length.

then maintained for several time instants. Median filtering will not reduce the level of such transitions because the values available are only those present in the neighborhood region, not an average between those values.[20] Longer filter lengths produce less degradation of the rapidly rising leading edge of an action potential as compared with boxcar averaging filtering. The effect on signal appearance as well as squared error is shown in Figure 10 for the same S/N = 3 signal shown in Figure 6. For the four median filter lengths provided in this figure, the error is seen to flatten out rather than to provide a clear minimal value as was observed for the boxcar filter. Additionally, the gradual flattening of the action potential rise time is not observed as was apparent with boxcar averaging. Figure 11 is a summary diagram for the dependence of error on median filter length. Now note that for all four S/N ratios examined, a filter length of approxi-

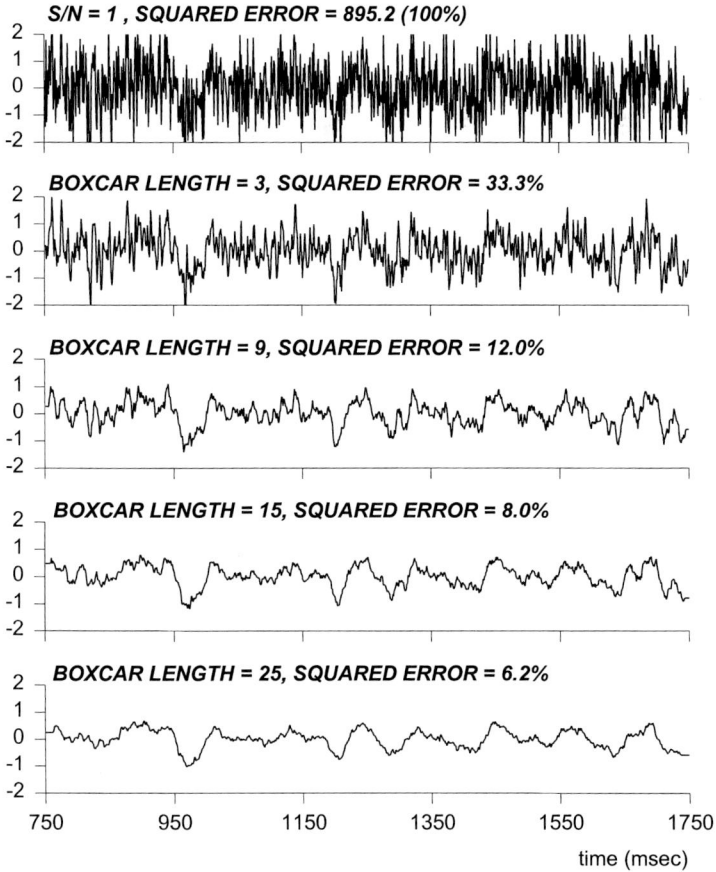

Figure 8. Waveforms similar to those in Fig. 6 but now degraded to a signal-to-noise ratio of 1.0. Note that now no minimal error value is readily observed at the four boxcar averaging lengths depicted.

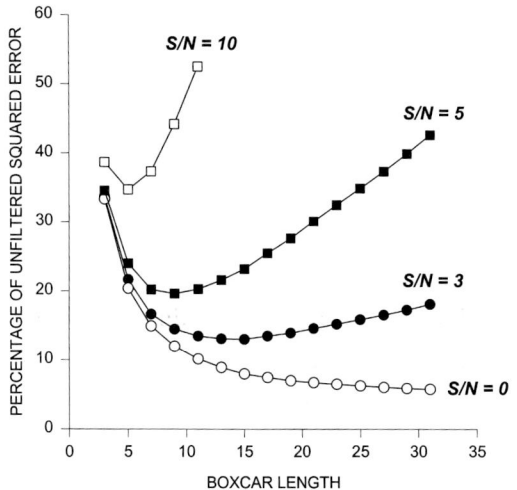

Figure 9. Summary diagram of percentages in cumulative squared error referenced to the unfiltered error term as a function of boxcar length for boxcar lengths from 3 to 31 for four different levels of signal degradation. Note that for signals with signal-to-noise (S/N) ratios in excess of 5, certain boxcar lengths can yield errors that exceed the minimally filtered signals.

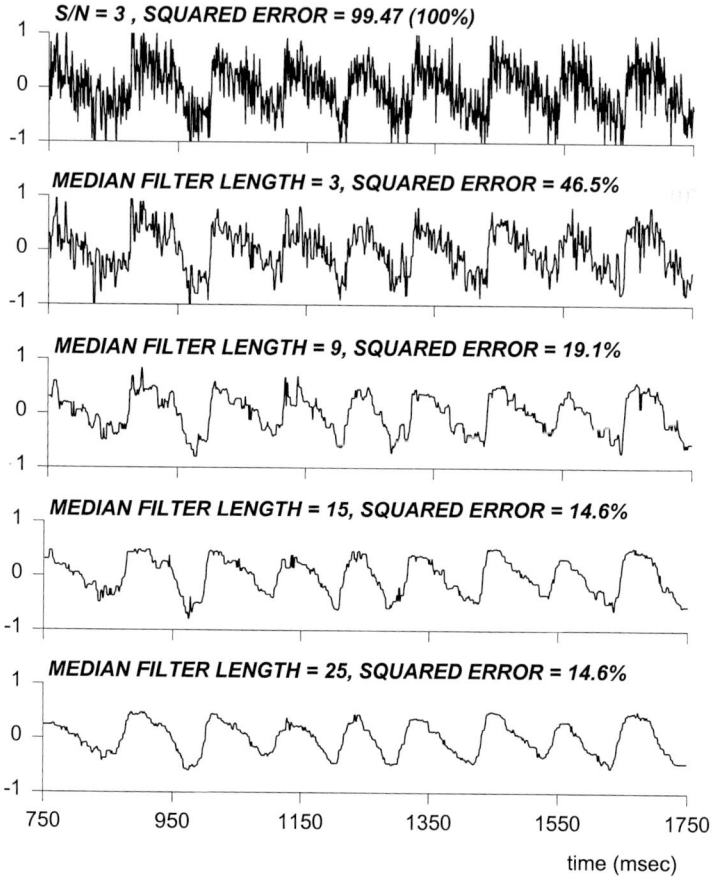

Figure 10. Waveforms similar to those in Fig. 6, with the same initial signal for processing degraded to a signal-to-noise ratio of 3 but now demonstrating the effects of varying lengths of median filtering.

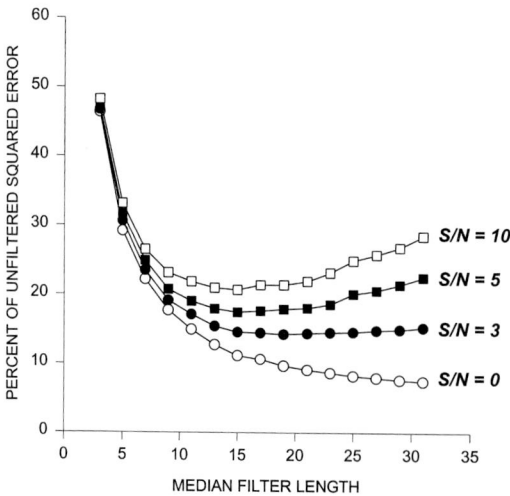

Figure 11. Summary diagram similar to that in Fig. 9 for median filter lengths from 3 to 31 for four different levels of signal degradation. Note that the minimal values occur over a broader range of filter lengths compared with the data presented in Fig. 9, and provide lower error values for signal-to-noise (S/N) ratios in excess of 5.

mately 21 provides a reasonable choice due to the extended and flattened minimal zone provided by median filtering as compared with boxcar averaging approaches.

Ideally, one attempts to improve the S/N ratio of experimentally derived data at the very first stage of data acquisition. This is true whether one is dealing with analog signals or CCD images. Hopefully tomorrow's CCD technology will provide S/N ratios of 50 from 20,000 sites at temporal resolutions faster than 1 ms for whole heart recordings, and at 20,000 frames per second for single cell examinations. It would be wonderful if voltage-sensitive dyes could be found that produced changes in fluorescence comparable in magnitude to those obtained with calcium-sensitive dyes. If this could be achieved, the choice of filtering would be more of academic interest than practical necessity. In the meantime, to attempt to optimally process the data from today's instruments, approaches such as the one we present have proven useful to interpret the electrophysiological complexity of rhythm disturbances such as VF.

References

1. Focus issue: Fibrillation in normal ventricular myocardium. Guest Editor: Winfree AT. *Chaos* 1998;8(1):1–241.
2. Chalfie M, Tu Y, Euskirchen G, et al. Green fluorescent protein as a marker for gene expression. *Science* 1994;263:802–805.
3. Takahashi M, Tsuchiya H, Hosoi S, et al. Development of 50x50 fiber-array photodiode camera. *SPIE* 1992;1757:111–114.
4. Bove RT, Dillon SM. Optically imaging cardiac activation with a laser system. *IEEE Eng Med Biol* 1998;Jan/Feb:84–94.
5. Pertsov AM, Davidenko JM, Salomonsz R, et al. Spiral waves of excitation underlie reentrant activity in isolated cardiac muscle. *Circ Res* 1993;72:631–650.
6. Baxter WT, Davidenko JM, Loew LM, et al. Technical features of a CCD video camera system to record cardiac fluorescence data. *Ann Biomed Eng* 1997;25:713–725.
7. Tuft RA, Bowman DS, Carrington WA, et al. High speed digital imaging microscopy with continuous focus scanning. *Biophys J* 1997;72(2):A215.
8. Witkowski FX, Leon LJ, Penkoske PA, et al. A method for visualization of ventricular fibrillation: Design of a cooled fiberoptically coupled image intensified CCD data acquisition system incorporating wavelet shrinkage based adaptive filtering. *Chaos* 1998;8(1):94–102.
9. Witkowski FX, Leon LJ, Penkoske PA, et al. Spatiotemporal evolution of ventricular fibrillation. *Nature* 1998;392:78–82.
10. Janesick JR, Klassen KP, Elliott T. Charge-coupled-device charge-collection efficiency and the photon-transfer technique. *Optical Eng* 1987;26(10):972–980.
11. Parsons TD, Kleinfeld D, Raccuia-Behling F, et al. Optical recording of the electrical activity of synaptically interacting Aplysia neurons in culture using potentiometric probes. *Biophys J* 1989;56:213–221.
12. Schaffer P, Ahammer H, Muller W, et al. Di-4-ANEPPS causes photodynamic damage to isolated cardiomyocytes. *Pflugers Arch* 1994;426:548–551.
13. Parsons TD, Salzberg BM, Obaid AL, et al. Long-term optical recording of patterns of electrical activity in ensembles of cultured Aplysia neurons. *J Neurophys* 1991;66(10):316–333.
14. Beeler GW, Reuter H. Reconstruction of the action potential of ventricular myocardial fibers. *J Physiol* 1977;268:177–210.
15. Drouhard JP, Roberge FA. Revised formulation of the Hodgkin-Huxley repre-

sentation of the sodium current in cardiac cells. *Comp Biomed Res* 1987;20:333–350.

16. Leon LJ, Roberge FA. Structural complexity effects on transverse propagation in a two-dimensional model of myocardium. *IEEE Trans Biomed Eng* 1991;38:997–1009.

17. Leon LJ, Roberge FA, Vinet A. Simulation of two-dimensional anisotropic cardiac reentry: Effects of the wavelength on the reentry characteristics. *Ann Biomed Eng* 1994;22:592–609.

18. Roberge FA, Vinet A, Victorri B. Reconstruction of propagated electrical activity with a two dimensional model of anisotropic heart muscle. *Circ Res* 1986;58:461–475.

19. Winfree AT. Electrical instability in cardiac muscle: Phase singularities and rotors. *J Theor Biol* 1989;138:353–405.

20. Russ JC. *The Imaging Processing Handbook.* 2nd ed. New York: CRC Press; 1994:166.

Section II

Microscopic Propagation

Introduction:

Unique Role of Optical Mapping in the Study of Propagation and Repolarization

David S. Rosenbaum

Multisite electrophysiological mapping is a powerful tool for investigating arrhythmia mechanisms in experimental animals and for guiding therapy for patients. Although mapping systems vary considerably in design and implementation, the principles underlying electrical mapping of the heart are quite similar. The basic premise is that one can record electrical activity either simultaneously or sequentially from multiple focal sites on the heart's surface. Typically, a local activation time is estimated from an extracellular electrogram recorded from each electrode recording site. Subsequently, a series of activation times (i.e., time domain) are then mapped onto the location of each electrode in space (i.e., space domain), and these two fundamental pieces of information are used to construct activation maps. Most often, activation maps are plotted as isochrone or contour plots. Such plots can be used to depict propagating waves underlying normal and abnormal cardiac rhythms.

The advent of optical mapping has provided the opportunity to overcome several of the limitations inherent to extracellular mapping. Optical cardiac mapping provides an additional dimension that is not attainable by conventional mapping techniques: i.e., the voltage domain. In optical mapping, the time course of membrane potential is registered at every recording site. Therefore, it is possible to relate complex propagation patterns to voltage changes occurring at the level of individual cells. This has many important implications. For instance, the timing of local propagation can be determined directly from the upstroke of the cardiac action potential, eliminating nearly all ambiguity in estimating local activation time. Also, the amplitude of local responses can be related in a meaningful way to biophysical principles that underlie impulse propagation in the heart. Finally, because optical mapping is an imaging modality, it obviates the need for physical electrodes, thereby permitting essentially limitless spatial resolution.

This section of the book reviews some of the innovative approaches investigators have used to exploit the unique capabilities of optical mapping to reveal novel mechanisms of impulse propagation in the heart. In chapters 6 and 7, Windisch, Rohr, and Kucera review the special considerations involved in designing an optical recording system used to measure propagation on a microscopic scale. They demonstrate how one can use the optically coupled recording to achieve resolution of membrane potential on the cellular and subcellular level. An elegant application of such techniques to uncover fundamental processes governing propagation in multicellular tissue is discussed in chapter 8, which is by Kleber, Rohr, and Fast. In chapter 9 Mazgalev and Efimov, and in chapter 10 Salama and Choi, discuss how optical mapping has also created new frontiers for investigating physiology of very small but important structures such as the atrioventricular node. Finally, in chapter 11 Waldo reviews practical and clinical applications of these recent innovations.

Chapter 6

Optical Mapping of Impulse Propagation within Cardiomyocytes

Herbert Windisch

Propagation Phenomena

The functioning heart depends on the generation and proper distribution of the cardiac impulse, which provides, beat by beat, the synchronized activity of the whole organ. The spread of excitation takes place in the syncytium, which is formed by electrically connected myocytes with various degrees of coupling. Each individual cell receives and provides electrical currents and keeps the cardiac impulse propagating. Intracellular propagation depends strongly on the tissue structure and on the power and direction of the excitation wave as it approaches the cell, as a distinct electrical event in space and time.[1,2] By means of the gap junctions between cells, electrical sources and loads develop and the active ionic membrane currents contribute to the discharge of the membrane and to local currents, which spread out and continue the excitation wave. In close relationship with the tissue structure and with the direction and power of the excitation wave, the speed of propagation varies wildly in ventricular tissue from approximately 0.1 to 1 m/s. These values are mean values that include the propagation within the cell as well as the delays at the gap junctions. In tightly coupled cablelike structures in a longitudinal direction, the wave propagates smoothly with a quite uniform velocity. The same structure, when carrying a wave in a transverse direction, may yield a very different appearance of excitation: despite a decreased mean velocity, the intracellular propagation is faster, but at the gap junctions prominent delays will occur, hence slowing down the movement of the wave.[3] In the case of a weak connection to the neighbors, due to intercellular uncoupling the whole cell may depolarize highly synchronized within a few microseconds. This resembles an isolated cell that has been stimulated by a current pulse applied via a patch electrode: there is no longer a propagating active wave but the applied current spreads out all over the cell and

This work was supported by the Austrian Science Research Fund, grant no. 6829-Med, 8729-Med, and 12294-Med.
From Rosenbaum DS, Jalife J (eds): *Optical Mapping of Cardiac Excitation and Arrhythmias.* ©Futura Publishing Co., Inc., Armonk, NY, 2001.

depolarizes the membrane. If the rising phase occurs simultaneously within the cell, the speed of "propagation"—indeed a phase velocity—would appear to be infinity. An isolated cell has a length distinctly below the membrane length constant (approximately 100 μm compared with approximately 500 μm),[4] and is thus too small to provide a structure for an active cablelike propagation that is based on local currents. In addition, the time constant (which is responsible for equalizing membrane charges within the isolated cell) is in the order of microseconds and is thus much shorter than the development of ionic currents, which takes at least some 100 μs.[5] Even a most inhomogeneous spatial distribution of membrane currents (as it occurs during field stimulation) thus leads to highly synchronized changes of the cellular membrane potential.

To summarize: intracellular propagation can appear smooth and homogeneous with velocities typical for ventricular tissue in the range of approximately 0.1 to 1 m/s. In contrast, it can also appear as a membrane discharge event, discontinuous in nature, showing intracellular phase velocities that may appear to reach infinity.

How Can We Monitor Intracellular Propagation?

Measuring intracellular propagation, of course, requires a measuring system with a spatial resolution distinctly below the size of a single cell, offering at least some points of measurement within the cell. The required temporal resolution (i.e., the ability to detect time delays between characteristic electrical events, e.g., rising phases in different membrane areas) depends on the experimental condition. Based on the idea of a continuous propagation, the required temporal resolution needed is inverse to the size of the object under study. Considering a particular cell with 100-μm length and a velocity of 0.5 m/s, it will take the cardiac impulse 200 μs to travel through the cell. However, as structure-related discontinuities come into play, or even if the cell is isolated, intracellular electrical events may occur highly synchronized (within some microseconds), which would require a much higher temporal resolution. To meet all conditions, it is desirable to have a temporal resolution in the microsecond range.

At present, various methods are used to study propagation phenomena: extracellular electrodes and electrode arrays, magnetic field detection, intracellular microelectrodes and patch electrodes, and optical techniques.

Extracellular electrodes measure voltage drops along the path of extracellular currents, and thus allow for the monitoring of propagating active waves in tissues. This technique, most often used in large-scale objects such as the whole heart, with properly designed electrodes, is also capable of monitoring excitation events at a microscopic scale.[6] However, though electrode arrays with subcellular distances between the electrodes can be manufactured,[7] the signals are related to the sum of extracellular currents rather than to a particular one. In addition, ionic currents that discharge a cell membrane without spreading out (as is the case when a cell fires a synchronized action potential) are hidden by this technique. These facts, in addition to the technical problems that arise with extremely small sized electrodes, pose a severe limitation in the measurement of intracellular propagation.

Magnetic field detection is based on capturing the field of current loops that are related to the propagation process. This technique can yield interesting results in whole heart measurements, but seems, especially because of the lack of a proper spatial resolution, inappropriate.

In contrast to extracellular current measurements, microelectrodes and patch electrodes allow the measurement of the membrane voltage (to be more precise, the voltage between the impaled or attached tip of the electrode and a reference electrode somewhere). This technique, which is very useful in gaining absolute values of the membrane potential, is severely hampered by the fact that it is nearly impossible to apply more than two electrodes within a single cell. In addition, the electrodes themselves may disturb the measurement, especially if extracellular electrical fields are present. In this latter case, as an additional problem, severe interferences of the electrical field with the measurement circuit may lead to erroneous signals.

Of the methods mentioned above, optical mapping is the only one that can, at least in principle, fulfill all requirements for measuring intracellular propagation: the spatial resolution, depending on the detector size and the magnification of the microscope, can lead to spot sizes distinctly below the size of a single cell; several (or even many) measuring spots can be applied to a single cell, and the temporal resolution can approach the microsecond region.[8–10] Of course this method also has its limitations: only relative changes of the membrane potential—rather than absolute values—can be obtained, dye bleaching may cause baseline drifts in isolated cells or in cells grown in tissue culture, which must be considered, and phototoxic effects limit the total exposure of the preparation. Additionally, compared with electrically gained signals, the signal-to-noise (S/N) ratio is usually diminished. However, the possibility of obtaining many membrane-potential-related signals within one particular cardiomyocyte simultaneously makes this method unique.

Propagation at the Level of the Single Cell

When we discuss scientific questions related to intracellular propagation, we have to discern two major experimental situations: 1) the cardiomyocyte being part of the tissue, and 2) the isolated ventricular cell. This chapter focuses on the isolated cardiomyocyte, which is widely used in basic cardiac electrophysiology. There are three common experimental conditions: the current-clamped cell, the voltage-clamped cell, and the field-stimulated cell. Whole cell current- and voltage-clamping is mostly performed with sealed patch electrodes. The electrically insulated membrane patch within the mouth of the electrode is disrupted and thus allows the application of currents via the electrode or the measurement of the membrane potential. If current pulses are applied, action potentials can be elicited; if the voltage is controlled, currents can be measured. However, the current spreads throughout the whole cell and interacts with all parts of the membrane, which we can pick up with the same electrode, and consequently represents the resultant of all currents located in different areas of the cell membrane. The isolated cell is an electrically tightly coupled system, and the question is, to what extent are the membrane responses from different areas synchronized? This is also a crucial question when an attempt is made to control the membrane potential in a voltage-clamp experiment. In addition to the question of the synchronization of membrane activities, it is most important to know the quality of the clamp procedure, i.e., to reveal deviations between the wanted and the real membrane voltage. In field stimulation experiments, the cell is treated with extracellular electrical fields; different parts of the membrane are exposed to different voltages and the particular membrane currents contribute to a common response of the whole cell.[11] This complex situation is related to stimulation and defibrillation problems and is by far not yet fully understood.

Staining Procedure

Before going into the details of our set-up, some basic methodical aspects should be stressed. As mentioned above, optical potential measurements are based on dye molecules, which, when bound to cell membranes, change their optical properties depending on changes of the voltage across the membrane (i.e., the membrane potential). Letting them work as a molecular sensor, it is necessary to monitor these voltage-dependent properties. Usually this is done by measuring light absorption or fluorescence; correspondingly, we discern two types of dyes: absorption dyes and fluorescent dyes. In our preparation (guinea pig ventricular cardiomyocytes), the response of an absorption dye (NK2761) to a change of the membrane potential was only approximately 0.02% per 100 mV. In contrast, the fluorescent dye di-4-ANEPPS changed its fluorescence light intensity by more than 8% at the same voltage change.[8] With the absorption measurements, as compared with the fluorescence technique, easily a higher light intensity at the detector can be achieved which, per se, improves the S/N ratio; however, if the difference of the two percentage changes is as high as mentioned above, the S/N ratio obtained with the fluorescence method is by far better. For that reason, in our experiments we used the fluorescence method, usually with the styryl dye di-4-ANEPPS. The similar dye di-8-ANEPPS led to similar results; depending on the specimen, a comparative usage of these (and other) dyes may be advantageous.[9,10]

Optically obtained signals reflect only changes of the membrane potential and no absolute values. In addition, bleaching effects may cause signal drifts that cannot easily be distinguished from membrane potential changes. These problems, inherent to the optical method, are discussed later in the chapter. The most severe problem, however, is phototoxic side effects. In contrast to cardiac tissue, isolated cardiac cells after staining with a potential sensitive dye show pronounced phototoxicity when high light intensities are used during measurement: action potentials show prolongation, early afterdepolarizations occur, and finally the cell can be damaged, showing shrinking and hypercontracture.[12] To reduce these effects, the total exposure of a stained cell (i.e., light intensity, exposure time of a recording, the number of records, and the staining itself) should be minimized. The light intensity, on the other hand, is a main factor in determining the signal quality. In any case, the number of records obtained from a particular cell is limited by the total exposure. For example, isolated guinea pig ventricular cardiomyocytes, stained with the di-4-ANEPPS (6 to 12 μmol/L, 10 min), in our experiments allowed a total exposure of approximately 500 ms (light intensity about 200 W/cm^2). With a 40-ms exposure in each record we were sometimes able to take more than 10 recordings from a particular cell.[8] As has been shown by Schaffer and colleagues,[12] the relatively weak light from the microscope lamp (approximately 1 W/cm^2) was also sufficient to produce phototoxic effects. Consequently, in all experiments with stained cells, not only the light exposure during measurements, but also all other necessary exposures, e.g., during experimental manipulations or imaging, should be minimized. Based on the idea that primarily the light absorbed by the bound dye must be avoided, in our experiments we use only red light (the bound dye di-4-ANEPPS absorbs light in the blue-green region). When choosing a dye for a particular specimen, not only its sensitivity to membrane potential changes, but also phototoxic side effects should be considered.[10]

Cardiac cells, when stimulated, contract; this may disturb the optical measurement due to a mechanical movement. If only the rising phase of an action potential or a short time after stimulation is of interest, due to the electromechanical coupling latency of approximately 20 ms, these measurements will be undisturbed. In experiments in combination with patch electrodes, the presence of ethyleneglycoltetracetic acid in the pipette solution avoids mechanical movements. For other experiments the contraction can be suppressed by drugs.[13,14]

The Measuring System

Our measuring system (Fig. 1)[8] is primarily designed to work with voltage-sensitive fluorescent dyes. It is based on an inverted fluorescence microscope and uses a frequency-doubled continuous wave Neodymium-YAG laser as excitation light source (532 nm, 100 mW). The detector unit consists of a 10×10 photodiode array (PDA) that is connected to 100 individual amplifiers. The array and the amplifiers are situated in a common housing and are battery powered to minimize power line interferences. Data are stored in a 2-step procedure: the first step occurs in a 24-channel transient recorder with up to 200,000 samples per second in parallel (12 bit). With the use of plugs, up to 24 signals can be selected from the 100 photodiodes and stored simultaneously, or, alternatively, the whole array of signals can be stored in the same transient recorder by means of a multiplexing unit. The second step is the transfer of the data to a computer (IEEE-bus) for disk storage and data evaluation.

Of course the realization of such an experimental set-up depends not only on the requirements, but also (and mainly) on the technique available at the time. It may be less expensive—and perhaps better—to use a data acquisition board combined with a personal computer rather than an expensive transient recorder. Another type of detector and/or another light source may be used. However, a few rules must be taken into account:

1. The detector should have a high quantum efficiency (i.e., provide a maximal use of the available light), it must be able to handle a high dynamic range (the interesting part of the signal is

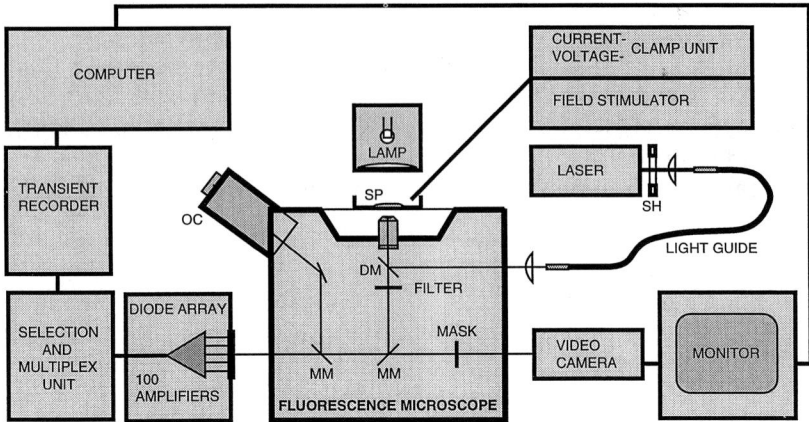

Figure 1. Schematic drawing of the set-up. The set-up is built around a conventional inverted fluorescence microscope. The light of a frequency-doubled Neodymium-Yag laser (100 mW, 532 nm), after passing a electromechanical shutter (SH) and guided by a light guide, enters the microscope and is reflected onto the specimen by a dichroic mirror (DM). The fluorescence light, emerging from the stained specimen (SP), passes through the dichroic mirror, then afterward a filter, and is then projected onto the 10 × 10 PDA which is followed by 100 individual current-to-voltage amplifiers. The selection and multiplexing unit allows to select up to 24 signals from 100 available, by using plugs. Alternatively, with use of multiplexing, all channels could be used. The signals are stored simultaneously in a fast 24-channel transient recorder with a sample rate of up to 200 kHz, 12 bit. For further storage and evaluation, data are stored on a computer via an IEEE data connection. Movable mirrors (MM) within the microscope allow the image to be seen through the ocular (OC), or to be projected to a video camera. In the optical path to the video camera a drawing of the diode matrix (mask) allows positioning of the specimen. In addition, the microscope allows photography of the image using a 35-mm camera (not shown). Depending on the experiment, a patch-clamp amplifier is used (current- and voltage-clamp experiments), or a current pulse generator for field stimulation.

only about 10% in amplitude of the total signal), and it should produce as little noise as possible.

2. The inverted fluorescence microscope must allow the projection of a sharp image onto the detector and guide the excitation light from an adequate light source (e.g., a laser).

3. The light source must provide a high intensity at a wavelength that is suitable for the selected potential sensitive dye. In addition, this light should be extremely quiet (noise <0.1%).

4. A fast (mechanical) shutter that can open and close within milliseconds, allowing one to switch the excitation light on or off very rapidly, thus minimizes phototoxic side effects.

Preparing and Running Experiments

Staining solutions were prepared for each experiment by diluting an ethanol stock solution of the potential-sensitive dye di-4-ANEPPS[15] in Tyrode's solution. The final concentration of the dye was approximately 6 to 12 μmol/L. The cells were stained for approximately 10 minutes at room temperature. During experiments the cells were superfused with dye-free Tyrode's solution. Optical potential mapping was performed during current-clamp and voltage-clamp experiments (using a sealed patch electrode and a conventional voltage-clamp amplifier) and (without attached electrode) during field stimulation.

Optical records were taken in the following manner: the periodic pulses of a pulse generator were used to stimulate the cell continuously at a chosen rate. When a recording was performed, a pulse from the same generator was used to trigger the fast storage device, which then stored signal samples from up to 24 channels simultaneously with a rate of up to 200 kHz. After a short delay, the shutter of the excitation laser was opened to evoke the fluorescence light. Shortly after this, the cell was stimulated as mentioned above. When the chosen time of measurement was over, the shutter was closed, and the transient recorder stopped when the selected number of samples was reached. In a second step, data were transferred to a computer for long-time storage and evaluation.

Optical Signals

Optical signals are obtained by illuminating the stained specimen with intense light (laser light, 532 nm, of approximately 200 W/cm^2) and detecting the fluorescence light. Isolated guinea pig ventricular cells show a T-tubular system with a 3-dimensional architecture. T-tubular membranes are also stained with the potential-sensitive dye and contribute to the total amount of fluorescence. Fluorescence images taken with a confocal laser-scan microscope show a regular pattern throughout the cell.[16,17] Figure 2 shows an optical section of an isolated ventricular cell. The section plane was through the center of the cell and the stained T-tubular membranes are clearly visible. We must consider that an optical measuring spot that rep-

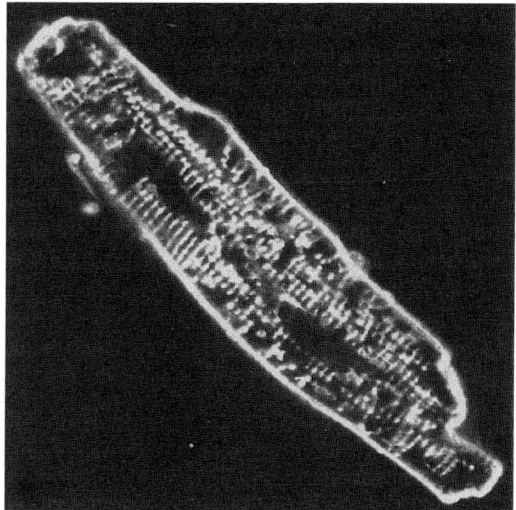

Figure 2. Optical cross-section of an isolated guinea pig ventricular myocyte. The fluorescence image was taken with a laser-scanning microscope, the section plane was through the center of the cell, the slice was 2.5 μm thick. The staining was di-4-ANEPPS, the size of the image is 115 μm × 115 μm. The periodic structure in the image is the optical appearance of the T-tubular system.

resents a particular image area (e.g., 14 μm × 14 μm) and is related to a particular detector element collects the fluorescence light from all membrane elements within this area. As can be seen in Figure 2, due to the tubular membranes the fluorescence light distribution is rather nonuniform, which will also lead to optical signals of different amplitudes.

In Figure 3 an optical signal that was obtained by a measuring spot of 14 μm × 14 μm is shown. The signal is scaled in nanoamperes and represents the photocurrent from the corresponding photodiode, the time is given in milliseconds. The excitation light was switched on for approximately 40 ms (the signal jumps up from 0 to about 2 nA and back again at the end). After about 10 ms, the cell was stimulated with a short current pulse, which was applied via a sealed patch electrode. The corresponding action potential rising phase is reflected in a sudden decrease of the optical signal by approximately 10%. Because the light was switched on for only 40 ms, the repolarization phase of the action potential (which would lead to an increase of the optical signal) is not visible. The decline of the signal (especially at the beginning) is an artifact that is caused by dye bleaching. The noise, prominent in this original signal, can easily be reduced by digital filtering.

Signal Processing and Evaluation

Normalization and Calibration of the Optical Signals

Stored signals were processed and evaluated depending on the type of experiment performed. Some steps, however, were frequently used: the data were digitally filtered. If necessary, a baseline drift resulting from dye bleaching was eliminated by subtracting a properly scaled optical signal that was gained from the cell at rest. Because of different bleaching

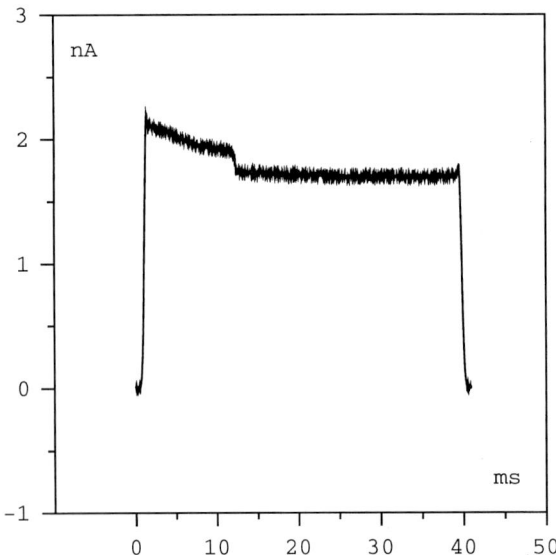

Figure 3. An original optical signal (the photo current of a particular photodiode from the detector matrix). The light was switched on for 40 ms. After stimulation of the cell, an action potential was elicited. The rising phase can be seen as a deflection in the optical signal.

processes, this method did not work perfectly but, within small deviations, a usable baseline could be obtained. Alternatively, the wavelength dependency of the voltage sensitivity of the dye[18] may be used to correct the optical signal for bleaching: a conventional optical signal shows both membrane voltage-related changes and changes caused by dye bleaching. Use of another excitation wavelength, where the dye shows no (or nearly no) voltage sensitivity, yields a signal that reflects only the drifting baseline. In a dual-wavelength procedure (changing the excitation wavelength periodically or on demand), signals with and without membrane voltage changes can be obtained and the baseline drift eliminated. In preliminary experiments in guinea pig papillary muscle, the voltage sensitivity of the dye di-4-ANEPPS dropped by a factor of 10 to less than 1% per 100 mV when the excitation wavelength was changed from the usual 532 nm to 457 nm. This allowed a satisfying correction of the bleaching artifact. Optical signals, even if they are related to the same electrical event in the cell, show different amplitudes due to spatially different fluorescence light intensities and to different percentage changes in response to the same voltage change at the membrane. In addition, these amplitudes vary from record to record. For comparison we often used a normalization procedure which unified the amplitudes of the optical signals: based on the idea that the cell at rest and in the plateau phase of an action potential (when only small membrane currents are present) must show a uniform membrane potential, we equalized selected data points of the signals in these regions. Optical signals can only reflect relative changes of the membrane potential, not the membrane potential itself. Despite this, often a partially or even a complete calibration of the optical signal is possible:

1. In experiments with simultaneously performed electrical recording via an electrode, in a normalization procedure as described above, the optical signals can be normalized to the electrical ones and can thus be calibrated in absolute voltage values. Figure 4 shows the final steep part of an action potential rising phase obtained with a patch electrode (the smooth trace)

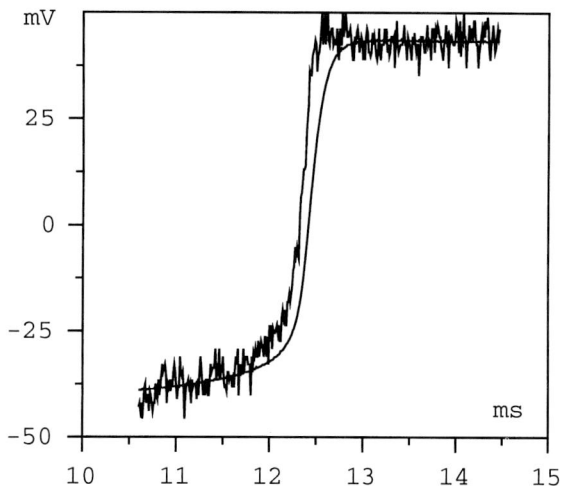

Figure 4. Comparison of an optical and a simultaneously obtained electrical signal. The optical signal (without any filtering) was normalized to the electrical signal, which was simultaneously recorded with a patch electrode. The optical signal occurred approximately 40 μs earlier and showed a steeper rising phase.

and an optical signal from a measuring spot with 14 μm × 14 μm. The amplitudes are normalized, calibrating the optical signal in absolute values. A comparison of the signals shows that the optically obtained rising phase is steeper and occurs earlier; it was shown that the electrical equipment was not able to follow the fast-changing membrane potential.[8,9]

2. In voltage-clamp experiments (whole cell voltage-clamping via a sealed patch electrode), also a complete calibration of the optical signal is possible. Figure 5 shows a voltage-clamp experiment with simultaneous optical monitoring. From a holding potential from −80 mV (the resting potential) a 50-mV clamp step was applied (panel A). Due to this step, the clamp current (panel B) developed, thus depolarizing the cell. A comparison with the command voltage (in panel A) shows a current spike that discharged the membrane, an ionic inward current due to membrane depo-

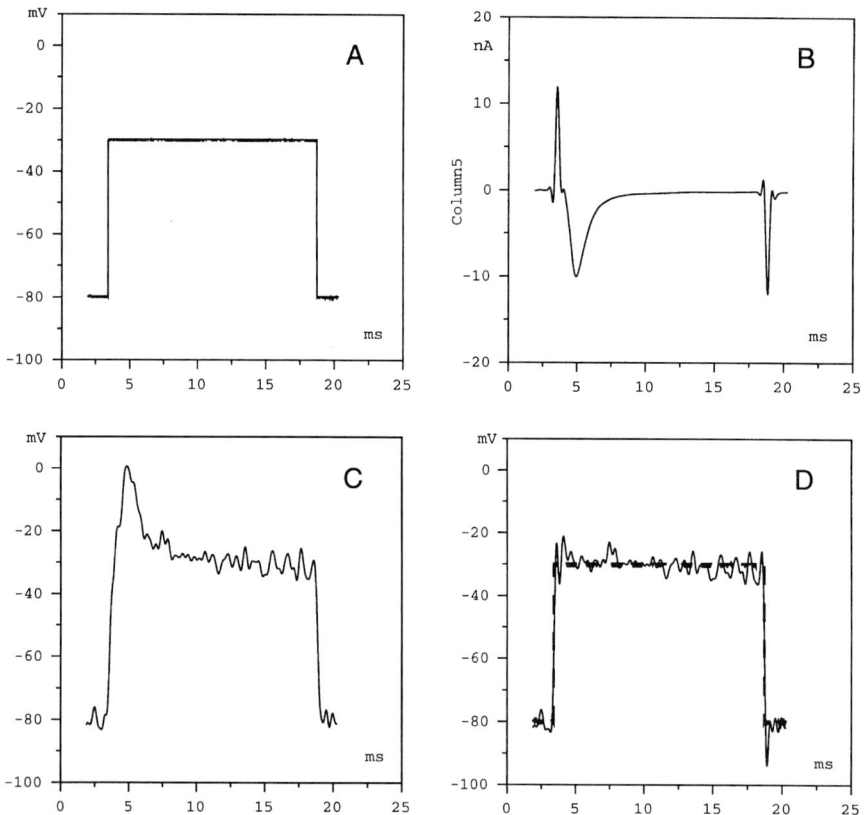

Figure 5. Voltage-clamp experiment with simultaneous optical recording. **A.** Command voltage, a 50 mV-step from the holding potential of −80 mV. **B.** Clamp current. **C.** Optical signal, which reflects the true membrane potential. **D.** Reconstruction of the command clamp step by adding the voltage drop at the access resistance (i.e., the current signal multiplied by the access resistance) to the proper scaled optical signal (the membrane voltage). The procedure allowed a calibration of the optical signal in absolute values (**C**) as well as the calculation of the actual cell access resistance (1.9 MΩ).

larization (the current peak in the negative direction), and the last current spike that recharged the membrane. The optical signal (panel C) did not follow the command voltage due to poor clamp control in this experiment: the deviation between the command voltage (panel A) and the optical signal (panel C) was caused by the voltage drop of the clamp current across the cell access resistance. When this voltage drop (the clamp current multiplied by the access resistance) was added to the properly scaled optical signal, the command voltage was reestablished (panel D). There is only one solution, which, when found, yields the proper access resistance and the calibration of the optical signal in absolute values. In addition, in previous voltage-clamp experiments we could show the linear response of the dye di-4-ANEPPS and the influence of series resistance compensation on the clamp control.[8]

3. If no simultaneous membrane potential measurement is performed via an electrode, true values of the resting potential and the action potential amplitude of the cell cannot be reestablished. Despite this, the optical signal (which shows an action potential rising phase) may be calibrated to well-known values of typical resting potentials and action potential amplitudes.[8]

4. In field stimulation experiments (the cell is stimulated with electrical field pulses), the amplitude of the optical signal can be calibrated with electrical test pulses of known field strength: the field pulse causes a voltage drop along the current path in the extracellular medium. This leads to location-dependent membrane potential changes in the cell (during the pulse, the cell membrane next to the anode shows a hyperpolarization and the membrane next to the cathode shows a depolarization whereas a neutral zone between shows no polarization).[11,19,20] Optical potential mapping yields signals from different areas of the cell membrane simultaneously which allows, in consideration of the known distances between measuring spots, the calibration of the pulse-induced membrane potential changes.

5. A comparison of optical signals with properly performed computer simulations can act as a tool that allows at least a suggestive calibration of the optical signal and a validation of the mathematical model (Fig. 6).[21]

Upstroke Velocities

Optical signals from action potential rising phases with unified or calibrated amplitudes allow one to gain upstroke velocities, in relative or even absolute values, by calculating the first time derivatives. A fast-responding measuring system (in our equipment the response time to a light pulse, taken from 10% to 90% of the pulse amplitude, was 70 μs) and a carefully applied digital filtering procedure allows one to approach the often high values of maximal upstroke velocities in single cells. In current-clamp experiments with simultaneously performed optical potential monitoring, we could show that the optically obtained upstroke velocities were significantly higher than those measured with a patch electrode.[8]

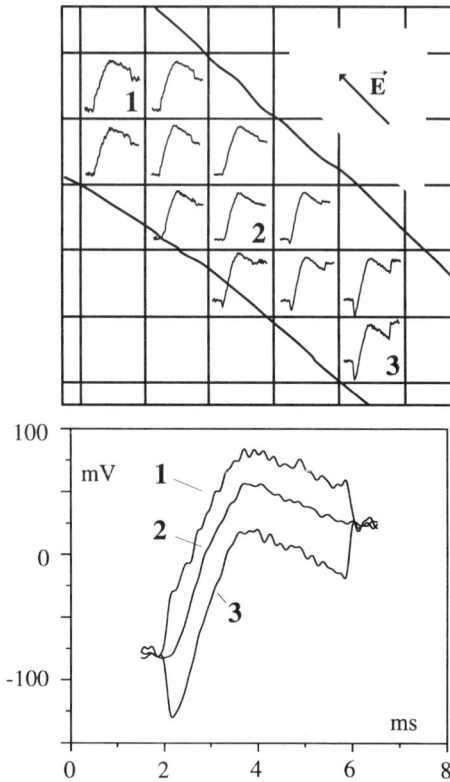

Figure 6. Optical potential mapping of a single cardiomyocyte during field stimulation. The outline drawing of the cell is shown with the projected photodiode matrix overlaid. One square represents a measuring spot with 15 μm × 15 μm. A 4-ms pulse was applied via platin electrodes situated in the tissue bath. The arrow indicates the direction of the electrical field. Individual optical signals are drawn within their corresponding measuring spots. In areas closer to the cathode, the pulse caused a membrane depolarization, in areas closer to the anode, a hyperpolarization. In the middle part of the cell, a zone remained neutral without field-induced polarization. During the pulse, a rising phase developed. *Lower panel:* Three selected signals (labeled 1, 2, and 3) are shown in an overlay plot. The calibration was obtained by comparison of the optical signals with a corresponding mathematical model.

Time Lags

As discussed above, an isolated cardiomyocyte is a tightly coupled system which synchronizes electrical events (e.g., an action potential upstroke) in the cell to within the microsecond range. Figure 7A shows three optical signals (selected from a dozen similar ones) from an action potential rising phase. All time lags between the signals were within approximately 10 μs, which demonstrates the high amount of synchronization. The tight electrical coupling was a common finding also in voltage-clamp and field stimulation experiments. In Figure 7B, again three similar optical signals from another cell are shown. In this exceptional case, the occurrence times of the maximal upstroke velocities of the signals, taken as a measure of the local membrane activation time, showed statistically significant time lags (within a 95% confidence interval) of up to about 30 μs.

Temporal Resolution

The temporal resolution determines the extent to which time lags between optical signals that are related to a characteristic electrical event within a cell, e.g., to an action potential rising phase, can be measured. It

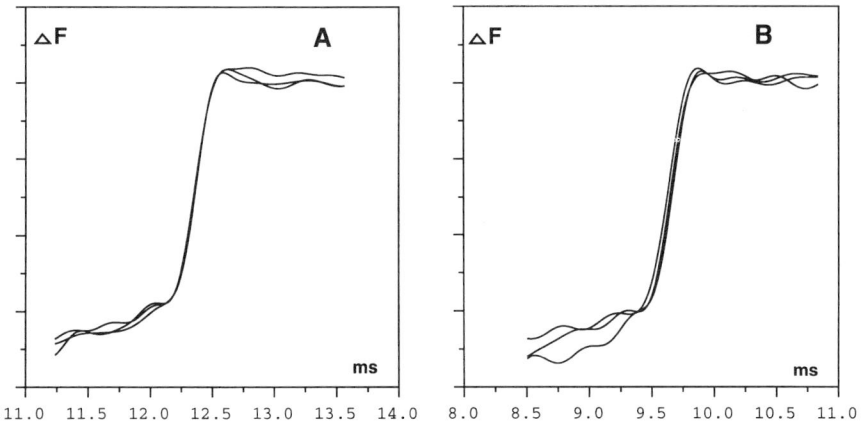

Figure 7. Three selected optical signals (out from about a dozen) from a single recording of action potential rising phases from isolated cells. ΔF = change of the fluorescence intensity. **A.** The usual finding (the signals showed no significant time lags within the cell). **B.** In another cell, as an exception, significant time lags between the signals were detected.

depends on the measuring system as well as the experimental condition which yields signals with a given shape and quality. When intracellular propagation phenomena in isolated cells are studied, usually the response time of the apparatus is much slower than occurring time lags within the cell. Despite this, time lags can be measured properly, provided that all measuring channels respond in the same manner. To avoid systematic errors related to different responses of the individual measuring channels, the apparatus should be calibrated or the individual intrinsic time lags should be measured, allowing for a correction of the results after the experiment.

The noise in the optical signals is the main factor that finally limits the temporal resolution. It distorts the shapes of the signals, making the measurement of time lags uncertain. The usual way to combat noise by repetitive measurement and averaging of the same signal is limited by phototoxic side effects. We have developed a method that is based on the assumption that the signal noise during a particular recording remains essentially the same and which allows us to calculate noise-induced uncertainties in measurements (a detailed description is given in reference 8). Basically, from an optical signal, which shows a region of interest and a region that contains only a baseline with the characteristic noise, the latter is cut out, shifted in time, and added to the interesting part of the signal. This procedure is repeated many times with increasing shift, which "moves" the noise when it is added to the interesting part of the signal. Each calculation leads to a somewhat differing result (e.g., a time lag), which finally allows us to calculate a standard deviation and a 95% confidence interval. The method can also be used in single-shot recordings and may be applied to all measurements that yield results that are influenced by noise (e.g., upstroke velocities).

Field Stimulation Experiments

In field stimulation experiments the isolated cell is exposed to an electrical field pulse, which, as mentioned above, yields to location-dependent membrane polarizations during the pulse. Optical potential mapping is the only method that allows one to monitor these effects in a single cell. In Figure 6, a field stimulation experiment is shown. The upper part shows the outline drawing of a cell together with the projected grid of the photodiodes. Individual optical signals are drawn within their corresponding measuring spots. An electrical pulse was switched on for 4 ms, the direction of the electrical field is indicated by the arrow. The signals reflect the local polarizations caused by the pulse as well as the depolarizations of the cell membrane during the pulse. Three selected signals (1, 2, and 3) are drawn in an overlay plot in the lower part of the figure. When the pulse was switched on (after 2 ms), trace 1, which was nearer to the cathode, showed a depolarization step and a step back again when the pulse was switched off (after 6 ms). In trace 3, which was nearer to the anode, the same electrical pulse caused a hyperpolarizing step at the beginning and a depolarizing step at the end. Trace 2, which was gained from an area somewhere in the middle of the cell, lacks any pulse-induced membrane polarization but shows the overall depolarization. During the pulse, each part of the cell membrane undergoes its own depolarization process and contributes membrane currents which, in sum, depolarize the cell. Despite different local membrane potentials and different local ionic currents, the traces are rather parallel, which again demonstrates the tight electrical coupling within the cell. The suggestive calibration of the optical signal, given in absolute voltages, was obtained by comparing the optically measured signals with hypothetic signals that were gained by modeling the same experiment on a computer.[21]

Conclusion

Measuring intracellular propagation means monitoring the spatial-temporal electrical events in cardiomyocytes that undergo an activation process. At present, optical potential mapping is the only method that provides, along with the ability to monitor many measuring spots simultaneously, the necessary spatial and temporal resolution. Several single cell experiments revealed the tight electrical coupling within the cell that synchronizes all electrical activities. Field stimulation experiments in which the cell membrane shows a location-dependent polarization demonstrated the high spatial resolution that allowed differences to be seen in the optically obtained membrane potential changes between adjacent measuring spots. In the future, confocal techniques may provide optical mapping with the same spatial and temporal resolution in complex 3-dimensional tissues.[22,23]

Optical potential mapping does not work on a "plug-and-play" basis; the same potential-sensitive dye may act differently in a different specimen, and phototoxic side effects must be considered. Rather than replacing conventional electrode techniques, optical mapping opens a new field that is not attainable by other methods. From the beginning of optical potential monitoring, comparative electrode measurements were performed to verify the optical signals. In addition, in our studies we could use the optical signals to show limitations of established electrode techniques.[8,24]

A combination of optical measurements and other techniques or properly designed mathematical models seems to be the best instrument to study intracellular propagation phenomena.

Acknowledgments: I would like to thank H. Ahammer, D. Dapra, and H. Köhler, for establishing the set-ups and performing experiments, D. Platzer for performing computer simulations, and T.T.J. DeVaney, for proofreading the manuscript.

References

1. Spach MS, Heidlage JF, Darken ER, et al. Cellular V_{max} reflects both membrane properties and the load presented by adjoining cells. *Am J Physiol* 1992;263:H1855–H1863.
2. Müller W, Windisch H, Tritthart HA. Fast optical monitoring of microscopic excitation patterns in cardiac muscle. *Biophys J* 1989;56:623–629.
3. Spach MS, Heidlage J. The stochastic nature of cardiac propagation at a microscopic level. Electrical description of myocardial architecture and its application to conduction. *Circ Res* 1995;76:366–380.
4. Brown AM, Lee KS, Powell T. Voltage clamp and internal perfusion of single rat heart muscle cells. *J Physiol (Lond)* 1981;318:455–477.
5. Ehrenberg B, Farkas DL, Fluhler EN, et al. Membrane potential induced by external electric field pulses can be followed with a potentiometric dye. *Biophys J* 1987;51:833–837.
6. Spach MS, Kootsey JM. Relating the sodium current and conductance to the shape of the transmembrane and extracellular potentials by simulation: Effects of propagation boundaries. *IEEE Trans Biomed Eng* 1985;32(10):743–755.
7. Hofer E, Urban G, Spach MS, et al. Measuring activation patterns of the heart at a microscopic size scale with thin-film sensors. *Am J Physiol* 1994; 266:H2136–H2145.
8. Windisch H, Ahammer H, Schaffer P, et al. Optical multisite monitoring of cell excitation phenomena in isolated cardiomyocytes. *Pflugers Arch* 1995;430:508–518.
9. Fast VG, Kleber AG. Microscopic conduction in cultured strands of neonatal rat heart cells measured with voltage-sensitive dyes. *Circ Res* 1993;73:914–925.
10. Rohr S, Salzberg BM. Multiple site optical recording of transmembrane voltage (MSORTV) in patterned growth heart cell cultures: Assessing electric behavior, with microsecond resolution, on a cellular and subcellular scale. *Biophys J* 1994;67:1301–1315.
11. Tung L, Borderies JR. Analysis of electric field stimulation of single cardiac muscle cells. *Biophys J* 1992;63:371–386.
12. Schaffer P, Ahammer H, Müller W, et al. Di-4-ANEPPS causes photodynamic damage to isolated cardiomyocytes. *Pflugers Arch* 1994;426:548–551.
13. Dillon SM. Optical recordings in the rabbit heart show that defibrillation strength shocks prolong the duration of depolarization and the refractory period. *Circ Res* 1991;69:842–856.
14. Pertsov AM, Davidenko JM, Salomonsz R, et al. Spiral waves of excitation underlie reentrant activity in isolated cardiac muscle. *Circ Res* 1993;72:631–650.
15. Loew LM, Cohen LB, Dix J, et al. A naphthyl analog of the aminostyryl pyridinium class of potentiometric membrane dyes shows consistent sensitivity in a variety of tissue, cell, and model membrane preparations. *J Membr Biol* 1992;130:1–10.

16. Stegemann M, Meyer R, Haas HG, et al. The cell surface of isolated cardiac myocytes—a light microscope study with use of fluorochrome-coupled lecitins. *J Mol Cell Cardiol* 1990;22:787–803.
17. Shacklock PS, Wier WG, Balke CW. Local Ca^{2+} transients (Ca^{2+} sparks) originate at transverse tubules in rat heart cells. *J Physiol* 1995;487(Pt. 3):601–608.
18. Müller W, Windisch H, Tritthart HA. Fluorescent styryl dyes applied as fast optical probes of cardiac action potential. *Eur Biophys J* 1986;14:103–111.
19. Windisch H, Ahammer H, Schaffer P, et al. Fast optical potential mapping in single cardiomyocytes during field stimulation. In Morucci JP, Plonsey R, Coatrieux JL, Laxminarayan S (eds): *Proceedings of the 14th Annual Conference of the IEEE Engineering in Medicine and Biology Society.* New York: IEEE Inc.; 1992:634–635.
20. Knisley SB, Blitchington TF, Hill BC, et al. Optical measurements of transmembrane potential changes during electrical field stimulation of ventricular cells. *Circ Res* 1993;72:255–270.
21. Platzer D, Windisch H. Simulation of excitation of single cardiomyocytes under field stimulation. In Morucci JP, Plonsey R, Coatrieux JL, Laxminarayan S (eds): *Proceedings of the 14th Annual Conference of the IEEE Engineering in Medicine and Biology Society.* New York: IEEE Inc.; 1992:642–643.
22. Dapra D, Münzer T, Ahammer H, et al. A confocal setup to measure transmembrane potential in cardiac tissue with very high spatial and temporal resolution. In *Proceedings of the First Joint BMES/EMBS Conference Serving Humanity, Advancing Technology.* Oct. 13–16; Atlanta: IEEE; 1999:164.
23. Diaspro A, Robello M. Two-photon excitation of fluorescence for three-dimensional optical imaging of biological structures. *J Photochem Photobiol B* 2000;55:1–8.
24. Windisch H, Müller W, Tritthart HA. Fluorescence monitoring of rapid changes in membrane potential in heart muscle. *Biophys J* 1985;48:877–884.

Chapter 7

Optical Mapping of Impulse Propagation between Cardiomyocytes

Stephan Rohr and Jan P. Kucera

The Question

It is well recognized that both the macroscopic and the microscopic structure of cardiac tissue are important determinants of impulse propagation, as illustrated by the following selected experimental findings: 1) It was shown several decades ago that conduction in the anisotropically structured myocardium is faster along the fiber axis, i.e., in the direction of the parallel aligned cells, than perpendicular to them.[1,2] 2) It was observed that impulse propagation can be delayed or even blocked at the transition from narrow tissue strands to the bulk of the myocardium (e.g., Purkinje fiber ventricular junction)[3,4] because of the imbalance between the size of the current source (small: narrow tissue strand) and the size of the current load (large: bulk of the myocardium). 3) Slow conduction velocities were observed in both chronically infarcted and aged ventricular tissue, which showed, histologically, an increase in collagenous septa. These septa caused a reduction in the spatial frequency of lateral electrical coupling of muscle bundles. When these preparations were activated in a direction perpendicular to the bundles, this infrequent lateral coupling resulted in a zigzag course of activation and, thus, in macroscopically slow conduction.[5-7] 4) It was shown that surviving tissue in an infarct scar can exhibit a highly complex microarchitecture with small tissue strands connecting islands of intact tissue ("mottled myocardium"), and it was suggested that such structures are likely to form the substrate underlying the generation of life-threatening cardiac arrhythmias.[8]

While all of these findings stressed the importance of the cellular architecture of cardiac tissue for impulse propagation, they were based on experiments that were conducted with spatial resolutions considerably larger than the dimensions of single cells. Thus, it remained elusive how exactly individual cardiomyocytes were involved in the respective acti-

This work was supported by the Swiss National Science Foundation.
From Rosenbaum DS, Jalife J (eds): *Optical Mapping of Cardiac Excitation and Arrhythmias.*
©Futura Publishing Co., Inc., Armonk, NY, 2001.

vation patterns. This question was advanced in the past nearly exclusively by computer simulation studies whose numerous predictions, to name just a few, included 1) that impulse propagation in a chain of single cells is discontinuous at the cellular level due to the recurrent increases in axial resistances at the cell-to-cell borders[9,10]; 2) that the calcium inward current can be crucial for supporting conduction at sites of an impedance mismatch[11,12]; and 3) that the safety of conduction can be increased by partial gap-junctional uncoupling.[9]

How can the relationship between cellular network architecture and impulse propagation be investigated with cellular/subcellular resolution, i.e., which preparations and which measurement techniques are suitable to tackle this interdependence? Regarding the preparation, it would obviously be desirable to use intact tissue in order to perform the experiments under as physiological conditions as possible. However, considering available recording techniques, it is presently not possible to assess the spread of activation in 3-dimensional tissue with microscopic resolution. A possible alternative consists of reducing the dimensionality of the preparation, i.e., of using 2-dimensional monolayer cultures of cardiomyocytes instead. There, each and every cell involved in the propagation process can be identified and impulse propagation can be followed at the single cell level with use of appropriate techniques. "Appropriate" in this context means 1) that the recording system is fast enough to permit the exact determination of propagation at the microscopic level, and 2) that the spatial resolution is high enough to allow several recording sites to be situated in each cell involved in the conduction process. Considering the dimensions of cultured ventricular myocytes (approximately 15×60 μm),[13] the spatial resolution, i.e., the interdetector distance, should be at least 10 μm, as shown schematically in Figure 1A. At this level of resolution, activation delays between adjacent detectors at normal conduction velocities ($\theta = 0.5$ m/s) become very small and amount to 20 μs for the case of continuous ("axonlike") conduction (Fig. 1B). If, however, macroscopic conduction velocities of 0.5 m/s are based on microscopically discontinuous conduction, the minimal values for interdetector activation times within the cells will be further reduced: according to previous computer simulation studies of conduction along a chain of single cardiomyocytes,[9,10,14] it can be expected that propagation times along individual cells are similar to propagation times across cell-to-cell borders under conditions of normal gap-junctional coupling. Thus, for $\theta = 0.5$ m/s and for an interdetector distance of 10 μs, intracellular activation delays will be approximately 10 μs, as schematically illustrated in Figure 1C. This value will further decrease if gap-junctional resistance and therefore the degree of discontinuity increases. In order to resolve such small temporal differences, it must be known with very high precision (approximately 1 μs) when activation of a given recording site is occurring. Summarizing these prerequisites, the investigation of the characteristics of propagation at the cellular/subcellular level requires a spatial resolution in the micrometer range and a temporal resolution permitting the tracking of activation delays between neighboring detector sites with microsecond precision.

In the past, three types of recording techniques have been commonly used to determine patterns of activation in cardiac tissue: 1) measurement

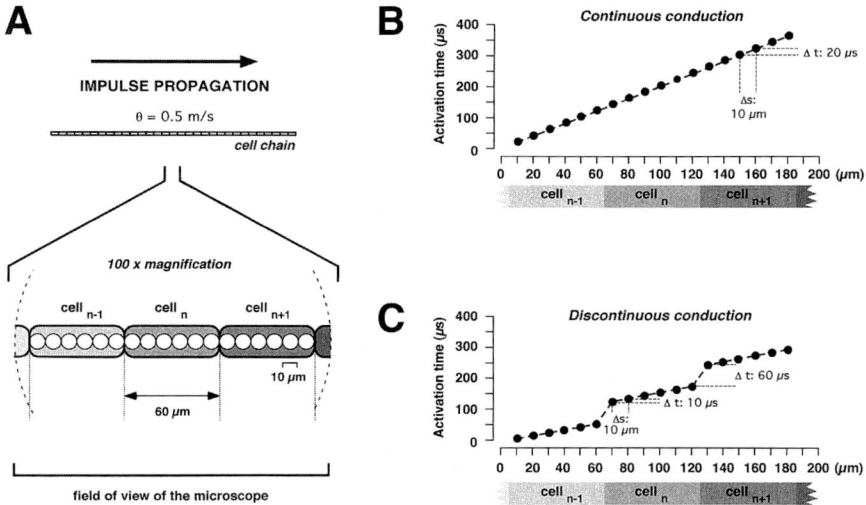

Figure 1. Spatiotemporal requirements for the measurement of impulse propagation at the cellular level. **A.** Spatial requirements: assuming a typical diameter of the intermediate image plane of the microscope of 20 mm, a magnification of 100× permits the imaging of three full cell lengths (shaded in gray; cell length = 60 μm). In order to resolve both intracellular and intercellular activation, individual recording sites (indicated by white discs) should be considerably smaller than the dimensions of individual cells (≤10 μm, which corresponds to a diameter of the detector of 1 mm at 100× magnification). **B.** Temporal requirements for the case of continuous conduction: under the assumption of an overall conduction velocity (θ) of 0.5 m/s and an interdetector distance of 10 μm, activation delays between adjacent recording sites during continuous conduction are 20 μs. **C.** Temporal requirements for the case of discontinuous conduction: for this type of conduction, which is due to recurrent increases in axial resistance at the cell-to-cell borders, minimal intracellular activation delays of 10 μs or less are to be expected.

of conduction between two or more intracellular electrodes, 2) multiple-site extracellular recordings; and 3) multiple-site optical recording of transmembrane voltage (MSORTV). While it is immediately obvious that multiple intracellular recordings cannot be used for assessing conduction at the cellular/subcellular level in monolayer cultures because simultaneous insertion of multiple electrodes into these fragile cells is virtually impossible, the use of multiple-site extracellular recording seems to be a viable alternative. There, photolithographic techniques permit the construction of closely spaced extracellular electrodes that can report activation patterns from the monolayer cultures growing on top of the electrodes.[15–17] The major disadvantages of this method in the context of measuring impulse propagation on the cellular scale are twofold: first, even the smallest interelectrode distance of 20 μm achieved so far is not small enough for obtaining a detailed picture of impulse propagation within single cells and across cell-to-cell borders. Second, computer simulations have suggested that, even at a hypothetical interelectrode spacing of 5 μm, extracellular electrodes might fail to detect propagation delays across cell-to-cell borders.[10] These disadvantages can be overcome by optical recording methods that offer sufficiently high spatial and temporal resolution if appropriate dyes and recording techniques are used. Their spatial resolution is only limited by the optical magnification, the size of the detectors, and signal-to-noise (S/N) considerations, while their temporal resolution is limited solely by the bandwidth of the detector-amplifier combinations and the sampling rate of the data acquisition system, because fast voltage-sensitive dyes react instantaneously to changes of the electrical field across cell membranes.[18] Further important advantages of optical recording techniques over extracellular electrode arrays include 1) the circumstance that they report transmembrane voltage changes instead of extracellular potentials; 2) the freedom to map any region of interest in a given preparation; and 3) the possibility to change, at any time, the spatial resolution according to given experimental goals. Thus, given the present state of the art in recording technologies, the combination of MSORTV and monolayer cultures of cardiomyocytes seems to represent an adequate approach to address questions related to action potential propagation from cell to cell in multicellular cardiac tissue and to investigate, in the case of patterned cultures, the relationship between cellular network architecture and impulse propagation.

The Experimental Approach

The Preparation

As briefly outlined above, the investigation of impulse propagation at the cellular level under conditions of steady-state conduction requires that 1) each cell contributing to the conduction process can be exactly identified, and that 2) the size of the preparations exceed a certain minimal length permitting the establishment of steady-state conduction in a given region of interest. While common monolayers of cultured cardiac cells are suitable for addressing basic questions regarding impulse propagation in uniform 2-dimensional cell networks, questions regarding the relationship between specific tissue geometries and impulse propagation can be addressed with so-called patterned growth cell cultures. In these cultures, a photolithographic patterning process permits the reproducible construction of predefined 2-dimensional tissue geometries, and the resulting preparations, by virtue of being only one cell thick, permit the unambiguous determination of individual cardiomyocytes involved in impulse propagation. While it is outside the scope of this chapter to describe the procedures involved in producing patterned growth cultures of neonatal rat ventricular myocytes (see reference 13), it must be mentioned that the resulting preparations display basic electrophysiological characteristics that are close to those exhibited by intact tissue of the same species in respect to both action potential shapes[13] and conduction velocities.[19,20]

The Recording System

As outlined in more detail in previous chapters of this book, optical recording of transmembrane voltage in excitable tissues is based on the use of fast potentiometric dyes which, after being incorporated into the sarcolemma, report changes in transmembrane voltage by changes in their absorption or fluorescence properties. While the general recording techniques for these optical signals are similar for both macroscopic and microscopic measurements, answering questions related to impulse propagation on the cellular scale requires addressing the following additional issues: 1) While, in intact multicellular tissue, many stained membranes stacked on top of each other contribute to the overall signal, only two membranes contribute to the signal in the case of monolayer cultures. This results, under the assumption of a constant baseline noise, in considerably reduced S/N ratios. Therefore, ample consideration must be given to both the detector design and the illumination strategies in order to achieve S/N ratios high enough to permit the precise characterization of activation at the cellular level. 2) Because impulse propagation should be followed at the level of single cells, adequate spatial and temporal resolution is required. This implies that minimal interdetector distances should be ≤10 μm (i.e., smaller than the width of individual cells) and that activation delays between neighboring detector elements as small as few microseconds must be detectable (cf. Fig. 1). In the following section, we describe a system that was developed to fulfill these requirements, i.e., that permits optical recordings of propagated action potentials with sufficiently high S/N ratios, spatial resolution, and temporal resolution to permit the characterization of both intracellular and intercellular propagation.[21]

System Overview. As illustrated in Figure 2, the recording system is built around a commercially available inverted microscope equipped for epifluorescence (Axiovert 135 M, Zeiss, Switzerland). The excitation light for the stained preparations is provided by a 150-W short arc xenon lamp, which is connected to a low ripple power supply (Optiquip, New York, NY). A shutter (D122, Vincent Assoc., Rochester, NY) mounted between the lamp housing and the microscope permits illumination of the preparations to be kept as short as possible in order to minimize phototoxic damage. Because the opening of the shutter induces vibrations that tend to distort the initial phase of the optical recordings, a custom-built vibration isolator is inserted between the lamp housing and the microscope. This isolator consists of an aluminum cage holding the spring-suspended shutter. After passing a cut-off filter, the excitation light is deflected toward the objective by the dichroic mirror of the microscope. Generally, objectives with high numerical apertures (NA) are used during the experiments in order to increase the S/N ratio by maximizing light throughput (Fluar 5×, NA 0.25; Fluar 10×, NA 0.5; Fluar 20×, NA 0.5; Fluar 40×, NA 1.3; Plan-Apochromat 100×, NA 1.4, all from Zeiss, Switzerland). After it passes the emission filter, the image of the preparation can be enlarged beyond the specifications of a given objective by a built-in magnifying lens (additional magnification by a factor of 1.6× or 2.5×).

The microscope used is equipped with an optical port at the bottom, which, in essence, converts the instrument into a straight optical bench, therefore offering an efficient light throughput because of the absence of additional deflecting optical elements in the light path. A custom-built attachment to this port permits the emitted light to be filtered according to the goals of a given experiment and to relay the image of the preparation to separate detector arrays. This port attachment is composed of two ver-

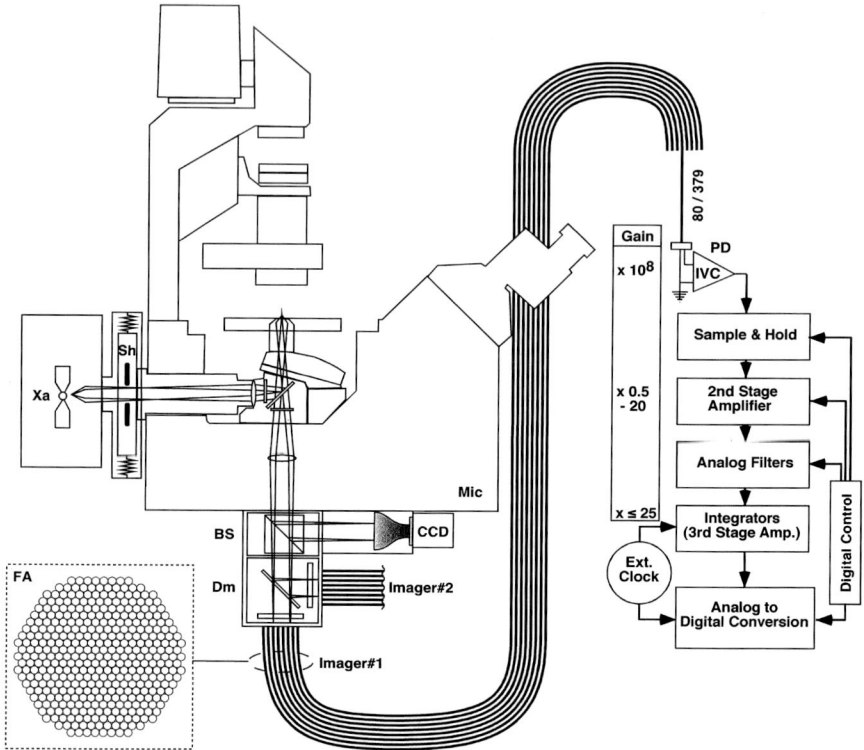

Figure 2. Schematic drawing of the optical recording system. BS = beam splitter; CCD = charge-coupled device (video camera); Dm = dichroic mirror; FA = arrangement of fibers in the faceplate of fiberoptic imager; IVC = current-to-voltage converter; Mic = inverted microscope equipped for epifluorescence; PD = photodiode; Sh = shutter; Xa = xenon short arc lamp. For further explanation see text.

tically stacked sliders, each of which offers three positions for the insertion of optical elements into the light path. A charged coupled device (CCD) camera facing the upper slider permits the recording of either a full (silver mirror) or a 50% (cube beam splitter) intensity picture of the preparation. In order to obtain images of the entire microscopic field of view, a fiberoptic taper is attached to the 2/3″ CCD sensor, which reduces the size of the field of view by a factor of 4 while retaining a highly efficient light throughput. The third position of the upper slider is empty, allowing all light to reach the slider below. There, the light is relayed to one or two photodetector arrays after being split into appropriate wavelengths by suitable combinations of dichroic mirrors and emission filters. From there, the signals reach the optical detectors of choice.

Choice of Detector Type for MSORTV.   Basically, there exists a whole range of photodetectors that are suitable for recording signals produced by voltage-sensitive dyes. Among these, CCD cameras and photodiode arrays (PDAs) are the most widely used. While CCD cameras offer high pixel counts, PDAs have the advantage of high temporal resolution. As illustrated in other chapters of this book, CCD cameras can be used for recording macroscopic activation in cardiac tissue because signal sizes are relatively large as many stacked cell layers contribute to the signal and because activation times are relatively long thereby permitting the determination of activation patterns at the slow frame rates typical for these devices (50 to 60 Hz). As briefly outlined above, both of these typical features of macroscopic recordings, i.e., large signals and comparably long activation times between adjacent detectors, are absent during microscopic determinations of conduction in cultured heart cells: cells form a monolayer with the consequence that available fluorescence is minimal and, if recordings are performed at high spatial resolution, the frame rate of even the fastest CCD cameras presently available (<2 kHz[22]) is too slow to accurately track the activation process at the cellular level. Under these circumstances, detectors with a higher temporal resolution must be used to accurately determine spatial activation patterns. Such devices are typically based on arrays of photodiodes, where the signals of all detectors are individually amplified and read out in parallel. Commercially available PDAs are fabricated on a single chip with pixel counts ranging up to 34×34.[23] Alternatively, they consist of many individual photodiodes coupled rigidly to optical fibers which form the input window of the detector.[24] While PDAs have a low overall number of pixels compared with CCD cameras, they can be operated at much higher frame rates, i.e., they display a much higher temporal resolution thus rendering them the detectors of choice for answering questions related to impulse propagation and repolarization at the cellular scale.

Fiberoptic Signal Conduit.   PDAs are either constructed on a single chip or they are custom-assembled from discrete photodiodes which are rigidly coupled to the image plane of the microscope by fiberoptic cables. In either case, the layout of the detectors is fixed, i.e., each element records changes in light from a defined region within the field of view of the microscope. In the set-up presented, a variation of the fiberoptic approach was implemented. Instead of a fixed attachment between fiberoptic cables and detectors, each detector was equipped with a connector, which permitted fiberoptic cables and photodiodes to be freely combined. This approach has the following advantages: 1) The useful spatial resolution is not limited by the physical dimensions of the photodetectors used but is defined solely by the diameter of the individual optical fibers, by the optical magnification used, and by S/N ratio considerations. 2) The possibility of rearranging the spatial pattern of detectors has the unique advantage that the location of recording sites can be adjusted to regions of interest in a given preparation, thereby circumventing the problem of "wasted" photodetectors (i.e., detectors that lie outside the preparation). 3) Because the photodetectors are noncommitted, it is possible to assign individual detectors to different ports of the microscope, thus enabling dual-emission wavelength measurements. Furthermore, it is possible to simultaneously monitor other parameters relevant for a given experiment, such as light intensity fluctuations of the lamp, which might serve to correct the optical signals for light ripple or arc wander. 4) Finally, the use of discrete photodetectors permits the most appropriate types of photodiodes to be selected during construction of the recording system.

In the system presented, the fiberoptic signal conduit consists of a custom-built hexagonal array of plastic fiberoptic cables comprising 379 fibers with an active diameter of 1 mm each (for layout see Fig. 2 "FA"; for fabrication details see reference 21). The array is attached to the bottom port of the microscope and its positioning relative to the field of view of the microscope is determined as follows: the 50% beam splitter in the upper slider is inserted into the light path and the loose ends of four optical fibers located at the periphery of the array are connected to light-emitting diodes (LEDs). The outputs of these fibers are recorded by the CCD camera after being reflected from a sheet of aluminum placed in the object plane of the microscope. The resulting image of the four illuminated light guides permits the determination of the exact position of the entire fiberoptic array relative to the field of view of the microscope.

Signal Conditioning: Theoretical Considerations and Implementation. Three electronic stages serve to convert and amplify the minute photocurrents produced by the photodiodes into signals of suitable size for the digital data acquisition system:

1. Current-to-voltage conversion stage: most of th e overall gain of the system is achieved in the first amplification stage, i.e., in the current-to-voltage converters (IVCs) connected to the photodiodes. This stage is critical for overall system performance in regard to both bandwidth and noise. Ideally, the bandwidth of the system extends from direct current (DC) to at least the maximal signal frequency generated by the preparation under investigation. In cardiac cell cultures, this maximal frequency corresponds to the maximal upstroke velocity (dV/dt_{max}) of the propagated action potential, and can be expected to be in the range of 100 to 200 V/s.[13] As shown experimentally below, a corner frequency (f_o) of 1.6 kHz, which corresponds to a time constant of approximately 100 μs, was sufficient to record values of dV/dt_{max} up to 500 V/s. Why is this stage also essential for the noise performance of the system? Because most (10^8) of the maximal overall gain $(1 \times 10^9$ to $5 \times 10^{10})$ is delivered by this stage, it is obviously also the major contributor to overall system noise (dark noise). Using sufficiently quiet operational amplifiers, a fundamental limit for the noise performance of an IVC is the Johnson noise arising from the feedback resistor (FR). The current noise amplitude produced by this resistor is $i_J = (4kTB/FR)^{1/2}$, where k is the Boltzmann constant, T the absolute temperature, and B the bandwidth.[25] From this formula, it can easily be seen that the noise is minimized by a reduction of the bandwidth and by an increase in the value of FR. Therefore, it would obviously be advantageous for the noise performance of the system to choose an FR that is sufficiently large as to obtain the entire desired gain in the first amplification stage (2 of 50 GΩ for the system presented). However, an increase in the value of the FR is accompanied by a substantial decrease in the bandwidth of the amplifier due to the increasing susceptibility of large FRs to stray capacity effects $(f_o$ typically around 400 Hz for 5 GΩ.[24]) Thus, FRs with values that do not exceed 100MΩ , which offer a reasonable compromise between bandwidth and

noise requirements, must be chosen. When measured at full bandwidth (f_o = 1.6 kHz) and full gain (5×10^{10}), overall peak-to-peak dark noise of the combination of components used for building the IVC (photodiode S2164, 1.4 mm × 1.4 mm photo-diode, Hamamatsu Corp., Bridgewater, NJ, and operational am-plifier OPA121KU, Burr-Brown Corp., Tucson, AZ) amounted to 75 ± 25 mV (mean±SD of a 10-ms-long recording period, n = 75). This value translates into approximately twice the theoret-ically predicted current noise level produced by the Johnson noise of the FR (for a more comprehensive discussion of noise in dye recording systems see references 24, 26, and 27). All of the components of the IVC are assembled on individual printed circuit boards that are mounted into individual brass casings in order to minimize noise pick-up. One end of the brass casing is designed as a fiberoptic connector that permits the reversible coupling of the optical fibers to the photodiodes.

2. Analog signal conditioning stage: The second amplification stage serves to further condition the raw signals produced by the IVCs. Sample-and-hold amplifiers at the input of this stage permit the subtraction of background fluorescence before the signal size is further adjusted (additional gain of 0.5×, 1×, 2×, 5×, or 20×) by use of either a DC or an alternating current (AC) coupling mode (time constants for AC coupling of 60 ms, 750 ms, or 9 s). Finally, the signals are passed through RC low pass filters (f_o of 0.5, 1, 2, or 3 kHz).

3. Integrator stage: The final amplifier stage consists of integrators (ACF2101BP, Burr-Brown) with gains inversely proportional to their driving frequency. Usually, experiments are performed at 20 kHz and result in an additional gain of 25×. The outputs of the integrators are fed to sample-and-hold stages, which store the signals during the scanning cycle of the analog-to-digital (A/D) converters.

The detectors and their circuitries are mounted in groups of 12 on printed circuit boards, which are connected to a digital control bus. This modular design permits the upgrading of the total number of channels by simply adding boards to the bus and by expanding the digitization capa-bilities of the system. The signals of the 80 detectors are acquired by two 12-bit A/D converters (PC20501C, Burr-Brown, installed in a personal computer), which scan 40 channels each with a frame rate of 20 kHz, re-sulting in 1.6 million samples/s (3.2 MB/s of data).

Temporal Accuracy of the System. In order to achieve the temporal pre-cision that is necessary for the determination of intracellular and intercel-lular propagation delays, the following prerequisites must be met: 1) the sampling frequency of the A/D conversion system should be high enough to permit an accurate tracking of the action potential upstroke; 2) each point in time, at which a single data acquisition is performed, must be ex-actly defined; 3) because the bandwidth of the amplifiers is, due to noise considerations (see above), close to the bandwidth of fast-rising action po-tential upstrokes, the frequency responses of all amplifiers should be identical, because otherwise the time course of the measured action potential upstrokes will vary from detector to detector thereby resulting in inaccurate determinations of the respective activation times. If all of these prerequisites are met, the rising phase of each signal is exactly defined in time, and delays between signals of interest can be calculated with microsecond precision. In other words, despite the relatively slow response of the amplifiers ($\tau = 100$ µs), their identical bandwidths in conjunction with a simultaneous sampling scheme permits us to obtain accurate phase information on the action potential upstrokes and, thus, to calculate delays between signals of interest with a temporal precision that is considerably smaller than τ (few µs range, see below). The three requirements mentioned above are addressed in the recording system as follows: 1) The sampling frequency of the A/D conversion is 20 kHz. This value is well above the Nyquist criterion (twice f_o) and corresponds to approximately 10 measurement points along the action potential upstroke under the assumption of a duration of the upstroke of 500 µs. 2) Because the A/D conversion is initiated with the same clock driving the sample-and-hold output stages of the integrators, all signals recorded originate from exactly the same point in time. Therefore, it is known with submicrosecond precision when each data point is acquired. 3) During construction of the IVC, τ ranged from approximately 70 µs to 90 µs. This variability was compensated for by the introduction of an adjustable stray capacitance, i.e., a fine Teflon insulated wire was soldered to one terminal of the FR and the distance between the wire and the resistor was varied such that the time constant of each amplifier reached 100 µs ($f_o = 1.6$ kHz). Based on these measures, it was expected that temporal delays in the microsecond range could be detected between fast-rising optical signals. This assumption was tested by applying a square pulse of an LED to the array and by measuring the dispersion of "activation times" for each recording site. Activation times were determined as the point at which the signals reached 50% of their full amplitude, at_{50} (calculation based on interpolation, see reference 19; for discussion of differences between this type of determination of activation time versus the determination based on the maximal upstroke velocity of the signal see reference 21). Figure 3A shows the results of such an experiment: despite the measures taken, there remained a dispersion of at_{50} with a standard deviation of ±2.1 µs (range −6 to 6 µs; n = 75). In order to compensate for this dispersion, which was most likely due to slight inaccuracies in the "Teflon wire" procedure and to variations in the temporal responses of the second amplification stage, a short LED pulse was routinely recorded with each experiment. This permitted the determination of the temporal deviation of each individual channel and, subsequently, the correction of activation times obtained in biological preparations. By use of this procedure on an LED pulse simulating an action potential upstroke, the standard deviation of activation times was reduced to ±0.4 µs (n = 75; range −0.8 to 1.2 µs; Fig. 3B).

Based on these characteristics, it could be expected that propagating events in the range of 1 m/s could be resolved with a spatial resolution of ≤10 µm. In order to test this prediction, a propagating light intensity change was simulated by placing a rotating steel blade (2000 rotations/min) into the object plane of a 20× objective and by recording, in transillumination mode, the shuttering of the field of view. The result of such an

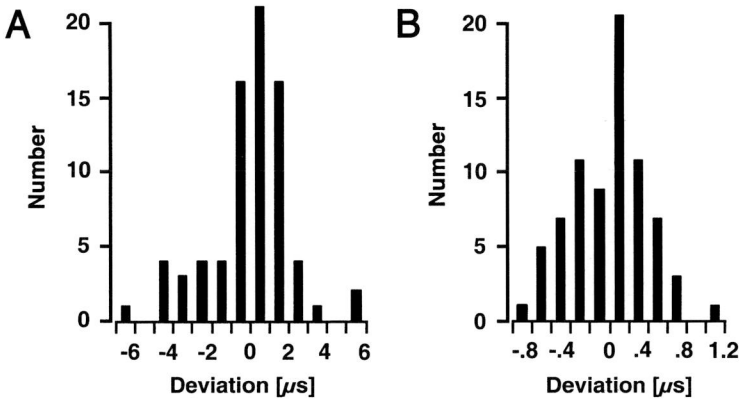

Figure 3. Histograms of the temporal deviations of all optical amplifiers in response to the edge of a square pulse of a light-emitting diode (LED). The light pulse was applied simultaneously to all opto-amplifiers and the point at which the signals reached 50% of their full amplitude (at$_{50}$), was determined for each channel. **A.** In the absence of a digital correction, the deviations ranged from -7 µs to $+6$ µs. **B.** When the values obtained in A were used for correction of a second LED pulse, the range of deviations was substantially reduced to ± 1 µs. Reproduced, with permission, from reference 21.

experiment is illustrated in Figure 4. Signals were recorded with the spatial arrangement of detectors shown in panel A. Panel B depicts the isochrones of the light intensity change as the blade swept over the objective. The isochrones were parallel because the distance between the axis of rotation and the center of the objective (20 mm) was large compared with the diameter of the field of view (1 mm); this resulted in a virtually parallel shuttering of the recording area. Individual signals recorded along the center row of detectors are shown in Figure 4C. A linear fit of the at$_{50}$ values of these signals yielded a velocity of the blade of 4.25 m/s, which closely matched the theoretically predicted value of 4.19 m/s. From this finding, namely that a light intensity change propagating with a velocity of 4.25 m/s can be measured with a spatial resolution of 50 µm (20× objective), it can be inferred that the system is capable of tracking events propagating at up to 0.8 m/s with a spatial resolution of 10 µm or less, i.e., with cellular/subcellular resolution. Finally, if it is assumed that the signals shown in Figure 4C correspond to a transmembrane voltage change of 100 mV, the resulting maximal upstroke velocities shown in Figure 4D would have been in the range of 500 V/s, which illustrates the upper limit of the frequency response of the recording system.

Spatial Resolution. In order to determine the useful optical resolution experimentally, propagated action potentials were recorded in linear strands of cultured neonatal rat ventricular myocytes (width: 50 to 100 µm) at magnifications ranging from 5× to 250×. These recordings were obtained using experimental protocols described in detail elsewhere.[21] In short, the preparations were mounted in a temperature-controlled chamber[28] and were superfused with Hanks' balanced salt solution (HBSS) at 36°C. Then a region of interest was identified and an extracellular stimulation electrode was positioned at a distance greater than 1 mm from the prospective optical recording site. This minimal distance prevented elec-

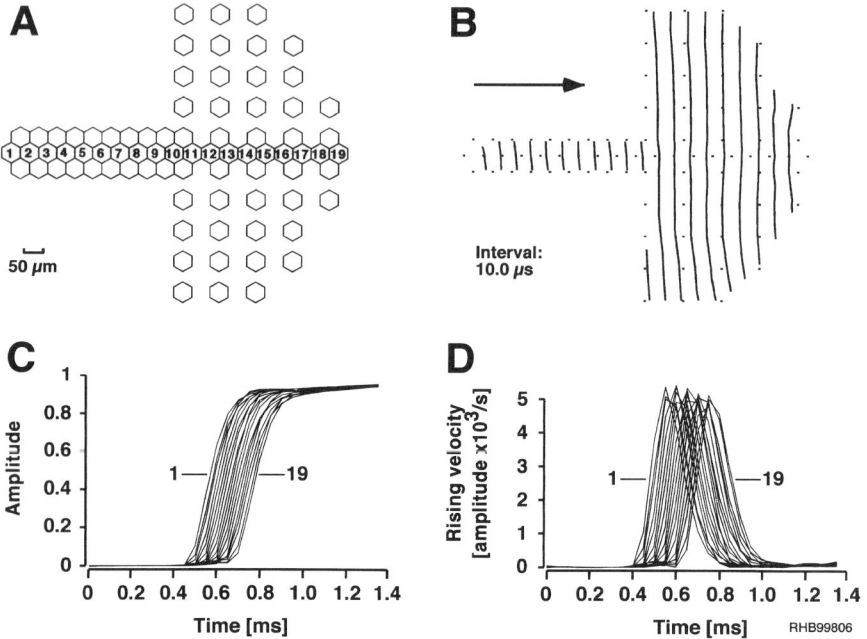

Figure 4. Test of the temporal resolution of the recording system by tracking a fast moving shutter in the object plane of the microscope (rotating steel blade). **A.** Spatial placement of the detectors. **B.** The parallel and evenly spaced isochrones correspond to the shuttering of the field of view and indicate that a moving light signal with a velocity of approximately 4 m/s can be accurately tracked with a spatial resolution of 50 µm. **C.** Plot of individual signals along the center row of detectors. The numbers correspond to the numbering in A. **D.** First derivative of the signals shown in C. Reproduced, with permission, from reference 21.

trotonically mediated stimulation artifacts from distorting the signals of interest and, furthermore, it permitted activation to reach steady-state conditions at the measurement site. After successful stimulation was established, superfusion was stopped and the preparations were stained with 135 µmol/L of the voltage-sensitive dye di-8-ANEPPS (Molecular Probes Inc., Eugene, OR) in HBSS for 3 to 4 minutes (for an extended discussion of the choice of dye see reference 19). Thereafter, superfusion was resumed and experiments were started following an equilibration period of 10 minutes. The experiments were completely under software control, i.e., the acquisition of control parameters (resting fluorescence, determination of frequency response of each amplifier) and the experiment itself (illumination, timing of stimulation, and data acquisition) were controlled by the digital I/O ports of the computer system. The results of these experiments are shown in Figure 5. While signals could be recorded at all magnifications corresponding to spatial resolutions ranging from 4 µm to 200 µm, signals at either extreme yielded poor S/N ratios of approximately 30 because light levels and, therefore, signal amplitudes were minimal: at low magnification (200 µm; panel A), this was primarily due to the small NA of the objective (signals size ~ proportional to the fourth power of NA[29]) while, at high magnification (4 µm; panel G), light intensities were

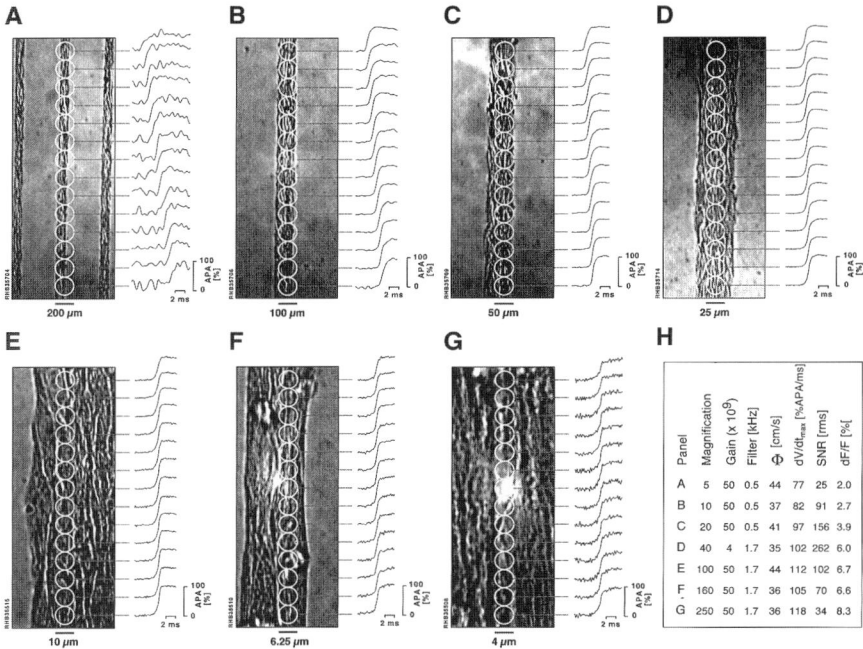

Panel	Magnification	Gain (x10^9)	Filter [kHz]	Θ [cm/s]	dV/dt$_{max}$ [%APA/ms]	SNR [rms]	dF/F [%]
A	5	50	0.5	44	77	25	2.0
B	10	50	0.5	37	82	91	2.7
C	20	50	0.5	41	97	156	3.9
D	40	4	1.7	35	102	262	6.0
E	100	50	1.7	44	112	102	6.7
F	160	50	1.7	36	105	70	6.6
G	250	50	1.7	36	118	34	8.3

Figure 5. Useful spatial resolutions of the optical recording system. **A** through **G**. Illustration of action potential upstrokes recorded along linear cell strands at increasing spatial resolutions. The optical magnifications used, together with other relevant parameters of the experiments, are summarized in **H**. θ = conduction velocity; dV/dt$_{max}$ = maximal upstroke velocity; SNR = signal-to-noise ratio; dF/F = fractional fluorescence change. For further explanation see text. Reproduced, with permission, from reference

low due to the small size of the area imaged. Between these two extremes, objectives offering highly efficient light throughputs improved S/N ratios substantially. The highest values (between 200 and 300) could be recorded with the 40× objective as illustrated by the example shown in panel D. During experiments using objectives with a large light throughput, the predominant source of noise changed from dark noise to noise dominated by the small ripple of the light source (<0.1%). These experiments illustrate that the recording system is capable of resolving transmembrane voltage changes with spatial resolutions ranging from the subcellular to the multicellular level.

Optical Motion Artifact Subtraction. A disadvantage of optical recordings of transmembrane voltage changes in contractile tissues is that the contraction-induced light scattering distorts the repolarization phase of the action potentials. For cultured cells, this effect is especially pronounced if the region monitored by a given detector contains brightly stained debris that adheres to the cell monolayer and therefore moves with every contraction. For intact cardiac tissue, three main strategies were used in the past to overcome this disadvantage of optical recordings: 1) motion was restricted by pressing the tissue onto a glass window[30–32]; 2) the end of repolarization was identified by a maximum in the second derivative of the optical signal[33]; and 3) contraction was suppressed with suitable drugs (butanedionemonoxime,[34,35] verapamil,[36,37] or, more recently, cytochalasin-D[38,39]). Because these methods are either unsuited for cultured cells (#1), do not permit the visualization of the entire repolarization phase (#2), or rely on drugs that potentially interfere with the excitability of cardiac tissue (#3), we tried to implement yet another method,[21] which is based on the observation, that the "ANEPPS" class of voltage-sensitive dyes contains two distinct regions that react either with a decrease (longer wavelengths) or an increase (shorter wavelengths) of fluorescence intensity to depolarizations of the membrane.[40,41] Because, obviously, the motion artifact (MA) is not dependent on the wavelength, it seemed feasible to use a dual-emission wavelength approach to correct optically for MAs. The result of such an experiment is illustrated in Figure 6. The preparation was broadly excited (excitation: <500 nm, dichroic mirror: 505 nm, emission: >515 nm) and the emitted light was split by a dichroic mirror (590 nm) and directed to two fiberoptic arrays that were spatially exactly matched. Accordingly, one array recorded light with wavelengths >590 nm (Fig. 6B) while the other received light with wavelengths between 515 and 590 nm (Fig. 6C). Signals of both wavelengths were scaled to the resting fluores-

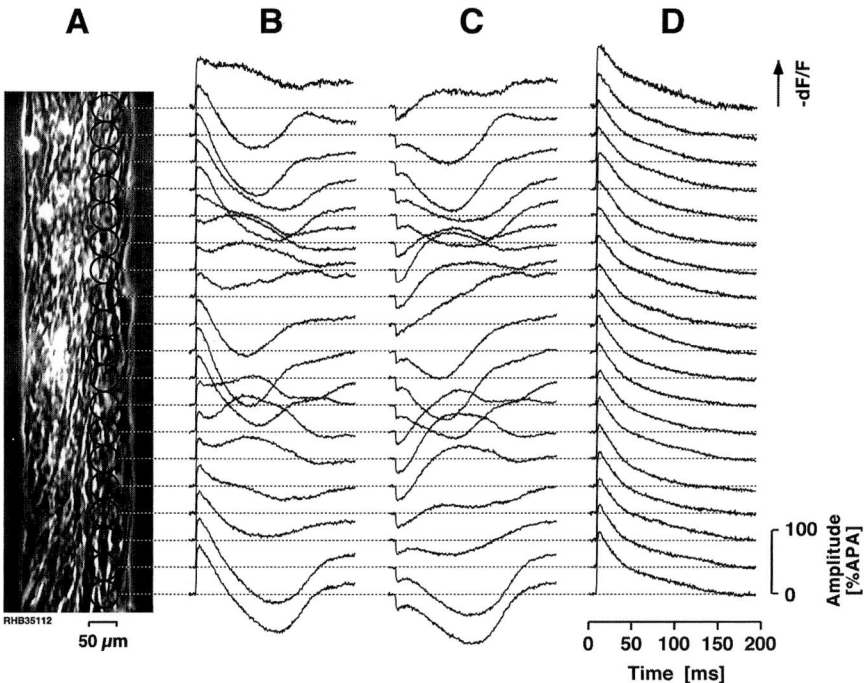

Figure 6. Optical motion artifact (MA) subtraction. **A.** Phase contrast image of the preparation with overlaid black circles indicating the positions of the photodetectors. **B.** Signals recorded at wavelengths at which the potentiometric dye di-8-ANEPPS responded with upward-going deflections to the action potential upstrokes. **C.** Signals recorded simultaneously at the same sites but at wavelengths at which the action potential upstrokes resulted in a negative-going deflections. **D.** Subtraction signals: signals shown in B and C were subtracted from each other after having been normalized to their respective resting fluorescence values. This resulted in action potentials that were virtually free of MAs (all normalized to 100%). Reproduced, with permission, from reference 21.

cence recorded at the respective wavelengths and sites. As expected, di-8-ANEPPS reacted with opposite changes in fluorescence to the change in membrane potential as indicated by upstrokes going up (panel B) or down (panel C). Signals recorded at either wavelength showed a considerable distortion of the action potential due to the MA. As shown in Figure 6D, this distortion was completely eliminated after subtraction of the signals in panel C from those in panel B. In addition to the elimination of MAs, dual-emission wavelength measurements also tended to increase the S/N ratio because the signal sizes and the level of common mode noise rejection were increased. These results illustrate that it is feasible to record optically, with cellular resolution, spatial patterns of action potential repolarization without using drugs that might interfere with the normal electrophysiological characteristics of the tissue.

Measurements of Intercellular Propagation

Intercellular Propagation during Normal Gap-Junctional Coupling. One of the first problems ever tackled with the combination of patterned growth myocyte cultures of neonatal rat ventricular myocytes and high-resolution optical mapping of impulse propagation was the question of whether impulse propagation in chains of single cardiomyocytes is discontinuous at the cellular level due to recurrent increases in longitudinal resistance at the sites of cell-to-cell appositions as shown previously in computer simulation studies.[9,10,14,42] This question was investigated with preparations that were patterned so that they formed "monolines" of cardiomyocytes, i.e., they consisted of strands of cardiomyocytes one cell wide. In these strands, impulse propagation was followed at high spatiotemporal resolution permitting the determination of activation delays both within individual cardiomyocytes and across cell-to-cell borders. An example of such a measurement is shown in Figure 7. As schematically shown in panel A, the region of the monoline preparation selected for the optical recording consisted of cardiomyocytes being abutted in the center of the field of view. During action potential propagation from left to right, the simultaneously recorded action potential upstrokes revealed an activation gap between detectors #5 and #7, thus demonstrating that conduction was, as predicted, discontinuous at the cellular level. The action potential upstroke recorded by detector #6 showed an intermediate timing, which is explained by the circumstance that this detector received input simultaneously from the left and the right cell.

When the same type of measurement was conducted with strands that were several cells wide, discontinuities at the sites of cell-to-cell appositions could no longer be observed.[20] An example for such a recording is shown in Figure 8. Activation of the 3- to 4-cell-wide strands occurred in a mostly continuous manner as indicated by the even spacing between the isochrones of activation, as in Figure 8A and by the absence of any major gaps as in Figure 8B, in which all recorded action potential upstrokes are shown separately for each row of detectors. The difference in activation patterns between monolines of cardiomyocytes and wider cell strands can be explained by the rather intense lateral gap-junctional coupling observed in several-cell-wide strands.[43] This lateral coupling smoothes out

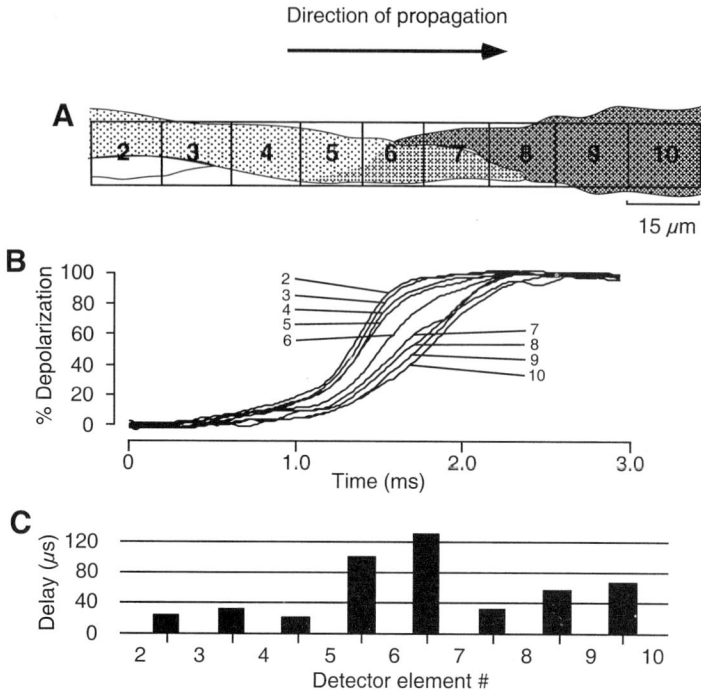

Figure 7. Discontinuous conduction in "monolines" of cardiomyocytes. **A.** Schematic drawing of the imaged region of the preparation consisting of two slightly overlapping cardiomyocytes (light gray and dark gray). The squares indicate the positions of individual photodetectors. **B.** Action potential upstrokes recorded during propagation from left to right. Numbers correspond to the numbering of photodetectors in A. **C.** Activation delays along the preparation. Reproduced, with permission, from reference 44.

differences in local activation times ("lateral averaging"[14,44]) because, as shown in a computer simulation study,[14] the staggered arrangement of laterally connected myocytes offers the excitatory current a collateral pathway around a given end-to-end connection thereby delaying conduction along the cytoplasm while speeding up conduction across cell junctions situated end to end.

Intercellular Propagation Delays during Partial Electrical Uncoupling. While, as shown above, activation in several-cell-wide strands under conditions of normal intercellular coupling is continuous, this situation is expected to change significantly during gap-junctional uncoupling. Computer simulations have shown that a reduction of intercellular conductance results in an increase of activation delays across the cell-to-cell borders and in the confinement of depolarizing current to individual cells.[9,42] In order to investigate this type of conduction experimentally, impulse propagation was mapped in several-cell-wide strands which were electrically uncoupled to a degree that nearly induced conduction blocks.[20] The results of such an experiment are shown in Figure 9. The 4- to 5-cell-wide preparation (Fig. 9A) was partially uncoupled with palmitoleic acid, and action potential upstrokes recorded during propagation from left to

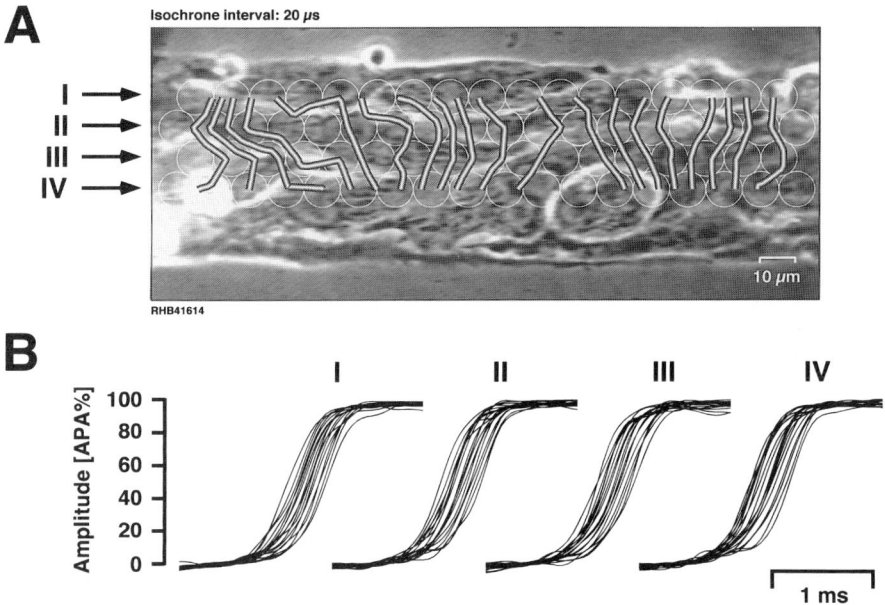

Figure 8. Microscopic impulse propagation in a several cell wide linear strand . **A.** Phase contrast picture of the preparation with overlaid white circles indicating the positions of the photodetectors and isochrones of activation (spacing: 20 μs) during impulse propagation from left to right. **B.** Plot of action potential upstrokes recorded simultaneously from the four rows of photodetectors numbered I through IV in panel A. Reproduced, with permission, from reference 20.

right are shown, in superimposed form, in panel B. Compared with control recordings obtained in several-cell-wide strands (Fig. 8B), conduction was not only substantially slowed during partial uncoupling (decrease of Θ from 43 cm/s to 1.1 cm/s) but activation became highly discontinuous as indicated by the clustering of optically recorded action potential upstrokes, which pointed to a stepwise advancement of excitation. Activation delays among the clustered action potential upstrokes ranged from 0.5 to 4.5 ms while the activation of the clusters themselves took 80 μs to 450 μs to complete. The origin of the clustered signals within the preparation is illustrated in Figure 9C, which shows the projection of all recording sites onto a schematic drawing of the preparation with highlighted borders of individual cells. The correlation of sites reporting clustered activation (same color coding as in panel B) with the cellular structure of the preparation reveals that clustered activity originated from small patches of the preparation consisting of one to three cells, i.e., conduction invaded the preparation in a saltatory fashion where the patches were activated sequentially with variable delays. As indicated qualitatively by the dashed arrows, the activation path was tortuous due to the presence of a central obstacle consisting of a single cell (cross-hatched outline). This cell, which was still completely uncoupled at the time of the measurement, forced the activation to take a turn, resulting in a region of the preparation exhibiting backward propagation.

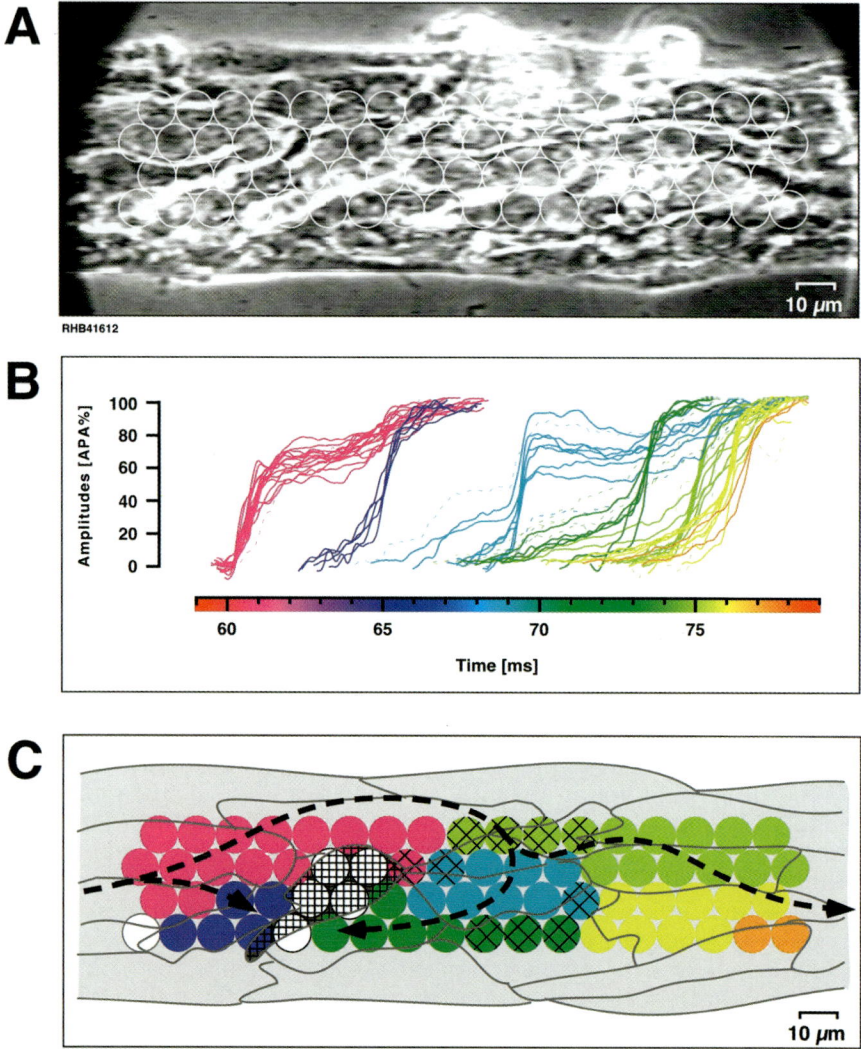

Figure 9. Highly discontinuous microscopic conduction during critical gap-junctional uncoupling. **A.** Phase contrast picture of the preparation with overlaid white circles indicating the positions of individual photodetectors. **B.** Plot of all action potential upstrokes recorded simultaneously from all photodetectors during impulse propagation from left to right under conditions of critical gap-junctional uncoupling. **C.** Schematic drawing of the cellular architecture of the imaged region of the preparation. The overlaid discs are color coded according to the colors used for the clustered upstrokes in B and indicate regions of the preparation being activated nearly simultaneously. The dashed line describes qualitatively the path of activation of the preparation. Reproduced, with permission, from reference 20.

Limitations and Perspectives

In summary, the system presented fulfills the basic requirements for measuring the spread of activation at the cellular/subcellular scale because it permits measurements with a spatial resolution of ≥ 4 μm and because it is fast enough to track delays between fast-rising signals with an uncertainty of ± 1 μs. Due to its modular design, the recording system offers a flexible approach to the spatially resolved measurement of fast optical signals with subcellular resolution and it can be easily upgraded in terms of the number of photodetectors. The use of an exchangeable fiberoptic image conduit between the microscope and the detectors opens the possibility to design higher resolution imagers by using smaller fiber diameters and/or to use two or more fiberoptic arrays to simultaneously record signals at different emission wavelengths. Because the optical amplifiers are spatially noncommitted, they can arbitrarily be assigned to 1) measure signals from freely selectable regions of the preparations; 2) measure signals from identical sites in the preparation at different emission wavelengths; or 3) record other signals of interest, e.g., light intensity fluctuations of the lamp that might serve to correct the optical signals for light ripple or arc wander. Despite these attractive features, there remain a number of disadvantages inherent to optical determinations of transmembrane voltage changes that must be taken into account when pursuing optical experiments at high spatiotemporal resolution:

1. The most important drawback in comparison to, for example, arrays of extracellular electrodes, consists in the phototoxicity exerted by the potentiometric dyes. While this poses a negligible problem for low-resolution measurements (≤ 50 μm), it becomes highly pronounced when propagation is to be followed with cellular/subcellular resolution (≤ 10 μm) as discussed in this chapter. In this case, it is imperative to use high NA optics in order to achieve sufficient S/N ratios. This in turn results in large illumination intensities at the level of the preparations with the consequence that the function of the imaged cells is often highly compromised even after a single-shot recording lasting approximately 100 ms or even less. While this damage often precludes the use of the same sites in a preparation for both control experiments and interventions, it is our experience that the first recording itself at a given site is not compromised by the high-intensity illumination. Thus, it seems that the damage to the cell function lags behind the actual light exposure by several seconds. Even though this lag period has never been investigated, it might be explained by the time it takes for free radicals, which are generated during high-intensity illuminations, to exert their damaging effects on the cells.
2. Another drawback of optical recording techniques using voltage-sensitive dyes consists of their inability to support long-term experiments (hours to days) in order to follow, for example, developmental aspects of impulse conduction in the patterned growth myocyte cultures. This inability is caused

primarily by the problem of phototoxicity and, furthermore, by the circumstance that the dye concentration in the sarcolemma progressively decreases with time (internalization of the dyes into the cells and washout). This results in a progressive reduction of S/N ratios which would require repeated restaining of the preparations, thus making it difficult to maintain stable culture conditions for the cells.

3. Finally, even though ratiometric approaches permitting the determination of absolute voltage changes from signals of potentiometric dyes have been reported,[41,45,46] these techniques have not found wide acceptance because their precision is hampered by the modest S/N ratios normally encountered with fast voltage-sensitive dyes. Thus, unless new dyes are being developed that are more suited for a ratiometric approach, it seems that the interpretation of fast signals from voltage-sensitive dyes will remain mostly qualitative in the sense that they do not easily permit one to assign absolute voltages to the recorded signals.

Based on the general features of the recording system described, one might think of a range of future developments that would extend the use of "fiberoptic imagers" to experimental situations that are different from mapping intracellular and intercellular propagation:

1. It could be envisaged to extend the capabilities of the system into the macroscopic range not only by replacing the microscope with a tandem-lens macroscope,[29] but by placing the fiber inputs directly onto a given preparation. As an example, it should be possible to shape the optical front end in such a way as to form a cavity into which an entire heart could be placed and where the entire surface could be imaged simultaneously in three dimensions. In such an experiment, part of the fibers could be assigned to deliver the excitation light to the preparation while the other fibers could be used to record from the tissue in a manner similar to the "optrode" design described earlier.[36,47,48]

2. The sensitivity of the system could be increased by replacing the photodiode detectors with devices that offer less dark noise at comparable gains, i.e., with photomultipliers or avalanche photodiodes. These devices could be inserted between the outputs of the fiberoptic array and the integrators, thereby still making use of both the fiberoptic input and simultaneous digitization capabilities of the system. Such an approach would possibly extend the range of useful resolutions to both smaller and larger magnifications than the ones presently used and, moreover, it would permit weaker signals to be recorded from other types of optical indicators.

3. Finally, it could be envisaged to assemble the optical fibers in such a way that they form a linear array serving as a fast and sensitive detector for slit-hole confocal microscopes. Such a linear array should theoretically result in an increase of both

the temporal resolution and S/N ratios of this type of confocal microscope, thus rendering it more suitable for the detection of fast and propagated events in intact excitable tissue.

Acknowledgments: We are grateful to Dr. H.-P. Clamann for his comments on the manuscript.

References

1. Sano T, Takayama N, Shimamoto T. Directional difference of conduction velocity in the cardiac ventricular syncytium studied by microelectrodes. *Circ Res* 1959;7:262–267.
2. Clerc L. Directional differences of impulse spread in trabecular muscle from mammalian heart. *J Physiol (Lond)* 1976;255:335–346.
3. Mendez C, Mueller WJ, Merideth J, et al. Interaction of transmembrane potentials in canine Purkinje fiber-muscle junctions. *Circ Res* 1969;24:361–372.
4. Overholt ED, Joyner RW, Veenstra RD, et al. Unidirectional block between Purkinje and ventricular layers of papillary muscle. *Am J Physiol* 1984; 247:H584–H595.
5. Gardner PI, Ursell PC, Fenoglio JJ, et al. Electrophysiologic and anatomic basis for fractionated electrograms recorded from healed myocardial infarcts. *Circulation* 1985;72:596–611.
6. Spach MS, Dolber PC, Heidlage JF. Influence of the passive anisotropic properties on directional differences in propagation following modification of the sodium conductance in human atrial muscle. A model for re-entry based on anisotropic discontinuous propagation. *Circ Res* 1988;62:811–832.
7. de Bakker JMT, van Capelle FJL, Janse MJ, et al. Slow conduction in the infarcted human heart. 'Zigzag' course of activation. *Circulation* 1993;88:915–926.
8. Ursell PC, Gardner PI, Alabla A, et al. Structural and electrophysiological changes in the epicardial border zone of canine myocardial infarcts during infarct healing. *Circ Res* 1985;56:436–451.
9. Shaw RM, Rudy Y. Ionic mechanisms of propagation in cardiac tissue: Roles of the sodium and L-type calcium currents during reduced excitability and decreased gap-junction coupling. *Circ Res* 1997;81:727–741.
10. Rudy Y, Quan W. Propagation delays across cardiac gap junctions and their reflection in extracellular potentials: A simulation study. *J Cardiovasc Electrophysiol* 1991;2:299–315.
11. Joyner RW, Kumar R, Wilders R, et al. Modulating L-type calcium current affects discontinuous cardiac action potential conduction. *Biophys J* 1996; 71:237–245.
12. Sugiura H, Joyner RW. Action potential conduction between guinea pig ventricular cells can be modulated by calcium current. *Am J Physiol* 1992; 263:H1591–H1604.
13. Rohr S, Schölly DM, Kléber AG. Patterned growth of neonatal rat heart cells in culture. Morphological and electrophysiological characterization. *Circ Res* 1991;68:114–130.
14. Fast VG, Kléber AG. Microscopic conduction in cultured strands of neonatal rat heart cells measured with voltage-sensitive dyes. *Circ Res* 1993;73:914–925.
15. Israel DA, Edell DJ, Mark RG. Time delays in propagation of cardiac action potentials. *Am J Physiol* 1990;258:H1906–H1917.
16. de Bakker JMT, van Capelle FJI, Tasseron SJA, et al. Load mismatch as a cause of longitudinal conduction block in infarcted myocardium. *Circulation* 1997;96:I497. Abstract.
17. Kucera JP, Heuschkel MO, Renaud P, et al. Power-law behavior of beat rate

variability in monolayer cultures of neonatal rat ventricular myocytes. *Circ Res* 2000;86:1140–1145.

18. Salzberg BM, Obaid AL, Benzanilla F. Microsecond response of a voltage-sensitive merocyanine dye: Fast voltage-clamp measurements on squid giant axon. *Jpn J Physiol* 1993;43:37–41.

19. Rohr S, Salzberg BM. Multiple site optical recording of transmembrane voltage in patterned growth heart cell cultures: Assessing electrical behavior, with microsecond resolution, on a cellular and subcellular scale. *Biophys J* 1994;67:1301–1315.

20. Rohr S, Kucera JP, Kléber AG. Slow conduction in cardiac tissue: I. Effects of a reduction of excitability vs. a reduction of electrical coupling on microconduction. *Circ Res* 1998;83:781–794.

21. Rohr S, Kucera JP. Optical recording system based on a fiber optic image conduit: Assessment of microscopic activation patterns in cardiac tissue. *Biophys J* 1998;75:1062–1075.

22. Iijima T, Witter MP, Ichikawa M, et al. Entorhinal-hippocampal interactions revealed by real-time imaging. *Science* 1996;272:1176–1179.

23. Hirota A, Sato K, Momose-Sato Y, et al. A new simultaneous 1020-site optical recording system for monitoring neural activity using voltage-sensitive dyes. *J Neurosci Methods* 1995;56:187–194.

24. Chien CG, Pine J. An apparatus for recording synaptic potentials from neuronal cultures using voltage-sensitive fluorescent dyes. *J Neurosci Methods* 1991;38:93–105.

25. Horowitz P, Hill W. *The Art of Electronics.* Cambridge: Cambridge University Press; 1989.

26. Salzberg BM. Optical recording of electrical activity in neurons using molecular probes. In Barker JL, McKelvy JF (eds): *Current Methods in Cellular Neurobiology. Vol. 3. Electrophysiological and Optical Recording Techniques.* New York: John Wiley & Sons, Inc.; 1983:139–187.

27. Cohen LB, Lesher S. Optical monitoring of membrane potential: Methods of multisite optical measurement. In DeWeer P, Salzberg BM (eds): *Optical Methods in Cell Physiology.* New York: John Wiley & Sons, Inc.; 1986:71–99.

28. Rohr S. Temperature-controlled perfusion chamber suited for mounting on microscope stages. *J Physiol (Lond)* 1986;378:90.

29. Ratzlaff EH, Grinvald A. A tandem-lens epifluorescence macroscope: Hundred-fold brightness advantage for wide-field imaging. *J Neurosci Methods* 1991;36:127–137.

30. Rosenbaum DS, Kaplan DT, Kanai A, et al. Repolarization inhomogeneities in ventricular myocardium change dynamically with abrupt cycle length shortening. *Circulation* 1991;84:1333–1345.

31. Kanai A, Salama G. Optical mapping reveals that repolarization spreads anisotropically and is guided by fiber orientation in guinea pig hearts. *Circ Res* 1995;77:784–802.

32. Girouard SD, Laurita KR, Rosenbaum DS. Unique properties of cardiac action potentials recorded with voltage-sensitive dyes. *J Cardiovasc Electrophysiol* 1996;7:1024–1038.

33. Efimov IR, Huang DT, Rendt JM, et al. Optical mapping of repolarization and refractoriness from intact hearts. *Circulation* 1994;90:1469–1480.

34. Pertsov AM, Davidenko JM, Salomonsz R, et al. Spiral waves of excitation underlie reentrant activity in isolated cardiac muscle. *Circ Res* 1993;72:631–650.

35. Gray RA, Jalife J, Panfilov A, et al. Nonstationary vortexlike reentrant activity as a mechanism of polymorphic ventricular tachycardia in the isolated rabbit heart. *Circulation* 1995;91:2454–2469.

36. Dillon SM. Optical recordings in the rabbit heart show that defibrillation

strength shocks prolong the duration of depolarization and the refractory period. *Circ Res* 1991;69:842–869.

37. Kwaku KF, Dillon SM. Shock-induced depolarization of refractory myocardium prevents wave-front propagation in defibrillation. *Circ Res* 1996; 79:957–973.

38. Wu J, Biermann M, Rubart M, et al. Cytochalasin D as excitation-contraction uncoupler for optically mapping action potentials in wedges of ventricular myocardium. *J Cardiovasc Electrophysiol* 1998;9:1336–1347.

39. Jalife J, Morley GE, Tallini NY, et al. A fungal metabolite that eliminates motion artifacts. *J Cardiovasc Electrophysiol* 1998;9:1358–1362.

40. Fromherz P, Lambacher A. Spectra of voltage-sensitive fluorescence of styryl-dye in neuron membrane. *Biochim Biophys Acta* 1991;1068:149–156.

41. Bullen A, Saggau P. High-speed, random-access fluorescence microscopy: II. Fast quantitative measurements with voltage-sensitive dyes. *Biophys J* 1999; 76:2272–2287.

42. Murphy CR, Clark JW, Giles WR, et al. Conduction in bullfrog atrial strands: Simulations of the role of disc and extracellular resistance. *Math Biosci* 1991;106:39–84.

43. Darrow BJ, Fast VG, Kléber AG, et al. Functional and structural assessment of intercellular communication: Increased conduction velocity and enhanced connexin expression in dibutyryl cAMP-treated cultured cardiac myocytes. *Circ Res* 1996;79:174–183.

44. Rohr S, Salzberg BM. Discontinuities in action potential propagation along chains of single ventricular myocytes in culture: Multiple site optical recording of transmembrane voltage (MSORTV) suggests propagation delays at the junctional sites between cells. *Biol Bull Mar Biol Lab* 1992;183:342–343.

45. Montana V, Farkas DL, Leow LM. Dual-wavelength ratiometric fluorescence measurements of membrane potential. *Biochemistry* 1989;28:4536–4539.

46. Beach JM, McGahren ED, Xia J, et al. Ratiometric measurement of endothelial depolarization in arterioles with a potential-sensitive dye. *Am J Physiol* 1996;270:H2216–H2217.

47. Neunlist M, Zhou SZ, Tung L. Design and use of an 'optrode' for optical recordings of cardiac action potentials. *Pflugers Arch* 1992;420:611–617.

48. Witkowski FX, Plonsey R, Penkoske PA, et al. Significance of inwardly directed transmembrane current in determination of local myocardial electrical activation during ventricular fibrillation. *Circ Res* 1994;74:507–524.

Chapter 8

Role of Cell-to-Cell Coupling, Structural Discontinuities, and Tissue Anisotropy in Propagation of the Electrical Impulse

André G. Kléber, Stephan Rohr,
and Vladimir G. Fast

Introduction

Knowledge about the mechanisms governing propagation of the electrical impulse from the sinoatrial node to the ventricular myocardium is important for the understanding of the normal electrocardiogram and the mechanisms of cardiac arrhythmias. The basic patterns of cardiac macroscopic excitation through the atrial and ventricular myocardium were described early in this century in the dog heart,[1] and were later confirmed in the isolated, perfused human heart.[2] With the possibility to record transmembrane action potentials from isolated cardiac tissue,[3] and the accumulation of knowledge about the ionic nature of the main depolarizing and repolarizing ionic currents involved in the generation of the action potential, it became important to establish models that explained the propagation of the cardiac impulse at a cellular level. Early models of cardiac propagation were adapted from models developed for nerve tissue and involved so-called continuous cables.[4,5] In such a cable, the intracellular space and, optionally, the extracellular space are represented by a series of equal resistors, which symbolize the lumped resistances of the cytoplasmic space and the gap junctions. The passive and excitable properties of the cell membranes are represented by a membrane capacitance arranged in parallel with resistors representing the time- and voltage-dependent carriers of transmembrane ionic current flow (channels, exchangers, and pumps). Although it was known early on that cardiac tissue involves a complex network of cells connected by gap junctions, experi-

Supported by the Swiss National Science Foundation and the Swiss Heart Foundation.
From Rosenbaum DS, Jalife J (eds): *Optical Mapping of Cardiac Excitation and Arrhythmias.*
©Futura Publishing Co., Inc., Armonk, NY, 2001.

mental work carried out in tissues selected for their "ideal cablelike" geometry has shown that such selected tissues indeed behave similarly to a cablelike structure at normal or only moderately impaired cell-to-cell coupling. Such models were taken to describe the effects of, for example, hypoxia, ischemia, or antiarrhythmic drugs on conduction velocity.[6–8]

Over the past years it has become evident that models involving a continuum of intracellular and/or extracellular resistances do not suffice to explain 1) conduction in part of the hearts with a marked discontinuous structure in the normal state (e.g., trabeculated atrial tissue, midmural ventricular layers); 2) conduction in aged hearts exhibiting marked fibrosis; and 3) conduction in diseased states involving remodeling of tissue architecture (chronic infarction, hypertrophy, and failure).[9,10] Importantly, in continuous models, the changes in the resistive properties of the cellular network modulate propagation velocity independently of changes in membrane ionic currents. In contrast in *discontinuous* structures, the effects of changes in membrane properties and the role of ionic currents on conduction depend on the underlying state of cell-to-cell coupling. This interaction makes the mechanism of the propagation process more complex than previously anticipated.

Over the past several years, two types of studies have added significantly to the understanding of cardiac impulse propagation and its relation to cellular electrical activity and the discontinuous cellular architecture: 1) simulation studies including sophisticated models of cardiac excitation and cellular networks,[11,12] and 2) multisite high-resolution optical mapping of transmembrane potential.[13] This chapter attempts to review the recent work on the basic mechanisms of discontinuous conduction involving optical mapping.

Conduction in Cell Strands and 2-Dimensional Networks

A main interest in the investigation of propagation in a single cardiac cell chain involves the separation of the role of the cytoplasmic resistance from the role of the gap-junctional connexins. Both computer simulations and experimental studies, which have been carried out to assess this relation, have provided similar results.[14,15] As illustrated in Figure 1, neonatal rat hearts were grown in single cell chains by means of a patterned growth technique[14,16] and electrical propagation was measured by positioning two light-sensitive diodes (diameter 6.5 mm, interdiode distances 30 mm) within a single cell and a third diode across the adjacent end-to-end cell connection. In such a way, cytoplasmic conduction times were obtained and compared with the time needed for the electrical impulse to cross the cell border. As shown in Figure 1, the mean cytoplasmic conduction time in cultured neonatal rat cells chains amounted to approximately 38 μs, and the mean conduction time across a cell-to-cell connection 118 μs. Accordingly, the conduction delay at the gap junctions was 80 μs, or approximately 50% of overall conduction time. The observation that the conduction delay located at the gap junctions is a relatively large fraction of the overall conduction time was also made in the simulation

A

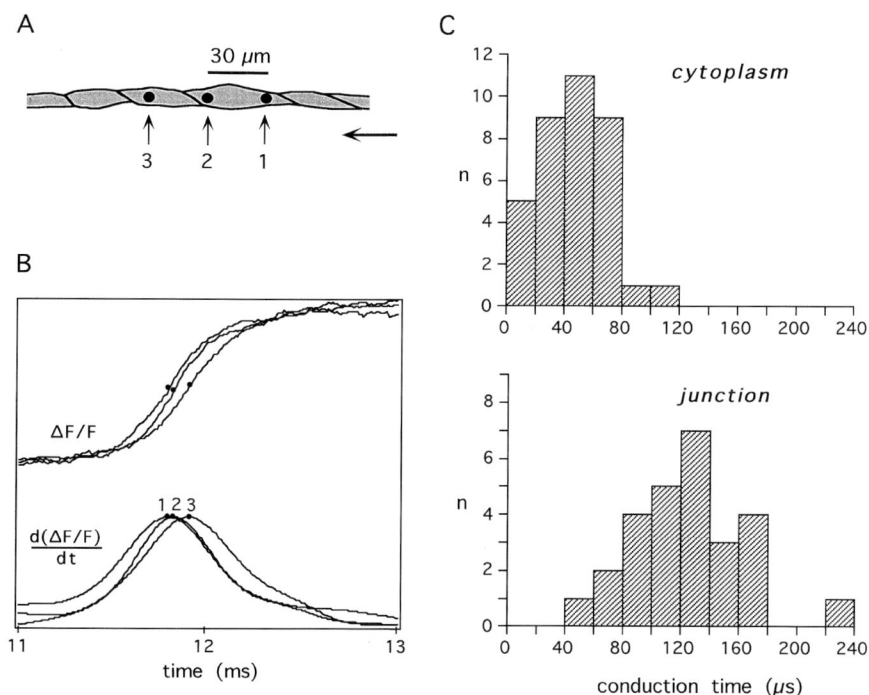

B

C

Figure 1. Experimental determination of conduction in a single cell chain. **A.** Reproduction of the microscopic appearance of a cultured cell chain. Dots and numbers denote positions of three light-sensitive diodes (6.5 μm in diameter) separated by a distance of 30 μm. **B.** Optical recording of action potential upstrokes from diodes 1 to 3, measured as fluorescence change ΔF/F of a voltage-sensitive dye (RH237, *upper traces*) and the first time derivatives (*lower traces*). Numbers 1 to 3 denote times of local activation. Note that the conduction delay across the cell border (2 to 3) is larger than delay within the cytoplasm (1 to 2). **C.** Histograms of cytoplasmic (*upper graph*) and junctional (*lower graph*) conduction times. The difference between the mean conduction times amounts to approximately 80 μs and reflects the mean conduction time across the end-to-end cell junctions. Reproduced, with permission, from reference 14.

study by Rudy and Quan.[15] They simulated conduction in cell chains with parameters taken from experimental results obtained in guinea pig hearts. In this simulation, a value of approximately 800 Ωcm for the specific gap-junctional resistance, R_j, between two cells produced equal conduction times across the cytoplasm and the intercellular connection. This value is situated within the higher range of values obtained from measurements in cell pairs using the double voltage-clamp technique.[17]

From the observation that gap junctions significantly delay conduction in single cell chains, two questions emerged: 1) Is the effect in single cell chains different from the effect in 2- and 3-dimensional cellular networks? 2) How does an increase in R_j or, equivalently, a decrease in gap junction expression consequent to remodeling (as observed in many pathological situations: myocardial ischemia, hypoxia, infarction, failure) affect conduction? The first question was answered by comparing conduction in a single chain (Fig. 1) with conduction in a cell strand where several chains were coupled by gap junctions laterally. Interestingly, the presence of lateral coupling increased cytoplasmic conduction time and concomitantly decreased junctional conduction time, the contribution of gap-junctional delay to overall conduction time decreasing to 22% (versus 50% in single cell chains). The effect of lateral coupling to decrease microscopic inhomogeneities in conduction, which was also observed in models simulating anisotropic propagation,[18,19] is illustrated in Figure 2. During longitudinal propagation, local excitatory current through lateral junctions between an individual cell and the neighboring cells will flow whenever the cells are activated out of phase. If a neighboring cell is activated earlier, lateral current will act to speed up propagation in the cell concerned and to slow down propagation in the neighboring cells, i.e., lateral current will smoothen propagation ("lateral averaging"), or, inversely, if a cell concerned is activated earlier than the neighboring cells, lateral current of opposite polarity will delay propagation in the cell concerned and accelerate propagation in the neighboring cells, again with the overall effect of smoothing propagation. As shown in Figure 2, lateral averaging is critically dependent on the lateral coupling resistance: a very high degree of lateral coupling is predicted to cancel almost totally the delaying effect of individual end-to-end cell connections.[14]

As mentioned above, electrical cell-to-cell uncoupling or remodeling involving a change in gap junction expression is a process that occurs in many important cardiac diseases. Experimental studies on electrical un-

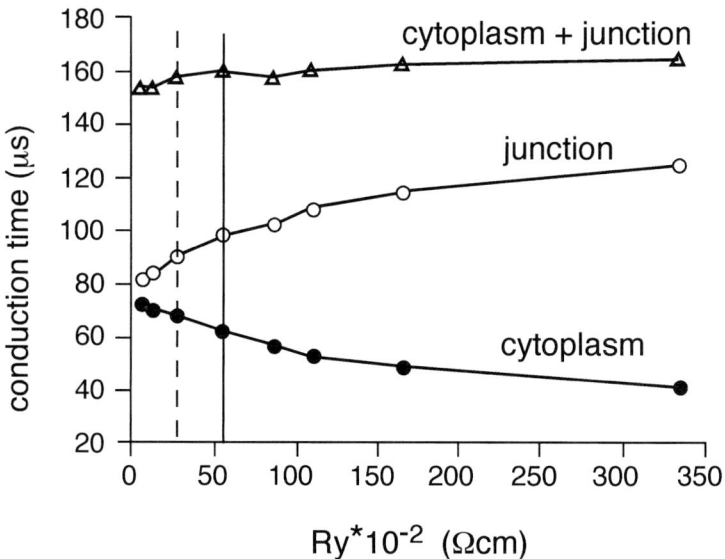

Figure 2. Cytoplasmic and cell-to-cell conduction times in a simulated cell strand consisting of five cell chains coupled laterally. With very low lateral resistance (Ry), the system behaves like a functional syncytium and conduction times are equal. Progressive lateral uncoupling prevents lateral electrical cross-talk. With total lateral uncoupling, each chain behaves as if it is insulated from its neighbor. In this case conduction times correspond to the experimental values shown in Fig. 1. Reproduced, with permission, from reference 14.

coupling have been carried out mostly with relatively large specimens (whole hearts, isolated tissue) by means of the so-called cable analysis (see above). Only recently did it become possible to measure the effect of uncoupling on propagation at a cellular level, with the use of high-resolution optical mapping of transmembrane potential.[20] Both experimental and simulation studies demonstrated that conduction velocity, θ, can decrease to very low values with reduced electrical coupling, in the order of a few cm/s or even less than 1 cm/s, until conduction block takes place. Since θ is a key determinant of the size of reentrant circuits, decreasing θ to 1 cm/s predicts an excitation wavelength in the order of 1 mm (with the assumption of a refractory period of 100 s). Projecting this length on the circumference of a circuit in microreentry yields a diameter of approximately 300 μm. The pronounced decrease of θ *contrasts* with the only moderate decrease and the early occurrence of propagation block observed with a *reduction in membrane excitability.* Thus, the lowest velocities observed in myocardial ischemia or in elevated extracellular K^+_o in isolated, perfused pig hearts, conditions well known to depress I_{Na}, amounted to approximately 15 cm/s (in longitudinal direction of the cardiac fibers).[21] Similarly, inhibition of I_{Na} by terodotoxin (TTX) in guinea pig trabeculae produced lowest velocities of approximately 15 cm/s. Also, conduction depending on I_{Ca} in the presence of normal cell-to-cell coupling amounted to approximately 15 cm/s.[20,21] Although Ca^{2+}-dependent conduction is generally considered to be slow, this value is still 10-fold higher than the lowest values observed during cell-to-cell uncoupling and significantly higher than the values observed in the atrioventricular node. Comparison of the role of membrane excitability with the role of gap-junctional coupling in propagation therefore suggests that *conduction safety* is affected differently by changes in these two parameters, and that only cell-to-cell uncoupling or a high degree of discontinuity in tissue architecture[22] can lead to very slow conduction. Although the notion of the *margin of safety* seems to be intuitively clear, several quantitative formulations do exist in the literature. Shaw and Rudy[12] have recently presented a definition (see appendix of reference 12) that can account for most basic observations made with either reducing excitability or cell-to-cell uncoupling. As illustrated in Figure 3, the initial decrease of θ with cell-to-cell uncoupling is associated with an increase in the margin of safety (single chain of equal cells). Only in the end stage of uncoupling does the margin of safety decrease rapidly, concomitantly with a further rapid decrease of θ and formation of conduction block. Figure 3 also indicates that the very low velocities reached with cell-to-cell uncoupling are critically dependent on the presence of I_{Ca} (see discussion below).

As suggested in early studies by Joyner[23] and Rudy and Quan,[15] the *marked* change in θ with cell-to-cell uncoupling and the transient increase in the margin of safety is related to the *discontinuous nature* of propagation, i.e., to the fact that the increased resistance in the intracellular space during uncoupling is confined to the connexins while the cytoplasmic resistance remains low. The basic principles of discontinuous conduction were simulated early on by Joyner[23] with a chain of excitable elements. In this chain, as illustrated in Figure 4, a number of N elements were coupled to each other by low resistances R', and each group of N elements was cou-

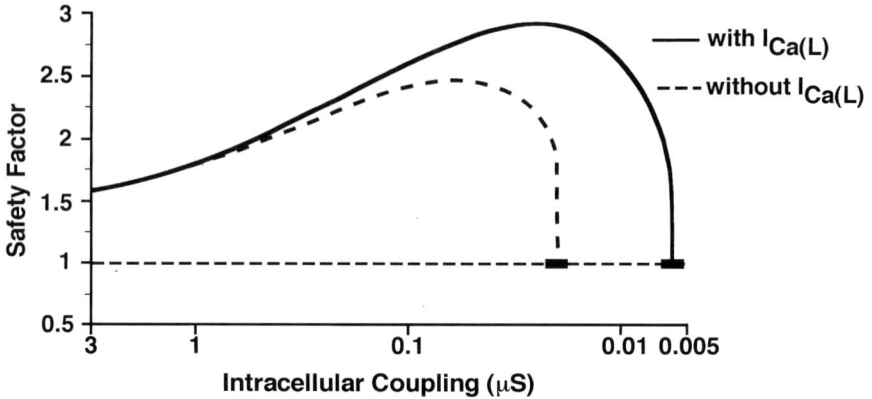

Figure 3. Change of the safety factor (SF) of propagation with increasing cell-to-cell uncoupling. Results of computer simulation of propagation in a cell chain. Change of SF as a function decreasing cell-to-cell conductance. Note initial increase of SF and subsequent decrease until block occurs (at very low velocities of a few cm/s). Note that in absence of I_{Ca}, block occurs at a higher degree of cell-to-cell coupling, demonstrating that I_{Ca} is necessary to maintain propagation in a markedly uncoupled state. Reproduced, with permission, from reference 12.

pled to the next group by a higher resistance R'. In such a system, the macroscopic or overall longitudinal resistance R per unit length (given by all high and low resistors in series) can be changed independently from the degree of discontinuity. The changes of θ^2 in such a system, as a function of the overall resistance R, is shown in the lower panel of Figure 4 for three different degrees of discontinuities. If discontinuities are absent, the θ^2 decreases linearly, as predicted by the square root relationship for propagation along continuous cables (see introduction). With a relatively low degree of discontinuity, the decrease of θ is qualitatively similar, but, for a given overall resistance R, the value of θ is less. Importantly, increasing the degree of discontinuity beyond a critical point by rising R' changes the conduction behavior (lowest curve on Fig. 4): in this case, conduction is only present within a certain range of overall resistances R while the parameters determining the left and the right extremes of the curves lead to propagation block. In the case of the left extreme, the left position on the abscissa is determined by a very high value of the resistance R' and a large number of N. In this case, R' is so high that the local current flow from one element of low resistance of length N to the other (see inset of Fig. 4) is too low to maintain propagation. Leaving the value of R' constant and decreasing the number of excitable elements N (which is also equivalent to decreasing the distance between two subsequent high resistors) suddenly establishes successful propagation, although the overall value of longitudinal resistance R has increased. This seemingly paradoxical behavior occurs because of electronic interaction between the high-resistance obstacles formed by R', which augments with decreasing N. This electrotonic interaction partially prevents the local current from flowing through the subsequent R'. As a consequence, in a given low-resistance compartment, more local current will flow through the membrane elements and exert an

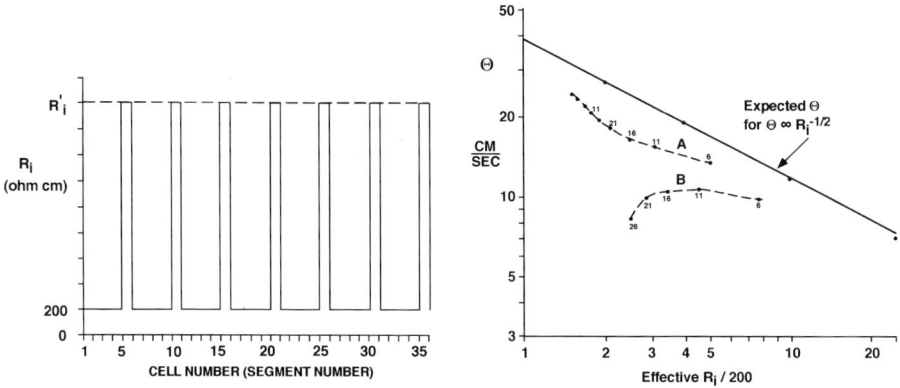

Figure 4. Effects of resistive discontinuities on propagation. *Left:* A row of simulated excitable elements (abscissa denotes element number) is separated by resistors. A number (N) of elements is connected by resistors of low value (200 Ωcm). In turn, each group of N elements is connected to the next group by a single resistor, R'_i, of high value. Discontinuity at a constant value of effective longitudinal resistance can be changed by the simultaneous increase of N and R'_i. *Right:* Effects of resistive discontinuities on conduction velocity (θ). Propagation is simulated in the model shown in the upper panel as a function of the overall or effective resistance R_i. The solid line depicts the decrease of δ in *a continuous cable* where $\theta^2 \sim 1/R_i$ (so-called "square root relationship"). In *curve A,* the value for the high resistor, R'_i, is 5000 Ωcm. The numbers on the curve denote the number of elements N. Decreasing the number N in each element simply moves the high resistors closer together, thereby increasing overall resistance R_i, and consequently, decreasing θ. In *curve B,* the degree of discontinuity is higher, because R'_i is 10,000 Ωcm. Note that the behavior of curve B is biphasic. Similarly to the other curves, θ decreases if the number N is lowered. In contrast to the other curves, block also occurs at the left extreme, that is if N is greater than 26. This seemingly paradoxical behavior, i.e., that a leftward movement on the abscissa or a lowering of the overall resistance can produce block, is explained by interaction of the repetitively spaced high-resistance obstacles. Reproduced, with permission, from reference 23.

excitatory action. Up to a given limit, therefore, decreasing the interval between R′ or increasing overall resistance R produces safer, albeit slower conduction. Beyond this limit, the decrease of N within a given low-resistance compartment decreases the local current flowing through R′ so much that inactivation of depolarizing currents and block results (right extreme of curve III on Fig. 4). As mentioned above, discontinuous conduction is also associated with a change in the activation profile of excitable elements. Increasing the degree of discontinuity, e.g., by increasing gap-junctional resistance in a cell chain, concentrates activation delays to the gap junctions while the excitable elements representing a cell are activated almost simultaneously. Since this process is associated with an overall decrease of propagation velocity, large activation delays result between single cells. These delays can exceed the duration of the upstroke of a transmembrane action potential. In this case, the action potentials in a given element ("driver" element) may already be shifted to their plateau level at the instant the threshold for activation in the next element ("follower" element) is reached.[24] During this early plateau phase, I_{Ca} is necessary to maintain local current flow (and to assure propagation) because I_{Na}

is already largely inactivated during this phase of the action potential. This explains why propagation becomes dependent upon I_{Ca} at advanced stages of electrical cell-to-cell uncoupling (see Fig. 3, lower panel). It illustrates a basic feature of discontinuous excitable systems, namely that membrane properties (membrane currents) and network properties (cell-to-cell coupling) *interact.*

In this section, the main features of discontinuous conduction in a cellular network are discussed on the basis of simple models related to the discontinuous electrical properties of cell chains or strands. Importantly, such theoretical models are scale-independent, i.e., they can be applied not only to cellular networks, but also to interactions between groups of cells (cell strands, cell layers), as discussed in the next paragraph.

Discontinuous Conduction: Role of Obstacles and Expansions

Discontinuities in cardiac structure that have an impact on propagation occur in many regions of the heart. The atria are characterized by marked trabeculation, the specific ventricular conduction system is composed of a network of excitable tissue, and the ventricles are organized in layers of tissue bridged by muscle strands with each showing a distinct fiber orientation.[25] In pathological settings, discontinuities are present in tissue surviving infarction[10] and are also likely to have an impact on propagation in fibrosis associated with age[9] and, probably, hypertrophy and failure. Although such tissue discontinuities may assume multiple shapes, their impact on propagation is likely to be similar. Figure 5 shows schematically the types of tissue discontinuities that have been studied in both theoretical and experimental studies and that are considered important for explaining initiation and maintenance of cardiac arrhythmias.[26–32] Common to all these discontinuities is the fact that, within the distance of electrotonic interaction, the geometrical properties of the tissue change in a way that results in either convergence or divergence of local current. The lower panel of Figure 5 illustrates the simulated changes in conduction velocity at a so-called expansion site and at an "isthmus site." In both cases, the current-to-load mismatch at such tissue discontinuities results in a marked divergence of local circuit current with "*curved*" isochrones beyond the site of current-to-load mismatch and an associated depression of conduction velocity. At a critical geometry and, accordingly, a critical degree of current-to-load mismatch, conduction block results.[33] If the geometrical discontinuity is asymmetrical (Fig. 5), conduction block will be unidirectional. Conduction block will not be located at the site of the abrupt geometrical discontinuity but at a small distance beyond, where the critically small curvature of the wave front will exclude maintenance of propagation. This indicates that the biophysical rules governing wave rotation in continuous excitable structures (devoid of obstacles) and in discontinuous tissue share close similarities. For conduction block to occur, the critical diameter of a 2-dimensional strand emerging into a large tissue area (in the presence of a small "taper" at the transition site) was approximately 50 μm in both experimental and theoretical studies.[30,31,34]

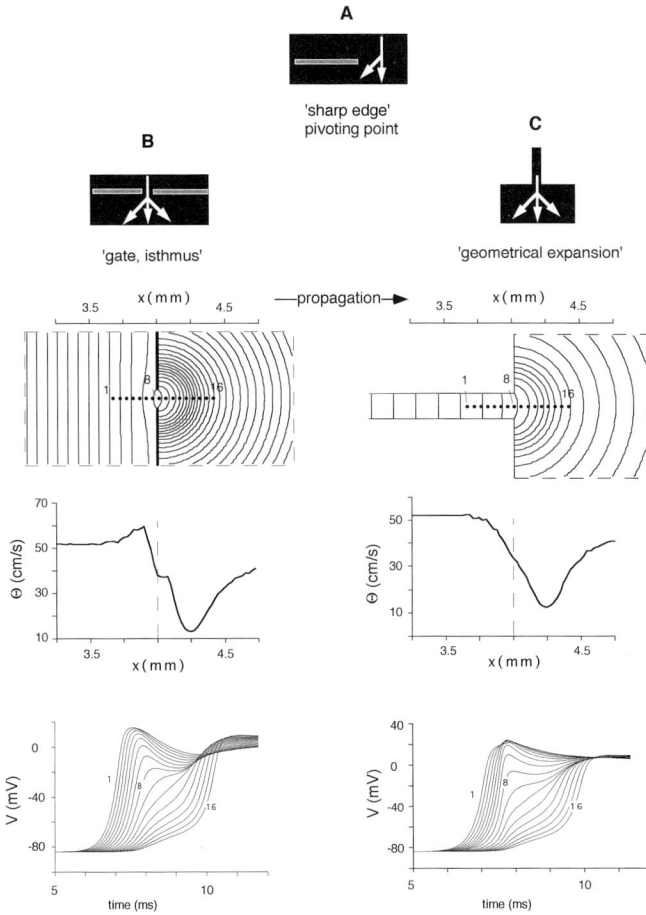

Figure 5. *Top:* Schematic presentation of different types of 2-dimensional tissue discontinuities. Arrows denote spread of local circuit current in the wave front of propagation with divergence at the discontinuity. *Bottom left:* Simulation of propagation through *isthmus*. *Bottom right:* Simulation of propagation across *geometrical expansion*. In both parts the upper graphs illustrate propagation spread by means of isochrones. The middle graphs depict the conduction velocity profile along the axis given by the dotted line in the upper part, and the lower graphs show the simulated action potentials from the dots (sites 1 through 16) in the upper graph. Reproduced, with permission, from reference 31.

Importantly, the propagation behavior across tissue discontinuities is not static, i.e., not solely a function of the geometrical arrangement of the cellular network per se, but it also depends on the underlying state of excitability and cell-to-cell coupling. Obviously with decreasing depolarizing strength of the excitation wave front (decreasing I_{Na}) the critical strand width or critical isthmus width diminishes.[31] This is likely to explain the finding of Cabo et al.[27] that the occurrence of propagation block at an isthmus or, accordingly, the critical isthmus width for occurrence of block, is dependent on excitation frequency. During a tachycardia, a wave front arriving at an isthmus will conduct or block the impulse depending on the state of excitability of the cells, which in turn will depend on the previous excitation intervals. According to whether an impulse conducts across such an isthmus, the next pathlength of the reentry circle and, concomitantly, the duration of the next circle will change. Consequently to this change in frequency of the tachycardia, propagation at the particular isthmus during the subsequent cycle, and accordingly at all other tissue discontinuities, will be changed further. This scenario emphasizes the contribution of *interactions* between membrane properties and structure to electrical instability.

Interaction between discontinuous propagation and cell-to-cell coupling has been shown in both computer simulations and experiments and is illustrated in Figure 6.[30,35] In these experiments, abrupt tissue expansions were grown by patterning cell cultures in such a way that narrow strands produced unidirectional block under conditions of normal superfusion. Subsequently, the cultures were superfused with the uncoupling agent palmitoleic acid. During superfusion, bidirectional conduction was established, which then, at the point of total cell-to-cell uncoupling, resulted in complete bidirectional conduction block. During washout of the uncoupling agent, the propagation behavior of the discontinuity again changed from total bidirectional block to transient bidirectional conduction block and, eventually, to control unidirectional block. Both experiments and simulations showed that the effect was produced by the partial uncoupling of the cells at the expansion which prevented the local current from being dispersed laterally (see also Fig. 4), thereby reducing the degree of current-to-load mismatch. These seemingly paradoxical findings suggest that the effects of cell-to-cell uncoupling on propagation and on arrhythmias are difficult to predict. First, reduction of propagation velocity by cell-to-cell uncoupling decreases the wavelength of excitation. Accordingly, it reduces the size of a reentrant circuit and enhances the likelihood that reentry will occur. Second, partial cell-to-cell uncoupling in tissue exhibiting marked geometrical discontinuities (e.g., increased trabeculation, fibrosis, scars, branching fibers, etc.) is predicted to attenuate the role of these discontinuities in the establishment of unidirectional conduction blocks and, consequently, to decrease the propensity for arrhythmias.

The degree of tissue discontinuity (very similarly to the degree of cell-to-cell coupling, as discussed above) also determines the role of depolarizing currents (I_{Na} versus I_{Ca}) in propagation.[34] This is shown for an abrupt tissue expansion, in Figure 7. In expansions with a moderate current-to-load mismatch (conduction delay <1 ms during control conditions), localized superfusion of the strand segment with TTX produced unidirectional, anterograde propagation block, while superfusion with nifedipine had no effect. By contrast, in expansions with marked current-to-load mismatch (conduction delay >1 ms during control conditions), conduction was produced by blocking $I_{Ca,L}$ with nifedipine but leaving I_{Na} unaffected. Accordingly, in expansions with extreme discontinuities which exhibited unidirectional block during control conditions, bidirectional conduction was established by enhancing $I_{Ca,L}$ with Bay K. This indicates that, very similarly to the state of advanced cell-to-cell uncoupling, flow of $I_{Ca,L}$ is essential for successful propagation at sites of local conduction delays

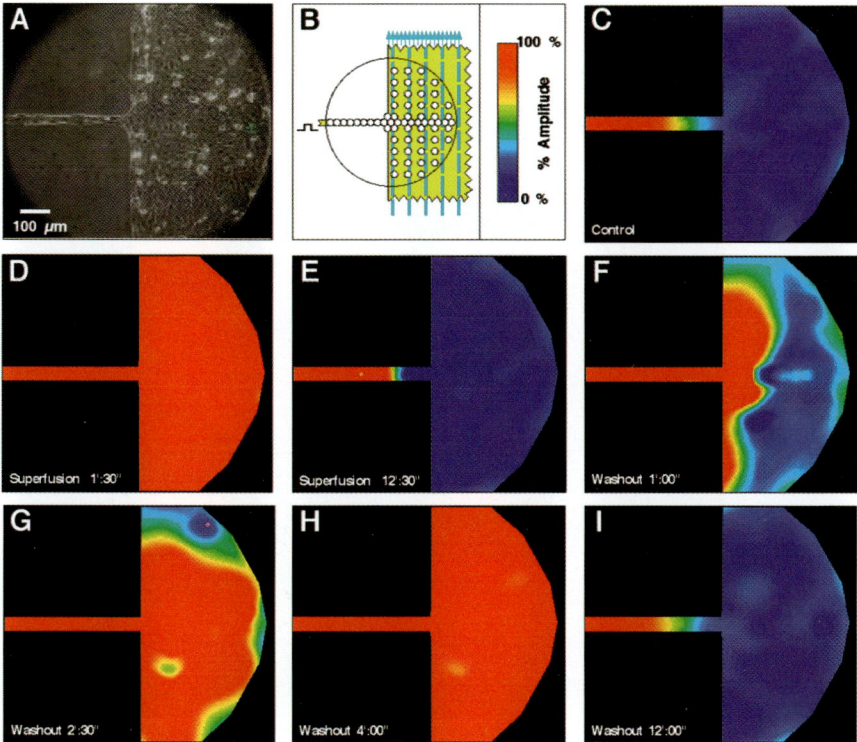

Figure 6. Reversal of unidirectional block to bidirectional conduction by partial cell-to-cell uncoupling. Unidirectional block in patterned cell cultures (**A**) is produced by current-to-load mismatch at a geometrical expansion, i.e., an insertion of a small cell strand into a large tissue mass. The degree of electrical cell-to-cell coupling in the large area can be changed by application of a blocking agent (palmitoleic acid, 10 µmol/L) through local superfusion (yellow area, **B**). During control (**C**), excitation (red) after stimulation of the strand is observed only in the small strand, while the unidirectional block leaves the large area at rest (blue), because of current-to-load mismatch at the expansion. Application of the uncoupling agent reverses block to bidirectional conduction during partial cell-to-cell uncoupling (**D**) and block is obviously observed again after total uncoupling (**E**). Washout of the uncoupling agent establishes conduction again transiently (**F** through **H**), while unidirectional block is observed after completion of washout. Recordings were performed using the optical dye 8-di-ANEPPS. Reproduced, with permission, from reference 35.

caused by tissue discontinuities. Such findings may also attribute a new role to drugs that inhibit $I_{Ca,L}$ in tissue with marked discontinuities, e.g., in infarct scars.

Anisotropic Conduction

The anisotropic architecture of the heart has important impacts on its electrical properties. Propagation velocity is higher in the longitudinal (θ_L) than in the transverse (θ_T) direction, the anisotropy velocity ratio, θ_L/θ_T ranging from about 10 to 2.2 in different regions of the hearts (see refer-

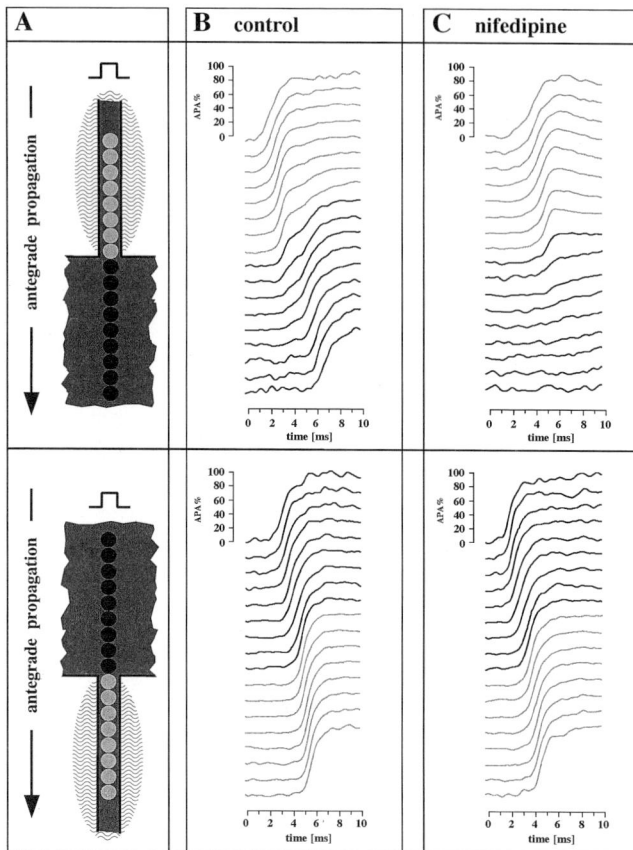

Figure 7. Unidirectional block at a geometrical tissue expansion: the role of Ca^{2+} inward current. **A.** Schematic representation of a cultured cell monolayer with geometrical expansion and overlaid photodiodes during antegrade (*top*) and retrograde (*bottom*) conduction. **B** and **C.** Action potential upstrokes recorded using a voltage-sensitive dye in control conditions (B) and after administration of 5 μmol/L nifedipine. In control conditions, the antegrade propagation was characterized by biphasic upstrokes and local slowing of conduction at the expansion (B). The blockage of Ca^{2+} current with nifedipine produced antegrade conduction block (C), indicating that flow of $I_{Ca,L}$ was essential for maintaining propagation at the site of the discontinuity. The retrograde propagation was successful in both cases. Reproduced, with permission, from reference 34.

ences 36 and 37). In most regions of the adult normal heart, gap junctions are concentrated at the end while the lateral connections are more scarce.[38,39] Moreover, most connective tissue and the larger portion of the microvascular tree is oriented in parallel to the long axis of cardiac fibers. This predicts that all the specific features of discontinuous propagation, as discussed above, will become more prominent during transverse than during longitudinal propagation. A further effect of anisotropy is related to the observation that the resistance of the *intracellular space* (r_i) is strongly dependent on the angle of current flow relative to fiber orientation while this is less the case for the extracellular resistance (r_o). As discussed in chapter 19 of this book, the dependence of the ratio r_i/r_o on fiber direction is important to explain the effects of extracellular stimuli and field shocks on the myocardium.[40]

Anisotropic Propagation in Cellular Networks. The effects of cellular anisotropy on propagation have been studied in cell cultures and in computer simulations. In a theoretical study[19] parameters simulating networks, properties were derived from a structural analysis in the dog heart.[41] In the cell culture studies,[42,43] the anisotropic structure was obtained by directed growth of neonatal rat myocytes and propagation was assessed by high-resolution optical mapping of transmembrane potential. While connectivity in such cultures (number of cells connected in average to an individual myocyte) is close to connectivity in vivo, the cells differ in shape (fusiform versus brick-stonelike) and gap junction pattern (regular gap junction distribution along cell circumference) from adult tissue (see reference 43). In computer simulations, the subcellular changes in excitation pattern, activation of I_{Na}, and maximal upstroke velocity (dV/dt_{max}) of the action potential upstroke changed according to the rules of discontinuous conduction[19]: during longitudinal conduction, activation was slower and dV/dt_{max} was lower at the proximal cell pole (relative to the propagation wave front) than at the distal pole. Moreover, more I_{Na} was activated at the proximal cell pole than at the distal pole. Similar observations were made during transverse propagation, where dV/dt_{max} was lowest at the insertion points of the lateral junctions and highest at the site of intracellular wave collision. Overall undulating profiles of dV/dt_{max} were observed at a cellular level along and in transverse direction to the main fiber axis.

In an early work, Spach and Dolber.[44] showed that discontinuous conduction expressing itself either in discontinuities in action potential upstroke or in the extracellular electrogram can occur with age. The morphological counterpart of this phenomenon is a relatively dense and fine fibrosis leading to separation of lateral gap junctions. This remodeling, which, by virtue of the alignment of the connective tissue with the myocytes, is highly anisotropic, is thought to underlie the phenomenon of anisotropic reentry observed in the atrial crista terminalis.[9,45] With multisite optical recording of transmembrane potentials, it became possible to study experimentally the effect of small, anisotropically oriented, resistive obstacles on propagation, as illustrated in Figure 8.[43] In this figure, longitudinal propagation in an anisotropically grown tissue culture across a culture segment including a large obstacle (>100 μm) produced only a minor effect on the isochronal pattern, on the pattern of dV/dt_{max}, and on the shape of the action potential upstroke. By contrast, current-to-load mismatch during transverse propagation at the end of the obstacle produced local slowing of propagation (wave front curving), a discontinuity in the action potential upstroke, and a decrease in dV/dt_{max}. Very similar observations were made in experiments in which the resistive obstacles were present because of localized inhomogeneous gap junction expressions.[43] An example of such a case is shown in Figure 9. Panel A shows a dense tissue culture in which one of the myocytes is connected to its neighbors by only a single detectable junction at the left cell pole, as illustrated by the immunohistochemical staining of connexin43. Accordingly, during

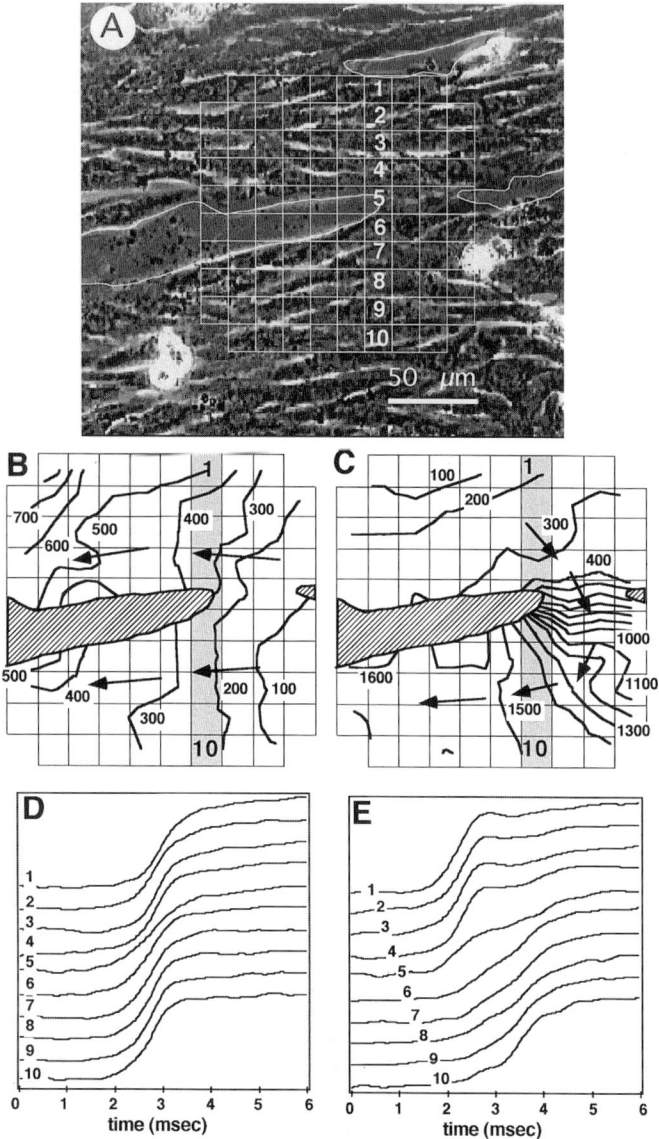

Figure 8. Effect of microscopic resistive barriers on propagation. **A.** Phase-contrast image of a cell culture (neonatal rat myocytes) with the overlaid diode array. Action potential upstrokes are measured at each diode location. The numbers 1 through 10 on the diode array correspond to the locations of the signals shown in **D** and **E**. In **D** and **C**, the location of these signals is indicated by the gray area. The two clefts in the central area (outlined in white) form a narrow isthmus of 40 μm. Activation maps of longitudinal and transverse conduction are shown in panels **B** and **C**, respectively. Note slowing and deviation of the wave front at the isthmus. Numbers denote separation of isochrones by 100 μs. Selected recordings of action potential upstrokes during longitudinal and transverse conduction are shown in panels **D** and **E**, respectively. Discontinuities in the action potential upstrokes occur at the expansion site during transverse propagation. Reproduced, with permission, from reference 43.

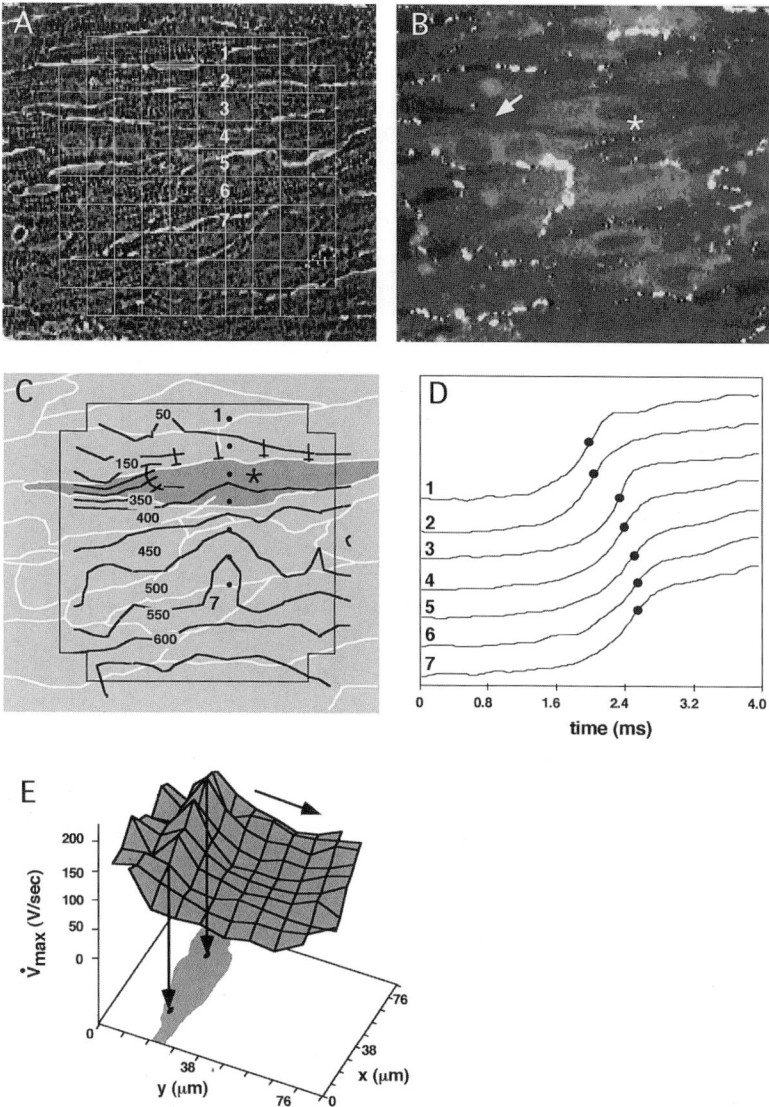

Figure 9. Effect of inhomogeneous gap junction distribution on activation spread. **A** and **B.** Phase-contrast and fluorescent images (connexin43 [Cx43] immunolabeling) of the same cell region. Asterisk depicts a central myocyte with almost no expression of Cx43. The only Cx43 fluorescence can be seen at the left end of this cell (arrow). **C, D,** and **E.** Isochronal activation map, selected optical recordings (voltage-sensitive dye: RH237), and distribution of dV/dt_{max} during transverse propagation. Dark area corresponds to the myocyte with no Cx43 expression. Note block of propagation at the upper cell border and excitation of the myocyte from the left end. The highest values of dV/dt_{max} are recorded within this myocyte where ionic depolarizing current cannot escape because of the lack of gap junctions. Reproduced, with permission, from reference 43.

transverse propagation, the impulse was deviated, it collided with the upper cell border, and it entered the cell from only one side. Since the membrane current produced by the cell was prevented from flowing to its neighbors because of the almost entire lack of gap junctions, all the current was used to charge the membrane capacity locally, and accordingly, dV/dt_{max} values of these cells were highest.

Although measurements performed with high-resolution optical mapping can elegantly demonstrate wave front deviation and current-to-load mismatch, extrapolation to microreentry must be made with care. As mentioned in the first section of this chapter, the lowest velocities associated with a decrease in membrane excitability are in the order of 15 cm/s. With a refractory period of 100 ms, this yields a wavelength of excitation of 15 mm, which would require relatively long obstacles (several millimeters) for reentry to occur. In the case where there is enough I_{Ca} activated, uncoupling of gap junctions may reduce velocity to approximately 1 cm/s or even below. In this case the critical length of such obstacles to produce microreentry would amount to a few hundred micrometers. However, uncoupling, as previously mentioned, would also reduce the effect of such obstacles to produce unidirectional block,[35] a key requirement for the initiation of reentry. Certainly, other effects of tissue anisotropy, such as the production of virtual electrodes and wave front singularities with relatively high local stimulus strengths, should be considered as a cause of reentry as well.

Summary

The combined the use of 2-dimensional patterned cultures of neonatal myocytes and multisite high-resolution optical mapping of transmembrane potential allows the experimental assessment of the role of gap junctions and tissue geometry in impulse conduction and of the mechanisms of unidirectional conduction block and microreentry. Such studies are especially suited for comparison with computer modeling of propagation, because of the possibility of varying the geometrical arrangement of the cultured cells and adopting it to various simulated shapes. However, distinct differences exist between tissue cultures and real tissue (2-dimensional versus 3-dimensional tissue, absence of microvasculature, neonatal cell type and connexin pattern, etc.) Therefore, conclusive knowledge about arrhythmia mechanisms should be drawn from experiments carried out with a variety of experimental models including measurements in isolated tissue and whole hearts.

Acknowledgments: We would like to thank Mrs. Lilly Lehmann-Bircher for her help with the figures.

References

1. Lewis T. *The Mechanism and Graphic Registration of the Heart Beat/* London: Shaws & Sons; 1920.
2. Durrer D, Van Dam RT, Freud GE, et al. Total excitation of the isolated human heart. *Circulation* 1970;41:895–912.

3. Coraboeuf E, Weidmann S. Potentiel de repos et potentiel d'action du muscle cardiaque, mesures a l'aide d'électrodes intracellulaires. *Comptes Rendus des Séances de la Société de Biologie* 1949;143:1329–1331.
4. Jack JJB, Noble D, Tsien RW. *Electric Current Flow in Excitable Cells.* Oxford: Clarendon Press; 1975.
5. Walton MK, Fozzard HA. The conducted action potential: Models and comparison to experiments. *Biophys J* 1983;44:9–26.
6. Kléber AG, Riegger CB, Janse MJ. Electrical uncoupling and increase of extracellular resistance after induction of ischemia in isolated, arterially perfused rabbit papillary muscle. *Circ Res* 1987;61:271–279.
7. Riegger CB, Alperovich G, Kléber AG. Effect of oxygen withdrawal on active and passive electrical properties of arterially perfused rabbit ventricular muscle. *Circ Res* 1989;64:532–541.
8. Buchanan JW, Saito T, Gettes LS. The effects of antiarrhythmic drugs, stimulation frequency, and potassium-induced resting membrane potential changes on conduction velocity and dV/dt_{max} in guinea pig myocardium. *Circ Res* 1985;56:696–703.
9. Spach MS, Josephson ME. Initiating reentry: The role of nonuniform anisotropy in small circuits. *J Cardiovasc Electrophysiol* 1994;5:182–209.
10. De Bakker JMT, Van Capelle FJL, Janse MJ, et al. Slow conduction in the infarcted human heart—zigzag course of activation. *Circulation* 1993;88:915–926.
11. Luo CH, Rudy Y. A dynamic model of the cardiac ventricular action potential. 1. Simulations of ionic currents and concentration changes. *Circ Res* 1994;74:1071–1096.
12. Shaw RM, Rudy Y. Ionic mechanisms of propagation in cardiac tissue. Roles of the sodium and L-type calcium currents during reduced excitability and decreased gap junction coupling. *Circ Res* 1997;81:727–741.
13. Rohr S. Determination of impulse conduction characteristics at a microscopic scale in patterned growth heart cell cultures using multisite optical mapping of transmembrane voltage. *J Cardiovasc Electrophysiol* 1995;6:551–568.
14. Fast VG, Kléber AG. Microscopic conduction in cultured strands of neonatal rat heart cells measured with voltage-sensitive dyes. *Circ Res* 1993;73:914–925.
15. Rudy Y, Quan W. Propagation delays across cardiac gap junctions and their reflection in extracellular potentials: A simulation study. *J Cardiovasc Electrophysiol* 1991;2:299–315.
16. Rohr S, Schölly DM, Kléber AG. Patterned growth of neonatal rat heart cells in culture: Morphological and electrophysiological characterization. *Circ Res* 1991;68:114–130.
17. Weingart R, Maurer P. Action potential transfer in cell pairs isolated from adult rat and guinea pig ventricles. *Circ Res* 1988;63:72–80.
18. Leon LJ, Roberge FA. Directional characteristics of action potential propagation in cardiac muscle. A model study. *Circ Res* 1991;69:378–395.
19. Spach MS, Heidlage JF. The stochastic nature of cardiac propagation at a microscopic level—electrical description of myocardial architecture and its application to conduction. *Circ Res* 1995;76:366–380.
20. Rohr S, Kucera JP, Kléber AG. Slow conduction in cardiac tissue: I. Effects of a reduction of excitability versus a reduction in cell-to-cell coupling on microconduction. *Circ Res* 1998;83:781–794.
21. Kléber AG, Janse MJ, Wilms-Schopmann FJG, et al. Changes in conduction velocity during acute ischemia in ventricular myocardium of the isolated porcine heart. *Circ Res* 1986;73:189–198.
22. Kucera JP, Kléber AG, Rohr S. Slow conduction in cardiac tissue: II. Effects of branching tissue geometry. *Circ Res* 1998;83:795–805.
23. Joyner RW. Effects of the discrete pattern of electrical coupling on propagation through an electrical syncytium. *Circ Res* 1982;50:192–200.

24. Sugiura H, Joyner RW. Action potential conduction between guinea pig ventricular cells can be modulated by calcium current. *Am J Physiol* 1992; 263:H1591-H1604.
25. Le Grice IJ, Smaill BH, Chai LZ, et al. Laminar structure of the heart: Ventricular myocyte arrangement and connective tissue architecture in the dog. *Am J Physiol* 1995;38:H571–H582.
26. Dillon SM, Allessie MA, Ursell PC, Wit AL. Influences of anisotropic tissue structure on reentrant circuits in the epicardial border zone of subacute canine infarcts. *Circ Res* 1988;63:182–206.
27. Cabo C, Pertsov AM, Baxter WT, et al. Wave-front curvature as a cause of slow conduction and block in isolated cardiac muscle. *Circ Res* 1994;75:1014–1028.
28. Cabo C, Pertsov AM, Davidenko JM, et al. Vortex shedding as a result of turbulent electrical activity in cardiac muscle. *Biophys J* 1996;70:1105–1111.
29. Girouard SD, Pastore JM, Laurita KR, et al. Optical mapping in a new guinea pig model of ventricular tachycardia reveals mechanisms for multiple wavelengths in a single reentrant circuit. *Circulation* 1996;93:603–613.
30. Fast VG, Kléber AG. Cardiac tissue geometry as a determinant of unidirectional conduction block: Assessment of microscopic excitation spread by optical mapping in patterned cell cultures and in a computer model. *Cardiovasc Res* 1995;29:697–707.
31. Fast VG, Kléber AG. Block of impulse propagation at an abrupt tissue expansion: Evaluation of the critical strand diameter in 2- and 3-dimensional computer models. *Cardiovasc Res* 1995;30:449–459.
32. Rohr S, Salzberg BM. Characterization of impulse propagation at the microscopic level across geometrically defined expansions of excitable tissue: Multiple site optical recording of transmembrane voltage (MSORTV) in patterned growth heart cell cultures. *J Gen Physiol* 1994;104:287–309.
33. Fast VG, Kléber AG. Role of wavefront curvature in propagation of cardiac impulse. *Cardiovasc Res* 1997;33:258–271.
34. Rohr S, Kucera J. Involvement of the calcium inward current in cardiac impulse propagation: Induction of unidirectional conduction block by nifedipine and reversal by Bay K 8644. *Biophys J* 1996;72:754–766.
35. Rohr S, Kucera JP, Fast VG, Kléber AG. Paradoxical improvement of impulse conduction in cardiac tissue by partial cellular uncoupling. *Science* 1997; 275:841–844.
36. Goodman D, van der Steen ABM, van Dam RT. Endocardial and epicardial activation pathways of the canine right atrium. *Am J Physiol* 1971;220:1–11.
37. Spear JF, Michelson EL, Moore EN. Cellular electrophysiologic characteristics of chronically infarcted myocardium in dogs susceptible to sustained ventricular tachyarrhythmias. *J Am Coll Cardiol* 1983;1:1099–1110.
38. Saffitz JE, Kanter HL, Green KG, et al. Tissue-specific determinants of anisotropic conduction velocity in canine atrial and ventricular myocardium. *Circ Res* 1994;74:1065–1070.
39. Kanter H, Saffitz J, Beyer E. Cardiac myocytes express multiple gap junction proteins. *Circ Res* 1992;70:438–444.
40. Wikswo JP, Lin S-F, Abbas RA. Virtual electrode effect in cardiac tissue: A common mechanism for anodal and cathodal stimulation. *Biophys J* 1995; 69:2195–2210.
41. Hoyt RH, Cohen ML, Saffitz JE. Distribution and three-dimensional structure of intercellular junctions in canine myocardium. *Circ Res* 1989;64:563–574.
42. Fast VG, Kléber AG. Anisotropic conduction in monolayers of neonatal rat heart cells cultured on collagen substrate. *Circ Res* 1994;75:591–595.
43. Fast VG, Darrow BJ, Saffitz JE, Kléber AG. Anisotropic activation spread in heart cell monolayers assessed by high-resolution optical mapping: Role of tissue discontinuities. *Circ Res* 1996;79:115–127.

44. Spach MS, Dolber PC. Relating extracellular potentials and their derivatives to anisotropic propagation at a microscopic level in human cardiac muscle. Evidence for electrical uncoupling of side-to-side fiber connections with increasing age. *Circ Res* 1986;58:356–371.
45. Spach MS, Dolber PC, Heidlage JF. Influence of the passive anisotropic properties on directional differences in propagation following modification of the sodium conductance in human atrial muscle. A model of reentry based on anisotropic discontinuous propagation. *Circ Res* 1988;62:811–832.

Chapter 9

Optical Mapping of Impulse Propagation in the Atrioventricular Node: 1

Todor N. Mazgalev and Igor R. Efimov

Introduction

There are several novel modalities of imaging, which revolutionized biomedical research during the last decades of the 20th century. These modalities are based on different principles such as x-ray and positron emission tomography, ultrasound, nuclear magnetic resonance, and optical methods. Novel contrast agents allowed the extension of various imaging modalities from sophisticated structural imaging to dynamic functional imaging. Yet, only optical imaging has so far been able to shed light on intracellular- and cellular-level physiology, due to availability of a wide range of effective fluorescent dyes, and due to their spectroscopic methods of functional readout. These agents are designed to sense various parameters of biological systems, such as ion concentrations, proteins, functional states of the proteins, and local electrical fields within the cell and on its membrane. The latter are known as voltage-sensitive dyes.[1,2]

Voltage-sensitive dyes and optical imaging techniques[3] have become a commonly accepted tool in cardiac electrophysiological studies. These techniques excel due to the high spatial and temporal resolution, usually unachievable by alternative recording methods. On the other hand, the high degree of light scattering and absorption by cardiac tissue and blood has limited the depth of penetration, theoretically to 1 to 2 mm or less. Ideally, the techniques are most suitable to study electrical activity in thin layers of epicardial cells[4] or isolated cells and cellular cultures,[5] which can be considered 2 dimensional. Yet, in some cases, 3-dimensional information can be derived from the fluorescent images. The atrioventricular (AV) node is such a case due to its limited depth. The propagation of

This modified chapter was published in its original form in Atrial-AV Nodal Electrophysiology: A View from the Millennium, edited by Todor N. Mazgalev, PhD and Patrick J. Tchou, MD© 2000 Futura Publishing Company, Inc., Armonk, NY, and is published with permission.

From Rosenbaum DS, Jalife J (eds): *Optical Mapping of Cardiac Excitation and Arrhythmias.* ©Futura Publishing Co., Inc., Armonk, NY, 2001.

electrical impulses through the AV node has been intensively studied for many years in the basic electrophysiology laboratory.[6] In addition to the traditional electrocardiographic approach, direct catheter recordings from the endocardial surface along with the bundle of His electrogram have been used to study functional AV node properties in the clinic. Numerous studies have been also performed on isolated heart preparations. The advent of the glass microelectrodes permitted recording action potentials from individual AV node cells.[7] The addition of the cellular electrophysiological properties to the overall picture was of utmost importance and helped to describe in greater detail and depth the complexity of AV node propagation.

The application of microelectrodes and the parallel intensive morphological investigations shaped the modern view of the AV node as a multilayer 3-dimensional structure that contains several distinctly different types of cells. However, the pattern of propagation from one cellular subgroup to another and ultimately to the bundle of His is still not well understood. It might be surprising that almost 100 years after the fundamental morphological work of Tawara[8] we are still debating such "basic" questions as: Does the AV node conduct or oscillate? Where is the site of the predominant AV node delay? How exactly is the AV node engaged by the atrial wave fronts? The difficulties in answering these and many other questions are, in part, related to methodological limitations. Thus, while microelectrodes can record individual cellular responses, the simultaneous impalement of multiple (even more than two) microelectrodes is extremely difficult. Therefore, the global picture of AV node excitation is still unclear despite the persistent efforts of many investigators. The need for a new tool that would permit multisite cellular recordings and, ultimately, mapping of propagation has always been acknowledged. It was therefore logical to expect that optical imaging that has been successfully applied in other cardiac tissues would eventually be also applied in studies of AV nodal electrophysiology.

Since the majority of the cellular electrophysiological studies of the AV node have been performed on rabbit hearts, the techniques for preparing and maintaining flat-endocardial-surface preparations are well developed. Normal AV node conduction can be maintained in such preparations for many hours, and well-characterized reversible pharmacological interventions are routinely used, along with all standard pacing protocols similar to those applied clinically. Autonomic effects, both vagal and sympathetic, can also be evoked. Thus, optical imaging appears to be easily adaptable in such a well-established experimental framework.

The major challenge to an optical mapper of the AV node is the complex 3-dimensional structure of the node. Most of the electrical AV node mystery is hidden below the endocardial surface and this could be a major obstacle in studies of large animal hearts, e.g., dog, sheep, and human. The rabbit heart is a lucky exception. Not only is it reasonably well studied by other conventional methods, but its AV node is located just under the endocardial surface and, according to evidence from microelectrode and histological studies,[9] the deepest cellular layers are less than 500 μm from the endocardial surface. Therefore, we decided to explore the feasibility of recording optical signals from the rabbit AV node and to correlate them with the currently known electrophysiological properties. The goal of this chapter is to describe our initial experience with AV node optical imaging.[10,11] We hope that this will be useful for the future refinement of the techniques and as a guide for others who will be tempted to visualize the electrical propagation in this as important as amazing minute structure in the heart.

Methods for Investigating AV Node Physiology

The Atrial-AV Nodal Preparations

We performed experiments in vitro on atrial-AV nodal preparations obtained from the hearts of white New Zealand rabbits. The dissection procedure has been described previously.[10] The resulting preparation is shown in Figure 1. The preparation was superfused with modified oxygenated Tyrode's solution of the following composition (in mmol/L): NaCl 128.2, $CaCl_2$ 1.3, KCl 4.7, $MgCl_2$ 1.05, NaH_2PO_4 1.19, $NaHCO_3$ 25, and glucose 5.0. The temperature and pH were continuously maintained at $35 \pm 0.5°C$ and 7.30 ± 0.05, respectively.

Staining of the preparation was conducted using two different methods. Initially we used the coronary perfusion method. In this case, the heart before dissection was placed on a modified Langendorff apparatus and perfused retrogradely via the coronary arteries. A stock solution of the

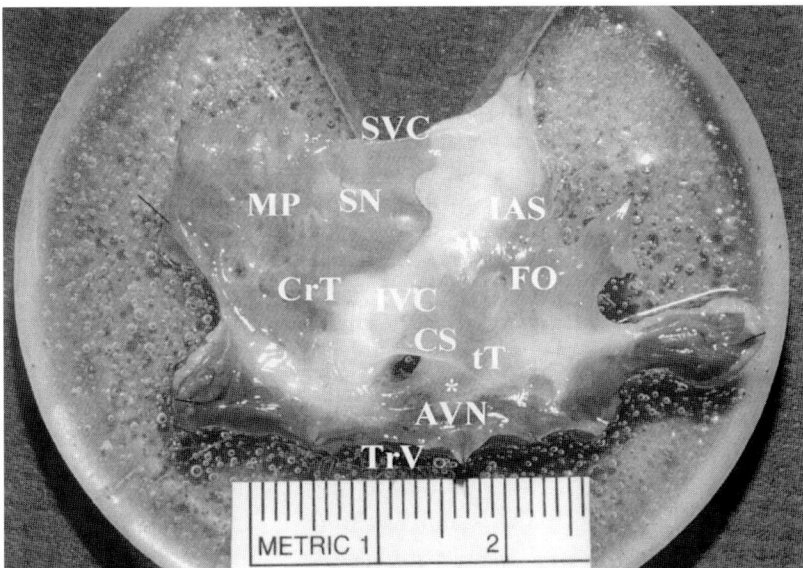

Figure 1. Photograph of the rabbit atrial atrioventricular nodal preparation. Shown are the sinoatrial node (SN), the atrioventricular nodal (AVN) region with the compact nodal region of the AV node (asterisk), the tricuspid valve (TrV), the superior vena cava (SVC), the interatrial septum (IAS), the right atrial appendage with the musculi pectinati (MP), the fossa ovalis (FO), the inferior vena cava (IVC), the crista terminalis (CrT), the opening of the coronary sinus (CS), and the tendon of Todaro (tT).

dye di-4-ANEPPS was prepared at concentration of 1 mg/mL and kept frozen at −20°C. The solvent was dimethyl sulfoxide (DMSO) + pluronic (4:1 weight ratio). The final staining solution was prepared immediately prior to staining. Following gentle warming, 1 mL of the dye stock solution was dissolved in 100 mL of oxygenated Tyrode's solution, yielding a final concentration of 20 μmol/L, and delivered to the heart via the aorta over 5 to 10 minutes. Alternatively 0.5 to 1 mL of the stock solution was gradually injected into the bubble trap above the cannula over 5 to 10 minutes, yielding a 10 to 20 μmol/L final concentration of the dye. The quality of staining was verified by acquiring optical action potentials from the epicardium of the atria and ventricles of the intact hearts.

We initially chose the staining procedure using coronary perfusion since it is well known that the AV nodal area is covered with a thin layer of connective tissue, which would make the staining by superfusion difficult. Indeed, Hewett et al.,[12] using a superfusion method of staining, had to apply the voltage-sensitive dye di-4-ANEPPS in concentration of 2 mmol/L. This concentration is 100 to 1000 times higher than concentrations used in other laboratories, which are in the range of 2 to 20 μmol/L.[13–16] Our experience shows that coronary perfusion allows the AV node to be stained with concentrations at which the toxic effects of the dye are acceptable while the quality of the optical signals (see later) is manageable.

Following the staining procedure and verification of optical signal quality, the heart was removed from the Langendorff apparatus and placed into a horizontal dissection chamber filled with oxygenated Tyrode's solution. Following a cross-sectional cut above the cardiac apex, a probe was inserted in the opening and guided upward through the right ventricle, the tricuspid valve, the right atrium, and the superior vena cava. Using the probe as a guide, the heart was opened with a pair of scissors along the atrial appendage to expose the endocardial surface of the right atrium. The ventricles were removed by a cut just below the AV ring and, by careful trimming, the left atrial and any remaining attached tissues were also discarded. The final preparation, shown in Figure 1, contained right atrial tissues consisting of the interatrial septum, the right atrial appendage with the musculi pectinati, the septal leaflet of the tricuspid valve, the central fibrous body, and small portion of the ventricular septum just below the bundle of His. Also depicted in Figure 1 are the fossa ovalis, inferior vena cava, the sinus node region, the crista terminalis, the opening of the coronary sinus, and the tendon of Todaro. The dotted line defines the triangle of Koch and the asterisk indicates the compact nodal region of the AV node. This preparation was pinned down on a thin silicon disk with the endocardial surface oriented up. It was transferred into a thermostatically controlled glass superfusion chamber, continuously superfused at a flow rate of 30 mL/min with the same Tyrode's solution as previously described, except for the addition of 10 to 12.5 mmol/L 2,3-butanedione monoxime (BDM), added to suppress contraction-induced distortion of optical action potentials. It is worth stressing that the use of BDM as an electromechanical uncoupler has frequently been discussed. Although it is being widely used in optical imaging studies, the possible side effects of BDM should not be ignored. We have performed separate studies to evaluate dose-dependent effects of BDM on AV node electrophysiology.[17] It has been concluded that, in concentrations of 10 to 15 mmol/L, BDM has no detrimental effects on the conduction through the AV node and, in contrast, assures stable performance over extended periods while virtually eliminating the undesired mechanical contractions.

Recently, we have adopted a new staining procedure, which further reduced the toxic effects of the dye. Now we dissect first and then stain by superfusion. However, unlike Hewett et al.,[12] we use a lower concentration of 1 to 2 μmol/L, while staining for a longer period—40 to 60 minutes. We found that, due to a slow diffusion of the dye, it takes 20 to 30 minutes to stain deeper structures such as the compact node.[18]

Under these conditions the AV nodal preparations survived and conducted impulses in a stable manner for at least 8 hours. However, due to washout and/or photobleaching of the voltage-sensitive dye, imaging could best be performed during the first 1 to 3 hours. This was a problem at the initial stage of our research, since restaining by perfusion was impossible after dissection. Now this limitation is gone, because restaining by superfusion can be done when needed. In addition, some dye washout from the superficial layers, by reducing the optical signals generated there, allows obtaining better signals from deeper structures not masked by optical signals from the superficial structures.[18]

Electrode Recordings and Pacing

Small bipolar electrodes were custom made from Teflon-isolated silver or platinum-iridium wire with an interelectrode distance of 0.5 mm. The two bipoles were mounted 1 mm apart on a common carrier, forming a compact quadruple recording/stimulating electrode. We recorded electrograms from the crista terminalis and interatrial septum inputs to the AV node as well as from the bundle of His. Pacing was applied at the recording sites or, in some experiments, at the high atrium or the mid septum.

Several pacing protocols were used. Typically, a basic drive at a 300-ms cycle length was applied for 20 beats (S1 beats) and then a premature beat S2 was delivered with variable S1-S2 coupling interval. Incremental pacing at progressively faster basic drive was used to observe Wenckebach periodicity. Finally, random atrial pacing was used to simulate atrial fibrillation. This was achieved by delivering a train of stimuli with coupling intervals randomly changing in the range 75 to 150 ms. The pacing protocols were executed by a computer-controlled programmable stimulator.

Standard glass microelectrodes were filled with 3 mol/L KCl and had resistance in the range of 20 to 30 MΩ. They were attached to the input probes of high-impedance amplifiers (AxoProbe, Axon Instruments, Foster City, CA) and were "floating"—mounted to permit stable long-term impalement. The input probes rested on precision step-motor micromanipulators permitting vertical movement in 5-μm steps.

Optical Mapping System

A schematic drawing of the system is shown in Figure 2. Fluorescence was excited by light produced by a 250-W quartz tungsten halogen

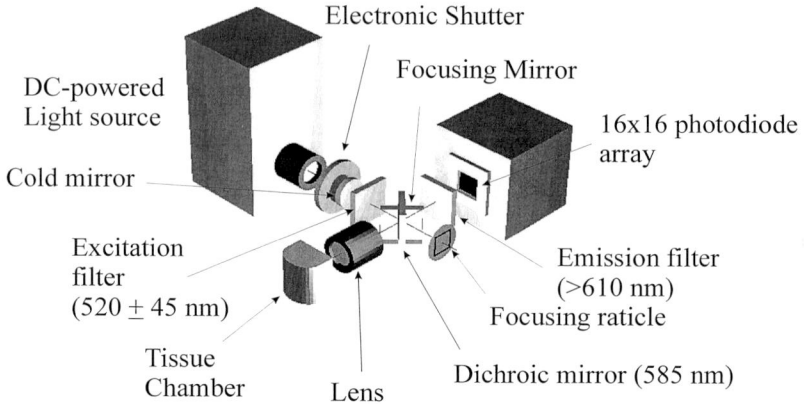

Figure 2. Schematic presentation of the optical set-up. The atrioventricular nodal preparation was stained with di-4-ANEPPS and was pinned down in a horizontal superfusion chamber. Fluorescence was induced by an excitation direct current light source (Oriel Corp.) with 520±45-nm filter. Emission light was collected by a lens and passed through a 610-nm cut-off filter. The light was then collected and converted into electric current by a 16x16 photodiode array (Hamamatsu). Each current signal was converted into voltage with 256 current-to-voltage converters (Hamamatsu), amplified with second stage amplifiers (Yale University, New Haven, CT), and fed into a PC-based data acquisition system (not shown).

direct current light source (Oriel Corp., Stratford, CT). Two variations of light delivery were explored. In an initial system (not shown) the excitation light passed through a 520±45-nm interference filter (Omega Optical, Battleboro, VT) and was guided by liquid-filled light guide to the surface of the preparation. In a later variation (shown in Fig. 2) the excitation light was reflected from a dichroic mirror and reached the preparation through the optical lens. The emitted light was collected by a 50-mm lens (1:1.4, AF Nikkor, Nikon, Torrance, CA). It was then passed through a cut-off filter (>610 nm, Schott Glass, Duryea, PA) and was focused on the sensing area of the 16×16 photodiode array (C4675, Hamamatsu, Bridgewater, NJ), either directly or after passing through the dichroic mirror (depending on which of the above variations was used). The optical apparatus and photodiode array were mounted on a rail that, in turn, was mounted on a heavy-duty ball-bearing boom-stand. This design permitted easy readjustment of focusing on necessary areas of the preparation with the required magnification. The magnification could be varied from 150×150 μm² to 750×750 μm² per diode. Since the photodiode array does not permit direct observation of the preparation, focusing was done using a black-and-white charge coupled device camera, which provided adequate spatial resolution. This optical system allowed correlation of fluorescent recordings with anatomical landmarks with an accuracy of about 100 μm.

The emitted light was collected by the 256 photodiodes and the current of each diode passed through its individual I/V converter (operational amplifiers with 10 MΩ or 50 MΩ feedback resistors, Hamamatsu). The outputs of the first stage amplifiers were connected to 256 second stage amplifiers,[19] with a programmable gain of 1, 50, 200, 1000, and with several alternating current coupling time constants (not shown). A time constant of 30 seconds and automatic resetting of the amplifiers prior to data acquisition was used in order to achieve a sample-and-hold operational mode and remove the direct current component of the optical signals caused by the background fluorescence. Signals were filtered at a cut-off frequency of 1000 Hz by built-in Bessell filters. After amplification the signals were fed to a multiplexor and an analog-to-digital converter. We used two types of analog-to-digital converters: 1) DAP 3200/415e from MicroStar Laboratories (Bellevue, WA), and 2) PCI-6031E or PCE-6033E from National Instruments (Austin, TX). The sampling rate was 1000 to 3000 frames per second. Custom-developed data acquisition and analysis software was used. Figure 3 shows user interface of the software. Activation time points in individual optical action potentials, corresponding to the upstroke, were automatically determined using $(-dF/dt)_{max}$ criteria, where F was the fluorescent signal measured by each photodiode. Based on the calculated activation times, isochronal or grayscale maps were generated and analyzed.[20,21]

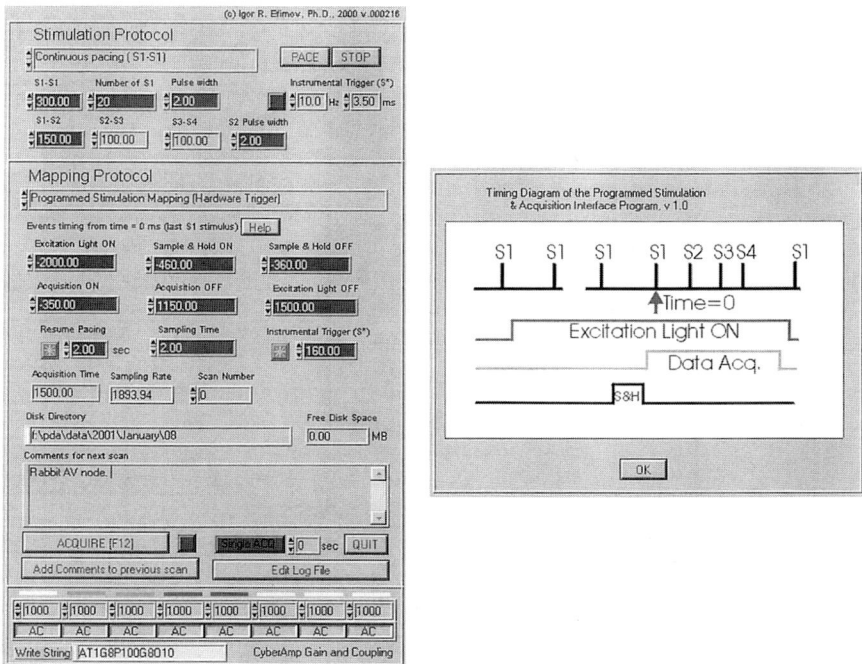

Figure 3. Data acquisition software interface. Computerized data acquisition system was controlled by a custom-made software based on LabVIEW (National Instruments). *Left:* The main interface with allowed controlling pacing protocol, data acquisition parameters, and signal conditioning (see text for detail). *Right:* Timing diagram of the system, which included premature pacing protocol (upper trace), excitation light trigger, data acquisition trigger preceded by amplifier resetting trigger.

Computer-Controlled Data Acquisition and Pacing

In order to reduce photobleaching effects, the preparation was illuminated only for a short period. An electronic shutter (Fig. 2) opened a few seconds before the start of the data acquisition and closed tens of milliseconds after it. The right panel of Figure 3 shows a timing diagram of these events. The opening of the shutter was synchronized with the activation of solenoid valves that stopped the perfusion of the preparation for the duration of the data collection. In addition, a glass window was placed at the surface of the bath to eliminate light scattering at wavelets of the water. These steps assured a still surface of the perfusate and greatly reduced movement/reflection artifacts. A computer was used for generation of the above synchronization signals that were a part of the pacing protocol program, written in LabVIEW language (National Instruments). Such computerized interface allowed full automation of series of recordings taken at various coupling intervals or at various time intervals of drug application. Each data record contained 256 optical signals and 8 additional channels of data with surface and microelectrograms, pacing triggers, and other control pulses used during data acquisition.

Atrial-AV Nodal Optical Signals
and Conduction Patterns

Optical Recordings from Different Areas of the Rabbit Heart

Figure 4 shows representative optical action potentials recorded from different regions of the same rabbit heart, stained with di-4-ANEPPS via coronary perfusion.[10] The first two optical recordings (top row, left to right) were taken before dissection from the ventricular and atrial epicardium of the intact Langendorff-perfused heart, 10 and 15 minutes after staining, respectively. In both cases, the signals were recorded from an area of 430×430 μm. The heart was then removed from the Langendorff apparatus and dissected according to the procedure described above. The atrial-AV nodal preparation was positioned in front of the optical apparatus. Four consecutive recordings were taken from this flat isolated preparation by focusing on the following regions: the interatrial septum, the central AV node region, the crista terminalis, and the distal AV node region toward the bundle of His. As seen from the traces in Figure 4, the signal-to-noise (S/N) ratio was higher in the epicardial recordings than in the recordings made from AV node area. Quantitatively, these signals had the following S/N ratio (peak-to-peak): left ventricular epicardium 29.3, left atrial epicardium 29.3, interatrial septum 18.6, AV node 7.6, crista terminalis 7.9, distal AV node and His bundle area 8.0.

This comparison of S/N ratios demonstrates that the area of the AV node presents a challenge for optical measurements. As demonstrated in Figure 4, signals recorded from atrial and ventricular cells approach the quality of microelectrode recordings. In contrast, signals recorded from the AV nodal area were typically 2 to 4 times smaller in amplitude. Although the AV nodal responses were more difficult to analyze, the signals had

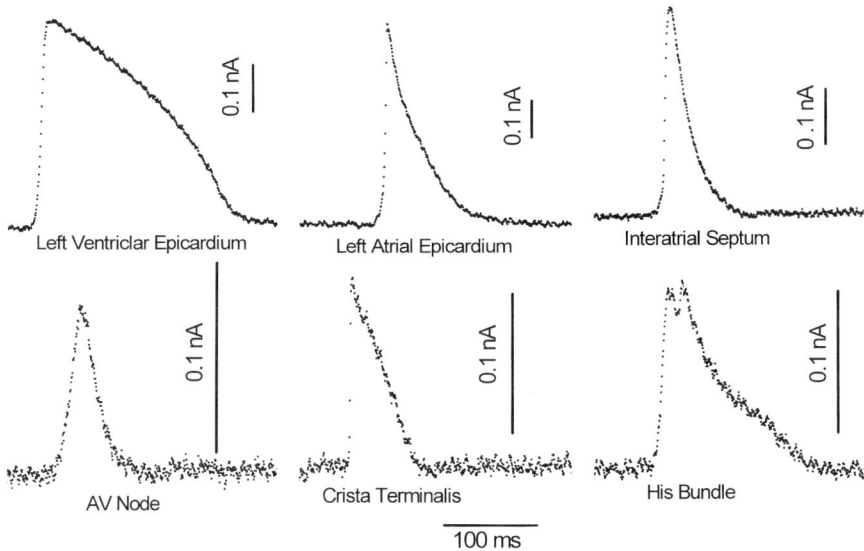

Figure 4. Optical recordings from a rabbit heart. The heart was stained on a Langendorff apparatus with voltage-sensitive dye via the coronaries. Action potentials were first recorded from two areas of the intact heart: left ventricular epicardium and left atrial epicardium. Then the heart was removed from the Langendorff apparatus and an atrial-atrioventricular (AV) nodal preparation was dissected (see Fig. 1). Action potentials were recorded from the interatrial septum, the AV node, the crista terminalis, and from the distal nodal area near the bundle of His. See the text for details. Reproduced, with permission, from reference 10.

morphology previously observed with microelectrode recordings. Specifically, optical action potentials from the central AV node had a slow upstroke rise time, whereas the crista terminalis action potentials exhibited the most rapid rise times.

The optical signals represent an average electrical activity from hundreds or even thousands of cells, depending on magnification. Obviously, the optical signal depends on the characteristics of responses of individual cells as well as on conduction velocity of propagation between them.[16] Therefore, recordings from areas composed of cells with different morphology of responses might yield complex optical responses, such as the double-humped optical action potential recorded from the area of transition between the distal AV node and the bundle of His, as shown in the right bottom trace in Figure 4. We presented this hypothesis in 1997, when we first observed such multiphasic optical signals.[10] Later these findings were further explored by us[11,18,22–24] and others.[25,26]

Morphology of Optical Action Potentials from the Triangle of Koch

Figure 5 shows a map of 256 optical action potentials recorded from the triangle of Koch in our first study.[10] The lower edge of the field of view was aligned with the tricuspid valve. The left edge was at the base of the trian-

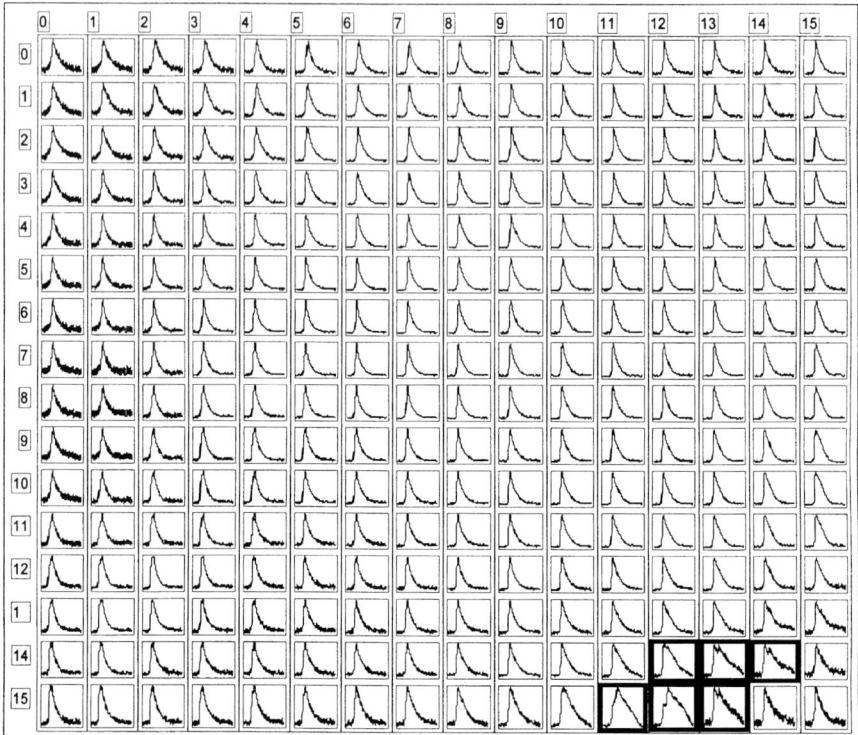

Figure 5. Map of 256 optical action potentials recorded from the atrioventricular nodal area of a rabbit heart. The 256 action potentials were recorded simultaneously at a sampling rate of 2 kHz per channel. Each signal represents the integral optical activity of an area of 430×430 μm. The "dead" space between neighboring diodes was 66 μm. Signals were normalized to the same amplitude. Reproduced, with permission, from reference 10.

gle of Koch. The tendon of Todaro was approximately along the diagonal of the field of view. The optical apparatus was adjusted to view 8×8 mm of tissue including the entire triangle of Koch area. The action potentials shown in Figure 5 do not represent actual amplitudes of signals; they were normalized to the same uniform maximum amplitude throughout the diagram. Typically we observed substantial differences in signal levels. For example, signals recorded from the opening of the coronary sinus (upper left corner in the map) had relatively low amplitude compared with the septal signals (right top corner). Importantly, one can clearly see that some signals in the lower bottom corner of the map had a complex morphology (see signals highlighted with black boxes). These signals were recorded from the distal AV node and the junction between the AV node and the bundle of His.[10]

Isochronal Maps of Activation

Traditional maps of activation can be easily constructed from atrial-AV nodal optical recordings. We defined activation time in each channel as a maximum of the first derivative of optical signal.[10] Then, using a matrix of activation times, we constructed a map of contour lines using Origin software (MicroCal, Northampton, MA). Figure 6 shows an example of isochronal activation maps for one rabbit preparation. The upper left panel depicts a simplified anatomical diagram. The three areas from which the isochronal maps were constructed are marked as squares and the arrows point to the corresponding maps. Different gray colors are used to mark timing of the activation process: each shade represents an area of cells activated within a 4-ms time frame, as indicated to the right of each map. Note that the zero reference point in each map has been assigned to the earliest depolarized site in the map. The map from the area of the crista terminalis (bottom left panel) shows rapid conduction with 0.5 m/s along the crista terminalis, which is blocked in the anterior direction near the coronary sinus opening. The activation turns slowly below the coronary sinus and then invades the AV nodal area.

The next map was taken from the region of the "slow pathway" entrance into the AV node (lower right panel). The activation propagated

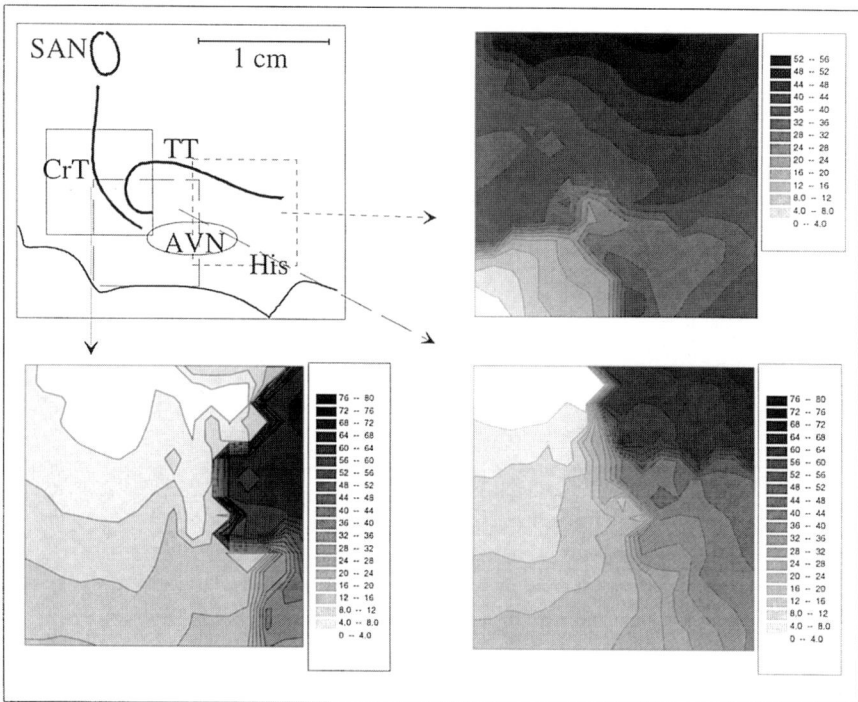

Figure 6. Activation maps of the atrioventricular (AV) node area. Three successive recordings were taken from a preparation in sinus rhythm (420-ms cycle length). The top left panel is a simplified diagram correlating maps with anatomical landmarks on the preparation. The solid box on the diagram represents the position from which the map shown in the bottom left panel was derived. The longer dashed box represents position of a map taken from the proximal AV node that is shown in the right bottom panel. The shorter dashed box shows an area for the map shown in the right top panel. It represents the activation pattern in the distal AV node. All maps were drawn with isochronal lines 4 ms apart. Reproduced, with permission, from reference 10.

with decreasing conduction velocity toward the region of the central node. Interestingly, it then turned counterclockwise, so that the area just below the tendon of Todaro was depolarized last.

The last map (top right panel) shows that the above-described retrograde pattern of septal activation persisted after leaving the AV nodal area.

We found that the above-observed unexpected pattern of activation of the septal approaches to the AV node was related to a substantial delay encountered during propagation between the sinus node and the septum. We observed a similar pattern of activation via the slow pathway in 7 out of 8 preparations used in this study.[10] In the remaining preparation, two activation wave fronts spread toward the AV node, one from the posterior approach (so-called slow pathway) and another from the anterior approach (so-called fast pathway).[10]

Combined Optical and Microelectrode Recordings

The above-described mapping procedure was not readily applicable in the most interesting area of the preparation, the AV node, where optical signals consistently exhibited multiple components. Which of the two components should be considered as a time-marker in the map? We hypothesized that both must be analyzed: the first represented depolarization of cells located in the superficial envelope of transitional cells, while the second represented the delayed depolarization of cells in the compact nodal region.

To test this hypothesis, we impaled a glass microelectrode to record AV nodal cellular action potentials. Fortunately, the narrow depth of field and large numerical aperture of the optical lens, as well as the transparency of the glass microelectrode, minimized optical interference from the electrode. Deeper impalement provided an action potential typical for a distal nodal cell (Fig. 7, lower-left panel). The upstroke of this action potential preceded the bundle of His electrogram activation and was absent when the latter was missing due to conduction block (in this example, a 3:2 Wenckebach cycle was observed and the second beat was blocked in the AV node). It is clear that the action potential of this deeper cell was always synchronous with the second component of the optical signal. AV node block was always associated with the absence of both the cellular action potential and the second component in the optical signal.

When the microelectrode was slightly withdrawn vertically, a more superficial transitional cell was impaled (Fig. 7, lower-right panel). This cell had a faster upstroke and depolarized earlier during the atrial activation in each beat. In addition, it was activated even when AV node block was present. Thus, this was a typical AV node transitional cell. Note that its action potential was synchronous with the first of the two components in the optical signal. In addition, both the cellular action potential and the first of the optical components in each beat were related to the atrial activation, and significantly preceded the bundle of His activation.

The above observations confirmed that the optical signal contained information from at least two wave fronts: one representing the activation of the superficial envelope of transitional cells, and a second one represent-

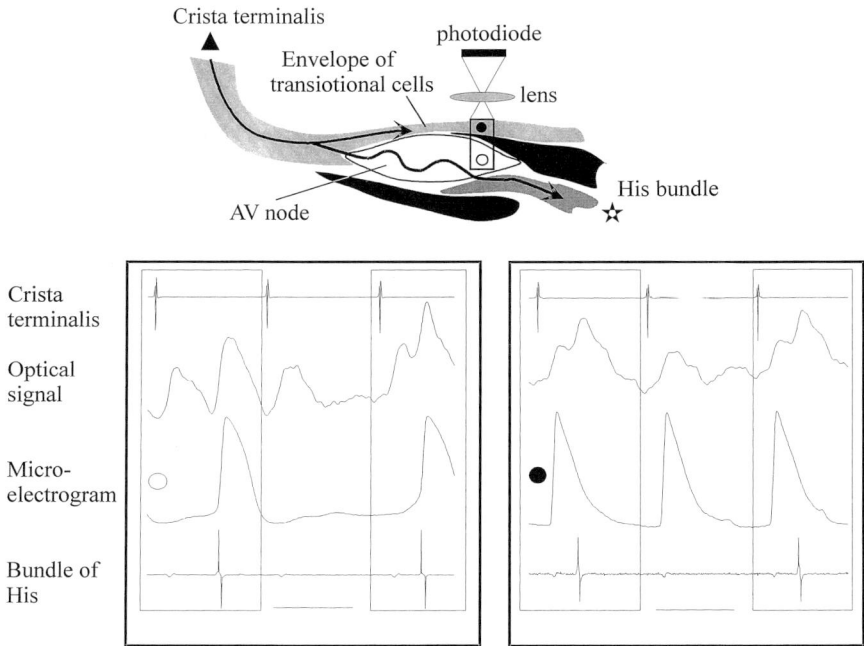

Figure 7. The nature of multiphasic optical recordings. A multilayer structure is schematically drawn in the upper panel to represent a simplified cross-section of the atrioventricular (AV) node perpendicular to the endocardial atrial surface. The compact AV node resembles a slightly flattened "football" covered with a superficial layer of transitional cells that form an envelope providing a connection between the atrial tissue and the compact node. The compact node connects to the bundle of His. Connective tissue protrusions are shown in black. The arrows show hypothetical wave fronts in the transitional and compact nodal fibers. Optical recordings obtained by a 16×16 photodiode array were accompanied by bipolar electrograms from the atrial input to the AV node (triangle) and from the bundle of His (star). In addition, a roving glass microelectrode was used to impale cells in different AV node layers (black and white circles). See text for details.

ing the ensuing depolarization of the deeper compact nodal layers.[11] Recently Wu et al.[26] presented similar observations from canine AV node, providing additional confirmation of our hypothesis.

Reconstruction of Multilayer Activation Patterns

Activation times derived from each of the two components can be used to reconstruct patterns of activation in the two layers, which are represented by these two components of optical signals. Figure 8 shows an example of such reconstruction during premature pacing protocol. As evident from Figure 8, two distinct wave fronts were present during the propagation of both the basic (left panels) and the premature (right panels) beats. The first wave front (upper maps) ran over the envelope of transitional cells and brought the excitation from the pacing site to the AV node

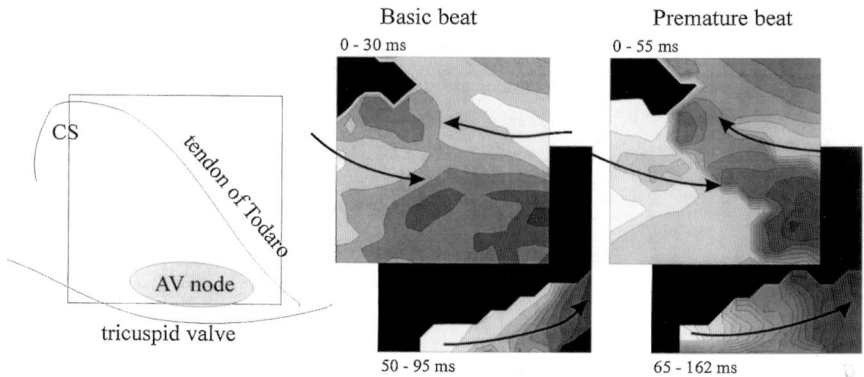

Figure 8. Activation maps during basic (left) and premature (right) beats. The activation times at each individual location were determined by -(dF/dt)$_{max}$ (F = fluorescence). The isochronal lines were drawn with a 5-ms resolution. Spread of activation is shown as white-to-gray gradient. The left pair of maps illustrates the conduction of a basic drive beat at a cycle length of 300 ms, while the right pair of maps was obtained during the propagation of a premature beat with a coupling interval of 180 ms. See the text for details.

region. This wave front encircled the opening of the coronary sinus (shown in black) and activated the viewing area within 30 ms during the basic beat and within 55 ms during the premature beat. The second wave front (bottom maps) was only traceable in a portion of the viewing field that corresponds with the location of the compact node and the more distal nodal region. Conduction in this deeper region of nodal fibers was initiated after and probably by the superficial wave front. It is clear that this conduction was substantially slower. This slowing of conduction was especially pronounced during premature beats. In Figure 8, it took 100 ms to traverse the deeper cellular layers, while the entire surface was activated within 55 ms. In addition, the area of slow conduction, defined by the presence of secondary components in the optical recordings, was consistently larger during propagation of premature atrial beats.

In the case of retrograde conduction, the sequence is reversed.[18,24] Figure 9 shows an example of such reconstruction performed during pacing applied at the bundle of His.[24] The upper right panel shows bipolar electrograms recorded at the bundle of His and crista terminals and four optical traces taken along the long axis of the hypothetical location of the AV node (see black boxes in lower-right panel). The left panel shows a pair of isochronal activation maps, which illustrates that the impulse first entered the AV node and then propagated across a bundlelike structure, which presumably is a part of posterior nodal extension.[27] At the 35th millisecond, the impulse broke through and appeared at the surface of the triangle of Koch, completing its activation with 12 ms in a radial fashion.

New Insights into AV Nodal Physiology from Optical Mapping

The application of voltage-sensitive dyes and optical imaging techniques to study the mechanisms of conduction through the AV node is just

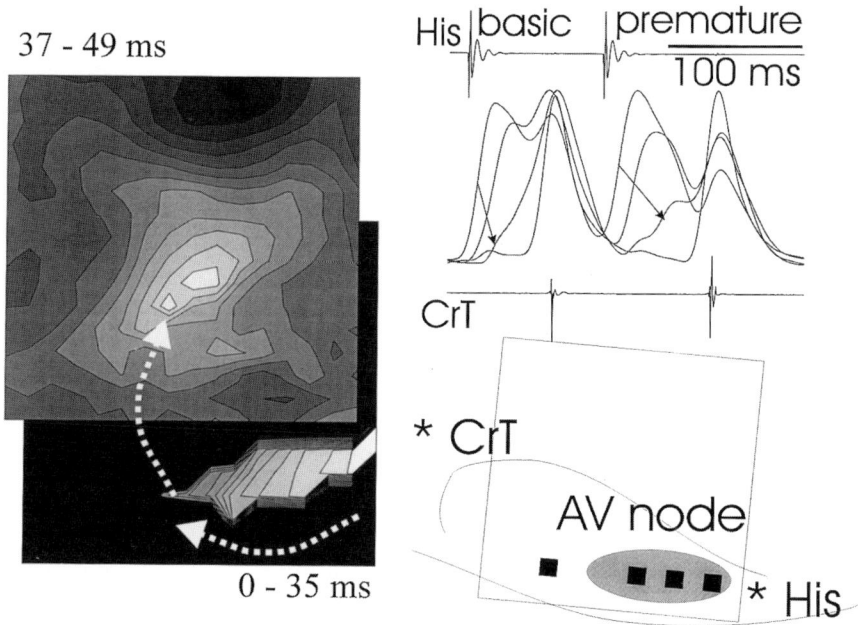

Figure 9. Double-layer activation pattern in the AV node during retrograde conduction. The left panel shows isochronal conduction maps. The lower and upper maps are drawn 3 ms and 1 ms apart, respectively. Electrograms and optical signals are shown in the upper left panel. The field of view and recording sites are illustrated in the lower-right panel.

emerging. It is difficult, at this early stage, to evaluate all the advantages and limitations of this new methodology. The initial results reported in this chapter, as well as observations by others (see chapter 10), confirm that optical imaging of the AV node is possible and is certain to bring new knowledge along with reevaluation and/or clarification of the previous knowledge.

The major power of the optical approach is its capability to provide maps of excitation, i.e., simultaneous recordings of electrical activity from multiple sites with a reasonable spatial and temporal resolution. Although the 256 photodiode array used in these studies may appear impressive as compared with the single microelectrode, it is worth stressing that an increased size of the array would be highly desirable. This is because of the need to "see" at the same time both the atrial approaches to the AV node and the nodal region itself. Moreover, the most important, deeper layer(s) of AV nodal propagation occupy only a fraction of the area of the triangle of Koch and detailed studies of this region will require high-density optical recordings.

Our studies have provided an important new insight into the electrophysiology of the atrial approaches to the AV node. In particular, in the rabbit heart preparation, it is common to observe the pattern of predominantly posterior AV nodal engagement. While it has been demonstrated that the pattern of the septal activation during normal sinus rhythm[28,29] is nonradial and anisotropic,[30-34] it is still not clear if the AV node is engaged via rather wide wave fronts or through well-defined electrically isolated pathways. The prevailing opinion, especially among the clinical electrophysiologists, is that the two main sites of atrial activation that are of specific interest are related to the posterior and anterior groups of the connections between the AV node and the atrium demonstrated histologically.[32–34]

By demonstrating that the anterior AV node approaches can be activated later and by the wave fronts that invade the posterior approaches, our observations bring a new argument in the ongoing debate about the nature of the dual nodal pathways.[35–37] Indeed, the classic view of dual-pathway electrophysiology[38] assumes that the fast pathway is an extension of the anterior septal input into the AV node. The experimental data suggest that the intranodal fast pathway may still be formed in the distal anterior node adjacent to the lower septum. However, the activation of this input may occur over the envelope of transitional cells that engulfs the compact node and is electrically connected with the posterior crista terminalis input.

An important step in optical imaging of the AV node is the novel combination of microelectrodes and high-resolution optical imaging with voltage-sensitive dyes. Such integration of techniques has helped to demonstrate directly the previously deduced pattern of multilayer AV node conduction, and to provide the first detailed 3-dimensional mapping of transmission of basic and premature beats through the AV node. This has been achieved by reconstructing a 3-dimensional pattern from 2-dimensional optical map assisted by the functional information obtained with micro- and macroelectrodes.

This creates an exciting possibility to gain a deeper understanding of the many still controversial properties of AV node conduction. Among those is the filtering role of the AV node during high-rate irregular rhythms such as atrial fibrillation, as well as the fundamental issue of whether or not the AV node truly conducts, or is an electrotonically modulated oscillator.[39] Furthermore, application of the optical imaging technique may help to visualize dual-pathway structures (if they exist) and to correlate specific bipolar potentials that were clinically described with the AV node cellular responses.

It is necessary to stress some important limitations in the application of voltage-sensitive dyes in the area of AV nodal electrophysiology. The optical imaging techniques do not eliminate problems associated with the complex 3-dimensional structure of the AV node. In fact, the optical signal of a given photodiode is generated not by one, but by hundreds (or thousands) of individual cells located within the depth of field of the optical apparatus. As our observations show, the optical signal obtained from the areas of the compact and the distal AV node carry the signatures of at least two functionally different processes. One represents the activation of the layer of the surface transitional cells, while the second appears associated with propagation in the deeper AV nodal structures. The fact that optical imaging can distinguish between these signals is both a great advantage and a source of possible misinterpretations. For example, it is tempting to suggest that the deeper propagating wave front is initiated by the earlier superficial wave front that may transversely invade the node. However, alternatively, the two wave fronts may have independent sources, so that the deeper wave front results from the connection between the inferior crista terminalis and the posterior approaches to the compact AV node. As evident from the maps reported in our studies, the origin of initiation of the late component of the optical signal, especially posteriorly, cannot be traced with certainty. Although the optical signals from this region of the AV node typically exhibit only one, early, component it is quite possible that the later component may still be present. It may be hidden in the "shadow" of the surface signal due to the small temporal dissociation between them at the beginning of the AV nodal propagation. Therefore, conclusions about the presence of discontinuous conduction over functional or anatomical barriers should be made with extreme caution.

The most attractive way, in our opinion, to solve these important problems of AV nodal electrophysiology is to carry out intensive studies that employ the combination of microelectrodes and optical imaging. While limited to recording the action potential of one cell at the time, the microelectrode has the advantage of demonstrating the arrival of two (or more) wave fronts at this same cell. Therefore, microelectrodes, guided by the gross-picture obtained with the voltage-sensitive dyes, would be the ideal tool for precise identification of sites of suspected discontinuity. Finally, the two techniques should be complimented by the use of complex pacing protocols executed from different atrial pacing sites in attempt to visualize the possible presence of specialized atrial-AV nodal entry sites, or, alternatively, to provide support for the predominantly intranodal nature of the dual-pathway AV nodal electrophysiology.

Future Directions

Fluorescent methods have revolutionized biomedical research, including both structural morphological and functional dynamic studies. Yet, unlike other imaging modalities, there is an important intrinsic limitation of optical techniques related to their inability of dynamic 3-dimensional functional reconstruction. Confocal microscopy methods have presented an opportunity to address this problem in structural studies, which allow slow rates of data acquisition in typically immobilized sections of biological tissue. These methods resulted in detailed 3-dimensional reconstructions of numerous biological phenomena. Yet, confocal methods are based on significant reduction of amounts of light collected by the sensor, which limits their application in functional studies.

Two new optical imaging methods appeared recently that are promising candidates for breaking the 3-dimensional barrier. These methods are 2-photon fluorescence[40] and optical coherence tomography (OCT).[41] The first method is based on nearly simultaneous absorption of two photons instead of one as in conventional single-photon fluorescence. The 2-photon method has already been successfully applied by several groups and resulted in 3-dimensional reconstruction of several phenomena, most remarkably the dendritic structure of rat brain neurons in vivo using calcium-sensitive fluorescent dyes.[42] Application of this method to voltage-sensitive dyes still presents a challenge, yet may be feasible.

OCT[43] uses the same principles as conventional ultrasound methods, except the carrier wave is light rather than sound. OCT has provided impressive 3-dimensional images of developing Xenopus cardiovascular system,[41] obtained noninvasively. Combination of this technique with absorption voltage-sensitive dye may prove feasible.

The future is likely to produce a major breakthrough in resolving the 3-dimensional barrier, which is an important limitation of studies of the conduction system of the heart.

References

1. Davila HV, Salzberg BM, Cohen LB, Waggoner AS. A large change in axon fluorescence that provides a promising method for measuring membrane potential. *Nat New Biol* 1973;241:159–160.
2. Salama G, Morad M. Merocyanine 540 as an optical probe of transmembrane electrical activity in the heart. *Science* 1976;191:485–487.
3. Grinvald A, Cohen LB, Lesher S, Boyle MB. Simultaneous optical monitoring of activity of many neurons in invertebrate ganglia using a 124-element photodiode array. *J Neurophysiol* 1981;45:829–840.
4. Davidenko JM, Pertsov AV, Salomonsz R, et al. Stationary and drifting spiral waves of excitation in isolated cardiac muscle. *Nature* 1992;355:349–351.
5. Fast VG, Kléber AG. Microscopic conduction in cultured strands of neonatal rat heart cells measured with voltage-sensitive dyes. *Circ Res* 1993;73:914–925.
6. Meijler FL, Janse MJ. Morphology and electrophysiology of the mammalian atrioventricular node. *Physiol Rev* 1988;68:608–647.
7. Watanabe Y, Dreifus LS. Inhomogenous conduction in the A-V node. A model for reentry. *Am Heart J* 1965;70:505–514.
8. Tawara S. *Das Reizleitungs System des Herzens*. Jena, Germany: Fisher; 1906.
9. Imaizumi S, Mazgalev T, Dreifus LS, et al. Morphological and electrophysiological correlates of atrioventricular nodal response to increased vagal activity. *Circulation* 1990;82:951–964.
10. Efimov IR, Fahy GJ, Cheng YN, et al. High resolution fluorescent imaging of rabbit heart does not reveal a distinct atrioventricular nodal anterior input channel (fast pathway) during sinus rhythm. *J Cardiovasc Electrophysiol* 1997;8:295–306.
11. Efimov IR, Mazgalev TN. High-resolution three-dimensional fluorescent imaging reveals multilayer conduction pattern in the atrioventricular node. *Circulation* 1998;98:54–57.
12. Hewett KW, Gillette PC, Buckles DS. Atrioventricular nodal conduction patterns recorded with voltage-sensitive dyes. *J Am Coll Cardiol* 1995;25:361A. Abstract.
13. Knisley SB. Transmembrane voltage changes during unipolar stimulation of rabbit ventricle. *Circ Res* 1995;77:1229–1239.
14. Efimov IR, Huang DT, Rendt JM, Salama G. Optical mapping of repolarization and refractoriness from intact hearts. *Circulation* 1994;90:1469–1480.
15. Cabo C, Pertsov AM, Baxter WT, et al. Wave-front curvature as a cause of slow conduction and block in isolated cardiac muscle. *Circ Res* 1994;75:1014–1028.
16. Girouard SD, Laurita KR, Rosenbaum DS. Unique properties of cardiac action potentials recorded with voltage- sensitive dyes. *J Cardiovasc Electrophysiol* 1996;7:1024–1038.
17. Cheng Y, Mowrey KA, Efimov IR, et al. Effects of 2,3-butanedione monoxime on the atrial-atrioventricular nodal conduction in isolated rabbit heart. *J Cardiovasc Electrophysiol* 1997;8:790–802.
18. Nikolski V, Efimov IR. Fluorescent imaging of a dual-pathway conduction system of the AV-node. *Circulation* 2000;102(18-II):3. Abstract.

19. Wu JY, Cohen LB. Fast multisite optical measurement of membrane potential. In Mason WT (ed): *Fluorescent and Luminescent Probes for Biological Activity: A Practical Guide to Technology for Quantitative Real-Time Analysis.* San Diego: Academic Press; 1993.

20. Efimov IR, Cheng Y, Van Wagoner DR, et al. Virtual electrode-induced phase singularity: A basic mechanism of failure to defibrillate. *Circ Res* 1998;82:918–925.

21. Cheng Y, Mowrey KA, Van Wagoner DR, et al. Virtual electrode induced re-excitation: A basic mechanism of defibrillation. *Circ Res* 1999;85:1056–1066.

22. Efimov IR, Mazgalev TN, Van Wagoner DR, Tchou PJ. Optical mapping reveals two-layer conduction pattern in the AV node. *PACE* 1998;21(4-II):824.

23. Mazgalev TN, Efimov IR. Fluorescent imaging of the AV node: A new frontier. *Ann Biomed Eng* 1998;26(1-S):17.

24. Efimov IR, Tchou PJ, Mazgalev TN. Optical mapping reveals two-layered conduction during retrograde activation in the atrio-ventricular node. *PACE* 1999;22(4-II):832.

25. Choi BR, Salama G. Optical mapping of atrioventricular node reveals a conduction barrier between atrial and nodal cells [see comments]. *Am J Physiol* 1998;274:H829-H845.

26. Wu J, Wu J, Olgin JE, et al. Mechanisms underlying the reentrant circuit of AV nodal reentry tachycardia in isolated canine AV nodal preparations using optical mapping. *Circulation* 2000;102(18-II):3

27. Medkour D, Becker AE, Khalife K, Billette J. Anatomic and functional characteristics of a slow posterior AV nodal pathway: Role in dual-pathway physiology and reentry. *Circulation* 1998;98:164–174.

28. Lewis T, Meakins J, White PD. Excitatory process in the dog's heart: I. The auricles. *Phil Trans Roy Soc Lond B* 1914;205:375–420.

29. Eyster JAE, Meek WJ. Experiments on the origin and propagation of the impulse in the heart: Point of primary negativity in the mammalian heart and the spread of negativity to other regions. *Heart* 1913;5:119–136.

30. Sano T, Yamagishi S. Spread of excitation from the sinus node. *Circ Res* 1965;16:423–430.

31. Schuessler RB, Boineau JP, Bromberg BI. Origin of the sinus impulse. *J Cardiovasc Electrophysiol* 1996;7:263–274.

32. Becker A, Anderson R. Morphology of the human atrioventricular junctional area. In Wellens H, Lie K, Janse M (eds): *The Conduction System of the Heart: Structure, Function and Clinical Implications.* Philadelphia: Lea and Febiger; 1976.

33. James T. The connecting pathways between the sinus node and the A-V node and between the right and left atrium of the human heart. *Am Heart J* 1963;66:498–508.

34. Racker DK. Atrioventricular node and input pathways: A correlated gross anatomical and histological study of the canine atrioventricular junctional region. *Anat Rec* 1989;224:336–354.

35. Spach MS, Lieberman M, Scott JG, et al. Excitation sequences of the atrial septum and the AV node in isolated hearts of the dog and rabbit. *Circ Res* 1971;29:156–172.

36. McGuire MA, Bourke JP, Robotin MC, et al. High resolution mapping of Koch's triangle using sixty electrodes in humans with atrioventricular junctional (AV nodal) reentrant tachycardia. *Circulation* 1993;88:2315–2328.

37. Sheahan RG, Klein GJ, Yee R, et al. Atrioventricular node reentry with 'smooth' AV node function curves: A different arrhythmia substrate? *Circulation* 1996;93:969–972.

38. Mendez C, Moe GK. Demonstration of a dual A-V nodal conduction system in the isolated rabbit heart. *Circ Res* 1966;19:378–393.

39. Meijler FL, Fisch C. Does the atrioventricular node conduct? *Br Heart J* 1989;61:309–315.

40. Helmchen F, Svoboda K, Denk W, Tank DW. In vivo dendritic calcium dynamics in deep-layer cortical pyramidal neurons. *Nat Neurosci* 1999;2:989–996.
41. Boppart SA, Tearney GJ, Bouma BE, et al. Noninvasive assessment of the developing Xenopus cardiovascular system using optical coherence tomography. *Proc Natl Acad Sci U S A* 1997;94:4256–4261.
42. Svoboda K, Helmchen F, Denk W, Tank DW. Spread of dendritic excitation in layer 2/3 pyramidal neurons in rat barrel cortex in vivo. *Nat Neurosci* 1999;2:65–73.
43. Huang D, Swanson EA, Lin CP, et al. Optical coherence tomography. *Science* 1991;254:1178–1181.

Chapter 10

Optical Mapping of Impulse Propagation in the Atrioventricular Node: *2*

Guy Salama and Bum-Rak Choi

In 1906 Tawara[1] proposed that the atrioventricular (AV) node serves as the electrical connection between the atria and the ventricles in mammalian hearts. The node is located between the right atrial and ventricular septum in a region called the triangle of Koch and provides an important filtering function by virtue of its rate-dependent properties.[2,3] Tawara investigated this structure in various species of hearts and found it to be similar in the dove, rat, guinea pig, rabbit, cat, sheep, calf, and human.[1] It is a heterogeneous 3-dimensional structure composed of a rod-shaped, ovoid, and spindle-shaped compact network of small cells.[4,5] Histological analysis of the AV node indicated that the node consists of five morphologically distinct cell types: 1) transitional cells; 2) atrial cells; 3) midnodal cells; 4) lower nodal cells; and 5) cells of the penetrating AV bundle embedded within the central fibrous body.[6] Transitional cells are distinguished from atrial cells by their smaller size, pale staining reaction, and extensive connective tissue. Midnodal cells are closely packed with little intervening connective tissue and form the "compact node," which corresponds to the Knoten of Tawara. Lower nodal cells are elongated and smaller than atrial cells, and form a bundle parallel to the AV ring.

The AV node of the rabbit heart has been extensively studied because of the following practical considerations: 1) Nodal cells in rabbit hearts are accessible from the surface, making it possible to impale individual cells with intracellular microelectrodes. 2) The AV nodal tissue can be isolated from the rest of the heart and presumably kept "healthy" by superfusion with oxygenated Tyrode's solution. 3) It can be stretched and pinned down to reduce movement due to muscle contractions to permit microelectrode impalements in these small cells. The dimensions of the rabbit AV node

These studies were supported by grants from the Western Pennsylvania Affiliate of the American Heart Association to B.-R. Choi and the National Institute of Health grants RO1 HL57929 and HL59614 to G. Salama.

From Rosenbaum DS, Jalife J (eds): *Optical Mapping of Cardiac Excitation and Arrhythmias.* ©Futura Publishing Co., Inc., Armonk, NY, 2001.

are estimated to be approximately 1.5 mm in width by 2 to 2.5 mm in length. The AV node dimensions are somewhat ambiguous because the posterior and anterior margins of the AV node cannot be clearly delineated, as changes in cell type occur gradually and different cell types are intermingled at border zones. AV nodal cells in various mammalian hearts were subdivided into three zones based on their electrophysiology: atrionodal (AN), nodal (N), and nodal-His (NH) cells.[7] The N zone is an area of slow conduction and slow action potential (AP) upstrokes; the AN zone is a transitional region between fast conducting atrial muscle and the N zone; and the NH zone is a transitional zone between N zone and His bundle. AN cells were further subdivided into AN and ANCO cells because at fast pacing rates, APs of ANCO cells exhibited two components or a "notch" on the AP upstroke.[8] Premature stimuli and pacing at faster rates were used to distinguish N from NH cells. The time course and shape of the AP responses were correlated to the morphology of the cell by recording APs with microelectrodes filled with potassium ferricyanide[9] or cobalt-containing KCl[10] to selectively stain cells that fired a particular type of AP. Such studies suggested that AN potentials emanate from transitional cells and NH potentials from lower nodal cells. Unfortunately, the diffusion of the stain to neighboring cells compromised the spatial resolution and made it difficult to demonstrate unequivocally that N cell APs originate from anatomically defined midnodal cells.[10]

Activation delays across the AV node were measured with intracellular microelectrodes.[8,11] However, a detailed map of impulse propagation within the midnodal and lower nodal zone could not be determined because at any location (but unknown depth) APs had markedly different characteristics and activation times, some activating early and others late in the same region. Thus, the complex 3-dimensional structure of the AV node and the difficulties of recording APs from a known depth with microelectrodes made it impractical to detect a wave of depolarization within the node or to measure conduction velocity.

Several hypotheses have been proposed to explain propagation delays at the AV node. The intracellular resistance of AV nodal cells and in particular N cells is markedly higher and the intercellular coupling is reduced compared with atrial and ventricular cells. The high coupling resistance could explain the basic conduction delay of the AV node if conduction is decremental such that the overall AV delay is gradual across the AV zone and is distributed across the cell network.[12] On the other hand, Billette[8] demonstrated that the conduction delay is not decremental in space following a premature stimulus but seems more localized in N cells where conduction stagnates. Such studies have led to the realization that slow conduction in the AV node cannot be solely explained by active properties of N cells such as $(dV/dt)_{max}$ and that both passive and active properties are responsible for the inhomogeneous potential spread in the AV node.[8,10,11,13] One of the earliest hypothesis of AV delay (1929) was based on the existence of a "step-delay" across an inexcitable gap as a major contributor to the total AV node delay.[14] D. Scherf pointed out that the relatively prompt conduction of the first response after a blocked impulse should not be expected because the tissue proximal to the block had been invaded by the blocked impulse and should be even more fatigued.[14] Rosenblueth expanded on this concept and showed that Wenckebach effects and AV node facilitation were consistent with a step-delay mechanism.[15–17] In the absence of direct evidence, Rosenblueth suggested that the step-delay occurred between mid and lower nodal cells and could account for numerous features of AV node conduction.[15,17] Thus, the mechanisms responsible for the AV delay remained unclear, in part due to the inability to map impulse propagation pathways using conventional electrode techniques.

Optical Mapping of AP Propagation across the AV Node

We refined voltage-sensitive dyes and optical imaging techniques to map impulse propagation across the AV node, and used optical sectioning of AV node signals in three dimensions to elucidate the mechanisms responsible for the AV node delay.[18,19] Voltage-sensitive dyes and imaging techniques have been used extensively to map APs optically in a variety of cardiac muscle preparations.[20–24] Simultaneous recordings of transmembrane potential by optical and microelectrode techniques have validated the high fidelity of optical APs compared with microelectrode recordings, and have demonstrated that optical APs detected the classic features of atrial, pacemaker, and ventricular APs.[20,22] Optical techniques also face limitations because the absolute value of the resting potential cannot be measured, the AP downstroke can be distorted by motion artifacts (MAs), and the optical AP represents the sum of APs from cells within a region of tissue, not the AP of a single cell. The latter property means that the optical APs represent the sum of APs from cells with very different time course, pharmacological responses, and phase delays. Despite these limitations, the technique offers important advantages to map inputs to the node, to detect the activation sequence in the compact node, and to identify zone(s) of conduction delay. Several features of the AV node pose unique challenges in applying optical techniques. 1) The AV node is a 3-dimensional structure sandwiched between atrial and transitional cells above and ventricular cells below, such that APs from these three cell types are superimposed on the voltage-dependent optical signals from the AV node. 2) The small dimension of AV nodal cells limits the amount of dye bound to the cells' membranes resulting in low-amplitude optical signals. 3) In order to immobilize the preparation to control movement artifacts required the design to a new chamber. Once these technical difficulties were overcome, it was possible to measure AP upstrokes from the AV node and thereby map the propagation pathways and velocity at high spatial and temporal resolution.

Methods and Procedures

AV Node Preparation

Rabbit hearts were continuously perfused in oxygenated (95% O_2 plus 5% CO_2) Ringer's solution containing (in mmol/L): NaCl 130, $NaHCO_3$ 12.5, $MgSO_4$ 1.2, KCl, 4.75, $CaCl_2$ 1.0, dextrose 20, at pH 7.4.[19] Coronary flow was controlled with a peristaltic pump and aortic pressure was continuously monitored to detect changes in coronary perfusion pressure. At the beginning of each experiment, the coronary flow rate was adjusted to obtain a mean aortic pressure of 80 to 100 cm H_2O and was kept constant thereafter. The free walls of the right ventricle and atrium were cut open and flipped to expose the AV node for optical recordings. No major coronary vessels were severed, as attested by a negligible decrease in coronary perfusion pressure. The intact heart was then pinned down to the bottom of a Sylguard-coated chamber. The Sylguard was carved in the shape of the heart, in which the left ventricle and atrium rested and the right endocardium lay horizontally and nearly flat. The chamber was water-jacketed to control temperature and temperature was continuously monitored with a thermistor placed near the optical field of view. A heating coil in the chamber regulated the temperature of the bath via a feedback system.[19] Electrograms were recorded with bipolar electrodes. Figure 1 illustrates the chamber, optical apparatus, and computer interface used for these measurements.

Staining Procedure. Several approaches were tested to deliver the voltage-sensitive dye to AV nodal cells and thereby maximize the signal-to-noise (S/N) ratio of optical APs.[19] The AV node was bathed in concentrated dye solution (1 to 10 mmol/L), or the dye was microinjected below the surface with syringe needle (100-μm diameter), or the dye was added to the coronary perfusate. In dozens of tests, the most effective staining procedure with respect to signal characteristics was obtained by perfusion with dye solution (10 to 30 μmol/L). Another important factor was the ability to restain the preparation by adding dye through the coronary perfusate. During the course of an experiment, the S/N ratio decreased due to dye washout and/or photobleaching but could be improved by restaining the heart. Thus, several advantages were derived from intact perfused hearts

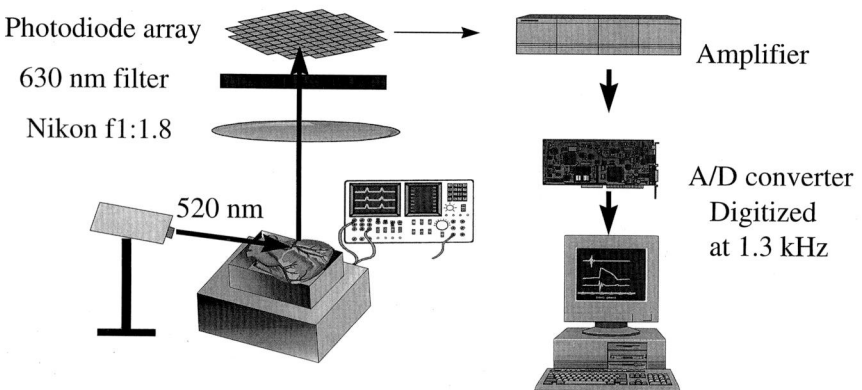

Figure 1. Schematics of the chamber and optical apparatus. The intact perfused heart (shown here before opened to expose the atrioventricular node) was pinned down in a Sylguard-coated horizontal chamber with a feedback system and heating coils to maintain temperature at $37 \pm 1°C$. A camera lens focused an image of the heart on the surface of a photodiode array. The photocurrents from each diode were passed through 124 parallel circuits, digitized, and stored in computer memory.

compared with the conventional superfused AV node preparation. 1) Maintaining the coronary perfusion made it possible to deliver the voltage-sensitive dye in a more effective way and gave us the option to restain the heart to improve S/N ratio of optical APs. 2) The heart was well oxygenated and remained metabolically healthy during experiments lasting 2 to 4 hours. 3) Perfusion was considerably more effective than superfusion to maintain a homogeneous and stable temperature throughout the AV node. Temperature regulation is critical to achieve stable conduction velocity and AV node delays and to compare results from heart to heart. 4) The dissection of the heart preparations caused considerably less trauma to the AV node tissue compared with cutting most of the ventricular and atrial tissues.

The best S/N ratio of optical APs was obtained from hearts stained with voltage-sensitive dye, di-4-ANEPPS (Molecular Probes Inc., Eugene, OR).[18,25] An aliquot (200 μL) of dye solution was injected (2 mmol/L dye in dimethyl sulfoxide) in the bubble trap above the aortic cannula, over a period of 5 to 10 minutes. AH and/or AV delays were measured with bipolar surface electrograms, before, during, and after staining the hearts, and showed that the staining procedure caused no detectable change in AV delay. AH delays averaged over 5 minutes before staining the hearts were 42.7±2.4 ms, and were 43.3±2.5 after staining the hearts.[18,19] Maps of electrical activation generated from activation time points were highly reproducible from beat to beat of the same heart and from heart to heart. In a spontaneously beating heart, the mean cycle length was 417.92±0.96 (SD) ms. The mean AV delay measured with surface electrograms was 88.75±0.37 ms (n = 5 beats).

Optical Apparatus. The optical apparatus has been described elsewhere and is shown in Figure 1.[19,21,22,26] The horizontal chamber was mounted on an X-Y-Z micromanipulator to select the zone of tissue viewed by the photodiode array (PDA) and to adjust the focal plane of the optics to different depths in the tissue. Light from two (100-W) filament lamps was collimated, passed through 530±30-nm interference filters, and focused on the triangle of Koch. Fluorescence from the stained tissue was collected with a camera lens (50 mm, f1:1.4, Nikon Corp., Torrance, CA), projected through a 630-nm cut-off filter (RG 645, Schott Glass, Duryea, PA), and focused on the surface of a 12×12 PDA (Centronic, Newbury Park, CA). The image of the AV node was focused on the array such that each diode detected fluorescence APs from a 0.46×0.46-mm area of epicardium. The depth of field of the collecting lens optimized the detection of fluorescence from a layer of cells ±100 μ from the focal plane. The depth of field of AP recordings was estimated from empirical calculations based on the magnification of the image, the effective numerical aperture of the lens, and the wavelength of the emitted light.[27] Precise focus and alignment of the heart with respect to the array was accomplished by focusing the image of the heart on a custom-made graticule, with the exact dimensions of the array (Graticules Ltd., Tonbridge, UK), located on a plane parafocal with the plane of the array. The photocurrents from 124 diodes were fed to a current-to-voltage converter, amplified, digitized (1.56 kHz per channel, 12-bit resolution per sample), and stored in a memory of buffer of IBM/PC Pentium-300 MHz computer. A scan of data acquisition consisted of 128 simultaneously recorded traces: 124 optical plus 4 instrumentation channels. A scan consisted of a continuous recording of these 128 channels for 1.2 to 3 seconds.

Inhibition of Force and MAs with Diacetyl Monoxime

Diacetyl monoxime (DAM) uncouples excitation from contraction in cardiac muscle primarily by inhibiting myosin ATPase activity and cross-bridge formation, and for this reason has been used extensively to block developed force and the resulting MA.[25,28,29] However, DAM influences other cellular systems involved in the regulation of myocardial contraction and electrical activity and thereby alters the substrate being studied. In rabbit and guinea pig ventricular myocytes, DAM inhibited the inward and delayed rectifier I_K currents and reduced L-type Ca^{2+} currents, resulting in a decrease in AP duration and refractory periods.[29,30] DAM at low concentrations (1 to 5 mmol/L) had no effect on intracellular Ca^{2+} transients (Cai) but inhibited Cai at higher concentrations (5 to 30 mmol/L). This effect of DAM does not involve a decrease in the Ca^{2+} affinity of troponin C but is due to a stimulation of Ca^{2+} release from the sarcoplasmic reticulum (SR).[31] The effect of DAM on the SR was confirmed in direct measurements of SR Ca^{2+} release induced by DAM from isolated canine SR vesicles.[32] Another severe pharmacological effect of DAM is a rapid, dose-dependent blockade of gap junction conductance in rat ventricular myocytes, which in principle reduces conduction velocity in heart muscle.[33] Most studies report the pharmacological effects of DAM in super-fused cardiac muscles and find that these effects are reversible upon washout. However, we found that when delivered through the coronary perfusate (in guinea pig and rabbit hearts), DAM (at 10 to 15 mmol/L for >30 min) causes a loss of electrical excitability, in a time- and dose-dependent manner. The effect is characterized by a gradual increase in stimulation threshold followed by a failure to trigger an AP or to detect AP propagation using extracellular electrodes.[19] The loss of electrical activity is consistent with an increase in gap junction conductance as observed with rat myocytes; but in perfused hearts this effect was not reversed after 30 to 45 minutes of DAM washout. In dog hearts, DAM changes the shape and time course of the "spike-and-dome" AP on the epicardium,[34] which is consistent with the DAM-induced inhibition of the transient outward K^+ current, I_{to}, in rat ventricular myocytes.[33]

In superfused rabbit AV node slices, DAM at 5 and 10 mmol/L produced a shortening of the effective and functional refractory period of the AV node and a slight increase in interatrial delay (6% and 14%, respectively).[35] At 20 mmol/L, DAM produced a further increase in the interatrial delay (up to 50%) and decreased AV node conduction (up to 16%) in the retrograde direction, but it improved anterograde conduction.[35] Similar findings were obtained in perfused rabbit hearts, in which DAM (10 mmol/L) had no detectable effects on atrial and ventricular conduction or AV delay for the first 20 to 30 minutes. However, after 30 minutes of perfusion, DAM first prolonged AV delays, produced Wenckebach effects, and then produced complete AV block. These time-dependent effects could be reversed if DAM was washed within 30 minutes but were irreversible once the heart became inexcitable.[19] The different findings regarding the pharmacological effects of DAM may be due to the efficiency of drug delivery in superfused preparations and to temperature (37°C versus 23°C). In superfused preparations, DAM diffuses in a time-dependent manner first in cells near the surface of the AV node preparation then gradually into cells located in deeper layers. The delivery of DAM and its multiple sites of action then produce heterogeneous effects, which depend on diffusion times of the drug. The cellular effects of DAM on AV nodal cells are a particular concern because of DAM-induced Ca^{2+} release from the SR and the inhibition of the inward Ca^{2+} currents. Thus, DAM must be used judiciously particularly when delivered for prolonged periods where it is likely to have time-dependent effects at different depths of the preparations.

MAs superimposed on the voltage-dependent optical recordings were reduced by perfusing the hearts with DAM (10 mmol/L) to inhibit contractions during data acquisition. Hearts were perfused in Tyrode's solution containing DAM for 10 to 12 minutes, then perfused with standard Tyrode's solution to avoid prolonged exposure to DAM, which produced time-dependent changes in conduction.

Isochronal Maps of Activation

Signals from the AV node region exhibited a set of three spikes or AP upstrokes separated by marked time delays (Fig. 2E). The first and third upstrokes were coincident with atrial and ventricular depolarizations, respectively. The second upstroke was only observed from the AV node region and was the smallest in amplitude. To elucidate the origins of the three spikes, isochronal maps of activation were generated as a wave front for each spike by use of a linear triangulation method. The region delineated by diodes that fired the second spike were identified in 12 to 18 diodes which overlay the AV node, and mapped impulse propagation across the node. With linear triangulation, 10 to 12 isochronal lines were generated in a 2- to 3-mm zone of nodal tissue (i.e., a matrix of 4×3 or 6×3 diodes).

Conduction velocity was determined from the time delays between isochronal lines and the distance traveled by the wave front, and represented an "apparent" conduction velocity, because it was a 2-dimensional approximation of propagation across a 3-dimensional structure (0.75 to 1.25 mm thick from histological analysis). Activation patterns of the three spikes represented atrial, nodal, and ventricular activation, respectively, as confirmed from the anatomical location of these regions of the heart.

AV Node Histology and Optical Maps. Histological analysis of the region identified from optical measurements as the AV node was obtained by first recording optical signals then placing silk sutures at the edges of the optical field of view to provide stable fiducial marks during histological processing.[18,19,26] The AV node region was excised, fixed overnight, and embedded in paraffin. Longitudinal cross-sections (5 μm thick) were taken serially from the endocardium to the epicardium, and every tenth section was mounted on a glass slide. Mounted sections were progressively stained with Mayer's hematoxylin-eosin or trichrome and placed under a

A. Optical recordings

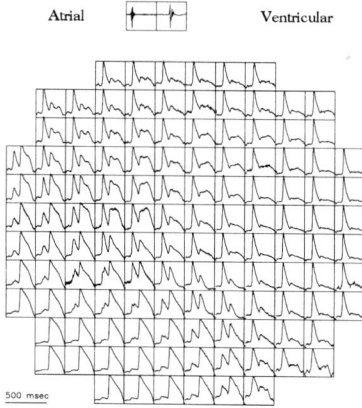

B. Orientation

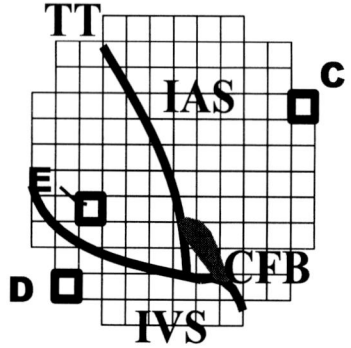

C. Atrium

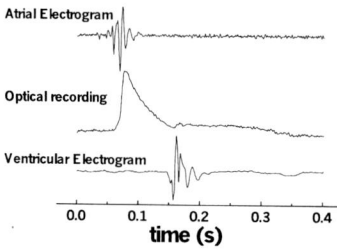

D. Ventricle

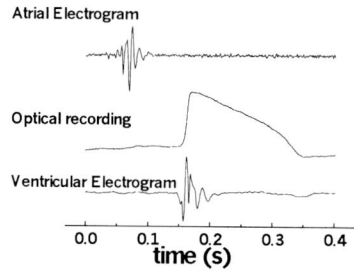

E. AV Node

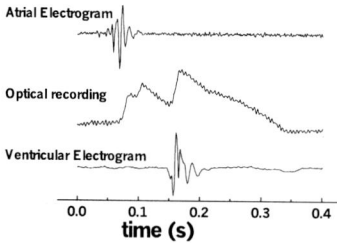

glass coverslip.[19,26,36] Stained sections were examined under a microscope and captured as TIFF images (in 24-bit true color) using a charged coupled device camera. Shrinkage caused by fixation (approximately 35%) was corrected by aligning the fiducial marks on the sections with the edges of the array. Isochronal maps derived from optical APs were superimposed on histological section using CorelDraw™ v7.0 (Corel Corp., Ontario, Canada).

Optical Signals from the AV Node.   Figure 2A shows a set of 124 optical signals recorded from the AV node region, and simultaneously recorded atrial (left) and ventricular (right) bipolar electrogram recordings (top traces). The AV node region is delineated by the tendon of Todaro, the *crista terminalis* forming the Triangle of Koch and the central fibrous body (Fig. 2B). A symbolic map of the array is superimposed on the AV node to identify the region of tissue mapped by the array. The orientation of the array relative to the AV node relative to the array was arbitrary but kept constant in the present study. Figures 2C through 2E illustrate three types of signals recorded from the AV node region and their temporal relationship relative to surface electrograms. Each of these panels shows three traces: the atrial (*top trace*) and ventricular (*bottom trace*) electrograms plus an optical recording from one of the diodes (C, D, E) (Fig. 2B). Diodes C and D detected atrial and ventricular APs, respectively (Figs. 2C, 2D). Electro-

---

Figure 2. Orientation of the atrioventricular (AV) node as viewed by the array and symbolic map of 124 simultaneously recorded action potentials (APs). A rabbit heart was perfused, stained with di-4-ANEPPS, and dissected to expose the AV node. **A.** Simultaneously recorded optical APs from 124 sites on the AV node zone. A symbolic map of the array is shown as 124 square boxes, each identifying the location of individual diodes. The region of tissue viewed by each diode is shown in panel B. The optical trace recorded by each diode is shown in its respective location (each diode being represented by a box) in compressed time base (400 ms). Bipolar electrograms were simultaneously recorded along with the 124 optical signals (*left* and *right* traces above the array). One located on the interatrial septum (IAS), 2 mm above the tendon of Todaro (TT), in B (outside the field of view of the array), the other on the interventricular septum (IVS) near the apex of ventricle. **B.** Sketch of the AV node preparation superimposed on a symbolic map of the array to delineate the AV node region viewed by the array. The anatomical landmarks of the AV node region are identified to correlate the optical signals obtained from each site with the origins of the signal. The "compact" node or midnodal region is bounded by the TT and the *crista terminalis,* and is surrounded by the IAS above and the IVS below, and is adjacent to the central fibrous body (CFB). The orientation of the array relative to the AV node zone was arbitrary but was kept the same for all the experiments shown here. The optical APs from the AV node region shown in A exhibited different characteristics depending on the location of the recording. Each class of optical AP was temporally correlated with the atrial and ventricular electrograms to illustrate the firing sequence of APs. Panels C, D, and E show a set of three traces: the atrial (*top trace*) and ventricular (*bottom trace*) electrograms plus an optical recording (*middle trace*) from one of the diodes (labeled C, D, and E) in panel B. **C.** The optical AP was recorded from atrial cells located on the IAS at diode C. **D.** The ventricular AP was recorded from the IVS by diode D. **E.** An optical recording from the node at diode E. The latter invariably consisted of three sequential upstrokes. The first and third upstrokes were coincident with the atrial and ventricular electrograms. The second fired at an intermediate time point and the AV node was the origin of the signals, which exhibited three sequential upstrokes.

gram recordings and the anatomical location of the recordings validated the origin of these signals (Figs. 2C, 2D). Moreover, the delay between the firing of the atrial and ventricular upstrokes was consistent with the expected AV delay. The most important feature of optical signals from the AV node region is a set of three sequential upstrokes per cardiac beat: peaks (Fig. 2E). The first and third coincided with atrial and ventricular depolarizations and the second fired at intermediate time points.

Impulse Propagation across the AV Node. Figure 3 illustrates the propagation pathway derived from the three spikes: spike 1 spreads across the atrial septum (left), spike 2 across the AV node (e.g., the zone of tissue detecting the second upstroke) (center), and spike 3 across the ventricular septum (right). Activation spread across the atrial septum in 15 ms (left), and after a 28-ms delay, a site in the AV node region fired an AP (spike 2) (center). AV node APs then spread across the node in 8 ms. A 1-second delay occurred between the last AV node AP and the first ventricular AP. The latter delay, τ_2, accounted for the time to propagate from the His bundle to the apex of the ventricles and back along the interventricular septum (IVS) to the base of the ventricle.

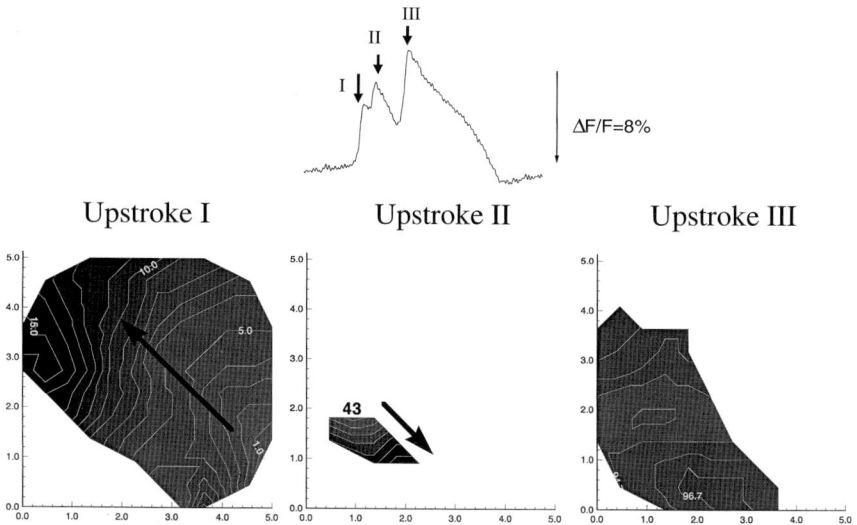

Figure 3. Isochronal maps of activation across the atrioventricular (AV) node. The time points of the first derivative, $(dF/dt)_{max}$, of all the action potential upstrokes were measured and used to determine the time points of activation at each site and to analyze the spread of activation across the AV node region. For signals from the AV node, $(dF/dt)_{max}$ identified three separate activation time points. From the activation time points obtained from all diodes, the depolarization sequence of the atrial (upstroke I), nodal (upstroke II), and ventricular (upstroke III) region were triangulated individually and isochronal lines of activation were drawn 1 ms apart. The gray scale from bright to dark represented "early" to "late" activation times and arrows depict the direction of impulse propagation. *Left:* Isochronal map generated from upstroke I mapped the depolarization sequence of the interatrial septum. *Middle:* Isochronal map generated from upstroke II mapped the activation sequence of the AV node. *Right:* Isochronal map generated from upstroke III mapped the activation sequence of the interventricular septum.

Figure 4 depicts the superposition of all three activation patterns, showing that the three maps overlap in a small region identified as the compact node. The ventricular septum fired APs at 93 ms and spread in the field of view in 4 ms. Maps of impulse propagation across the AV node were highly reproducible in their pattern and their temporal relationship. The average and standard deviation (n = 9 hearts) for the step-delay, τ_1, between AN and N cells and the delay, τ_2, between the second upstroke and the ventricular upstroke are also shown in Figure 4. These values were obtained for hearts under sinus rhythm, with a cycle length of 301.64 ± 8.41 ms (mean$\pm$SD). The time for AP propagation across the compact node was 10.33 ± 3.21 ms predicting a conduction velocity of 0.162 ± 0.024 m/s. The conduction velocity measured by optical techniques is faster than that inferred by intracellular microelectrode recordings because the latter measurements were not based on simultaneous multiple site recordings within the node and may have included a substantial component of the step-delay between AN and N cells.

Three-Dimensional Maps of AV Node APs

The majority of cells comprising the "compact node" are located approximately 0.06 to 0.5 mm below the surface of the atrial septum, and microelectrode studies have shown that transitional (AN) cells overlap zones of N and NH cells.[37] The 3-dimensional nature of the AV node implies that the focal plane of the imaging system must be located below the surface to maximize the amplitude of AV nodal APs. As shown in the schematic drawing in Figure 5 (*top right*), a diode on the array detects light

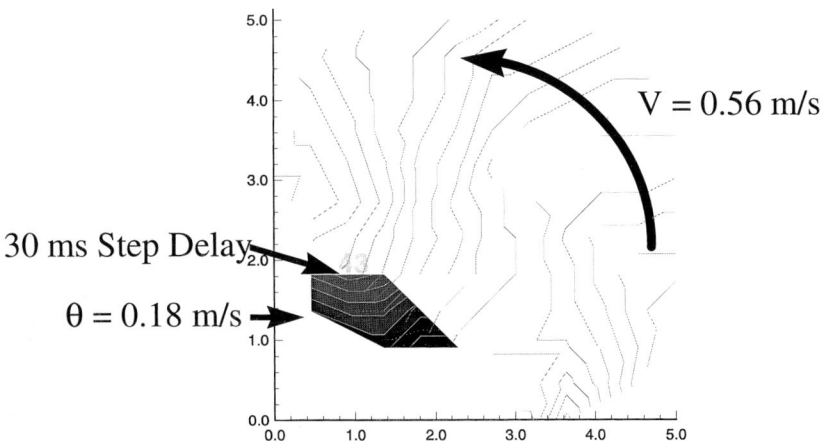

Figure 4. Analysis of atrioventricular (AV) node delay. Impulse propagation across the AV node region. The superposition of activation maps shown in panels A through C in Fig. 3 produced a composite isochronal map of the AV node region. It reveals details about activation across the interatrial septum, across the AV node, and across the interventricular septum. Note that from the last upstroke I to the first upstroke II, there is a 30- to 33-ms interval during which no action potential fired anywhere in the preparation.

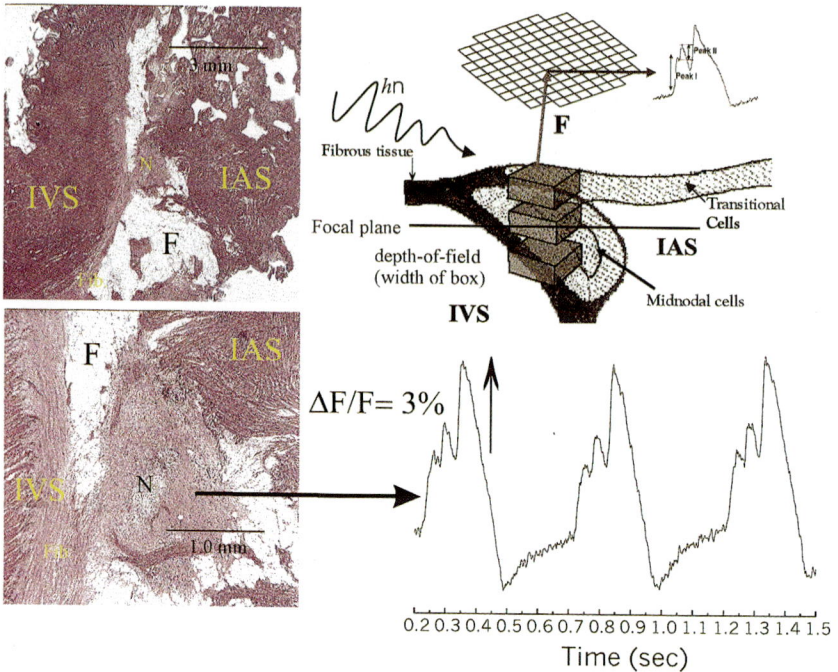

Figure 5. Histological analysis of the atrioventricular (AV) node confirms the origins of the second upstroke. Maps of action potentials were recorded from the AV node, then the preparation was labeled, fixed, embedded in paraffin, and sectioned for histological analysis, as previously described.[18] *Left panels:* Charge-coupled device images of a longitudinal cross-section of a rabbit AV node taken at a depth of 150 μm are shown at low (*top*) and high (*bottom*) magnification. Anatomical landmarks are the interatrial septum (IAS), the interventricular septum (IVS), fat deposits (F), fibrous tissue (Fib.), and the midnodal region (N). Note that under hematoxylin-eosin staining, nodal cells are pale compared with the more darkly stained ventricular and atrial cells. The compact node is surrounded by connective tissue and fat cell deposits, except for a continuum of excitable cells at inputs from the IAS. *Top right:* Schemas of a transverse histological section of the rabbit AV node indicating the different layers of cell types that are found as a function of depth in the tissue. Adapted from reference 37. Volumetric elements superimposed on the section represent the volume of cells which are the primary source of the signals detected by a diode when the focal plane is shifted in a stepwise manner, below the surface. At different focal planes, different layers of cells become the primary source of the fluorescence signal. *Bottom right:* Optical signal from a diode on the array, which detected voltage-dependent signals from the AV node. Signals from the node exhibited a sequence of three action potential upstrokes expected from the AV node (see text).

with maximum efficiency from a volume of tissue ($0.46 \times 0.46 \times 0.2$ mm). The dimensions of this volume are determined by the 2-dimensional magnification of the image (0.46×0.46 mm), two times the depth of field ($2 \times$ approximately 100 μm), and the location of focal plane of the optical apparatus. Cells "outside" this volume (i.e., ventricular cells below the node) contribute to the overall voltage-dependent signal but their contribution is reduced compared with cells close to the surface or when the focal plane is positioned on these cells. When the focal plane is displaced in a step-wise manner below the surface, light from cells located near the plane of focus is transferred to the diode with the highest efficiency, whereas light from cells above and below the focal plane is transferred with decreasing efficiency. This means that the location of the cells responsible for the second upstroke can be determined approximately by shifting the plane of focus until the maximum amplitude for the second upstroke is obtained. Optical sectioning of the AV node (i.e., shifting the focal plane in 100-μm steps) revealed that the ratio of the second to the first upstroke was dependent on the location of the focal plane, indicating that the two signals originate from different depths. The ratio reached a maximum when the focal plane was located approximately 0.5 mm below the surface of the IAS,[19] which implied that the second upstroke was generated by cells approximately 0.4 to 0.6 mm below the surface. Histological analysis of the AV node confirmed that the diodes detecting the second spike were suitably located to detect light from the compact node located 300 to 400 μm below the surface.[19] Figure 5 illustrates a longitudinal cross-section of the AV node region at low (*top left panel*) and high (*bottom left panel*) magnification, next to diode signals recorded from the center of the N zone. Several features of the histology allow us to identify the AV node with confidence. 1) The full slide shows the extent and dimensions of atrial and ventricular muscle and makes us confident of their identification. 2) Fat cell deposits are interposed in the picture between the atrial and ventricular tissue, as seen commonly in human (Dr. L. C. Nichols, personal communication, 1997) and rabbit hearts (see Fig. 12a in reference 34). 3) The location, shape, and dimensions of the zone are as expected for the rabbit AV node. 4) The tinctoral properties of these cells under hematoxylin-eosin stain cells are consistent with those expected for nodal cells.

Impulse Propagation in the Pacing AV Node. In the absence of SA node activity and atrial inputs, the AV node becomes the primary pacemaker due to the slow diastolic depolarization or pacemaker current of N or NH cells. The AP propagation pathway from the AV node to the atrial septum and ventricles was investigated by removing the SA node. Figure 6 illustrates, in a 3-dimensional graph, the sequence of depolarization detected via optical signals when pacemaker activity was initiated at the AV node. The x-y plane represents the AV node zone viewed by the array (5×5 mm), and the z-axis the level of depolarization (bright to dark). In Figure 6A, the node fired first and the upstroke is detected as a rise in signal from *bright to dark,* at the lower edge of the x-y plot. As a primary pacemaker, the AV node (or second upstroke) fired first and the atrial and ventricular electrograms were delayed (approximately 28 ms). When the AV node was the dominant pacemaker, the amplitude and slope of the first upstroke was markedly reduced since it now represented the second upstroke leading a wave of depolarization originating from the AV node. The signal spread in 10 ms within the node and, after a step-delay of 27.96 ms, activation spread across the IAS (Fig. 6B). The impulse then spread across the IAS and ventricle located in the upper and lower quadrants of the map, respectively. Interestingly, atrial depolarization did not begin at sites adjacent to the AV node region but appeared first 2 to 3 mm away in the IAS (Fig. 6B). This reproducible finding (n = 4) suggests that specialized path-

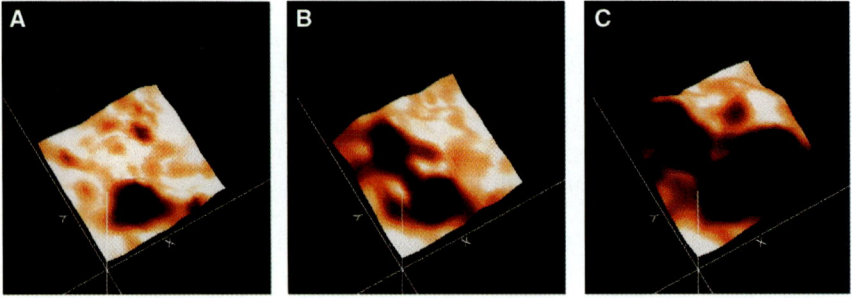

Figure 6. Spread of depolarization from a pacing atrioventricular (AV) node. The sinoatrial (SA) node was removed such that the AV node became the primary pacemaker. Atrial and ventricular electrograms were used to monitor the firing of the interatrial septum (IAS) and interventricular septum (IVS), and the optical wave of depolarization was depicted in 3-dimensional surface plots. The x-y plane represents the 2-dimensional surface of the AV node region with the same orientation as in Fig. 2B. The z-axis depicts the extent of depolarization correlated with optical action potentials (APs) from various regions of the preparation. **A.** Activation began in the proximal region of the AV node. **B.** Activation map taken 30 ms later depicts the spread of AP from the AV node to the IAS. Note that there exists a zone of polarized atrial tissue between the AV node and the first region to depolarize on the IAS. The data suggest that the impulse from the AV node to the IAS propagated through a specialized pathway from the AV node to approximately 2 mm in the IAS. **C.** Activation map, taken 45 ms after that in panel A, depicts the further spread of APs across the AV node and the IAS.

ways support electrical conduction between the AV node and the IAS. It is important to note that the AV node zone measured during sinus rhythm was the same as that delineated when the AV node became the pacemaker, which proves that spike 1 and 2 do not originate from the same cells but from different cells located at different depths.[19] The marked conduction delay from the AV node zone to the IAS (Fig. 6B) indicates that propagation is not smooth but discontinuous in both the anterograde and retrograde direction. This barrier to conduction between the compact node and the IAS is dramatically seen in all the activation maps (Fig. 6B)

A Step-Delay between AN and N Cells Regulates Total AV Delay. AV delay is physiologically regulated by heart rate and by parasympathetic and sympathetic activity. To investigate the mechanisms responsible for the physiological regulation of the AV node delay, activation maps across the node were analyzed as a function of cycle length. The SA node was removed and the right atrium was paced to control heart rate with bipolar electrodes placed near the SA node. The same activation patterns were measured across the AV node and the atrial and ventricular septa when heart rate was varied in a physiological range of cycle lengths (CL = 270 to 350 ms). AV delays varied as a function of CL and were highly correlated with the step-delay, τ_1, between atrial (AN) and nodal (N) cells, with a correlation coefficient of 0.98.[18,19] In contrast, AV delays correlated poorly with changes in the time to propagate across the AV node (see Figs. 3 and 4) and with τ_2 (correlation coefficient of 0.42), where τ_2 is defined as the delay between the second and third upstroke of signals recorded from the AV node region.[19]

AV delay is regulated by parasympathetic enervation, but the mechanism(s) involved in this regulation are poorly understood. Optical mapping techniques showed that perfusing the heart with acetylcholine ([ACh] 0.1 to 10 μmol/L) produced a significant increase in the step-delay, τ_1, by 19 ± 2.3 ms (30% increase). ACh also produced a slight decrease in conduction velocity across the node.[19] The prolongation of τ_1 and the slight decrease in θ_N is consistent with a hyperpolarization of N-cells by ACh, requiring that a greater atrial current be injected across a high-resistance barrier to reach threshold potential in the AV node.[19]

Discussion

Optical techniques provide detailed measurements of electrical propagation across the AV node and reveal that a conduction barrier produces a "step-delay" between atrial and nodal activation. These findings would not have been possible without the special features of optical mapping techniques that provided the spatial, temporal, and depth resolution needed to identify AV node APs as the second upstrokes sandwiched between the firing of transitional and ventricular cells. Optical sectioning is of critical importance to allow the identification of the AV node AP as a signal emanating from cells below the surface that fired with approximately 30 ms delay after the transitional cells on the surface. Several lines of evidence support the interpretation that the second upstroke represented AV nodal APs and could be used to map activation within the node.

The occurrence of the second upstroke was anatomically correlated with the location of the midnodal and lower nodal regions. The temporal relationship between the second upstroke and atrial and ventricular electrograms indicated that the second upstroke originated from cells firing in the correct time frame for AV nodal APs. Activation maps drawn separately for the three spikes confirmed the interpretation that the three spikes represented atrial, AV nodal, and ventricular depolarizations, respectively.

Intracellular microelectrode and optical APs were simultaneously recorded from the zone, which exhibited the sequence of three upstrokes. In all cases, the firing of the second spike was coincident with microelectrode AP recordings which had the characteristic shape of N and NH; that is, slow upstroke and/or slow diastolic depolarization.[19] Moreover, microelectrode recordings from atrial, AN, and ventricular APs were not coincident with the second upstroke.

Conduction velocities were calculated from spikes 1 and 2 and indicated that spike 1 propagates at atrial conduction velocities and spike 2 propagates slowly, as expected for an AV node velocity. The signal amplitude of the second upstroke as a function of depth of focus was consistent with the interpretation that it originated from the firing of APs by cells approximately 0.4 to 0.6 mm below the surface of the preparation.

Identification of Various AV Node Cell Types

Previous electrophysiological and morphological studies have identified at least five different cell types in the AV node zone. A major limitation of the optical technique is the difficulty of resolving single cell APs. However, interventions with drugs like terodotoxin proved to be useful to identify the cell types comprising the activation zone delineated by the second upstroke and His depolarization.[38] A limitation of the optical technique as applied to the intact heart was the inability to measure AP durations of compact node APs because these APs were preceded by APs fired by transitional cells and followed ventricular APs. As a result, the part of the plateau and the downstroke of AV node APs were obscured by the firing of APs from deeper ventricular fibers. This limitation was overcome by cutting the His bundle, which blocked ventricular APs and eliminated the third upstroke from signals recorded from the AV node.[19] The approach was effective in eliminating the ventricular APs but could change the time course of AV node APs by altering electrotonic coupling between N, NH, and His fibers and thereby alter N cell APDs. Despite these limitations, optical mapping techniques offer a new approach to study the organization and coupling of atrial, AN, N, NH, and His cells in ways that cannot be resolved by conventional electrode techniques.

Mechanism(s) Responsible for AH Delays

A number of important conclusions can be extracted from the present findings. One major finding is that the conduction through the AV node is not only decremental but also discontinuous in nature and that a conduction barrier exists between atrial and midnodal cells. Features of the barrier are consistent with the presence of an inexcitable gap across which activation proceeds electrotonically across a high-resistance pathway. Although a barrier consisting of resistive and capacitance components is consistent with the data, a barrier with more complex properties has not been excluded. The superposition of activation maps on longitudinal cross-sections of the AV node shows that the node is surrounded by a sheaf of fibrous and connective tissue (Fig. 5).[19] Fat deposits typically interposed between atrial and ventricular tissues in the AV node also contribute to the electrical isolation of these tissues in both human (Dr. L. C. Nichols, unpublished data, 1980–1995) and rabbit hearts.[39] Thus, the node is electrically insulated except for an electrical pathway consisting of a high-resistance electrical barrier which lies at the boundary of AN and N cells.

Decremental conduction did not appear to be the primary mechanism for AV delay because it is incompatible with the relatively fast conduction velocity, θ_N, across the node.[19] For instance, if conduction through the node is decremental (with no step-delay) and accounts for the total AV delay, then θ_N should be at least 10 times slower than in the atrium. From the analysis of optical signals, the conduction velocity in the node was 0.162 ± 0.024 m/s, approximately one third that of atrial tissue (0.76 ± 0.062 m/s).[19] The delay due to conduction through the node was ≤ 14 ms, an insufficient interval to account for the AV delay. In contrast, the step-delay due to discontinuous conduction between AN and N cells was 30.24 ms or approximately 50% of the total AV delay. In addition, when the AV node became the primary pacemaker, the conduction barrier at the posterior margin of AV node was still responsible for the major component of AV delay during retrograde as well as anterograde propagation (Fig. 6). On the basis of these results, the major AV nodal delay is primarily due to discontinuous conduction between AN and N cells.

The concept of an inexcitable gap in the node resulting in discontinuous conduction had been postulated from experimental[18] and theoretical studies[40–42] of AV node conduction. Discontinuous conduction was tested by applying a local perturbation (i.e., freezing,[43] a current,[44] high K+,[45] or a sucrose gap[46]) in otherwise uniform cardiac fibers (e.g., Purkinje or ventricular). In these experimental models, the perturbation produced a step change in delay and "stagnation" similar to that observed in the node. Step-delays were due to an interruption of active transmission of an impulse as it arrived at the inexcitable gap. The electrotonic transmission through the inexcitable gap slowly charged distal cells until the resting potential of the distal cells reached threshold and ignited active transmission in the distal cells. Of critical importance is that the step-delay is determined by the time needed to inject the electrotonic current necessary to induce active transmission in the distal cells. James et al.[47] argued against decremental conduction because AV delays were not proportional to the size of AV node in various mammalian hearts. They proposed that pacemaker cells were involved in the AV delay, as coupled relaxation oscillators modulated by electrotonic atrial inputs, across a resistive barrier.

Efimov et al.[48] used optical mapping techniques to map fast and slow pathways to the AV node and in the process reported measurements of optical APs from the rabbit AV node. In this study, AV node APs were identified because of their slow rise times but they did not overlap with APs from transitional or ventricular cells. The detection of AV node optical APs separate and without the overlap of signals from other cell types (see Fig. 3, in reference 48) is in conflict with our findings and is contrary to microelectrode studies that show extensive overlap of AN, N, and NH cells. In the absence of supporting pharmacological, histological, or microelectrode tests, the origins of their AV node APs cannot be appraised. However, their AV node APs most likely did not originate from N and/or NH cells (i.e., peak II) that lie below the surface and cannot be separated from AN or transitional cells lying on the surface. A more likely interpretation is that their AV node signals were generated by AN cells, which accounts for the unusually large dimension of their AV node zones ($\geq$6 mm instead of approximately 2 mm in length). Billette et al.[11] investigated the distribution of AN, N, and NH cells using intracellular microelectrode and found that APs from AN, N, and NH cells were commonly recorded from the same site. At any location (but unknown depth), APs had markedly different characteristics and activation times, with some cells activating early and others late in the same region. The superposition of these different cell types indicated that they are either intermingled or lie at different depth within the AV node region. In either case, optical recordings from such a distribution of cells represents the sum of their APs and, because of their temporal delays, will appear as a set of AP upstrokes separated by time delays. Thus, the detection of multiple upstrokes by a diode is the key to identify AV node APs by optical techniques. In optical studies with intact rabbit hearts under sinus rhythm, impulse propagation across the IAS traveled in a direction anterior to posterior before entering the AV node zone,[18,19] in agreement with maps in human hearts reported by McGuire et al.[49] In contrast, Efimov et al.[48] reported the opposite direction of propagation in the IAS, from posterior to anterior, and argued that the different directions could be due to species differences. The opposite findings obtained from isolated, superfused rabbit AV nodes indicate that the differences are most likely due to altered conduction pathways caused by the extensive dissection procedure used in the superfused preparation.[48]

The present study provides robust evidence for a step-delay in conduction across a resistive barrier. The regulation of the step-delay as a function of cycle length and ACh indicates that it plays a major mechanistic role in the physiological control of AV delay. Thus, optical mapping techniques have provided direct evidence for a conduction barrier and its location between AN and N cells, and have allowed us to measure the "step-delay" that is involved in the physiological regulation of AV delay. The study raises new questions regarding the mechanisms underlying total AV delay and demonstrates the potential of optical techniques to elucidate basic problems in AV node physiology and current clinical problems.

Acknowledgments: Thanks are due to Dr. Lawrence C. Nichols from the Department of Pathology at the University of Pittsburgh, for his technical advice and guidance regarding the analysis and interpretation of the AV node histology. The authors are indebted to William Hughes and Scott MacPherson, staff of the Departmental Machine Shop, for the construction of the heart chamber and manipulators to adjust the focal plane of the optical apparatus.

References

1. Tawara S. *Das Reizleitungs System des Herzens.* Jena, Germany: Fisher; 1906.
2. Lewis T, Masters AM. Observations upon conduction in the mammalian heart. A-V conduction. *Heart* 1925;12:209–269.
3. James TN. Anatomy of the cardiac conduction system in the rabbit. *Circ Res* 1967;20:638–648.
4. Anderson RH. Histologic and histochemical evidence concerning the presence of morphologically distinct cellular zones within the rabbit atrioventricular node. *Anat Rec* 1972;173:7–24.
5. Scherf L, James T, Wood WT. Function of the atrioventricular node considered on the basis of observed histology and fine structure. *J Am Coll Cardiol* 1985;5:770–780.
6. Meijler FL, Janse MJ. Morphology and electrophysiology of the mammalian atrioventricular node. *Physiol Rev* 1988;68(2):608–647.
7. Paes de Carvalho A, De Almeida DF. Spread of activity through the atrioventricular node. *Circ Res* 1960;8:801–809.
8. Billette J. Atrioventricular nodal activation during premature stimulation of the atrium. *Am J Physiol* 1987;252:H163-H177.
9. Sano T, Tasaki M, Shimamoto T. Histologic examination of the origin of the action potential characteristically obtained from the region bordering the atrioventricular node. *Circ Res* 1959;7:700–704.
10. Anderson RH, Janse MJ, Van Capelle FJL, et al. A combined morphological and electrophysiological study of the atrioventricular node of the rabbit heart. *Circ Res* 1974;135(6):909–922.
11. Billette J, Janse MJ, Van Capelle FJL, et al. Cycle-length dependent properties of AV nodal activation in rabbit hearts. *Am J Physiol* 1976;231:1129–1139.
12. Hoffman BF, Cranefield PF. *Electrophysiology of the Heart.* New York: McGraw-Hill; 1960.

13. Gettes LS, Buchanan JW Jr, Saito T, et al. Studies concerned with slow conduction. In Zipes DP, Jalife J (eds): *Electrophysiology and Arrhythmias*. Orlando: Grune & Stratton; 1985:81–87.
14. Scherf D. Über intraventrikuläre Störungen der Erregungsausbreitung bei den enckebachschen Perioden. *Wien Arch Inn Med* 1929;18:403–416.
15. Rosenblueth A. Mechanism of the Wenckebach-Luciani cycles. *Am J Physiol* 1958;194:491–494.
16. Zipes DP, Mendez C, Moe G. Some examples of Wenckebach periodicity in cardiac tissues, with an appraisal of mechanisms. In Rosenbaum MB (ed): *Frontiers of Cardiac Electrophysiology*. The Hague: Martinus Nijhoff; 1983:357–375.
17. Young M-L, Wolf GS, Castellanos A, Gelband H. Application of the Rosenblueth hypothesis to assess atrioventricular nodal behavior. *Am J Cardiol* 1986;57:131–134.
18. Choi B-R, Salama G. Optical mapping of atrioventricular (AV) node reveals a conduction barrier between atrial and nodal cells. *Circulation* 1997;70:83.
19. Choi B-R, Salama G. Optical mapping of the rabbit atrio-ventricular node reveals a conduction barrier between atrial and nodal cells. *Am J Physiol* 1998;274:H829-H845.
20. Salama G, Morad M. Merocyanine-540 as an optical probe of transmembrane electrical activity of the heart. *Science* 1976;191:485–487.
21. Salama G, Lombardi RA, Elson J. Maps of action potential and NADH fluorescence in intact working hearts. *Am J Physiol* 1987;252:H384-H394.
22. Salama G. Optical measurements of transmembrane potentials in heart. In Lowe L (ed): *Spectroscopic Probes of Membrane Potential*. Boca Raton: CRC Uniscience Publications; 1988:132–199.
23. Davidenko JM, Pertsov AV, Salomonz R, et al. Stationary and drifting spiral waves of excitation in isolated cardiac muscle. *Nature* 1992;355:349–351.
24. Loew L, Cohen L, Dix J, et al. A naphthyl analog of the aminostyryl pyridinium class of potentiometric membrane dyes shows consistent sensitivity in a variety of tissue, cell and model membrane preparation. *J Membr Biol* 1992;130:1–10.
25. Wiggins JR, Reiser J, Fitzpatrick DF, Bergey JL. Ionotropic actions of diacetyl monoxime in cat ventricular muscle. *J Pharmacol Exp Ther* 1980;212:217–224.
26. Kanai A, Salama G. Optical mapping reveals that repolarization spreads anisotropically and is guided by fiber orientation in guinea pig hearts. *Circ Res* 1995;77:784–802.
27. Piller H. *Microscope Photometry*. Berlin, Heidelberg, New York: Springer Verlag; 1977:16.
28. Li T, Sperelakis N, Teneick RE, Solaro RJ: Effects of diacetyl monoxime on cardiac excitation-contraction coupling. *J Pharmacol Exp Ther* 1985;232:688–695.
29. Liu Y, Cabo C, Salomonz R, et al. Effects of diacetyl monoxime on the electrical properties of sheep and guinea pig ventricular muscle. *Cardiovasc Res* 1993;27:1991–1997.
30. Gwathmey JK, Hajjar RJ, Solaro RJ. Contractile deactivation and uncoupling of crossbridges. Effects of 2,3-butanedione monoxime on mammalian myocardium. *Circ Res* 1991;69:1280–1292.
31. Steele DS, Smith GL. Effects of 2,3-butanedione monoxime on sarcoplasmic reticulum of saponin-treated rat cardiac muscle. *Am J Physiol* 1993; 265:H1493–H1500.
32. Phillips RM, Altschuld RA. 2,3-Butanedione 2-monoxime (BDM) induces calcium release from canine cardiac sarcoplasmic reticulum. *Biochem Biophys Res Commun* 1996;229:154–157.
33. Verrechia F, Hervé JC. Reversible blockade of gap junctional communication by 2,3-butanedione monoxime in rat cardiac myocytes. *Am J Physiol* 1997;272:C875-C885.

34. Salama G, Restivo M, Choi B-R. Optical mapping of activation repolarization and re-entry patterns in arterially perfused canine ventricles. *Ann Biomed Eng* 1995;23(1):527.
35. Cheng Y, Mowrey K, Efimov IR, et al. Effects of 2,3-butanedione monoxime on atrial-atrioventricular nodal conduction in isolated rabbit heart. *J Cardiovasc Electrophysiol* 1997;3:790–802.
36. Luna LG. *Manual of Histological Staining Methods of the Armed Forces Institute of Pathology*. 3rd ed. New York: Blakiston Division, McGraw Hill; 1968:36–38.
37. DeFelice J, Challice CE. Anatomical and ultrastructural study of the atrioventricular region of the rabbit heart. *Circ Res* 1969;24:457–474.
38. Zipes DP, Mendez C. Action of manganese ions and tetrodotoxin on A-V nodal transmembrane potentials in isolated rabbit hearts. *Circ Res* 1973;32:447.
39. Tranum-Jensen J. The fine structure of the atrial and atrio-ventricular (AV) junctional specialized tissues of the rabbit heart. In Wellens HJJ, Lie KI, Janse MJ (eds): *The Conduction System of the Heart: Structure Function and Clinical Implications*. Philadelphia: Lea & Febiger; 1976:55–81.
40. Kinoshita S, Konishi G. Mechanisms of atypical atrioventricular Wenckebach periodicity. A theoretical model derived from the concepts of inhomogeneous excitability and electrotonically mediated conduction. *J Electrocardiol* 1989;22(3):227–233.
41. LeBlanc AR, Dube B. Propagation in the AV node: A model based on a simplified two-dimensional structure and a bidomain tissue representation. *Med Biol Eng Comput* 1993;31:545–565.
42. Malik M, Ward D, Camm AJ. Theoretical evaluation of the Rosenblueth hypothesis. *Pacing Clin Electrophysiol* 1988;11(9):1250–1261.
43. Waxman MB, Downar E, Wald RW. Unidirectional block in Purkinje fibers. *Can J Physiol Pharmacol* 1980;58:925–933.
44. Wennemark JR, Ruesta VJ, Brody DA. Microelectrode study of delayed conduction in the canine right bundle branch. *Circ Res* 1968;23:753–769.
45. Cranefield PF, Kein HO, Hoffman BF. Conduction of the cardiac impulses. 1. Delay, block, and one way block in depressed Purkinje fibers. *Circ Res* 1971;28:199–219.
46. Antzelevitch C, Moe GK. Electrotonically-mediated delayed conduction and reentry in relation to 'slow response' in mammalian ventricular conduction tissue. *Circ Res* 1981;49:1129–1139.
47. James TN, Kawamura K, Meijler FL, et al. Anatomy of the sinus node, AV node, and His bundle of the heart of the sperm whale (Physeter macrocephalus), with a node on the absence of an os cordis. *Anat Rec* 1995;242:355–373.
48. Efimov IR, Fahy GJ, Cheng YN, et al. High resolution fluorescent mapping of rabbit heart does not reveal a distinct atrioventricular nodal anterior input channel (fast pathway) during sinus rhythm. *J Cardiovasc Electrophysiol* 1997;8:295–306.
49. McGuire MA, Bourke JP, Robotin MC, et al. High resolution mapping of Koch's triangle using sixty electrodes in human with atrioventricular junctional (AV nodal) reentrant tachycardia. *Circulation* 1993;88(1):2315–2328.

Chapter 11

Optical Mapping of Microscopic Propagation:
Clinical Insights and Applications

Albert L. Waldo

Mapping of cardiac propagation has been of interest to the physiologist and clinician since it was recognized that electrical impulses spread over heart muscle to generate the heartbeat. Over the years, progress in this area has been importantly related to advances in technology. It is all the more remarkable, therefore, that the initial principles of propagation as they relate to reentry established by Mayer[1,2] in the first decade of the 20th century were derived simply from watching contraction patterns in the jellyfish muscular ring. Subsequent studies in the early era of mapping cardiac propagation were performed with use of a lever attached at one end to cardiac tissue and at the other end to a smoked drum to record relative cardiac contraction time as a reflection of cardiac activation time. For instance, it was from such studies that the old, long-taught but now discredited concept of upper, middle, and lower nodal rhythms was formulated.[3,4]

The ability to record electrical activity directly from cardiac tissues using a cotton wick electrode, i.e., an electrode in which the tip was made of cotton and was dipped in saline and attached to a wire to record electrical signals on a string galvanometer, provided a major technological advance. It served to produce the initial electrophysiological studies of activation mapping, which helped establish, among other things, the concept of primary negativity for the study of localization of impulse initiation of the cardiac activation sequence (e.g., as in sinus rhythm).[5] This technique was also used in the mapping of reentrant rhythms such as atrial flutter in the canine heart.[6] An important advance was the subsequent development of metal electrodes (as opposed to a cotton wick dipped in saline) to record directly from cardiac tissue. Nevertheless, recording to establish the sequence of cardiac activation was usually performed by recording sequentially from selected sites. Primarily due to limitations in technology, recording from only a small number of sites simultaneously was sometimes possible as well. It was clear that the spatial and temporal resolution of the sequence of activation maps obtained in this fashion was limited. Nevertheless, for stable rhythms, much useful information was obtained.

From Rosenbaum DS, Jalife J (eds): *Optical Mapping of Cardiac Excitation and Arrhythmias.* ©Futura Publishing Co., Inc., Armonk, NY, 2001.

This includes recording from the specialized atrioventricular (AV) conduction system, in particular, the His bundle and the bundle branches.[7] The latter led directly to the clinical use of recording directly from cardiac tissues using catheter electrode techniques. In fact, the first clinical "breakthrough" using catheter electrode techniques for the study of cardiac propagation was when it was demonstrated that recordings could be made directly from the His bundle.[8,9] This first led to a systematic examination of AV conduction in humans, and despite inherent limitations of this technique, there was an explosion of interest and data of all sorts, which continues to this day. We now can even recognize potentials recorded from accessory AV connections, and have come to understand unique recordings such as fractionated potentials and double potentials.[10,11] These epicardial and endocardial recording techniques have been used principally for study of propagation rather than repolarization.

When microelectrodes to record transmembrane action potentials were introduced,[12,13] they provided yet another important leap forward in our ability to study not only impulse propagation but also repolarization, principally at the cellular level, in a manner not previously available with other techniques. Although this technology was and continues to be an important part of our understanding of impulse propagation and repolarization, it has been principally limited to in vitro studies of small-size tissue, as cardiac superfusion of the tissue with oxygenated physiological solutions limits thickness of the preparation, and contraction usually makes it very difficult to record from the whole heart, whether in situ or in vitro. Nevertheless, this technology has been and remains very important to our continued study and understanding of propagation and repolarization.

The next major advance, the development of the simultaneous multisite mapping from a very large number of electrodes using computer-aided multisite mapping techniques, was again the result of technology[14]; and with time, further advances in this technique have permitted simultaneous recording from large numbers of electrodes from cardiac tissue both in situ and in vitro. It has also permitted recording from epicardium, endocardium, and even intramyocardium, the latter in the ventricles using needle (plunge) electrodes.

The search for noninvasive mapping techniques has included body surface potential mapping.[15] The latter is largely still investigational. By means of the so-called inverse solution, it uses mathematical computation from signals recorded from numerous sites on the body surface to determine the activation sequence on the surface of the heart. In fact, there are now techniques that use the mathematics of the inverse solution to record from an endocardial cavity in order to compute the endocardial activation sequence.[16] These techniques have been of particular interest not only for study of cardiac propagation (depolarization), but also for studies of cardiac repolarization. All the above-described techniques have advantages and disadvantages but, in toto, have advanced our understanding of propagation of the cardiac impulse and of repolarization. This short chapter sets the stage for consideration of optical mapping.

As is well described in Section II of this text, optical mapping fills a very important niche in mapping of propagation in and repolarization of the heart. The several chapters in this section tell the story of the many advantages and exciting future of optical mapping. Nevertheless, a few comments are in order. Among its chief assets is the ability of optical mapping to record action potentials from groups of cells. In so doing, it not only provides a very accurate method to perform sequence of activation mapping, but also it makes available considerably more data than previous techniques used to study repolarization, if only because it can be easily applied to the whole heart. In fact, optical action potential mapping makes it possible to measure high-fidelity action potentials simultaneously from hundreds of sites with high temporal and spatial resolution.

Another important advantage to optical mapping is that it is relatively "noninvasive," thereby avoiding potential injury associated with placement of electrodes onto or into cells. Another benefit related to the lack of requirement of physical electrodes is that there is essentially no limit to the degree of spatial resolution of membrane potential that can be achieved. Hence, as described in this section of the book, it is possible to integrate microscopic propagation across the sarcolemma of individual cells and discontinuous propagation between cells. This already has and will continue to provide important new insights on the most fundamental aspects of impulse propagation in the heart. Also, because its recorded signals are not distorted by stimulation artifact, it has enormous advantages when studying stimulated tissue, in particular, following defibrillation shocks. It is also invaluable for the study of action potentials in circumstances in which more traditional electrode recordings are difficult or impossible, e.g., during studies, as just mentioned, using defibrillation shocks. In addition, optical dyes can be used as probes for the study of calcium, potassium, and sodium transients, as well as for study of pH. Inevitably, there are also limitations of optical mapping. These, too, are well discussed in the several chapters in Section II. They include such things as the need to greatly minimize or prevent movement of heart muscle with the artifact it introduces, phototoxicity exerted by the potentiometric dyes, inability to support long-term experiments, problems with signal-to-noise ratio, inability to measure the absolute value of the resting potential, the distortion of the action potential downstroke, and the fact that the optical action potential represents the sum of action potential from several cells within the region of tissue being recorded, rather than a single cell.

In the end, investigators will choose from the several available techniques to obtain data as the situation requires. And probably, the several techniques will often be complementary. But undoubtedly, optical mapping offers unique advantages and great opportunities to the investigator. In short, it is a relatively new and exciting technique that will greatly aid in advancing our knowledge of propagation and repolarization.

References

1. Mayer AG. *Rhythmical Pulsation in Scyphomedusae*. Washington, DC: Carnegie Institution of Washington, Publication 47. 1906:1–62.
2. Mayer AG. Rhythmical pulsation in scyphomedusae. II. In *Papers from the Tortugas Laboratory of the Carnegie Institution of Washington*. 1908;1:113–131.
3. Zahn A. Experimentelle Untersuchungen über Reizbildung im Atrioventrikularknoten und Sinus Coronarius. *Zbl Physiol* 1912;26:495.

4. Zahn A. Experimentelle Untersuchungen über Reizbildung and Reizleitung im Atrioventrikularknoten. *Arch Ges Physiol* 1913;151:247.
5. Erlanger J. The localization of impulse initiation and conduction in the heart. *Arch Intern Med* 1913;2:334.
6. Lewis T. Observations upon flutter and fibrillation. IV: Impure flutter: Theory of circus movement. *Heart* 1920;7:293–345.
7. Hoffman BF, Cranefield PF, Stuckey JH, et al. Direct measurement of conduction velocity in in situ specialized conducting system of mammalian heart. *Proc Soc Exp Biol Med* 1959;102:55.
8. Scherlag BJ, Helfant RH, Damato AN. Catheterization technique for His bundle stimulation and recording in the intact dog. *J Appl Physiol* 1968;25(4):425–428.
9. Scherlag BJ, Lau SH, Helfant RH, et al. Catheter technique for recording His bundle activity in man. *Circulation* 1969;39:13–18.
10. Waldo AL, Kaiser GA. A study of ventricular arrhythmias associated with acute myocardial infarction in the canine heart. *Circulation* 1973;47:1222–1228.
11. Shimizu A, Nozaki A, Rudy Y, Waldo AL. Characterization of double potentials in a functionally determined reentrant circuit—multiplexing studies during interruption of atrial flutter in the canine pericarditis model. *J Am Coll Cardiol* 1993;22:2022–2032.
12. Ling G, Gerard RW. The normal membrane potential of frog sartorius fibers. *J Cell Comp Physiol* 1949;34:383–396.
13. Weidmann S. Effect of current flow on the membrane potential of cardiac muscle. *J Physiol* 1951;115:227–236.
14. Boineau JP, Schuessler RB, Mooney CR, et al. Natural and evoked atrial flutter due to circus movement in dogs. Role of abnormal atrial pathways, slow conduction, nonuniform refractory period distribution and premature beats. *Am J Cardiol* 1980;45:1167–1181.
15. Taccardi B. Distribution of heart potentials on the thoracic surface of normal human subjects. *Circ Res* 1963;12:341.
16. Taccardi B, Arisi G, Macchi E, et al. A new intracavitary probe for detecting the site of origin of ectopic ventricular beats during one cardiac cycle. *Circulation* 1987;75:272–281.

Section III

Cardiac Arrhythmias

Introduction:

Unique Role of Optical Mapping in the Study of Cardiac Arrhythmias

José Jalife, MD

Cardiac arrhythmias are a major cause of morbidity and mortality throughout the world. Yet, despite many years of research, understanding of the precise mechanisms of the most complex arrhythmias, including atrial and ventricular fibrillation, remains elusive. Until recently, most experimental studies on the mechanisms of arrhythmias were based on single intracellular or multiple extracellular recording techniques. However, increased theoretical understanding of the dynamics and mechanisms of cardiac arrhythmias has augmented the need for highly sophisticated tools that are capable of recording cardiac excitation and recovery with very high spatial and temporal resolution. While far from ideal, optical mapping fulfills much of such a need. For example, recent application of optical mapping technology to the study of cardiac fibrillation has enabled investigators to test experimentally a number of predictions derived from the theory of wave propagation in excitable media, which significantly advanced our understanding of this life-threatening arrhythmia.[1–5] In fact, optical mapping has made it possible to demonstrate that fibrillation is a problem of self-organization whereby high-frequency reentrant sources generate spiraling waves that propagate throughout the ventricles in complex patterns.[6] In Section III of this book, contributions by some of the top experts in the optical mapping field illustrate the unique role of this powerful technology in the study of dynamics and mechanisms of arrhythmias.

One of the hallmarks of the vulnerability of the ventricles to reentrant arrhythmias is the highly heterogeneous spatial distribution of refractory periods. Before the advent of optical mapping, investigators had attempted, without much success, to determine the degree of a spatial dispersion of refractoriness and to provide a quantitative correlation between dispersion and the ability of the ventricles to undergo sustained arrhythmias. In chapter 12 Laurita, Pastore, and Rosenbaum address the problem of dispersion of repolarization from the optical mapping point of view. They use a photodiode array system to record action potentials from more than 100 sites simultaneously on the ventricular epicardial surface of the guinea pig heart, and measure action potential duration dispersion as a surrogate for refractory period dispersion. They demonstrate how the heterogeneous spatial distribution of electrophysiological properties that are inherent to the cardiac muscle result in complicated beat-to-beat temporal and spatial dynamics of action potential duration that lead to concordant and discordant alternans and ultimately reentrant arrhythmias. Then in chapter 13, Girouard and Rosenbaum look at the problem of action potential duration dispersion but during the process of reentry around a linear obstacle produced by a fine laser lesion on the ventricular epicardium of the guinea pig heart. They demonstrate that during sustained reentry action potential duration—and therefore wavelength—is not constant but changes depending on the position of the wave front with respect to the fiber orientation.

Reentrant cardiac arrhythmias may occur over various spatial scales, ranging from microreentry to rotors giving rise to spiral waves that encompass a whole atrium or ventricle. It is therefore desirable that a mapping system should cover a relatively large area with closely spaced recording sites. In chapter 14, Gray and Jalife provide direct demonstration of the power of high-resolution optical mapping to analyze the dynamics of cardiac fibrillation. Based on analytical tools (i.e., "phase mapping") used previously to study the mechanisms of reentry and ventricular fibrillation,[8] they present evidence for the existence of phase singularities during right atrial fibrillation and demonstrate the ephemeral nature of phase singularities occurring in the right atrium. Their results support the idea that normally atrial fibrillation in the isolated sheep heart is not sustained by events in the right atrial wall. Rather, it seems to be the of result activation by stable sources in the left atrium.[9–11] They also show that addition of acetylcholine shortens the wavelength and can result in rotor formation in right atrial preparations where the cut boundaries may influence the dynamics. In chapter 15, Baxter and Davidenko discuss the use of video imaging technology in the study of the dynamics and mechanisms of cardiac arrhythmias. They start by addressing the strengths and limitations of the various technologies that are currently used for optical mapping experiments, with particular attention paid to the use of charged coupled device (CCD) cameras. They then provide us with an illustrative example of the use of video imaging in the study of spiral wave activity as a mechanism of complex cardiac arrhythmias. In chapter 16, Samie et al. present previously unpublished results from an initial study on alterations in wave propagation on the ventricular epicardial surface of a transgenic mouse with familial hypertrophic cardiomyopathy caused by a mutation in the α-myosin heavy chain.[7] These mice exhibit the expected cardiac histopathology including hypertrophy, myocellular disarray, fibrosis, and small vessel disease. These authors postulate that when structural alteration present in the ventricles of these mice (e.g., fibrosis and myocellular disarray) are of the appropriate size, they result in changes in the electrical activation sequence and therefore serve as an arrhythmogenic substrate. They use a miniaturized video imaging system with high spatial and temporal resolution capable of recording complex patterns of activation in the adult mouse heart. Also, using new analytical tools they quantify propagation velocity and investigate the patterns of epicardial activation during sinus rhythm and during arrhythmias.

The preceding chapters do not deal explicitly with the relevance of optical mapping studies on arrhythmias in experimental animals to arrhythmology in human patients. For that, one needs the perspective of an expert clinical electrophysiologist. In chapter 17, Packer presents a realistic view of what all the results that are emerging from optical mapping experiments at an accelerating pace mean to the practicing clinician, and how that clinician can use the new information to more accurately diagnose arrhythmias seen in his or her patients. He identifies optical mapping as a powerful tool to help gain knowledge about mechanisms and dynamics of clinically relevant arrhythmias, including torsade de pointes, and ventricular as well as atrial fibrillation. Finally, he prudently discusses the limitations of these techniques, particularly in regard to our inability to use them in the clinic. He also looks into the future and identifies optical mapping as groundbreaking technology for the development of new imaging approaches that may have direct clinical application in the diagnosis and treatment of arrhythmias.

References

1. Davidenko JM, Pertsov AV, Salomonsz R, et al. Stationary and drifting spiral waves of excitation in isolated cardiac muscle. *Nature* 1992;355:349–351.
2. Pertsov AM, Davidenko JM, Salomonsz R, et al. Spiral waves of excitation underlie reentrant activity in isolated cardiac muscle. *Circ Res* 1993;72(3):631–650.
3. Cabo C, Pertsov AM, Davidenko JM, et al. Vortex shedding as a precursor of turbulent electrical activity in cardiac muscle. *Biophys J* 1996;70:1105–1111.
4. Gray RA, Jalife J, Panfilov AV, et al. Nonstationary vortexlike reentrant activity as a mechanism of polymorphic ventricular tachycardia in the isolated rabbit heart. *Circulation* 1995;91:2454–2469.
5. Gray RA, Jalife J, Panfilov AV, et al. Mechanisms of cardiac fibrillation. *Science* 1995;270:1222–1225.
6. Jalife J, Gray RA, Morley GE, Davidenko JM. Self-organization and dynamical nature of ventricular fibrillation. *Chaos* 1998;8:79–93.
7. Vikstrom KL, Factor SM, Leinwand LA. Mice expressing mutant myosin heavy chains are a model for familial hypertrophic cardiomyopathy. *Mol Med* 1996;2:556–567.
8. Gray RA, Pertsov AM, Jalife J. Spatial and temporal organization during cardiac fibrillation. *Nature* 1998;392:75–78.
9. Jalife J, Berenfeld O, Skanes AC, Mandapati R. Mechanisms of atrial fibrillation: Mother rotors or multiple daughter wavelets, or both? *J Cardiovasc Electrophysiol* 1998;9:S2-S12.
10. Skanes AC, Mandapati R, Berenfeld O, et al. Spatiotemporal periodicity during atrial fibrillation in the isolated sheep heart. *Circulation* 1998;98:1236–1248.
11. Mandapati R, Skanes A, Chen J, et al. Stable microreentrant sources as a mechanism of atrial fibrillation in the isolated sheep heart. *Circulation* 2000; 101:194–199.

Chapter 12

Mapping Arrhythmia Substrates Related to Repolarization:

1. Dispersion of Repolarization

Kenneth R. Laurita, Joseph M. Pastore, and David S. Rosenbaum

Numerous studies have established a close association between spatial heterogeneity of repolarization and cardiac arrhythmogenesis.[1–4] More recently, this association has been underscored by a growing interest in the spatial diversity of ion currents known to govern cellular repolarization. Many studies have focused on ion channel diversity that exists between juxtaposed ventricular muscle layers,[5–10] giving rise to functionally distinct regions within the ventricle. For example, the transient outward current (I_{to}), responsible for the prominent "notch" during early repolarization, is expressed almost exclusively in ventricular epicardial but not endocardial cells.[5–7] In contrast, M cells, present in the midmyocardial wall,[8–10] exhibit a reduced expression of the slow component of the delayed rectifier I_{Ks}.[11,12] Diminished I_{Ks} accounts for an enhanced sensitivity of M cells to interventions that prolong action potential duration (APD) (e.g., bradycardia, Class III antiarrhythmic drugs).[11] More recently, we have found that the cellular kinetics of repolarization also vary systematically between cells across the epicardial surface of the guinea pig heart, despite the presence of normal cell-to-cell coupling within the muscle layer.[13] It is apparent that cellular repolarization properties vary extensively within the heart and even within single myocardial layers. However, the implications of such diversity on repolarization heterogeneity and the formation of arrhythmogenic substrates in the heart was previously not well appreciated.

Critical components of the reentrant substrate such as spatial dispersion of repolarization[2,4,14] are classically thought of as static properties of the tissue that are either present or absent. However, because ion channels that govern repolarization are time-dependent,[15–18] one would predict that regional diversity of such channels is expected to significantly influence

From Rosenbaum DS, Jalife J (eds): *Optical Mapping of Cardiac Excitation and Arrhythmias.* ©Futura Publishing Co., Inc., Armonk, NY, 2001.

the pattern and spatial synchronization of ventricular repolarization on a beat-by-beat basis. Therefore, a suitable electrophysiological substrate for reentry (e.g., dispersion of repolarization) may not initially exist but may dynamically form, disappear, and reform in a heart-rate–dependent fashion. There is ample evidence that supports this concept. Bradycardia, which preferentially prolongs APD in M cells, enhances the formation of early afterdepolarizations and repolarization heterogeneities, which may presage intramural reentry and torsade de pointes.[19–22] Conversely, following an abrupt increase in heart rate, heterogeneity of APD across the guinea pig epicardium decreases significantly,[23] suggesting that repolarization gradients can decrease dynamically over several beats, significantly influencing synchronization of ventricular repolarization and, thus, the electrophysiological substrate for arrhythmias. This principle may have many important implications to the initiation and early maintenance of reentrant arrhythmias. For example, beat-to-beat changes in the electrophysiological substrate may explain the transition from atrial flutter to fibrillation and vise versa,[24] and determine if repetitive ventricular premature beats evolve to sustained or nonsustained ventricular tachycardia.

Conventional recording techniques make it difficult to track the dynamic beat-to-beat changes in spatial synchronization of repolarization and their effect on the electrophysiological substrate for reentry. On one hand, microelectrode and monophasic action potential (MAP) recordings faithfully reproduce beat-to-beat changes in cellular repolarization; however, it is nearly impossible to measure dynamic changes in the spatial gradients of cellular repolarization. On the other hand, extracellular mapping is capable of simultaneously recording from hundreds of sites, but direct information regarding repolarization is lost. In contrast to these techniques, optical action potential mapping with voltage-sensitive dye makes it possible to simultaneously measure high-fidelity action potentials from hundreds of sites with high temporal and spatial resolution. We used optical mapping to investigate how spatial diversity of cellular repolarization properties influence the spatial and temporal dynamics of ventricular repolarization that occur on a beat-to-beat basis and, more importantly, the role such changes have on the dynamic formation of arrhythmogenic substrates. In this chapter, we focus on two clinically relevant paradigms where heterogeneities of repolarization properties between cells directly influence dynamic changes in the underlying substrate for reentry. The first demonstrates how a single premature impulse systematically modulates spatial gradients of ventricular repolarization and, in turn, vulnerability to reentry.[25] The second demonstrates how heterogeneities of action potential alternans form steep gradients of repolarization that are responsible for the initiation of ventricular fibrillation (VF).[26]

Measurement of Repolarization Time

To quantify spatial heterogeneities of repolarization, we developed an algorithm that can accurately and reproducibly determine repolarization time from hundreds of optical action potentials.[23] Figure 1 is a schematic diagram of an action potential and its first and second derivatives. Depo-

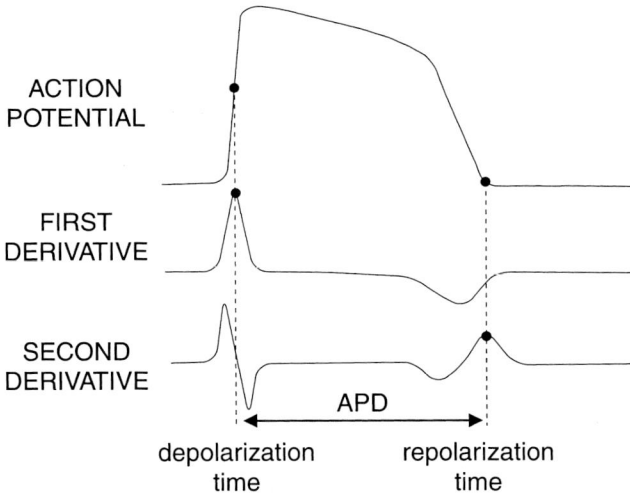

Figure 1. Schematic representation of an action potential and its first and second derivatives. Depolarization time is defined as the time at which the first derivative of the action potential is maximum (first dashed line). Repolarization time is defined as the time during final repolarization when the second derivative of the action potential is maximum (second dashed line). Repolarization time defined using this technique is less sensitive to the presence of motion artifact and baseline drift, unlike algorithms based on the absolute threshold or first derivative. APD = action potential duration.

larization time is defined as the time when the first derivative is at its maximum amplitude. Repolarization time, on the other hand, is defined as the time during final repolarization when the second derivative is at its maximum amplitude. Repolarization time, defined using this technique, corresponds to approximately 95% repolarization.[27] Unlike algorithms based on the absolute threshold or first derivative, this is a robust technique that is insensitive to the presence of motion artifact and baseline drift. It is important to note that repolarization time is defined by the time required for an impulse to propagate to and depolarize a cell (i.e., depolarization time) plus the cell's intrinsic APD. Therefore, in addition to heterogeneities of APD, heterogeneities of depolarization (i.e., conduction gradients) can also influence repolarization gradients.

Heterogeneity of Repolarization Kinetics in the Intact Heart

The kinetics of repolarization can be characterized, in part, by the response of APD to a premature stimulus, referred to as APD restitution.[28,29] As shown in Figure 2, restitution is defined by the relationship between APD of the premature stimulus (APD_p) and its preceding diastolic interval (DI). Typically, APD shortens exponentially as DI shortens.[16,30,31] Restitution is believed to reflect the time-dependent kinetics of several membrane and/or intracellular ionic currents that govern repolarization.[32,33] Thus, heterogeneity in the spatial distribution or expression of ion channel func-

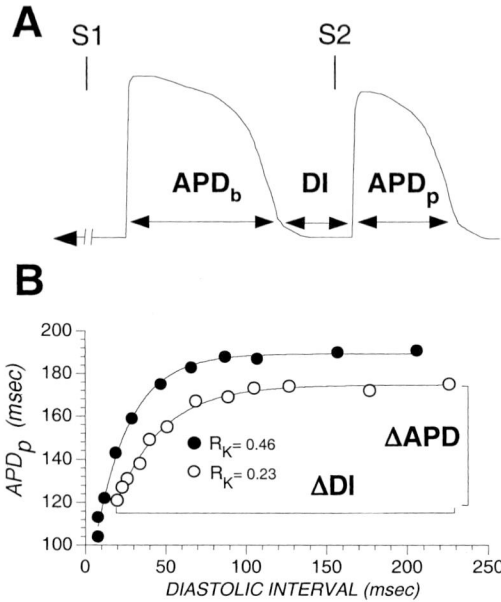

Figure 2. A. Schematic representation of an action potential during the last beat of a 50-beat baseline drive train (S1) and a single premature beat (S2). APD_b = action potential duration (APD) of the baseline beat; APD_p = APD of the premature beat; DI = diastolic interval. **B.** Two restitution curves calculated from action potentials recorded in guinea pig, one at a site where APD_b was longest (closed circles) and the other where APD_b was shortest (open circles). Shown are the parameters used to estimate the rate constant of restitution (R_K) at the site at which R_K was smallest, where ΔAPD is the extent of APD_p shortening over the range of diastolic intervals tested (ΔDI). R_K was also calculated (parameters not shown) at the site where R_K was greatest for comparison.

tion will be manifested as a heterogeneity of restitution properties between cells. Likewise, spatial heterogeneity of restitution kinetics is expected to influence significantly the spatial pattern of repolarization during stimulation of the heart.

Conventional electrophysiological recording techniques are limited to simultaneously measuring restitution at only a few sites, making it difficult to quantitatively determine the effect of cellular heterogeneities of restitution at the whole heart or tissue level. In contrast, optical mapping with voltage-sensitive dye can be used to measure action potentials, with high signal fidelity and spatial resolution, from hundreds of recording sites simultaneously. Moreover, optical mapping is well suited for measuring intrinsic (i.e., cellular) properties because it is insensitive to far field influences, and because each action potential represents an average local transmembrane potential that is less sensitive to biological variability between individual myocytes.[34] By focusing on restitution properties across the epicardial surface of the guinea pig ventricle, the direct influence *cellular* restitution heterogeneities have on the substrate for reentry could be investigated at the level of the *whole heart*. APD restitution was measured simultaneously from 128 recording sites by delivering a premature stimulus (i.e., S2) over a broad range of DIs as shown in Figure 2A. For the majority of recording sites, restitution followed a single exponential. However, since nonexponential behavior was also observed,[35–37] and since we have found that the characteristics of restitution curves vary when measured from hundreds of sites across the ventricular wall,[38] it is incorrect to assume a predefined mathematical relationship between APD and DI. Therefore, we defined an empirical restitution rate constant, R_K, which does not assume a predefined mathematical relation between APD and DI.[13] Greater values of R_K indicate a faster time course of restitution and a greater degree of APD shortening for any change in DI. Shown in Figure 2B are restitution curves measured from two ventricular sites, one where R_K was slow (0.23) and the other where R_K was fast (0.46). These restitution curves indicate the range of R_K observed across a 1-cm^2 region of epicardium.

The spatial variation of restitution across the epicardial surface is shown in Figure 3A. Within this 1-cm^2 area of epicardium, R_K varied by as much as 500% (range 0.04 to 0.24). Moreover, spatial heterogeneity of R_K was not random; rather, there was an organized pattern of R_K across the epicardial surface. In particular, the gradient of R_K was oriented parallel to cardiac fibers,[39] despite the fact that electrotonic coupling between cells is expected to minimize heterogeneities of repolarization in this direction.[40] These findings suggest the presence of considerable heterogeneity of cellular ionic processes across the epicardial surface.

In addition to ionic currents intrinsic to each cell, it is possible that restitution kinetics are also influenced by electrotonic loading from neigh-

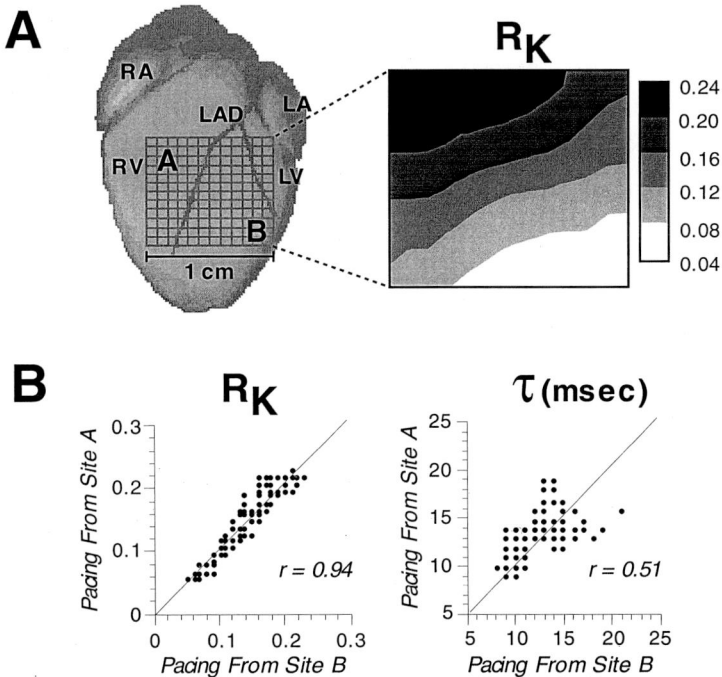

Figure 3. **A.** Diagram of the mapping field (1-cm^2 grid) and its position relative to the intact heart preparation (*top, left*), and spatial dispersion of restitution kinetics (R_K, *top right*). Shown to the right of the contour map is a gray scale with corresponding numerical values in normalized units (R_K). LA = left atrium; LAD = left anterior descending coronary artery; LV = left ventricle; RA = right atrium; RV = right ventricle. **B.** The effect of propagation direction on R_K and τ, determined by repeating the restitution protocol from opposite sides of the mapping field (sites A and B, *top right*). R_K was not dependent on propagation direction as evidenced by the alignment of data points along the line of identity (solid line), however, τ was dependent on propagation direction (see text). Reprinted from Laurita et al. *Can J Cardiol* 1997;13(11):1069–1076.

boring cells.[40–42] Since the direction of wave front propagation can influence cell-to-cell loading during repolarization,[42] it is possible that APD restitution measured in multicellular preparations can be influenced by the direction of propagation. As shown in Figure 3B (left), the magnitude of R_K at each site did not change when the site of pacing was changed to the opposite side of the heart (site B in Fig. 3A), reaffirming that spatial heterogeneities in R_K were caused by heterogeneities of repolarization properties intrinsic to each cell and independent of propagation.[13] In contrast, when the restitution curves were fit to a single exponential, the time constant of restitution (i.e., τ) changed at a significant number of sites when the pacing site was shifted from one side of the ventricle to the other (Fig. 3B, right). We have previously shown that subtle changes in the shape of the restitution curve occur at short coupling intervals. Using computer modeling studies in conjunction with optically recorded action potentials, we demonstrated that such pacing site induced changes in τ result from electrotonic current flow generated by intense spatial gradients of transmembrane potential that occur during final repolarization typically near the site of premature stimulation.[38] Therefore, in the intact heart, τ may not be the most appropriate measure of restitution properties intrinsic to each cell since it is influenced by electrotonic forces.[38]

Modulation of Ventricular Repolarization ("Modulated Dispersion") and Arrhythmia Vulnerability during Premature Stimulation of the Heart

Influence of Restitution Heterogeneity on Ventricular Repolarization Gradients

Heterogeneity of restitution kinetics across the epicardial surface is expected to alter significantly the sequence and pattern of repolarization during a premature beat. Figure 4 shows the patterns of depolarization and repolarization at a coupling interval equal to the baseline pacing cycle length (panels A,B), premature stimulation at an intermediate coupling interval (panels C,D), and at a coupling interval just longer than the effective refractory period of the baseline beat (panels E,F). During baseline pacing (panel A), the impulse propagated uniformly from the site of stimulation, and a significant gradient of repolarization was present, with latest repolarization occurring near the base of the heart and earliest repolarization occurring near the apex. In general, the repolarization gradient (solid arrow) during baseline pacing was oriented in an apex-to-base direction and parallel to cardiac muscle fibers of this preparation (dashed line).[39] Recent studies have substantiated these findings.[27,43]

A premature stimulus introduced at an intermediate coupling interval (Fig. 4B) produced no significant change in the pattern of depolarization; however, the repolarization gradient that was evident during baseline pacing was essentially eliminated. When a premature stimulus was intro-

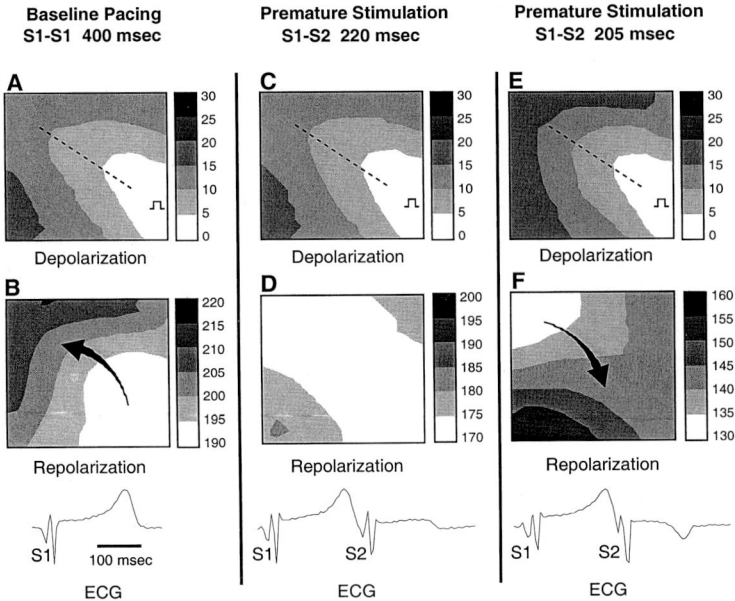

Figure 4. Contour maps of depolarization and repolarization at a coupling interval equal to the baseline pacing cycle length (**A, B**), a premature stimulus at an intermediate coupling interval (**C, D**), and a premature stimulus at a coupling interval near the refractory period (**E, F**) measured from the epicardial surface of a guinea pig. The electrocardiogram (ECG) recorded during the last two baseline beats (S1) and the premature stimulus (S2) is shown across the top. Depolarization and repolarization times are in milliseconds. The site of pacing (⊓ symbol) was identical for all recordings. The dashed lines indicate epicardial fiber direction. In contrast to depolarization, the gradient of repolarization (solid arrow) was markedly influenced by a premature stimulus. Reduced heterogeneity (D) and inversion of repolarization gradients (F) are reflected in the ECG by T wave flattening and a change in T wave polarity, respectively. Modified from reference 25.

duced at a very short coupling interval (Fig. 4E), conduction slowed somewhat, as evidenced by slight crowding of isochrone lines, but the overall pattern of depolarization remained unchanged. In contrast, repolarization changed substantially as the gradient of repolarization reappeared. However, the orientation of the repolarization gradient reversed and was completely opposite to repolarization at baseline. Also, note that the eradication and subsequent reversal of the repolarization gradient by intermediate and short premature coupling intervals were closely paralleled by flattening and inversion of the electrocardiographic (ECG) T wave of the premature beat. Since the ECG T wave amplitude and polarity reflect ventricular repolarization of the entire heart, similar coupling-interval–dependent changes in repolarization were most likely occurring throughout the heart and not just within the region of myocardium that was being mapped.

The initial decrease and subsequent increase (i.e., modulated dispersion) of repolarization gradients with shortening of premature stimulus cycle length can be explained by heterogeneity of cellular restitution kinetics across the epicardial surface. In general, where APD during baseline pacing (i.e., APD_b) is longest, R_K is fastest and where APD_b is shortest, R_K is slowest.[13] Since R_K is faster at sites having longer APD_b, APD of the premature beat (i.e., APD_p) shortens more rapidly at these sites compared to sites with shorter APD_b (i.e., smaller R_K), effectively eliminating repolarization heterogeneity across the epicardial surface. With further shortening of the S1-S2 coupling interval, cells initially having the longest APD now have the shortest APD because of their relatively fast R_K. Thus, the APD gradient is restored, but it is orientated in the opposite direction.

Since the timing of repolarization is dependent on conduction time plus APD, spatial heterogeneity of repolarization is determined by the combined effect of conduction gradients and spatial gradients of APD. We observed a much greater change in repolarization gradients compared with conduction gradients as the S1-S2 coupling interval was shortened, indicating that the magnitude and orientation of repolarization gradients are determined primarily by changes in APD. Kanai and Salama[43] made similar observations, in which the pattern of repolarization in guinea pig epicardium was dominated by APD and was essentially independent of the sequence of propagation. There is also evidence suggesting that this may be the case under conditions of abnormal repolarization. In experimental models of the congenital long QT syndrome, dispersion of repolarization is predominantly due to regional heterogeneity of APD.[19,20,22] Spatial heterogeneities of APD may also be enhanced in patients with sustained monomorphic ventricular tachycardia.[44] On the other hand, in the presence of marked conduction slowing caused by chronic myocardial infarction, propagation delays may also contribute to heterogeneity of ventricular repolarization.[45] Clearly, the factors that determine dispersion of repolarization in the heart are dependent on the specific pathophysiological substrate involved.

Modulation of the Substrate for VF by a Premature Stimulus

A premature impulse is traditionally viewed as a "trigger" for reentrant arrhythmias that, in the presence of a suitable arrhythmogenic "substrate,"[46] can provoke reentry. However, our data demonstrate that the trigger and the substrate are not necessarily independent, since a premature stimulus actively modulates the electrophysiological properties of the heart. Such modulation has several important effects. First, premature stimuli delivered at progressively shorter coupling intervals shorten refractoriness at the stimulus site, allowing capture of subsequent stimuli at increasing degrees of prematurity, shortening cardiac wavelength, and, thus, increasing the likelihood of inducing reentry (a concept similar to "peeling back" refractoriness[47]). However, an alternative hypothesis, referred to here as the modulated dispersion hypothesis, is that a premature beat, in addition to shortening refractoriness, also changes the underlying arrhythmogenic substrate by modulating spatial dispersion of repolarization in a manner that is dependent on the coupling interval. Such coupling-interval–dependent changes are an expected consequence of spatial heterogeneity of restitution properties. We tested this hypothesis using high-resolution action potential mapping with voltage-sensitive dye as a tool for measuring dispersion of repolarization that forms in the wake of a premature stimulus.[25] Vulnerability to VF following a premature beat was measured using a modified VF threshold (VFT) protocol,[25] where a train (100 Hz) of S3 pulses was applied during the T wave of the premature beat (S2). The minimum current strength that initiated VF defined the VFT (i.e., S3-VFT). The S3-VFT was measured as repolarization was modulated over a broad range of S1-S2 coupling intervals.

To quantitatively determine the relationship between S1-S2 coupling interval and repolarization properties of the ventricle, mean repolarization time (i.e., S2-RT) and dispersion of repolarization time (i.e., S2-DISP) were calculated for each S1-S2 coupling interval. Shown in Figure 5A are the mean (open circles) and dispersion (closed circles) of repolarization times generated during each prematurely stimulated beat in a representative experiment. Mean repolarization decreased monotonically from 221 ms to 145 ms as the S1-S2 coupling interval was shortened from 300 ms to 230 ms. These changes were attributed to coupling-interval–dependent changes in APD, which were most marked at short S1-S2 coupling intervals, as predicted from restitution properties of cardiac myocytes.[16] In contrast, dispersion of repolarization was modulated in a biphasic fashion as coupling interval was shortened. For S1-S2 coupling intervals near the baseline pacing rate, dispersion of repolarization was relatively high; however, as the S1-S2 coupling interval was shortened, dispersion of repolarization decreased until a critical coupling interval was reached (255 ms; Fig. 5, dashed arrow). With further shortening of the S1-S2 coupling in-

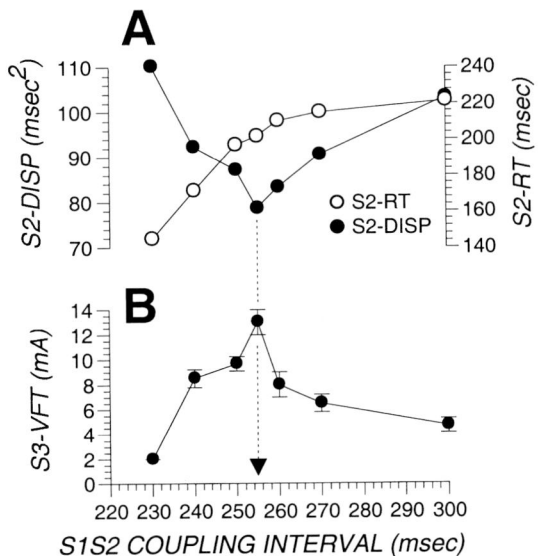

Figure 5. A. Mean repolarization (S2-RT, open circles) and dispersion of repolarization (S2-DISP, filled circles) of an S2 premature beat as a function of S1-S2 coupling interval. These values were calculated from 128 optical action potentials recorded from the epicardial surface of guinea pig ventricle. Dispersion of repolarization was calculated by the variance of repolarization times measured over the entire mapping field. **B.** Changes in vulnerability to ventricular fibrillation induced by an S3 pulse train (S3-VFT) in the wake of repolarization patterns induced by various S1-S2 coupling intervals. Dispersion of repolarization (A, filled circles) and vulnerability to fibrillation (B) were modulated in a similar biphasic fashion, with minimum vulnerability (i.e., maximum S3-VFT) and minimum dispersion occurring at the same S1-S2 coupling interval (255 ms, dashed arrow). Reprinted from reference 25.

terval, dispersion of repolarization rose sharply to a level slightly higher than that measured during baseline pacing.

The effect of cycle-length–dependent modulation of repolarization on susceptibility to VF is illustrated in Figure 5B. It is evident that vulnerability to VF, as measured by S3-VFT, was modulated in a biphasic fashion in parallel with dispersion of repolarization (filled circles, Fig. 5A). As the S1-S2 coupling interval was shortened to a critical value (Fig. 5, dashed arrow), S3-VFT increased (i.e., vulnerability decreased). With further shortening of S1-S2, S3-VFT decreased (i.e., vulnerability increased) to levels below those present at baseline pacing. These data indicate that the electrophysiological substrate for VF is not constant but can potentially form, disappear, and reform in a predictable fashion just by changing stimulus timing.

It is generally assumed that the effect of shortening the premature stimulus coupling interval is that the likelihood of inducing reentry is increased. Figure 5, however, illustrates a paradoxical decrease in arrhythmia vulnerability as the premature stimulus coupling interval was initially shortened over a broad range of coupling intervals. The attenuation of repolarization gradients by a premature stimulus may serve as a protective mechanism in electrophysiologically normal myocardium. On the other hand, the rapid increase in vulnerability at very short coupling intervals may explain why multiple, closely coupled premature stimuli are typically required to initiate VF in normal hearts. These findings also highlight the importance of accounting for changes in dispersion of repolarization throughout the heart, and not just the refractory period at one site, to develop a more comprehensive understanding of the underlying electrophysiological substrate for reentry. Inferences from these studies must be cautiously extrapolated to VF in patients since the mechanism of VF initiation during VFT testing is not completely understood. Because of these limitations, we also investigated the role of modulated dispersion in the formation of unidirectional block, a specific and necessary condition for reentry.

Modulation of the Electrophysiological Substrate for Unidirectional Block by a Premature Stimulus

To determine if modulation of repolarization gradients can directly influence the electrophysiological requirements of unidirectional block, we examined the characteristics of propagation of an S3 stimulus in the wake of repolarization gradients established by a premature (i.e., S2) beat.[48] To confine propagation to the epicardial surface and avoid the confounding influence of subepicardial breakthrough from the His-Purkinje system, the endocardial muscle layers were eliminated by use of a cryoablation procedure described previously.[39] To control the trajectory of propagation, a linear lesion containing a 1-mm isthmus (Fig. 6, white bar) was "etched" precisely (± 1 μ) onto the epicardial surface by use of a computer-driven 5-W argon ion laser. The lesion created a line of anatomical block that was parallel to the left anterior descending coronary artery and perpendicular to the orientation of repolarization gradients typically found on the guinea pig epicardium.[13] Baseline pacing (S1-S1 = 600 ms) and a

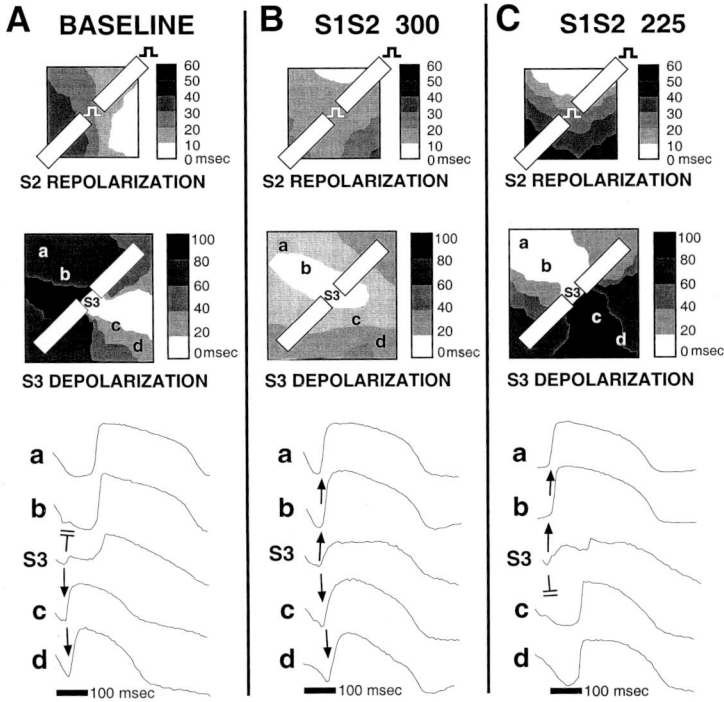

Figure 6. Dependence of unidirectional block of an S3 impulse delivered from the center of an isthmus within a linear lesion (white rectangles) on repolarization gradients formed by a single, S2, premature stimulus. Three different S1-S2 premature coupling intervals were tested: baseline pacing (**A,** S1-S2 = S1-S1 = 600 ms), an intermediate coupling interval (**B,** S1-S2 = 300 ms), and a short coupling interval (**C,** S1-S2 = 225 ms). Contour maps on top show the pattern of repolarization of the S2 beat surrounding the isthmus. Contour maps in the middle show propagation of the S3 beat in the wake of repolarization gradients established by the S2 beat. The S3 stimulus was always introduced just beyond the effective refractory period of an S2 beat. *Bottom:* Action potentials of the S3 beat recorded from equally spaced sites on either side of the lesion. A gradient of repolarization with sufficient magnitude to produce unidirectional block across the isthmus was present during baseline pacing (A). However, repolarization gradients were eradicated and then reformed in the opposite direction following an intermediate (B) and short (C) S1-S2 coupling interval, respectively. The reappearance of repolarization gradients at short coupling intervals was sufficient to produce unidirectional block (C). Reprinted from Laurita KR, Pastore JM, Rosenbaum DS. How restitution, repolarization, and alternans form arrhythmogenic substrates: Insights from high-resolution optical mapping. In Zipes DP, Jalife J (eds): *Cardiac Electrophysiology: From Cell to Bedside.* 3rd ed. Philadelphia: W.B. Saunders Co.; 2000:239–248.

single premature stimulus (S2) were delivered from the same site near the basal end of the laser lesion (black stimulus symbol). For each S1-S2 coupling interval tested, a second premature stimulus (S3) was delivered just beyond (<2 ms) the effective refractory period of the S2 beat at 2× diastolic threshold from the center of the isthmus (white stimulus symbol). Thus, propagation out of the isthmus encountered an abrupt tissue expansion that was equal on both sides of the isthmus.

Shown in Figure 6 are data from a representative experiment in which the S1-S2 coupling interval was sequentially shortened from 600 ms to 225 ms. Shown across the top are contour maps of repolarization of each S2 beat in the vicinity of the isthmus. Below the repolarization maps are contour maps of propagation of the S3 beat in the wake of repolarization gradients established by the S2 beat. For an S1-S2 coupling interval equal to the baseline cycle length (Fig. 6A), a gradient of repolarization was present that delayed repolarization time on the left side of the isthmus. In the wake of this repolarization pattern, the S3 impulse failed to propagate to the left side of the isthmus against the repolarization gradient, but successfully propagated to the right (i.e., unidirectional block) and continued around both ends of the lesion meeting on the other side of the isthmus in a pattern resembling figure-of-eight reentry. This is also reflected in the action potentials shown at the bottom of Figure 6, which were recorded from equally spaced sites perpendicular to the lesion. Propagation failed in the direction of site b but was successful in the direction of sites c and d continuing around the lesion, much later, to sites a and b. Thus, during baseline pacing, the electrophysiological requirements for unidirectional block (i.e., isthmus and a critical repolarization gradient) were present. We know that the isthmus was important since unidirectional block was not observed in the absence of an isthmus, even when repolarization gradients of similar magnitude were present. Likewise, repolarization gradients are also an essential condition for unidirectional block, because when these gradients were eradicated by a premature stimulus delivered at an intermediate coupling interval (Figure 6B), unidirectional block could not be produced.

Finally, at a short S1-S2 coupling interval (Figure 6C), the repolarization gradient is restored to a magnitude similar to that seen during baseline pacing; however, the orientation of the gradient is reversed. This pattern of repolarization gradient modulation was completely analogous to that shown in Figure 4. The S3 impulse once again failed to propagate against the repolarization gradient, which was now oriented in the opposite direction compared with baseline. The premature impulse successfully propagated to the left and continued around both ends of the lesion, meeting on the other side of the isthmus, again, in a pattern resembling figure-of-eight reentry. Consequently, at a short S1-S2 coupling interval the electrophysiological requirements for unidirectional block were restored. Therefore, these data demonstrate how the underlying substrate for unidirectional block and reentry are critically influenced by the trigger used to initiate it. Such dynamic beat-to-beat alterations of repolarization may explain how the substrate for reentry forms or disappears in a manner which ultimately determines the initiation and stability of reentry.

Role of Repolarization Alternans in the Formation of Arrhythmogenic Substrates

There are other mechanisms by which regional heterogeneities of membrane repolarization properties can influence the electrophysiological substrate for reentry. From the aforementioned discussion, it is clear that the time course of repolarization is highly sensitive to perturbations in heart rate (i.e., premature stimulation) and can be explained by regional heterogeneities of repolarization kinetics. Such heterogeneities may also alter the time course of repolarization from beat to beat even as heart rate is maintained constant. One common pattern is repolarization alternans, which is defined as a periodic change in the time course of repolarization (i.e., either the action potential or ECG T wave) which repeats once every other beat. Repolarization alternans is of particular interest because T wave alternans is a marker of vulnerability to ventricular arrhythmias in humans,[49] and often immediately precedes ventricular arrhythmias in many pathological conditions.[50–54] It is now evident that microvolt-level T wave alternans, which is generally unrecognized on clinical ECG tracings, is quite common in patients at risk for sudden cardiac death.[49,55] There is considerable evidence from single site action potential recordings suggesting that T wave alternans of the surface ECG arises from alternans of repolarization occurring at the level of the single cell.[56–63] Theoretically, spatial heterogeneity of repolarization, the primary source of the ECG T wave, is a likely target for investigation. Currently, optical mapping is the only technique available that is capable of tracking beat-to-beat changes in repolarization heterogeneity, making it ideal for investigating the cellular mechanisms of T wave alternans. Recently, we have found that repolarization alternans occurring between cells that have different restitution properties is a novel mechanism for the formation of arrhythmogenic substrates.[26]

Spatial Heterogeneity of Action Potential Alternans Parallels Heterogeneity of Restitution

We applied the technique of high-resolution optical mapping to the endocardial cryoablated Langendorff-perfused guinea pig model to investigate repolarization alternans.[26] At a time when T wave alternans was induced by steady-state pacing, action potentials were recorded simultaneously from 128 epicardial sites encompassing the majority of the anterior left ventricular surface. We found that an alternans threshold heart rate is present in action potentials recorded from cells in the intact heart. This is not surprising since electrocardiographic T wave alternans[64] and APD alternans from single ventricular myocytes[56] have been shown to occur above a critical threshold heart rate. We also found that the heart rate threshold for repolarization alternans varied between cells across the epicardial surface of the heart.[26] In addition, the magnitude and phase of repolarization alternans were also heterogeneously distributed across the surface of the heart in a systematic pattern. The distribution of local repolarization time alternans is plotted in Figure 7A. Interestingly, the pattern of repolarization alternans closely followed the typical distribution of cellular restitution properties (Fig. 7B). Local repolarization time alternans was calculated from the difference in cellular repolarization time measured during sequential beats. Therefore, positive and negative values indicate relative prolongation and abbreviation of local repolarization on a particular beat, respectively. Note that during the same beat, repolarization is prolonging near the base of the heart while shortening near the apex, indicating regional differences in the phase of alternation between

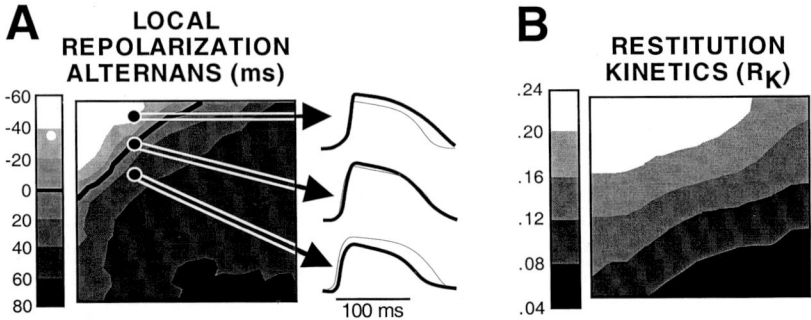

Figure 7. Distribution of action potential alternans in the intact ventricle. Shown is a plot of local repolarization alternans measured as the difference in repolarization time between consecutive beats at each ventricular recording site. Local repolarization alternans varies from apex to base according to known distribution of cellular restitution properties across the epicardial surface of guinea pig (**B**). Note the change in phase of repolarization alternans denoted by the thick black line, and demonstrated by action potential recordings shown for selected sites (**A**). These action potentials were recorded from two sequential beats (depicted by bold and thin traces) to illustrate the relative phase of repolarization alternans between cells. The alternation of action potentials with opposite phase is called discordant alternans.

epicardial cells. Such disruption of the phase relationship between cells has been referred to as discordant alternans.[61,65,66] Discordant alternans occurred despite the presence of normal intercellular coupling, and was most likely explained by regional heterogeneities in membrane restitution kinetics. Discordant alternans was consistently observed above a critical threshold heart rate, was always preceded by concordant alternans (action potential alternations having the same phase), and, in contrast to concordant alternans, produced marked changes in the pattern and sequence of ventricular depolarization and repolarization (see next section). Such inhomogeneous alternations of repolarization time occurring between neighboring regions of cells suggest that the ionic currents that determine repolarization differ substantially between these regions so as to overcome electrotonic forces which ordinarily act to synchronize repolarization.

Role of Discordant Alternans in the Initiation of Reentry

The initiation of repolarization alternans during constant cycle length pacing caused a reproducible cascade of events leading to reentrant VF.[26] First, above a threshold heart rate, alternation of repolarization with the same phase between all cells (i.e., concordant alternans) was induced and typically manifested as microvolt-level T wave alternans on the surface ECG (not shown). Concordant alternans was associated with only subtle beat-to-beat alternation in the magnitude of repolarization, with no change in the orientation of repolarization gradients. In addition, essentially no changes in beat-to-beat propagation occurred. As pacing rate was further increased, a critical heart rate was achieved at which cells within neighboring regions of myocardium alternated with opposite phase (i.e., discordant alternans). As shown in Figure 8, discordant alternans produced several key changes

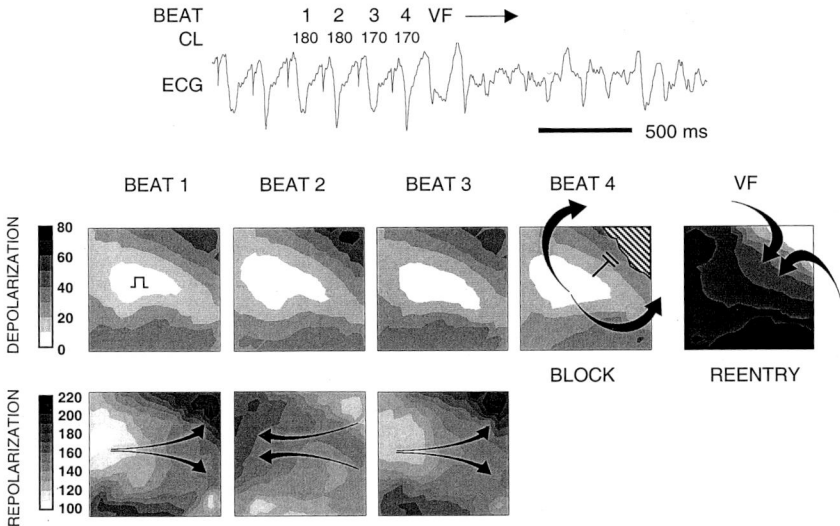

Figure 8. Representative example demonstrating the mechanism linking repolarization alternans to the genesis of reentrant ventricular fibrillation (VF). Contour maps indicate the patterns of depolarization and repolarization across the epicardial surface of guinea pig ventricle (times shown in milliseconds). As pacing rate is increased, discordant alternans develops producing complete reversal in the direction of repolarization gradients from beat to beat and, most importantly, steep gradients of repolarization that were not present during concordant alternans (not shown). These gradients formed a suitable substrate for reentry, as a slight shortening of stimulus cycle length (beat 4) causes local propagation failure against a repolarization gradient established during the previous beat (upper right corner of beat 3 repolarization map). Discordant alternans produces conditions necessary for unidirectional block after which reentrant VF immediately ensued. The electrocardiogram across the top is shown for reference.

in the pattern and sequence of propagation and repolarization of the heart. First, steep gradients of repolarization formed as evidenced by marked crowding of repolarization isochrone lines (Fig. 8, bottom). Differences in the phase of action potential alternations across the epicardium directly accounted for the magnitude of these gradients. Second, the orientation of repolarization gradients underwent nearly a complete reversal in direction from beat to beat. Although repolarization patterns are complex, they are highly reproducible on alternate beats (Fig. 8, compare repolarization maps on beat 1 versus beat 3). Finally, conduction begins to alternate as impulses slow when propagating against steep gradients of repolarization created by the previous beat. Under these conditions, a small reduction of stimulus cycle length (10 ms in Fig. 8, beat 4) resulted in conduction block into a region having most delayed repolarization from the previous beat (Fig. 8, beat 3 repolarization map). The impulse then propagated around either side of the line of block (hatched area), and 90 ms later the zone of block regained excitability allowing the impulse to reenter from outside the mapping field, forming the first spontaneous beat of reentrant VF. Importantly, in these experiments the initiation of VF was always preceded by discordant alternans, closely linking it to the mechanism of reentry.

Therefore, in the presence of regional heterogeneities of cellular restitution, discordant repolarization alternans could transform relatively minor gradients of repolarization into critical gradients, which were directly responsible for the development of unidirectional block and reentrant VF. This concept was supported by elegant studies in isolated myocytes that showed that the timing of membrane depolarization relative to the kinetics of membrane repolarization determined the phase of alternation.[56] One would predict, therefore, that pathological conditions that either increase spatial heterogeneity of repolarization or impair coupling between cells may facilitate the development of discordant alternans. Therefore, it is not surprising that discordant alternans has been observed in clinical conditions associated with marked spatial dispersion of repolarization properties, such as the congenital long QT syndrome.[63] Similarly, discordant alternans was also observed during interventions that reduce cell-to-cell coupling, such as ischemia[65] and hypoxia.[66]

Clearly, a large number of questions remain unanswered regarding the role of repolarization alternans in the mechanism of sudden cardiac death. Based on currently available data, we propose one possible mechanism in Figure 9. First, it is apparent that patients with structural heart disease who are at risk for life-threatening ventricular arrhythmias develop microvolt-level T wave alternans at significantly lower heart rates (typically 90 to 100 bpm) compared with patients in lower risk groups.[49,55,64] Microvolt-level T wave alternans is most likely associated with concordant patterns of repolarization alternans (i.e., alternations that occur with the same phase) of cells within the heart. Then, a critical trigger is required in the transformation from concordant to discordant alternans, providing a suitable substrate for reentry. Although we cannot determine from our data the

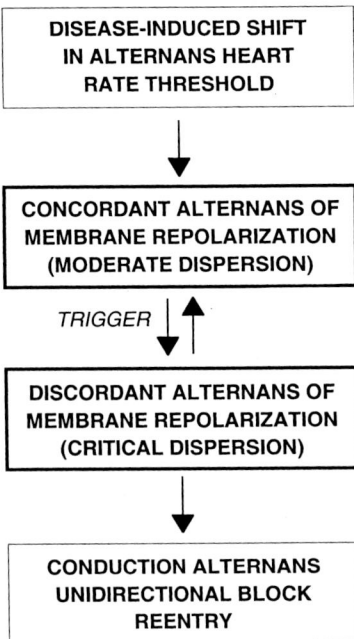

Figure 9. Proposed mechanism linking T wave alternans to arrhythmogenesis.

exact mechanisms responsible for triggering discordant alternans in patients, physiological perturbations such as transient ischemia, premature ventricular beats, or sympathetic stimulation are known to affect the phase and magnitude of repolarization alternans. Further studies aimed at delineating these mechanisms are expected to improve our ability to understand and potentially prevent the complex sequence of events that precipitate sudden cardiac death episodes in patients.

Summary

Using high-resolution optical action potential mapping with voltage-sensitive dye, we have demonstrated how spatial heterogeneity of cellular restitution kinetics across the epicardial surface of guinea pig heart influence the spatial and temporal dynamics of ventricular repolarization on a beat-to-beat basis. Due to limitations of conventional electrophysiological recording techniques, the influence that such heterogeneities of repolarization have on arrhythmia vulnerability in the intact heart has previously not been well appreciated. We demonstrated that during premature stimulation, repolarization gradients are modulated in a systematic and predictable manner that is highly dependent on premature coupling interval. Importantly, such changes critically influence vulnerability to fibrillation and the formation of unidirectional block, a fundamental requirement for reentry. Therefore, these findings indicate that the electrophysiological substrate for reentry is not necessarily static, but can potentially form, disappear, and reform in a predictable fashion. Thus, a premature stimulus not only serves as a "trigger" of arrhythmias, but also importantly modulates the electrophysiological substrate for reentry.

Spatial heterogeneities of repolarization also appear to play a critical role in the development of arrhythmogenic substrates during repolarization alternans. Heterogeneous ion channel function and expression, as manifest by regional variation in cellular restitution properties, create a situation in which cellular repolarization within separate regions of myocardium alternate with differing amplitude and phase. Regional differences in the phase of alternans (i.e., discordant alternans) produce critical gradients of repolarization that form a suitable substrate for unidirectional block and reentrant ventricular arrhythmias. These findings demonstrate the complexity of arrhythmogenic substrates that are dependent on dynamic and heterogeneous processes such as repolarization. Obviously, the factors that determine dispersion of repolarization in the heart are dependent on the specific pathophysiological substrate involved. Further studies are required to increase our understanding of how heterogeneities of repolarization in the presence and absence of cardiac pathology influence the electrophysiological substrate for reentry. Undoubtedly, optical mapping will play an important role in these investigations.

References

1. Mines GR. On dynamic equilibrium in the heart. *J Physiol (Lond)* 1913; 46:349–383.

2. Allessie A, Bonke FI, Schopman FJG. Circus movement in rabbit atrial muscle as a mechanism of tachycardia. II. The role of nonuniform recovery of excitability in the occurrence of unidirectional block as studied with multiple microelectrodes. *Circ Res* 1976;39:169–177.

3. Han J, Moe G. Nonuniform recovery of excitability in ventricular muscle. *Circ Res* 1964;14:44–60.

4. Gough W, Mehra R, Restivo M, et al. Reentrant ventricular arrhythmias in the late myocardial infarction period in the dog: 13. Correlation of activation and refractory maps. *Circ Res* 1985;57:432–442.

5. Litovsky SH, Antzelevitch C. Transient outward current prominent in canine ventricular epicardium but not endocardium. *Circ Res* 1988;62:116–126.

6. Furukawa T, Myerburg RJ, Furukawa N, et al. Differences in transient outward currents of feline endocardial and epicardial myocytes. *Circ Res* 1990; 67:1287–1291.

7. Fedida D, Giles WR. Regional variations in action potentials and transient outward current in myocytes isolated from rabbit left ventricle. *J Physiol (Lond)* 1991;442:191–209.

8. Sicouri S, Antzelevitch C. A subpopulation of cells with unique electrophysiological properties in the deep subepicardium of the canine ventricle: The M cell. *Circ Res* 1991;68:1729–1741.

9. Drouin E, Charpentier F, Gauthier C, et al. Electrophysiologic characteristics of cells spanning the left ventricular wall of human heart: Evidence for presence of M cells. *J Am Coll Cardiol* 1995;26:185–192.

10. Sicouri S, Quist M, Antzelevitch C. Evidence for the presence of M cells in the guinea pig ventricle. *J Cardiovasc Electrophysiol* 1996;7:503–511.

11. Liu D-W, Antzelevitch C. Characteristics of the delayed rectifier current (I_{Kr} and I_{Ks}) in canine ventricular epicardial, midmyocardial, and endocardial myocytes: A weaker I_{Ks} contributes to the longer action potential of the M cell. *Circ Res* 1995;76:351–365.

12. Gintant GA. Two components of delayed rectifier current in canine atrium and ventricle. Does I_{Ks} play a role in the reverse rate dependence of class III agents? *Circ Res* 1996;78:26–37.

13. Laurita KR, Girouard SD, Rosenbaum DS. Modulation of ventricular repolarization by a premature stimulus: Role of epicardial dispersion of repolarization kinetics demonstrated by optical mapping of the intact guinea pig heart. *Circ Res* 1996;79:493–503.

14. Kuo C, Munakata K, Reddy CP, Surawicz B. Characteristics and possible mechanisms of ventricular arrhythmia dependent on the dispersion of action potential durations. *Circulation* 1983;67:1356–1367.

15. Hauswirth O, Noble D, Tsien RW. The dependence of plateau currents in cardiac Purkinje fibres on the interval between action potentials. *J Physiol (Lond)* 1972;222:27–49.

16. Boyett MR, Jewell BR. A study of the factors responsible for rate-dependent shortening of the action potential in mammalian ventricular muscle. *J Physiol* 1978;285:359–380.

17. Carmeliet E. K^+ channels and control of ventricular repolarization in the heart. *Fundam Clin Pharmacol* 1993;7:19–28.

18. Varro A, Nanasi PP, Lathrop DA. Voltage-clamp characteristics of ventricular myocytes in rabbit. *Cardioscience* 1991;2:233–243.

19. Akar FG, Yan G, Antzelevitch C, Rosenbaum DS. Optical maps reveal reentrant mechanism of torsade de pointes based on topography and electrophysiology of mid-myocardial cells. *Circulation* 1997;96(8):I555.

20. El-Sherif N, Caref EB, Yin H, Restivo M. The electrophysiological mechanism of ventricular arrhythmias in the long QT syndrome—tridimensional mapping of activation and recovery patterns. *Circ Res* 1996;79:474–492.

21. Antzelevitch C, Nesterenko VV, Yan G-X. Role of M cells in acquired long QT syndrome, U waves, and torsade de pointes. *J Electrocardiol* 1995; 28(Suppl):131–138.
22. Antzelevitch C, Sicouri S. Clinical relevance of cardiac arrhythmias generated by afterdepolarizations. Role of M cells in the generation of U waves, triggered activity and torsade de pointes. *J Am Coll Cardiol* 1994;23:259–277.
23. Rosenbaum DS, Kaplan DT, Kanai A, et al. Repolarization inhomogeneities in ventricular myocardium change dynamically with abrupt cycle length shortening. *Circulation* 1991;84:1333–1345.
24. Ortiz J, Niwano S, Abe H, et al. Mapping the conversion of atrial flutter to atrial fibrillation and atrial fibrillation to atrial flutter: Insights into mechanisms. *Circ Res* 1994;74:882–894.
25. Laurita KR, Girouard SD, Akar FG, Rosenbaum DS. Modulated dispersion explains changes in arrhythmia vulnerability during premature stimulation of the heart. *Circulation* 1998;98:2774–2780.
26. Pastore JM, Girouard SD, Laurita KR, et al. Mechanism linking T wave alternans to the genesis of cardiac fibrillation. *Circulation* 1999;99:1385–1394.
27. Efimov IR, Huang DT, Rendt JM, Salama G. Optical mapping of repolarization and refractoriness from intact hearts. *Circulation* 1994;90:1469–1480.
28. Bass BG. Restitution of the action potential in cat papillary muscle. *Am J Physiol* 1975;228:1717–1724.
29. Carmeliet E. Repolarisation and frequency in cardiac cells. *J Physiol (Paris)* 1977;73:903–923.
30. Saitoh H, Bailey J, Surawicz B. Action potential duration alternans in dog Purkinje and ventricular muscle fibers. *Circulation* 1989;80:1421–1431.
31. Bjornstad H, Tande PM, Lathrop DA, Refsum H. Effects of temperature on cycle length dependent changes and restitution of action potential duration in guinea pig ventricular muscle. *Cardiovasc Res* 1993;27:946–950.
32. Sanguinetti MC, Jurkiewicz NK. Two components of cardiac delayed rectifier K+ current: Differential sensitivity to block by class III antiarrhythmic agents. *J Gen Physiol* 1990;96:195–215.
33. Varró A, Lathrop DA, Hester SB, et al. Ionic currents and action potentials in rabbit, rat, and guinea pig ventricular myocytes. *Basic Res Cardiol* 1993;88:93–102.
34. Girouard SD, Laurita KR, Rosenbaum DS. Unique properties of cardiac action potentials recorded with voltage-sensitive dyes. *J Cardiovasc Electrophysiol* 1996;7:1024–1038.
35. Franz MR, Swerdlow CD, Liem LB, Schaefer J. Cycle length dependence of human action potential duration in vivo. *J Clin Invest* 1988;82:972–979.
36. Kobayashi Y, Peters W, Khan SS, et al. Cellular mechanisms of differential action potential duration restitution in canine ventricular muscle cells during single versus double premature stimuli. *Circulation* 1992;86:955–967.
37. Watanabe M, Otani NF, Gilmour RF Jr. Biphasic restitution of action potential duration and complex dynamics in ventricular myocardium. *Circ Res* 1995;76:915–921.
38. Laurita KR, Girouard SD, Rudy Y, Rosenbaum DS. Role of passive electrical properties during action potential restitution in the intact heart. *Am J Physiol* 1997;273:H1205-H1214.
39. Girouard SD, Pastore JM, Laurita KR, et al. Optical mapping in a new guinea pig model of ventricular tachycardia reveals mechanisms for multiple wavelengths in a single reentrant circuit. *Circulation* 1996;93:603–613.
40. Lesh MD, Pring M, Spear JF. Cellular uncoupling can unmask dispersion of action potential duration in ventricular myocardium: A computer modeling study. *Circ Res* 1989;65:1426–1440.
41. Toyoshima H, Burgess MJ. Electrotonic interaction during canine ventricular repolarization. *Circ Res* 1978;43:348–356.

42. Osaka T, Kodama I, Tsuboi N, et al. Effects of activation sequence and anisotropic cellular geometry on repolarization phase of action potential of dog ventricular muscles. *Circulation* 1987;76:226–236.
43. Kanai A, Salama G. Optical mapping reveals that repolarization spreads anisotropically and is guided by fiber orientation in guinea pig hearts. *Circ Res* 1995;77:784–802.
44. Yuan S, Wohlfart B, Olsson SB, Blomstrom-Lundqvist C. The dispersion of repolarization in patients with ventricular tachycardia: A study using simultaneous monophasic action potential recordings from two sites in the right ventricle. *Eur Heart J* 1995;16:68–76.
45. Vassallo J, Cassidy D, Kindwall E, et al. Nonuniform recovery of excitability in the left ventricle. *Circulation* 1988;78:1365–1372.
46. Myerburg RJ, Kessler KM, Castellanos A. Sudden cardiac death: Structure, function, and time-dependent risk. *Circulation* 1992;85(Suppl I):I2–I10.
47. Moe GK, Childers RW, Merideth J. An appraisal of supernormal A-V conduction. *Circulation* 1968;38:5–28.
48. Laurita KR, Rosenbaum DS. The interdependence of modulated dispersion and tissue structure in the mechanism of unidirectional block. *Circ Res* 2000;87:922–928.
49. Rosenbaum DS, Jackson LE, Smith JM, et al. Electrical alternans and vulnerability to ventricular arrhythmias. *N Engl J Med* 1994;330:235–241.
50. Cheng TC. Electrical alternans: An association with coronary artery spasm. *Arch Intern Med* 1983;143:1052–1053.
51. Salerno JA, Previtali M, Panciroli C, et al. Ventricular arrhythmias during acute myocardial ischaemia in man. The role and significance of R-ST-T alternans and the prevention of ischaemic sudden death by medical treatment. *Eur Heart J* 1986;7:63–75.
52. Wayne VS, Bishop RL, Spodick DH. Exercise-induced ST segment alternans. *Chest* 1983;83:824–825.
53. Reddy CVR, Kiok JP, Khan RG, El-Sherif N. Repolarization alternans associated with alcoholism and hypomagnesemia. *Am J Cardiol* 1984;53:390–391.
54. Platt SB, Vijgen JM, Albrecht P, et al. Occult T wave alternans in long QT syndrome. *J Cardiovasc Electrophysiol* 1996;7:144–148.
55. Rosenbaum DS, Albrecht P, Cohen RJ. Predicting sudden cardiac death from T wave alternans of the surface electrocardiogram: Promise and pitfalls. *J Cardiovasc Electrophysiol* 1996;7:1095–1111.
56. Rubenstein DS, Lipsius SL. Premature beats elicit a phase reversal of mechanoelectrical alternans in cat ventricular myocytes: A possible mechanism for reentrant arrhythmias. *Circulation* 1995;91:201–214.
57. Saitoh H, Bailey J, Surawicz B. Alternans of action potential duration after abrupt shortening of cycle length: Differences between dog Purkinje and ventricular muscle fibers. *Circ Res* 1988;62:1027–1040.
58. Karagueuzian HS, Khan SS, Hong K, et al. Action potential alternans and irregular dynamics in quinidine-intoxicated ventricular muscle cells: Implications for ventricular proarrhythmia. *Circulation* 1993;87:1661–1672.
59. Kléber AG, Janse MJ, van Capelle FJL, et al. Mechanism and time course of S-T and T-Q segment changes during acute regional myocardial ischemia in the pig heart determined by extracellular and intracellular recordings. *Circ Res* 1978;42:603–613.
60. Dilly SG, Lab MJ. Electrophysiological alternans and restitution during acute regional ischemia in myocardium of anesthetized pig. *J Physiol (Lond)* 1988;402:315–333.
61. Kurz RW, Mohabir R, Ren X-L, Franz MR. Ischaemia induced alternans of action potential duration in the intact heart: Dependence on coronary flow, preload, and cycle length. *Eur Heart J* 1993;14:1410–1420.

62. Sutton PMI, Taggart P, Lab M, et al. Alternans of epicardial repolarization as a localized phenomenon in man. *Eur Heart J* 1991;12:70–78.
63. Shimizu W, Yamada K, Arakaki Y, et al. Monophasic action potential recordings during T-wave alternans in congenital long QT syndrome. *Am Heart J* 1996;132:699–701.
64. Hohnloser SH, Klingenheben T, Zabel M, et al. T wave alternans during exercise and atrial pacing in humans. *J Cardiovasc Electrophysiol* 1997;8:987–993.
65. Konta T, Ikeda K, Yamaki M, et al. Significance of discordant ST alternans in ventricular fibrillation. *Circulation* 1990;82:2185–2189.
66. Hirata Y, Toyama J, Yamada K. Effects of hypoxia or low pH on the alteration of canine ventricular action potentials following an abrupt increase in driving rate. *Cardiovasc Res* 1980;14:108–115.

Chapter 13

Mapping Arrhythmia Substrates Related to Repolarization:

2. Cardiac Wavelength

Steven D. Girouard and David S. Rosenbaum

With the advent of optical action potential mapping with voltage-sensitive dyes it became possible to study cellular electrophysiology at the level of the intact heart. Knowledge of membrane potential at hundreds of sites simultaneously allows insight to the cellular mechanisms responsible for the initiation and perpetuation of arrhythmias. This chapter focuses on the use of optical mapping techniques to better understand reentrant arrhythmia substrates, with particular emphasis on the role of cardiac wavelength, excitable gap, and pathlength changes in the development and maintenance of reentry. Discussed is the dynamic equilibrium between wavelength, pathlength, and excitable gap, and its modulation by stimulus rate and prematurity, as well as structural factors, and the effects of pharmacological agents.

Arrhythmias and Cardiac Wavelength: Historical Perspective

One of the earliest observations made on reentry was that the circulating wave must somehow fit into the available reentrant circuit pathlength.[1] The spatial dimension, or length of a wave propagating in a reentrant circuit, was first expressed schematically by Mines,[1] and his original depiction has been adapted as Figure 1. This figure shows the perpetuation of reentry where an absolutely refractory wave (black) propagates into fully recovered and relatively refractory tissue. Therefore, the black band graphically represents the wavelength, which extends from the leading edge of depolarization to the trailing edge of refractoriness. Similarly, the white and speckled regions graphically depict the spatial dimensions of the fully excitable gap and partially excitable gap, respectively.

From Rosenbaum DS, Jalife J (eds): *Optical Mapping of Cardiac Excitation and Arrhythmias.*
©Futura Publishing Co., Inc., Armonk, NY, 2001.

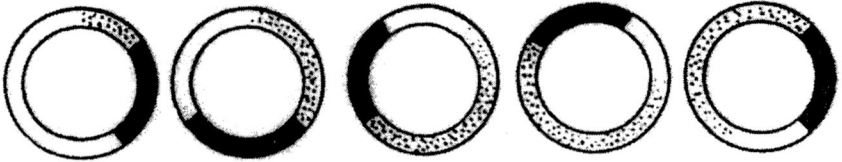

Figure 1. Figure adapted from reference 1. Wavelength is depicted as a nonvarying parameter as the wave (black) propagates in a clockwise manner around an anatomical obstacle. The wavelength extends from the leading edge of depolarization to the tail of absolutely refractory tissue. Relatively refractory tissue (stippled) graphically depicts the partially excitable gap. Similarly, the fully excitable gap is represented by the white region in advance of the propagating head. In this conceptual framework, reentry can persist only when wavelength is less than pathlength.

Two key questions arise from Mines' illustrations. First, wavelength is depicted as a single valued parameter and only its position within the circuit varies. *What are the factors that determine the magnitude of wavelength in the myocardium?* Second, the magnitude of wavelength is less than the reentrant path it occupies. *How does wavelength dynamically change during the initiation of reentry to allow it to fit within the circuit?*

In order to take wavelength from a concept to a measurable entity, it was necessary to define and quantify this parameter. Wiener and Rosenbleuth[2] first proposed the term "wavelength" and its mathematical treatment in the 1940s.

> *"Behind every wave front moving freely there will be a band of fixed width within which the recovery process is taking place. This may be spoken of as a wavelength."*

In their theoretical work, wavelength (λ) was represented by the product of the tissue refractory period (RP) and the conduction velocity (CV) of the wave.

$$\lambda = RP*CV$$

Their formulation assumed that 1) waves propagate at constant velocity through the tissue, and 2) the tissue has homogeneous refractory periods. These two assumptions are rarely valid, particularly in hearts that are susceptible to arrhythmias where spatial heterogeneities in conduction and refractoriness are known to be crucial. Therefore, despite being conceptually straightforward, quantitative experimental measurements of cardiac wavelength have been difficult to achieve. The accurate depiction of the spatial and temporal behavior of wavelength requires that both the depolarizing head and repolarizing tail of the propagating wave be recorded simultaneously. This can only be accomplished by simultaneously recording cellular action potentials from multiple sites in the heart. Herein lies the rationale for using optical action potential mapping for the measurement of the spatiotemporal dynamics of cardiac wavelength.

System to Investigate the Role of Wavelength in Reentry

We have developed a unique experimental system that applies high-resolution optical action potential mapping to a small mammalian model of anatomical reentry.[3] The details of the optical mapping system are described elsewhere.[4] Briefly, a photodiode array-based system is used to record cardiac action potentials from 128 sites on the anterior surface of the guinea pig ventricle. In studies of reentrant propagation, the guinea pig endocardium is cryoablated, leaving only a thin epicardial rim of surviving tissue.[3,5] This serves to restrict propagation to the surface from which action potentials are recorded, assuring that the dimensions of a propagating wave front can be fully assessed at any point of time. On this essentially 2-dimensional surface, a computer-controlled argon ion laser is used to "etch" a 2×10-mm obstacle onto the epicardial surface. Reentrant ventricular tachycardia (VT) caused by a circuit that circulates around the anatomical obstacle can be readily induced (approximately 90% of preparations).[3] Importantly, the model provides precise control of the size, trajectory, and location of the reentrant circuit with respect to cardiac fibers and important anatomical structures.

Our optical mapping system is used to record transmembrane activity from 128 sites encompassing the anatomical obstacle, with temporal (0.5 ms) and voltage (0.5 mV) resolutions required to measure in detail the time course of membrane potential.[4] Action potentials, conduction velocity, and wavelength can be monitored continuously throughout the entire reentrant circuit during steady-state reentry and during the critical events leading to the initiation of reentry.[3,6]

Measuring Cardiac Wavelength

As mentioned above, the measurement of cardiac wavelength is best achieved by monitoring transmembrane action potentials from multiple closely spaced sites across the heart. Techniques are now well established and validated for the detection of local activation and recovery times from optically recorded action potentials (see chapter 12). Activation is typically defined as the point of maximum positive first derivative[7] dF/dt_{max}, or a relative membrane potential threshold such as F_{50}.[8] Repolarization time has been shown experimentally and theoretically to correlate closely to the maximum positive second derivative of the fluorescence signal dF^2/dt^2_{max}.[7,9]

Measurement of wavelength in *space* at an instant in time is analogous to measuring action potential duration (APD) in *time* at a single site in space. The distance between the spatial location of dF/dt_{max} and the dF^2/dt^2_{max} can be directly measured with an accuracy that depends on the spatial, temporal, and voltage resolutions of the imaging system. When the entire wave is contained within the mapping field, wavelength can be measured at any point of time as the distance between the head of the wave front (i.e., point of dF/dt_{max} at the head of the wave) and the recovering tail (i.e., point of

dF^2/dt^2_{max} at the tail of the same wave). In this manner, wavelength can be measured directly as a function of time and space. In general, whenever the head of the wave accelerates relative to its tail, wavelength increases. Conversely, if the head of the wave decelerates relative to its tail, wavelength shortens. When the entire wave is not contained within the recording area, wavelength can be estimated using the Wiener and Rosenbleuth[2] formulation, if APD is known throughout the wave and an average conduction velocity in the direction of propagation can be calculated.

Steady-State Wavelength: Rate and Cardiac Structure

To date, wavelength has not been well characterized in ventricular myocardium, and only limited data exist for atrial tissues.[10,11] We have determined the basic relations governing wavelength in normal ventricular myocardium by use of plane wave stimulation along and across fibers over a wide range of pacing cycle lengths. As shown in Figure 2, wavelength shortens exponentially with increased stimulation frequency as a result of APD accommodation to rate[12] and concomitant reductions in conduction velocity.[13] Shortening of wavelength with increased rate was also ob-

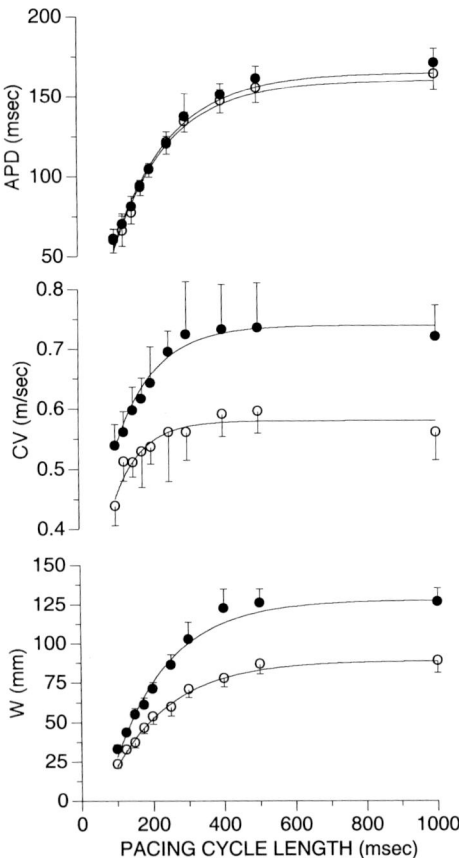

Figure 2. Influence of heart rate and fiber orientation on wavelength. Shown are action potential duration (APD), conduction velocity (CV), and wavelength (W) during plane wave stimulation in the guinea pig ventricle. Filled circles represent longitudinal propagation (relative to cardiac fiber orientation), and open circles represent transverse propagation. Values are mean ±SEM. Reproduced from reference 3.

served in rabbit[11] and canine[10] atria when wavelength was calculated based on the product of effective refractory period and conduction velocity measured from a limited number of sites.

Previous measurements of wavelength from canine atria did not take anisotropy into account, rather average values across all fiber angles were measured.[10] However, wavelength measured during plane wave propagation was dependent on both stimulation rate and fiber structure (Fig. 2, solid versus open cicles). Cardiac fiber structure resulted in anisotropic conduction velocities, however, APD was not dependent on the direction of propagation or fiber orientation. As a result, wavelength was consistently longer during propagation in the longitudinal direction compared with the transverse direction because of anisotropic conduction properties. These findings may have particular significance to structurally remodeled atrial and ventricular muscle where highly anisotropic tissue may support reentrant propagation.[14–16] The data in Figure 2 indicate that wavelength adapts to the local electrophysiological environment and can contract or expand dynamically as conditions change.

During steady-state reentry, wavelength is readily obtained from isopotential maps constructed from optically recorded action potentials, as depicted in Figure 3. By computing the wavelength at discrete times throughout a reentrant cycle, we demonstrated that the wavelength of a reentrant impulse varies considerably as it traverses a circuit.[3] Since wavelength varies as a continuous function of time (i.e., position within the cir-

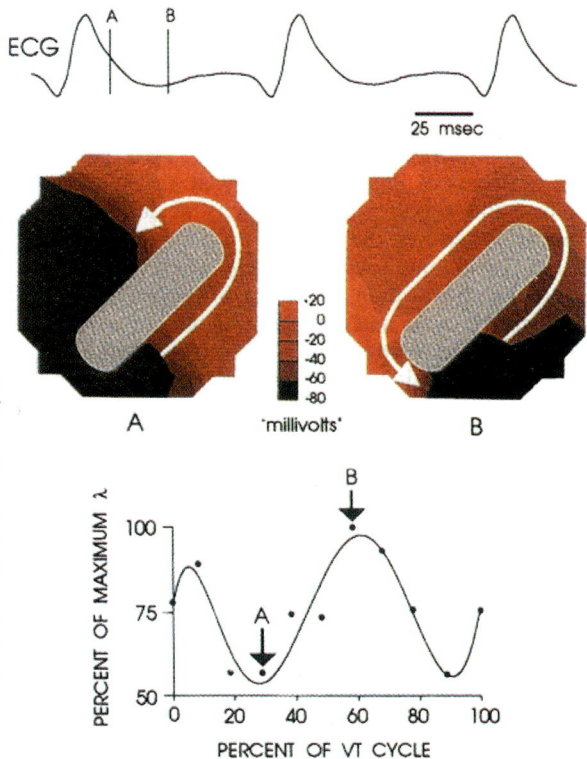

Figure 3. Graphic representation of wavelength from transmembrane potential maps generated by optical mapping. *Top:* Electrocardiographic recording for three beats of sustained monomorphic ventricular tachycardia (VT) in the guinea pig ventricle. *Middle:* Two snapshots taken at two time points (A and B) during a single reentrant cycle. The action potential amplitude is mapped to a pseudo-voltage color scale. As the leading edge of the wave front propagates around the reentrant circuit, the magnitude of wavelength changes. *Bottom:* Plots of the cyclic variation of wavelength during one beat of VT. Reproduced from reference 3.

cuit), the excitable gap also varies within the circuit. Direct measurement revealed approximately 50% variation in wavelength during a single reentrant cycle. Such a finding may explain why responses of clinical VT to artificial stimulation are often dependent on the region of the reentrant circuit where stimuli are delivered.

Optical Recordings Reveal Mechanism of Conduction Slowing at Pivot Points

In addition to the structure and rate dependence of wavelength, we found that conduction velocity slowing near pivot points of the reentrant circuit was an important factor in wavelength shortening during VT. At the cellular level slow conduction was associated with a reduction of action potential upstroke velocity at pivot points. This is illustrated in Figure 4 where action potential upstrokes recorded from five uniformly spaced sites around a typical pivot point are shown. As the wave front approaches the pivot point from the lower right, action potential upstrokes are rapid (potentials A and B) and are not different from upstrokes observed in other areas of the circuit where the wave front geometry was planar. However, as the wave rotates, action potential upstrokes become progressively slowed. Typically, multiple notches and slow upstrokes were observed (potentials C and D). In contrast, during plane-wave stimulation the action potentials recorded from sites C and D exhibited normal upstrokes, indi-

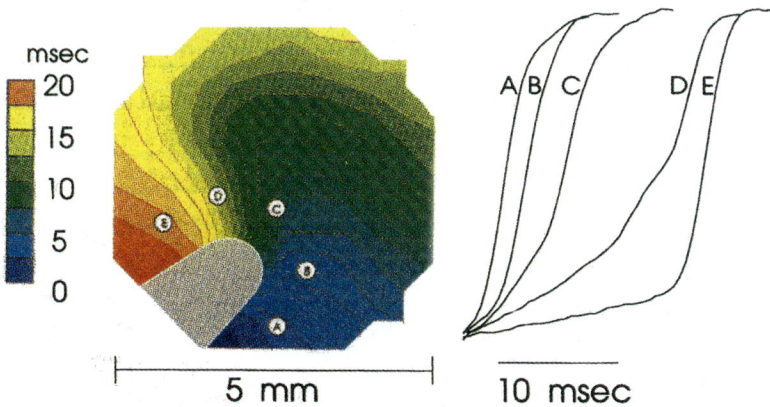

Figure 4. High spatial resolution map (400 μm resolution) of depolarization (1-ms isochrones) around the basal tip of the epicardial obstacle (hatched area) during established reentrant ventricular tachycardia. Pivoting around the obstacle requires that the reentrant wave front first propagate transverse to fibers (blue region), then turn parallel to fibers (blue > green > yellow), and finally turn transverse to fibers again (red region). As the wave front pivots, conduction slows (i.e., crowding of isochrones) paradoxically as propagation turns parallel to fibers. Action potential upstrokes recorded from five evenly spaced sites around the pivot point are shown to the right. While the wave front enters the pivot point (A, B), conduction is relatively fast and upstrokes are sharp. However, as the wave front pivots (C, D), action potential upstrokes become increasingly slowed. After pivoting is complete (E), conduction and action potential upstroke velocity are again normal. Reproduced from reference 3.

cating that conduction slowing was not due to intrinsically depressed excitability. These data are consistent with findings that link the curvature of a wave front to its propagation velocity.[17] As a reentrant wave front takes on increased curvature, the advancing depolarizing wave encounters a greater mass of downstream tissue, resulting in source-sink mismatch. Since all types of reentry, functional[16,18–20] and anatomical,[21,22] require wave fronts to rotate to form a complete circuit, slowing of conduction and wavelength reduction at pivot points may be a common phenomenon. Since the guinea pig VT model had only two pivot points, beat-to-beat variations of wavelength occurred with a sinusoidal variation that repeated twice every cardiac cycle (Fig. 3, bottom). It is important to emphasize how optical recordings of membrane voltage specifically led to such insights into the biophysical basis for pivot point conduction.

These data, derived from optical maps during pacing and spontaneous reentrant activation, suggest that the wavelength of a propagating impulse adapts to the local electrophysiological environment. Thus, wavelength can shorten or lengthen dynamically as local conditions change spatially or temporally. Wavelength dynamics are readily observed from isopotential plots obtained from optical mapping with voltage-sensitive dyes.

Wavelength Adaptation as a Mechanism of Reentry: Dynamic Arrhythmia Substrates

Because of difficulties in measuring wavelength with traditional extracellular mapping techniques, beat-to-beat changes of wavelength (i.e., wavelength adaptation) have not been quantified during the dynamic events leading to reentry. There is, however, ample evidence that supports the notion that wavelength adaptation must occur during the initiation of reentrant arrhythmias in humans. First, it is estimated that, at resting heart rates, wavelength is large, typically greater than the heart circumference and much greater than the dimensions of reentrant circuits thought responsible for most tachycardias. Second, faster stimulation rates (e.g., premature stimuli and tachycardia heart rates) are associated with marked shortening of ventricular refractoriness,[23] APD,[24] conduction velocity, and, hence, wavelength. Third, the termination of VT by antiarrhythmic drugs that prolong APD is attended by oscillations of QT interval and VT cycle length.[25,26] These data suggest that tachycardia is terminating because of "reversed" wavelength adaptation (i.e., wavelength increases until it exceeds the pathlength, forcing the head of depolarization to interact with the tail of refractoriness). Finally, it is common that multiple premature stimuli or a transitional polymorphic rhythm is observed before stable VT ensues, indicating that the initial electrophysiological conditions require substantial modification during the induction of reentry.[27–31]

The concept of wavelength adaptation and its potential importance to reentry mechanisms was alluded to by Mines[1] nearly 100 years ago.

"Ordinarily, in the naturally beating heart, the wave of excitation is so long and so rapid that it spreads all over the ventricle long before it has ceased in any one part. On increasing the frequency of excitation, the wave becomes slower and shorter. Under these circumstances it be-

comes possible for the whole wave to be present at one time on the muscle column."

The initiation of reentry is traditionally thought to require at least two conditions. First, there must be a spatial inhomogeneity or dispersion of membrane properties or tissue structure to create unidirectional block. The second requisite for reentry is "slow" conduction. These conditions can be stated more precisely in terms of wavelength. Following unidirectional block, the wavelength must be shorter than the reentrant pathlength in order for reentry to ensue. In fact, under this paradigm slow conduction is not a necessary condition for reentry.

The critical membrane events leading to the development of reentry are illustrated in Figure 5.[32] Isochrone lines (10 ms) depict the activation

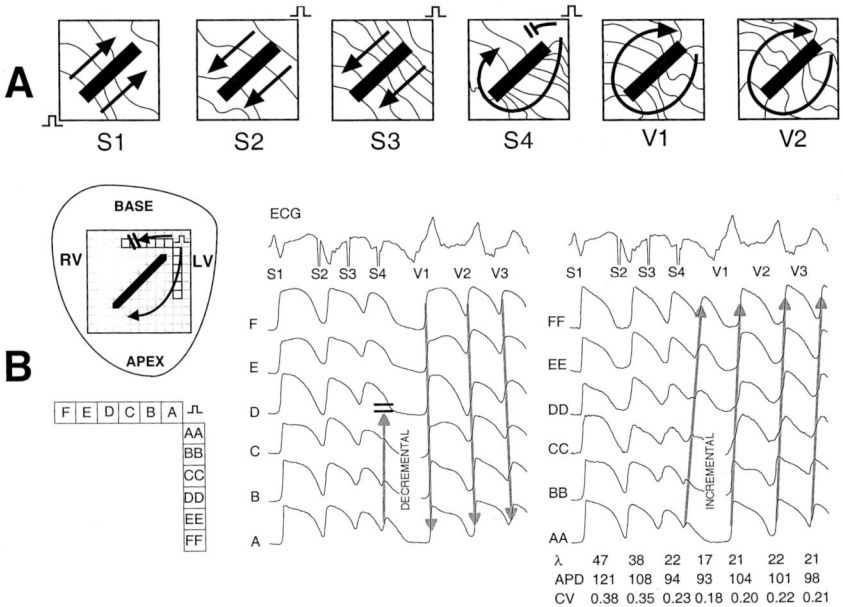

Figure 5. Initiation of reentry by three premature stimuli. **A.** Stimuli S1-S3 propagate with progressive slowing (note relative crowding of 10-ms isochrones) away from the pacing site. S4, however, encounters unidirectional block at the left ventricular (LV) base while the remaining wave propagates with sufficiently short wavelength that the head of depolarization reenters the circuit and stable reentry ensues (V1). **B** (*bottom*): Membrane responses leading to unidirectional block. Action potentials are shown along two orthogonal directions from the pacing site (shown schematically on the lower right) for propagation on the left hand side of the lesion (A through F), and propagation on the right hand side of the lesion (AA through FF). During baseline pacing, action potentials are relatively long and conduction is rapid in both directions. With increasing prematurity, action potential duration rapidly shortens at all sites, indicating wavelength adaptation. Following the S4 stimulus, unidirectional block develops. The S4 stimulus barely captures the tissue at the pacing site (A, AA). Propagation along the left side of the lesion proceeds decrementally (A through C), with decreased action potential amplitude and dV/dt, resulting in unidirectional block. Simultaneously, propagation along the right side of the lesion proceeds incrementally, and the wave front reenters the previous site of block (gray arrows). ECG = electrocardiogram; RV = right ventricular. Reproduced from reference 32.

patterns leading away from the stimulus sites for the S1-S4 paced beats and the first two spontaneous beats V1 and V2 (Fig. 5A). Unidirectional block developed following the S4 stimulus, and resulted in and stable VT. The membrane potential responses during the drive train, premature stimuli, and first reentrant beats are shown in Figure 5B for two orthogonal lines of recording sites leading away from the premature stimulus location. Action potentials following the S1 stimulus demonstrate normal characteristics (e.g., sharp upstrokes, plateau, and rapid repolarization phase). Following each additional premature stimulus, APD and conduction velocity decreased and wavelength shortened. The S4 stimulus captured the tissue closest to the pacing site (potentials A, and AA) and the impulse propagated in the orthodromic direction (potentials AA through FF). This propagation was characterized by a progressive increase in action potential amplitude and upstroke velocity at more distal sites (i.e., incremental conduction). In contrast, the antidromic wave (potentials A through F) propagated decrementally until conduction failed around site D. At sites where conduction previously failed, the returning orthodromic wave propagated through unimpeded (V1), since sufficient time passed for excitability to be restored (i.e., wavelength < pathlength). Indeed, because of the shortened wavelength following S4, on the first reentrant beat, the sites that previously blocked were the most excitable as evidenced by the long diastolic intervals at sites A though F prior to V1.

Pharmacological Modulation of Wavelength

Lewis[33] was the first to propose that an antiarrhythmic effect of a drug can be explained by its tendency to prolong cardiac wavelength by increasing refractoriness more than it slows conduction. We applied the I_{kr} blocking drug d-sotalol to the guinea pig model of reentry to investigate how drug-induced modulation of wavelength influenced the initiation of reentry.[32]

Figure 6 illustrates the response of wavelength to a single premature stimulus (S2) before and after perfusion with 15 μmol/L d-sotalol. Data are shown for propagation along the longitudinal and transverse fiber axes over a wide range of premature coupling intervals. As seen during steady-state pacing (Fig. 2), for each S1-S2 interval tested, wavelength was consistently shorter in the transverse direction compared with the longitudinal fiber direction because of relatively slow conduction transverse to fibers. However, the greatest absolute change in wavelength occurred in the longitudinal direction. This was due to a preferential slowing of conduction velocity in the longitudinal compared with the transverse direction. A shift in the restitution curve, upward and to the right, during d-sotalol perfusion limited the minimum S1-S2 achieved (control 128±13 ms; d-sotalol 167±18 ms; n = 5; P< 0.05). It should be noted that the two curves intersect (Fig. 6, arrow), indicating that in many instances (i.e., at shorter S1-S2 coupling intervals), wavelength was shorter during d-sotalol perfusion than in controls. This result is explained by the fact that diastolic intervals were shorter for the same S1-S2 interval during d-sotalol perfusion since baseline APD was prolonged. However, the minimum achievable wavelength was always prolonged by d-sotalol perfusion.

During plane-wave pacing, hearts were also stimulated with the four shortest premature stimuli that resulted in successful capture. The response of wavelength adaptation to multiple premature stimuli was characterized by two distinct phases (Fig. 7). The majority of wavelength reduction occurred during the initial phase of this response when the first (S2) and second (S3) stimuli were introduced, and was due to comparable reduction in both APD ($-29\pm3\%$) and conduction velocity ($-35.5\pm5\%$). In the latter phase of the response (i.e., beyond the S3 stimulus), wavelength adaptation continued, but at a slower rate. Wavelength changes during the slow phase were almost exclusively caused by persistent APD shortening over time.

As shown in Figure 7, d-sotalol was found to offset the rapid and slow phases of wavelength adaptation. On average, d-sotalol prolonged wavelength by 14 ± 4 mm during a steady-state pacing cycle length of 350 ms. During the S2 and S3, the mean difference between d-sotalol and control wavelength was 10 ± 6 mm and 14 ± 7 mm, respectively. These results indicate that, during the first two premature stimuli, d-sotalol acted to prolong wavelength substantially. In contrast, after 3 minutes of steady-state stimulation, the two curves converged such that, at a cycle length of 100 ms, d-sotalol prolonged wavelength by only 4 ± 2 mm. Therefore, after

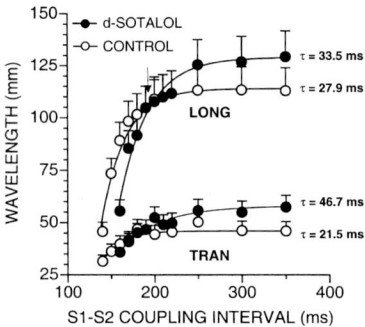

Figure 6. Restitution of cardiac wavelength in the guinea pig ventricle. Wavelength is plotted for two directions of propagation along (LONG) and transverse (TRAN) to cardiac fiber orientation. Wavelength dynamically shortens in an exponential manner as the premature stimulus (S2) is introduced at increasingly premature intervals (shorter S1-S2 coupling interval). Wavelength is greater during LONG compared with TRAN propagation at any coupling interval. Perfusion with d-sotalol resulted in an offset in the restitution curve (upward and to the right). Note the cross-over of the two curves (arrow) that results from the decreased diastolic interval for any applied S1-S2 coupling interval. Reproduced from reference 32.

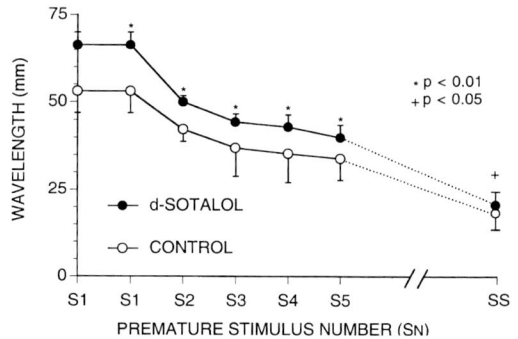

Figure 7. The process of wavelength adaptation shown during the introduction of four premature stimuli. Plotted is wavelength calculated at the shortest possible premature coupling intervals (S2-S5) in a representative heart before and after the addition of 15 μmol/L d-sotalol. Reproduced from reference 32.

abrupt shortening of cycle length, as occurs during premature stimulation or during the onset of VT, the wavelength-prolonging effect of d-sotalol is more than three times greater than during steady-state tachycardia. These results indicate that the reverse use-dependent properties of d-sotalol required many beats to fully develop, and, hence, after sudden acceleration of rate (e.g., onset of tachycardia) there is a window of time during which d-sotalol exerts its most significant antiarrhythmic effect.

Since the baseline wavelength was much larger than the reentrant pathlength, adaptation of the wavelength to dimensions shorter than the pathlength was necessary for initiation of VT. Figure 8 demonstrates wavelength adaptation quantitatively during the initiation of VT by premature stimuli in a representative experiment. The horizontal dashed line indicates the anatomical pathlength of the circuit. Note that following the S3 stimulus wavelength is less than pathlength, and when unidirectional block developed during the S4 stimulus (asterisk), reentry ensued. In contrast, during perfusion with d-sotalol, wavelength failed to shorten to the dimensions of the circuit and thus reentry could not be initiated.

To determine the effect of an antiarrhythmic drug on wavelength during the initiation of reentry with premature stimuli, important rate (use)-dependent effects of a drug must be considered. For example, I_{Na}-blocking drugs like flecainide have use-dependent properties such that conduction velocity slowing is more pronounced at faster rates. Flecainide has been found to have proarrhythmic effects,[34] which may be attributable to conduction velocity slowing[35,36] (i.e., wavelength shortening). Few studies have attempted to assess these proarrhythmic effects quantitatively.

In contrast to I_{Na}-blocking drugs, I_{Kr} blockers such as d-sotalol prolong APD without affecting conduction[37] and are therefore expected to lengthen wavelength. However, the effects of d-sotalol and several other I_{Kr}-blocking drugs are characterized by "reverse" use dependence resulting in a loss of APD-prolonging effects at rapid rates.[38–40] Therefore, at a

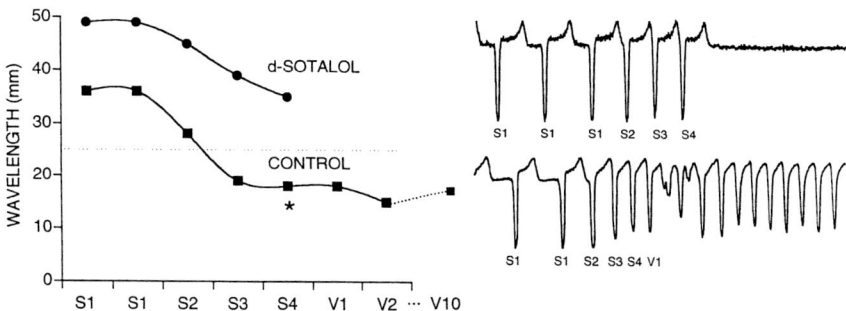

Figure 8. Wavelength adaptation during the initiation of reentry in the guinea pig ventricular tachycardia model. Shown are the wavelength responses in the heart during a successful initiation of reentry and in the same heart after addition of 15 μmol/L d-sotalol. Note that during control perfusion wavelength is shortened by the application of premature stimuli to a level less than the perimeter of the laser obstacle (horizontal stippled line) at the time of unidirectional block (*). Stable reentry ensues because wavelength has successfully adapted to the dimensions of the available reentrant path. Addition of d-sotalol alters wavelength adaptation (i.e., shifts curve upward), preventing wavelength from shortening to the reentrant path (horizontal stippled line). Reproduced from reference 32.

time when it is most desirable for d-sotalol to exert its greatest effect (i.e., during tachycardia), it is least effective. Nevertheless, d-sotalol appears to be among the most effective drugs for suppressing clinical VT.[41] This apparent paradox may be explained by the influence these drugs have on the time course of wavelength adaptation during the initiation of VT. Although d-sotalol may have little effect during fully developed tachycardia, it was recently found to exhibit slow-offset kinetics.[42] As a result, during an abrupt increase in rate (e.g., with premature stimuli), reverse use dependence may take many beats to develop. Hence, there may be a critical window during which time, in the presence of d-sotalol, a premature stimulus does not shorten wavelength sufficiently to induce reentry.

Optical Mapping Reveals Pathlength Expansion during Initiation of Reentry

Often during the initiation of VT a propagating wave does not necessarily adhere to the anatomical circuit defined by the laser lesion (i.e., pathlength > anatomical circuit). Therefore, the successful initiation of reentry based on adaptation of wavelength to the dimensions of the circuit's pathlength, as described above, is actually more complex because, in addition to wavelength, pathlength can also vary on a beat-to-beat basis. Fortunately, high-resolution optical mapping can also be used to measure dynamic changes in the pathlength of propagating wave fronts.

In particular, sites near both pivot points of the reentrant circuit were prone to transient functional block resulting in functional expansion of the anatomical pathlength. In these cases, reentry could potentially persist even when wavelength was greater than the anatomical pathlength since the actual reentrant path was partially extended by functionally unexcited tissue at pivot points. As before, during each beat of initiation of reentry, the actual pathlength must be longer than wavelength; hence, it is important to track both of these parameters on a beat-by-beat basis.

An example of transient pathlength expansion during the initiation of VT is depicted in Figure 9. Following the S3 and S4 stimuli, a region at the apical pivot point (A) became functionally unexcited. Action potentials recorded from within the apical pivot point (sites b and d) exhibited a loss of amplitude and a marked reduction in upstroke velocity compared with their baseline values. In contrast, sites that are located further from the pivot point (sites a and c) maintained sharp upstrokes and plateaus throughout the onset and perpetuation of VT. Thus, the pathlength functionally extended during premature stimulation. Similarly, during the initial beats of VT, sites h and f became functionally inexcitable at the basal pivot point. As a result, the wave trajectory left the anatomical path transiently (B). Action potentials recorded from the region of transient functional block (e and g) and neighbors outside this region (f and h) illustrate the spatial and temporal changes in the action potential configuration during detachment of the wave front from the anatomical obstacle.

Pathlength expansion always occurred during premature stimulation and/or during the early beats of reentry when the reentrant circuit was forming. The area of transient functional block was typically localized to

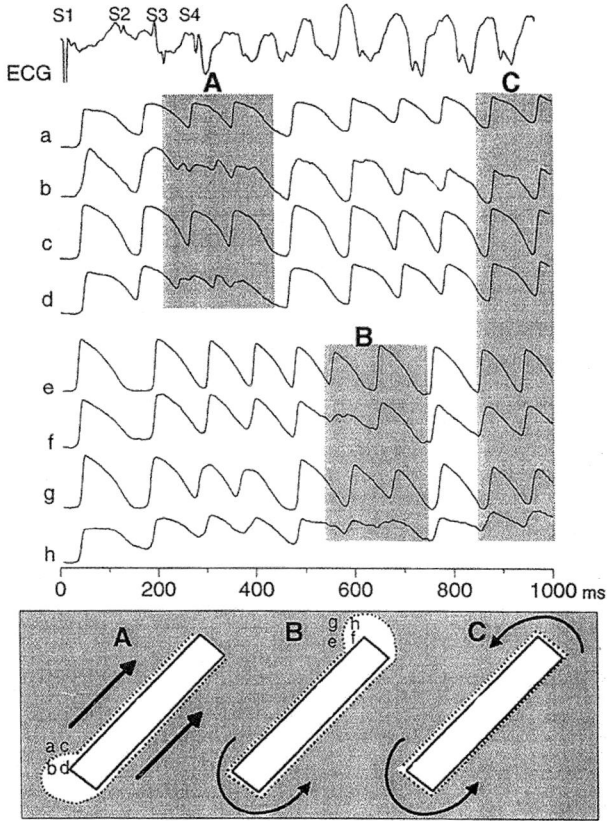

Figure 9. Pathlength expansion during the initiation and early beats of reentry. *Top:* Electrocardiogram and action potentials recorded during premature stimuli (S1-S4) and early beats of reentrant ventricular tachycardia which follow the third premature stimulus (S4). During baseline pacing (left most potentials at each recording site) action potential characteristics are normal everywhere. Premature stimulation resulted in a reduction of the action potential upstroke and amplitude as expected, since prematurely stimulated waves propagate into less excitable tissue. During the last prematurely stimulated beat (S4), action potentials recorded near the pivot point located near the apex of the ventricle (shaded region A, potentials b and d) exhibit multiphase low-amplitude depolarizations indicating failure of penetration of the depolarizing wave front into the pivot point with electronic depolarizations exclusively. During the early beats of reentry (shaded region B) a similar response was observed at the basal pivot point. Action potentials (sites f, h) exhibited a loss in amplitude and upstroke velocity compared with neighboring sites (g, e). Once stable reentry is established, all sites regained excitability and respond in a similar manner (shaded region C). Such failed depolarizations at pivot points result from the combined effect of reduced excitability to a premature stimulus coupled with source-sink mismatch caused by enhanced wave front curvature at each pivot point, and lead to functional expansion of the reentrant path beyond the anatomical line of block. After several beats of reentry, as action potential shortens refractoriness falls, excitability increases, and pathlength expansion resolves.

regions associated with high wave front curvature and occurred at times of reduced membrane excitability such as during the first several beats of reentry. In contrast, during established reentry, functional pathlength expansion was absent and the reentrant pathlength was determined solely by the perimeter of the anatomical obstacle (Fig. 9, C). Since action potential upstrokes were only transiently reduced, pathlength expansion could not be explained by an overall depressed excitability within the circuit. Rather, the tissue was excitable but unexcited possibly due to electrotonic loading imposed by wave front pivoting in the setting of relatively impaired excitability (before APD accommodated to the tachycardia rate). It was previously established that the maximum curvature a propagating impulse can achieve is directly related to tissue excitability.[17] Therefore, during periods of reduced excitability (i.e., longer wavelength) such as the first several beats of tachycardia, impulses fail to turn rapidly at pivot points of the circuit, resulting in functional expansion of the reentrant path. Detailed membrane potential maps obtained with optical mapping (Fig. 9) were key to developing insights into the biophysical basis for impulse propagation and antiarrhythmic drug effects in reentry.

Summary

Wavelength originated as a conceptual framework used to understand reentrant wave propagation and antiarrhythmic drug actions. Over the past century it has remained a useful concept; however, until recently it has been difficult to measure and quantify experimentally. Recent developments in optical action potential mapping techniques have made it possible to measure wavelength accurately during steady-state activation as well as during dynamically changing activation sequences that occur at the onset of arrhythmias.

Optical mapping with voltage-sensitive dyes has provided insight into how the arrhythmia substrate dynamically changes on a beat-to-beat basis. New insights directly attributable to the use of optical action potential mapping include the following: 1) Wavelength in the ventricle is highly dependent on stimulation rate, stimulus prematurity, tissue structure, and wave front topology. 2) Wavelength varies in space even during steady-state pacing and established reentry. 3) As a result of 1 and 2, the spatial excitable gap varies in a manner inversely proportional to wavelength. 4) Antiarrhythmic drugs may act on the process of wavelength adaptation to prevent adequate shortening of wavelength during premature stimulation. 5) Due to spatial and temporal variations in tissue excitability, the reentrant pathlength may functionally expand and contract transiently.

References

1. Mines GR. On dynamic equilibrium in the heart. *J Physiol (Lond)* 1913; 46:349–383.
2. Wiener N, Rosenblueth A. The mathematical formulation of the problem of conduction of impulses in a network of connected excitable elements, specifically in cardiac muscle. *Arch Inst Cardiol Mex* 1946;16:205–265.

3. Girouard SD, Pastore JM, Laurita KR, et al. Optical mapping in a new guinea pig model of ventricular tachycardia reveals mechanisms for multiple wavelengths in a single reentrant circuit. *Circulation* 1996;93:603–613.
4. Girouard SD, Laurita KR, Rosenbaum DS. Unique properties of cardiac action potentials recorded with voltage-sensitive dyes. *J Cardiovasc Electrophysiol* 1996;7:1024–1038.
5. Schalij MJ, Lammers WJEP, Rensma PL, Allessie MA. Anisotropic conduction and reentry in perfused epicardium of rabbit left ventricle. *Am J Physiol* 1992;263:H1466-H1478.
6. Pastore JM, Girouard SD, Laurita KR, et al. Mechanism linking T wave alternans to the genesis of cardiac fibrillation. *Circulation* 1999;99:1385–1394.
7. Rosenbaum DS, Kaplan DT, Kanai A, et al. Repolarization inhomogeneities in ventricular myocardium change dynamically with abrupt cycle length shortening. *Circulation* 1991;84:1333–1345.
8. Fast VG, Kléber AG. Cardiac tissue geometry as a determinant of unidirectional conduction block: Assessment of microscopic excitation spread by optical mapping in patterned cell cultures and in a computer model. *Cardiovasc Res* 1995;29:697–707.
9. Efimov IR, Ermentrout B, Huang DT, Salama G. Activation and repolarization patterns are governed by different structural characteristics of ventricular myocardium: Experimental study with voltage-sensitive dyes and numerical simulations. *J Cardiovasc Electrophysiol* 1996;7:512–530.
10. Rensma PL, Allessie MA, Lammers WJEP, et al. Length of excitation wave and susceptibility to reentrant atrial arrhythmias in normal conscious dogs. *Circ Res* 1988;62:395–410.
11. Smeets J, Allessie MA, Lammers W, et al. The wavelength of the cardiac impulse and reentrant arrhythmias in isolated rabbit atrium: The role of heart rate, autonomic transmitters, temperature, and potassium. *Circ Res* 1986;58:96–108.
12. Boyett MR, Jewell BR. A study of the factors responsible for rate-dependent shortening of the action potential in mammalian ventricular muscle. *J Physiol* 1978;285:359–380.
13. Hoffman BF, Suckling EE. Effect of heart rate on cardiac membrane potentials and unipolar electrogram. *Am J Physiol* 1954;179:123–130.
14. Spach MS, Dolber PC, Heidlage JF. Interaction of inhomogeneities of repolarization with anisotropic propagation in dog atria: A mechanism for both preventing and initiating reentry. *Circ Res* 1989;65:1612–1631.
15. Wit A, Allessie M, Bonke F, et al. Electrophysiologic mapping to determine the mechanism of experimental ventricular tachycardia initiated by premature impulses. *Am J Cardiol* 1982;49:166–185.
16. Spach MS, Josephson ME. Initiating reentry: The role of nonuniform anisotropy in small circuits. *J Cardiovasc Electrophysiol* 1994;5:182–209.
17. Cabo C, Pertsov AM, Baxter WT, et al. Wave-front curvature as a cause of slow conduction and block in isolated cardiac muscle. *Circ Res* 1994;75:1014–1028.
18. El-Sherif N, Scherlag B, Lazzara R, Hope R. Reentrant ventricular arrhythmias in the late myocardial infarction period: 1. Conduction characteristics in the infarction zone. *Circulation* 1977;55(5):686–702.
19. Ortiz J, Igarashi M, Gonzalez X, et al. Mechanism of spontaneous termination of stable atrial flutter in the canine sterile pericarditis model. *Circulation* 1993;88(4 Pt. 1):1866–1877.
20. Allessie A, Bonke FI, Schopman FJG. Circus movement in rabbit atrial muscle as a mechanism of tachycardia: The role of nonuniform recovery of excitability in the occurrence of unidirectional block as studied with multiple microelectrodes. *Circ Res* 1976;39:169–177.
21. Bernstein R, Frame L. Ventricular reentry around a fixed barrier. *Circulation* 1990;81:267–280.

22. Reiter MJ, Zetelaki Z, Kirchhof CJH, et al. Interaction of acute ventricular dilatation and d-sotalol during sustained reentrant ventricular tachycardia around a fixed obstacle. *Circulation* 1994;89:423–431.
23. Marchlinski FE. Characterization of oscillations in ventricular refractoriness in man after an abrupt increment in heart rate. *Circulation* 1987;75:550–556.
24. Franz MR, Swerdlow CD, Liem LB, Schaefer J. Cycle length dependence of human action potential duration in vivo. *J Clin Invest* 1988;82:972–979.
25. Duff HJ, Mitchell LB, Gillis AM, et al. Electrocardiographic correlates of spontaneous termination of ventricular tachycardia in patients with coronary artery disease. *Circulation* 1993;88:1054–1062.
26. Fei HL, Frame LH. d-Sotalol terminates reentry by two mechanisms with different dependence on the duration of the excitable gap. *J Pharmacol Exp Ther* 1996;277:174–185.
27. Gough W, Mehra R, Restivo M, et al. Reentrant ventricular arrhythmias in the late myocardial infarction period in the dog: 13. Correlation of activation and refractory maps. *Circ Res* 1985;57:432–442.
28. Kramer J, Saffitz J, Witkowski F, Corr P. Intramural reentry as a mechanism of ventricular tachycardia during evolving canine myocardial infarction. *Circ Res* 1985;56:736–754.
29. Bardy GH, Olson WH. Clinical characteristics of spontaneous-onset sustained ventricular tachycardia and ventricular fibrillation in survivors of cardiac arrest. In Zipes DP, Jalife J (eds): *Cardiac Electrophysiology: From Cell to Bedside.* Philadelphia: W.B. Saunders Co.; 1990:778–790.
30. Morady F, DiCarlo L, Winston S, et al. A prospective comparison of triple extrastimuli and left ventricular stimulation in studies of ventricular tachycardia induction. *Circulation* 1984;70:52–57.
31. Brugada P, Green M, Abdollah H, Wellens HJJ. Significance of ventricular arrhythmias initiated by programmed ventricular stimulation: The importance of the type of ventricular arrhythmia induced and the number of premature stimuli required. *Circulation* 1984;69:87–92.
32. Girouard SD, Rosenbaum DS. Role of wavelength adaptation in the initiation, maintenance, and pharmacologic suppression of reentry. *J Cardiovasc Electrophysiol* 2001; 12:697-707.
33. Lewis T: *Mechanisms and Graphic Registration of the Heart Beat.* London: Shaw & Son; 1925.
34. The Cardiac Arrhythmia Suppression Trial (CAST) Investigators. Preliminary report: Effect of encainide and flecainide on mortality in a randomized trial of arrhythmia suppression after myocardial infarction. *N Engl J Med* 1989; 321:406–412.
35. Restivo M, Yin H, Caref EB, et al. Reentrant arrhythmias in the subacute infarction period: The proarrhythmic effect of flecainide acetate on functional reentrant circuits. *Circulation* 1995;91:1236–1246.
36. Coromilas J, Saltman AE, Waldecker B, et al. Electrophysiological effects of flecainide on anisotropic conduction and reentry in infarcted canine hearts. *Circulation* 1995;91:2245–2263.
37. Carmeliet E. Electrophysiologic and voltage clamp analysis of the effects of sotalol on isolated cardiac muscle and Purkinje fibers. *J Pharmacol Exp Ther* 1985;232:817–825.
38. Schmitt C, Brachmann J, Karch M, et al. Reverse use-dependent effects of sotalol demonstrated by recording monophasic action potentials of the right ventricle. *Am J Cardiol* 1991;68:1183–1187.
39. Hondeghem LM, Snyders DJ. Class III antiarrhythmic agents have a lot of potential but a long way to go: Reduced effectiveness and dangers of reverse use dependence. *Circulation* 1990;81:686–690.

40. Cappato R, Alboni P, Codecà L, et al. Direct and autonomically mediated effects of oral quinidine on RR/QT relation after an abrupt increase in heart rate. *J Am Coll Cardiol* 1993;22:99–105.
41. Mason JW. A comparison of electrophysiologic testing with Holter monitoring to predict antiarrhythmic-drug efficacy for ventricular tachyarrhythmias. *N Engl J Med* 1993;329:445–451.
42. Weirich J, Hohnloser SH, Antoni H. D-sotalol and dofetilide exhibit slow offset kinetics: Significance for their antifibrillatory efficacy. *Pacing Clin Electrophysiol* 1994;17(Pt. II):824. Abstract.

Chapter 14

Video Imaging of Cardiac Fibrillation

Richard A. Gray and José Jalife

Introduction

Background

Fibrillation can occur in the atria or ventricles and is characterized by rapid, irregular electrical activity as recorded by an electrocardiogram (ECG) from the body surface.[1] Ventricular fibrillation (VF) is the leading cause of death in the industrialized world, claiming the lives of more than 1000 Americans each day.[2] VF leads to rapid and asynchronous contraction of the ventricles, which prevents the adequate pumping of blood through the body, resulting in death within minutes. Atrial fibrillation (AF) results in irregular contraction of the atria; AF is the most common sustained cardiac arrhythmia and often leads to stroke.[3]

The activity of the heart has been monitored for many years by recording the ECG. These recordings have led to many diagnostic advances in cardiology. However, since the ECG is recorded from the body surface at a distance from the heart, it reveals very little about the events occurring during complex cardiac rhythms. For example, during VF, ECG deflections continuously change in shape, magnitude, and direction; this has led to the idea that fibrillation is the result of disorganized, highly complex, perhaps even random, activation of the heart.

Mechanisms of Fibrillation

The inefficient and asynchronous contractions that occur during fibrillation are the result of spatiotemporal patterns of electrical activity in the heart. The detailed characteristics of the electrical activity throughout the heart during fibrillation have been debated for many years. Although the mechanisms of fibrillation have often been viewed as a single entity, fibrillation can result from a rapidly firing ectopic focus,[4] a single reentrant circuit,[5–7] or multiple meandering wavelets.[8,9] In addition, the substrate of the heart (e.g., ischemia,[10] fiber orientation,[11] wall thickness,[12] Purkinje

From Rosenbaum DS, Jalife J (eds): *Optical Mapping of Cardiac Excitation and Arrhythmias.* ©Futura Publishing Co., Inc., Armonk, NY, 2001.

fibers,[13] trabeculae,[14] and valves[15,16]) as well as its geometry[17] may play a role in the dynamics of fibrillation.

Cardiac Mapping

Many recordings from the heart surface are required to reveal the electrical activity throughout the heart during rapid cardiac rhythms (tachyarrhythmias). Nearly two decades ago, it became possible to measure electrical activity from many sites on the heart simultaneously,[18] a technique called cardiac mapping. "Traditional" cardiac mapping involves recording extracellular potentials (Fig. 1, top) and calculating activation times from up to 512 sites,[19] allowing a spatiotemporal description of the propagating waves of electrical activity in the heart. Under certain abnormal circumstances, the heartbeat can undergo dangerous transitions to rapid, irregular activity in the form of rotating waves of electrical activity. These rotating waves, which were first observed using extracellular cardiac mapping,[20] are thought to be responsible for the most dangerous tachyarrhythmias, including fibrillation. However, the detailed characteristics of these rotating waves remained speculative. Recently, a new form of cardiac mapping called video imaging has emerged, allowing the simultaneous recording from 10,000 to 100,000 sites. This high spatial resolution has led to some important findings regarding the characteristics of rotating waves in the heart. First, the shape of the wave front is curved, with increasing curvature toward the center of rotation resulting in a spiral shape.[21,22] Second, the propagation velocity in cardiac tissue is linearly related to the curvature of the wave front and a critical curvature for propagation exists.[23] Third, in the whole rabbit heart, rotating waves of electrical activity propagate in the ventricles during tachyarrhythmias.[24] In the ventricles, monomorphic tachycardias result from rotating waves that remain stationary and polymorphic tachycardias result when they move.[25] In fact, if a single reentrant wave moves rapidly through the heart, the ECG resembles fibrillation.[7] Typically, however, fibrillation is the result of multiple waves propagating throughout the heart.[9,10,26] Overall, these experimental results provided much needed support for the long-held belief of theoreticians that spiral waves occur in the heart.

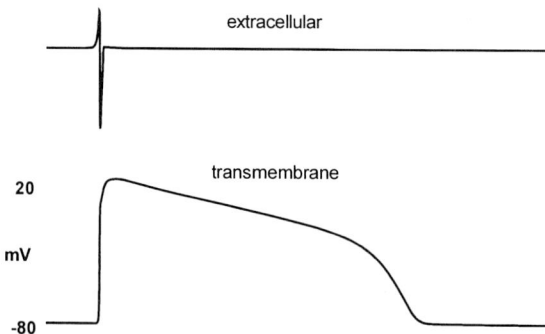

Figure 1. Extracellular versus optical mapping. An extracellular (*top*) and transmembrane (*bottom*) recording from a simulation of an action potential propagating in a cable. Typically, extracellular mapping allows the determination of activation times only, while optical recordings allow the mapping of both the depolarization and repolarization processes.

Optical Mapping

Video imaging, like other forms of optical mapping, records electrical activity from the heart using voltage-sensitive dyes that bind to cardiac cell membrane and that have optical properties that are altered due to changes in potential across the membrane, i.e., transmembrane potential (Fig. 1, bottom). The optical signal recorded by these dyes is linearly related to the true transmembrane potential.[27] A unique advantage of using voltage-sensitive dyes is that transmembrane activity is recorded, allowing the analysis of both depolarization (wave front) and repolarization (wave tail). The spatial distribution of action potential duration (APD) can be assessed only by optical mapping techniques.[28–30] Repolarization times and, hence, APDs can be determined by finding where the second temporal derivative is a maxima[31] or by using threshold methods.[28,32] In addition, the dynamics of the repolarization events can be studied.[27,31,33]

Cardiac Phase

The transmembrane signal alone does not accurately represent the "state" of each site. This is not surprising since the transmembrane signal does not uniquely describe the phase of the cardiac cycle; during one beat, the transmembrane signal is equal to a certain value (e.g., -20 mV) twice: once during depolarization and once during repolarization (see Fig. 1, bottom). At least one additional variable, such as dV/dt, is required to identify the state of the site.[34] Consider the multidimensional monodomain cable equation:

$$C \frac{\partial V}{\partial t} + \sum_i g_{i,\max} n_i^{k_i}(V - V_i) = C \, \nabla \cdot D \nabla V$$

(1)

$$\frac{\partial n_i}{\partial t} = f_i(n_i, V) \qquad i = 2 \text{ to } N$$

with N state variables: transmembrane potential (V) and N-1 gating variables (n_i's). In a computer model we have access to all state variables; however, in experiments we usually record only one state variable. For example, using optical mapping we record a measure of V(t) at many sites. Fortunately we can create a *reconstructed* state space that is *topologically* equivalent to the *true* state space[35]:

$$V, \frac{dV}{dt}, \frac{d^2V}{dt^2}, \dots \frac{d^{N-1}V}{dt^{N-1}} \text{ OR } V(t), V(t - \tau), V(t - 2\tau), \dots V(t - [N - 1]\tau) \quad (2)$$

By translating to a polar coordinate system using two reconstructed state variables (e.g., V and dV/dt), it is possible to create a phase variable (θ) that uniquely describes the phase of the cardiac cycle during the action potential (see below). Therefore, the spatiotemporal patterns of a single variable $\theta(x,y,t)$ can be used to study the phase dynamics in the heart. Surprisingly, at least to us, analyzing this phase variable (essentially throwing away the amplitude information) provided much new information regarding the events occurring during VF.[36]

Methods

Experimental Preparations

Experiments were carried out in a variety of animal preparations. The details have been described previously.[14,23,37] The preparations included in this chapter are: 1) isolated, perfused right atrium of the sheep[37]; 2) isolated whole sheep hearts[14]; and 3) isolated whole rabbit hearts.[23] The preparations were perfused with an oxygenated (95% O_2, 5% CO_2) Tyrode's solution buffered to a pH of 7.4. The solution consisted of the following (mmol/L): NaCl, 148; KCl, 5.4; $CaCl_2$, 1.8; $MgCl_2$, 1.0; $NaHCO_3$, 24.0; NaH_2PO_4, 0.4; glucose, 5.5. The temperature of the perfusate and the solution in the chamber were maintained at $36\pm1°C$. A bolus injection of 15 mL of the dye di-4-ANEPPS (10 µg/mL) dissolved in dimethyl sulfoxide was injected into the coronary arteries, and diacetyl monoxime was added to the Tyrode's solution (10 mmol/L) to stop the heart's contraction, thus eliminating mechanical artifacts.

High-Resolution Video Imaging

We used one or two complete video imaging systems to record from the various preparations. We used two systems to record simultaneously from the anterior and posterior surfaces of the rabbit heart or to record simultaneously from the epicardial and endocardial surfaces of the arterially perfused right atrium. Figure 2 shows a schematic diagram of the experimental set-up for the isolated, perfused right atrium. An image of the preparation is shown at the bottom, demonstrating the high spatial resolution of the video imaging system. Each system included a light source and associated optics, as well as a video camera system and computer. Briefly, for each recording system, the light from a 250-W tungsten-halogen lamp is passed through a collimator, an excitation filter (530 ± 30 nm), and a heat filter. The light is then reflected 90° from a dichroic mirror (560 nm) onto the epicardial or endocardial surface of the vertically hanging preparation. The emitted light is transmitted through an emission filter (590 nm) and projected onto the charged coupled device (CCD) camera (Cohu Inc., San Diego, CA). Each camera is connected to an analog-to-digital frame grabber (Epix, Inc., Buffalo Grove, IL) in a noninterlace mode acquiring data at speeds of 120 and 240 frames per second (fps), which results in sampling intervals (Δt) of 8.333 and 4.1667 ms, respectively. In noninterlaced mode the Cohu cameras could record from 739×240 (horizontal × vertical) CCD elements. The CCD elements (pixels) in the Cohu camera have an effective aspect ratio of 2.32 in noninterlaced mode. The Cohu camera is a line scan camera, so to achieve speeds of 120 and 240 fps we sent a vertical reset signal to trigger the frame readout, thus reducing the maximum vertical resolution to 120 and 60 pixels, respectively. An external trigger synchronized the beginning of acquisition of the two cameras. Details regarding the technical aspects of video imaging technology have been presented previously.[29]

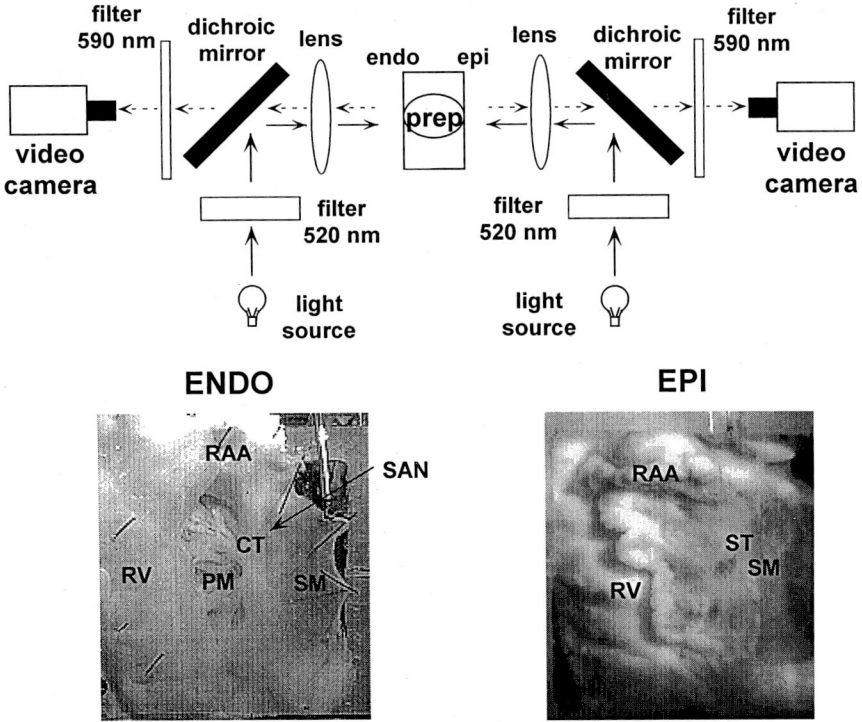

Figure 2. *Top:* Experimental set-up. Each video imaging set-up is composed of a light source, dichroic mirror, video camera, frame grabber, computer, and excitation and emission filters. See text for more details regarding the system. In some episodes video recordings were obtained from both endocardial and epicardial surfaces simultaneously. *Bottom:* Endocardial (168×95 pixels) and epicardial (166×95 pixels) images recorded by video camera. CT = crista terminalis; PM = pectinate muscle region; RAA = right atrial appendage; RV = right ventricle; SAN = sinoatrial node; SM = smooth muscle region; ST = sulcus terminalis.

Signal Processing

The signal recorded at each pixel (F_{raw}) is linearly related to the *change* in transmembrane potential (δV):

$$F_{raw}(x,y,t) = a(x,y) + b\,(x,y) \int_{t}^{t+\Delta t} \int_{y}^{y+\Delta y} \int_{x}^{x+\Delta x} \delta V\,(x', y', t')\,dx'\,dy'\,dt' \quad (3)$$

where x and y represent the horizontal and vertical location on the heart, t is time (t = nΔt; where n is frame number), a and b are parameters related to the excitation and emission properties at x,y, and Δx and Δy are the spatial dimensions of the area mapped by each pixel. The temporal integration, resulting from the iris of the video camera being open during the entire sampling interval, causes "blurring" of propagating waves perpendicular to the direction of movement.[29] The spatial extent of this smearing is equal to the conduction speed times the sampling interval (Δt).

The first digital processing step is to subtract the background fluorescence, a(x,y), from each frame.

$$F_{sub}(x,y,t) = F_{raw}(x,y,t) - a(x,y) \qquad (4)$$

Next, the signal from each site is stretched to 8 bits (256 levels) to reduce quantization effects[29] and to correct for spatial nonuniformities in fluorescence intensity, b(x,y), giving $F_{norm}(x,y,t)$. In some episodes where the activation patterns are repetitive, we average multiple beats (ensemble averaging).[14] Ensemble averaging significantly improves the signal quality because the noise decreases by a factor of $\sqrt{p}$ where p is the number of beats averaged together. If the period of activity is not a multiple of Δt, a sequence of k beats can be averaged such that k*(period of activity) is a multiple of Δt. Finally, spatial and temporal filters are applied, usually by convolving a filter kernel with the data set F_{norm}, to give the final data set F(x,y,t). The filters and the spatial and temporal integration inherent to the CCD can be completely characterized in the frequency domain, which allows one to assess the effect of the filters on the underlying signals. The frequency domain representation of boxcar and conical filters of various sizes are shown in Figure 3. Typically a 15×7 conical kernel was used for the spatial filter resulting in low pass spatial filtering with the 3-dB point of ~3 mm for the magnifications used here. A 3-point moving average (boxcar) temporal filter was applied to F to minimize the effects of noise on the repolarization tail.[28] It has been shown that blur, filtering, and quantization (number of levels in upstroke) do not affect the ability to localize wave fronts.[29] The effect of these quantities on repolarization parameters is less clear and certainly depends on the underlying signal.

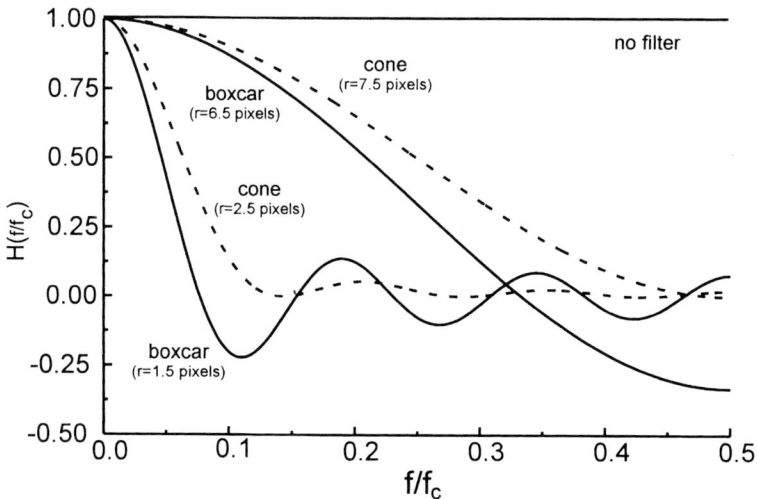

Figure 3. Filter characteristics. Frequency domain filter characterization for boxcar and conical kernels of various sizes. Normalized frequency is plotted on the abscissa (e.g., normalized frequency is pixels^{-1} for spatial filters and is frames^{-1} for temporal filters). The boxcar filters induce "ringing" in the frequency domain due to their high-frequency content.

Isochrone Maps

A point in the time plot was labeled as part of a wave front if F became greater than 128 in that frame (this cut-off corresponds to 50% of the action potential amplitude). The position of the wave front in subsequent frames is color coded and shown in a single image called a depolarization map.[31] Because of the motion-induced blurring, the depolarization maps are composed of isochrone bands rather than lines.[29] Here we use the term "depolarization map" instead of "isochrone map" because the repolarization process can also be mapped, which leads to ambiguity in the term "isochrone map."[31] Note that these bands derived from video images required no interpolation of data. A point in the time plot was labeled as part of a wave tail in frame *n* if F was greater than 128 in frame *n-1* and less than 128 in frame *n*. Hence, two successive frames are required to identify wave fronts and tails as well as their direction of propagation (see below).

Phase Mapping

Recently, a new signal processing technique called phase mapping provided new insights into the mechanisms and organization of VF.[35] An action potential recorded at 240 fps from the surface of the right atrium of an isolated, perfused sheep heart is shown in the left panel of Figure 4. The same data plotted in a 2-dimensional projection of a reconstructed state space (F,dF/dt) is shown in the right panel. In reconstructed state space, it is easy to differentiate the depolarization process (dF/dt > 0) and the repolarization events (dF/dt < 0) during the action potential. Alternatively, to avoid the difficulties with noise when taking derivatives, the reconstructed phase space can be determined using time delay embedding.[34] Here we compute the phase variable, θ, as:

$$\theta(x,y,t) = atan[F(x,y,t - \tau) - F_{mean}(x,y), F(x,y,t) - F_{mean}(x,y)]. \quad (5)$$

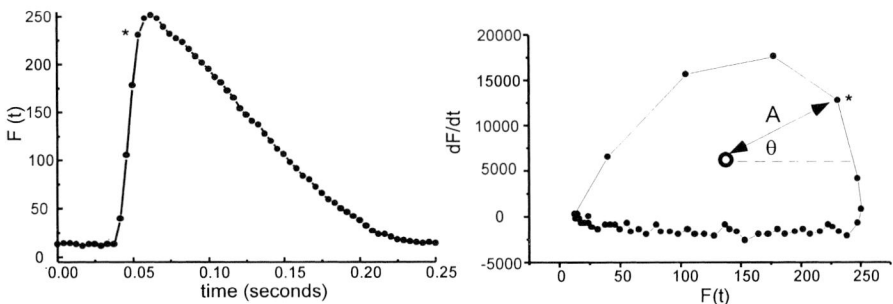

Figure 4. Cardiac phase. *Left:* An action potential recorded from the right atrial epicardial surface of an isolated sheep heart. *Right:* The same data plotted in *reconstructed phase space* by parameterizing time. The fluorescent time signal, F(t), shown on the left can be represented by its amplitude, A(t), and phase, θ(t). However, only the phase variable (θ) provides a unique description of the *state* of the site. Data were acquired at 240 frames per second and ensemble averaging of 27 beats was performed. Asterisk identifies same data point on both plots.

Although, our definition of phase differs slightly from earlier definitions[38,39] (they are equal in some cases) it allows us to compare experimental results with the theoretical basis of the dynamics of phase in individual cells[38] and spatially extended systems.[37] For example, the center of a rotating wave is a spatial phase singularity. A spatial phase singularity is a site in an oscillatory or excitable medium where its phase is arbitrary and its neighboring elements exhibit a continuous progression of phase equal to $\pm 2\pi$ around this site. The existence of a spatial phase singularity is a necessary, although not sufficient, condition for sustained rotation.[36]

Statistics

Data are presented as mean value $\pm$ standard deviation of the mean. Comparisons were performed using individual Student's t-tests.

Results

Simultaneous Mapping of Depolarization and Repolarization

In an effort to characterize the transmembrane activity in the heart more completely, we studied the dynamics of the depolarization and repolarization processes. Here, in Figures 5 and 6, we present wave fronts in white, wave tails in black, depolarized tissue in dark gray, and resting tissue in light gray. Results obtained during pacing from the posterior surface of the left ventricle of an isolated rabbit heart are shown in Figure 5. This heart was paced at a basic cycle length (BCL) of 200 ms (the pacing electrode is shown in black). Pacing resulted in a wave front of excitation (white) that propagated away from the stimulus site in an elliptical pattern with the long axis orientated along the fiber axis. The width of the wave front is wider along fibers compared with across fibers. The wave propagated away from the pacing site in all directions and the resulting wave fronts eventually collided on the anterior side of the heart. Only the wave front is seen in the top panel because the refractory period in the ventricle is sufficiently long that during pacing and sinus rhythm the repolarization process (wave tails: black) appears 100 to 300 ms after the wave front (depending on BCL).[40] In the lower panels (50 ms after the stimulus), the wave fronts are colliding on the anterior surface of the ventricles (right panel), and a wave tail has appeared on the left ventricle (left panel), and then has proceeded in an elliptical manner similar to the movement of the wave fronts. The distance between the wave front and wave tail is the wavelength and is a function of rate; here the wavelength is a few centimeters (the exact distance is difficult to measure due to the curved surface of the heart).

A unique property of spiral wave reentry is that the wave front touches the wave tail at a point[25] called a wavebreak or wave tip. By calculating the position of the wave front and tail during episodes of functional reentry, it is possible to identify and track the position of wavebreaks. A depolarization map of one period of activity during an episode of sustained stable reentry in the rabbit heart is shown in Figure 6, left. The convergence of isochrones near the center of rotation suggests that conduction speed is inversely related to wave front curvature consistent with

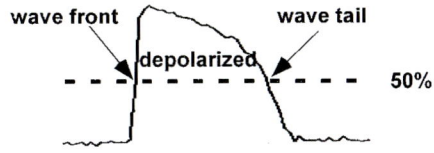

Figure 5. Mapping of depolarization and repolarization. Using a 50% threshold we calculated the position of the wave front and wave tail (*top*) to study the depolarization and repolarization processes, respectively. Here we used two cameras to record from the posterior (*left*) and anterior (*right*) surfaces of an isolated rabbit heart. Pacing the posterior epicardial surface of the left ventricle of a rabbit heart elicits a propagating wave front (white) that invades resting tissue (light gray). Later, the wave front has reached the anterior surface and collides in a "V shape" resulting from the curvature at the apex of the heart. At this time, most of the heart is depolarized (dark gray) and the wave tail (black) emerges on the epicardium and follows a pattern similar to the depolarization wave. Images from the posterior surface were 176×92 pixels (Δx = 0.160 mm) and images from the anterior surface were 208×106 pixels (Δx = 0.148 mm) acquired at 120 frames per second. Ensemble averaging of four beats was per-

t = S1 + 25 ms

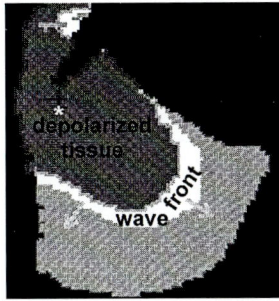
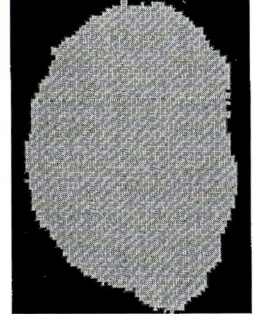

t = S1 + 50 ms

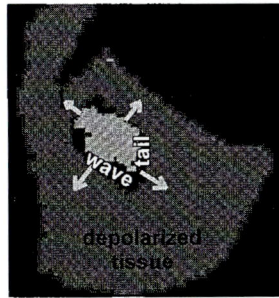
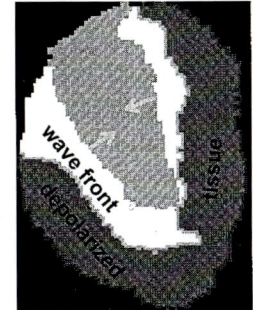

posterior   **anterior**

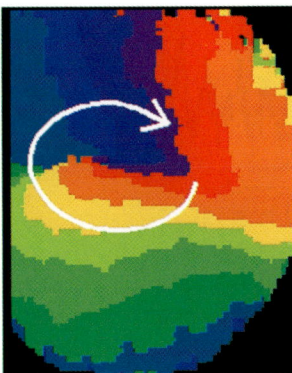
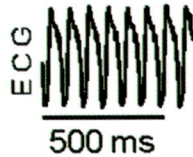
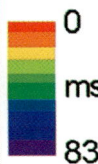
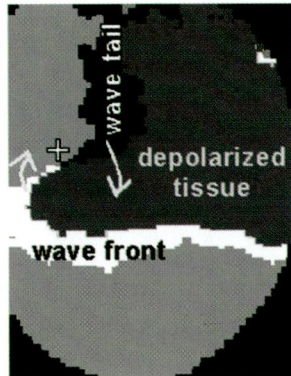

Figure 6. Monomorphic ventricular tachycardia (MVT). Addition of verapamil (1 mg/L) converted VF into MVT with a period of 79 ms. The images (168×100 pixels) were acquired at 120 frames per second. Due to the repeating patterns, ensemble averaging (P = 25) was accomplished by averaging every two beats (19 frames = 158 ms). Image size was 168×100 pixels with Δx = 0.120 mm. No diacetyl monoxime was used in this experiment; the heart was constrained between two Plexiglas rods.

spiral wave reentry.[41] This repeating pattern resulted in a monomorphic pattern in the ECG (middle panel). A snapshot of the wave front (white) and wave tail (black) during one frame shows that both the front and tail rotate clockwise around a wavebreak where wave front and tail meet. Wavebreaks can be classified depending on their chirality (+ for clockwise; −for counter-clockwise). According to this formulation, the "excitable gap" is the region ahead of the rotating wave front and behind the wave tail. The 50% cut-off value is arbitrary, however, and the extent of the excitable gap, the position, and perhaps the number of wavebreaks most certainly depend on this cut-off value. In addition, the action potential shape varies, and using a single measure for repolarization time is problematic. Therefore, a more robust method is required to determine the sites of wavebreaks.

Atrial Fibrillation

A more rigorous definition of the site of a wavebreak can be constructed in terms of this phase variable, which is useful to study fibrillation.[36] The fluorescence signals recorded from the surface of the right atrium of the isolated sheep heart during AF exhibit variation in action potential amplitude and duration[14] (Fig. 7) similar to those recorded during VF.[36] Although it is not possible to measure dV/dt from CCD recordings due to its spatial and temporal integration (see eq. 1), we found that dF/dt decreased by 45% during AF compared to pacing in the same preparation. It is not surprising that the phase variable gives a unique description of the phase of the cardiac cycle during sinus rhythm and pacing (see Fig. 4). The fact that the spatiotemporal dynamics of the phase variable obtained from a 2-dimensional projection of reconstructed phase space during fibrillation are consistent with the concepts of phase in spatially extended systems[36] appears remarkable. It seems that for some reason, still unexplained, the high dimensional state space of cardiac cells effectively reduces to two dimensions during fibrillation.

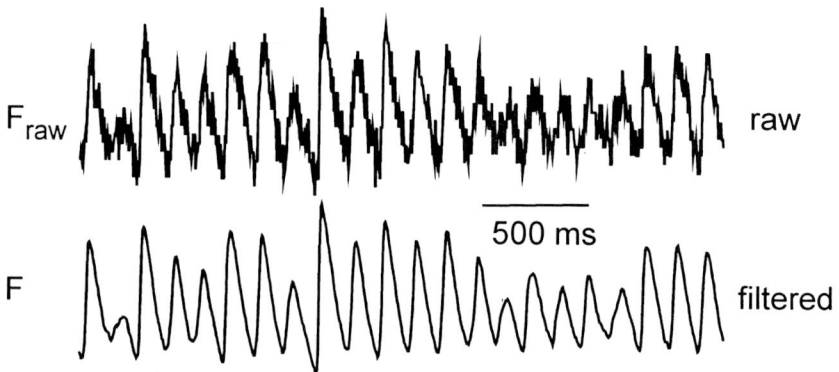

Figure 7. Transmembrane signals during atrial fibrillation. The fluorescent recordings obtained from the right atrial epicardial surface of isolated sheep hearts exhibited continual changes in action potential shape and duration. Raw (*top*) and spatially and temporally filtered (*bottom*) signals were recorded at 240 frames per second with an interpixel spacing (Δx) of 0.160 mm.

Two parameters must be chosen to calculate the phase variable. First, we must choose the length of time to calculate the mean value, $F_{mean}(x,y)$, which is used as the center point in phase space. This value should be chosen such that no major changes occur in the electrophysiology of the heart during this interval. Here we used 2 seconds, and since we were perfusing the heart during fibrillation, even longer values could be used. Second, we must choose the delay time (τ) to reconstruct the phase space at each site. Theoretically, any nonzero value of τ results in a reconstructed phase space that is topologically equivalent to the true phase space.[35] For real data, however, there are sophisticated methods for finding τ that optimize the calculation of embedding dimension and phase space reconstruction. Our aims are different, however, and involve calculating a new variable, θ, that represents the phase in the cardiac cycle; therefore it is not clear what value to choose for τ. Previously, for VF, τ was chosen to be approximately one fourth of the cycle length during fibrillation[36] (roughly corresponding to the first zero crossing of the autocorrelation of F, indicating linear independence). Here we study how the choice of τ influences the trajectories in reconstructed phase space during AF (Fig. 8). Of course, for $\tau = 0$ we get the identity line, and as τ is increased, the trajectories become more circular (see $\tau = 8$ ms and $\tau = 20$ ms). As τ becomes greater than the time of the upstroke (see Fig. 4), the trajectories "cross" in phase space (see $\tau = 40$ ms and $\tau = 60$ ms). To quantify this effect, we calculated the percentage of reconstructed phase space trajectories that rotated counterclockwise for delays (τ) ranging from 4 ms to 63 ms. This percentage showed a parabolic relationship with frame number, exhibiting a maxima at frame 6 as shown in Figure 8.

Snapshots of phase from the surface of the right atrium from an isolated sheep heart during AF are shown in Figure 9. The color presentation of the phase variable is chosen to represent the continuous yet periodic nature of phase (i.e., $\pi = -\pi$). For display purposes only, each color shade represents a range of 24 degrees. The pseudo ECG (PECG) shows irregular, rapid deflections characteristic of AF. Phase singularities were observed on the surface of the right atrium during sustained AF; however, unlike during VF,[36] sustained rotation (>1 cycle) around these phase singularities (i.e., rotors) did not occur in hearts perfused with Tyrode solution without acetylcholine. Panels A through D show snapshots of phase on the right atrial epicardium at various times (see PECG) throughout this episode of AF. Sometimes pairs of opposite chirality phase singularities were observed (panel D), other times only a single singularity was observed (panels A and B), and, finally, there were moments when no phase singularities were apparent (panel C). During AF, quiescent periods have been noted[14,42] in which no wave fronts are observed, meaning that no phase singularities are present within the recording array at that moment (see panel C, where orange wave fronts are absent). The converse is not true, since broad wave fronts can occur without a phase singularity.

Do the Atria Act as a 2-Dimensional Sheet?

The complex structure of the atria influences the patterns of propagation[37,43] and may play an important role during AF.[14,17,44,45] To study the 3-dimensional nature of conduction in the atria, we used two cameras to

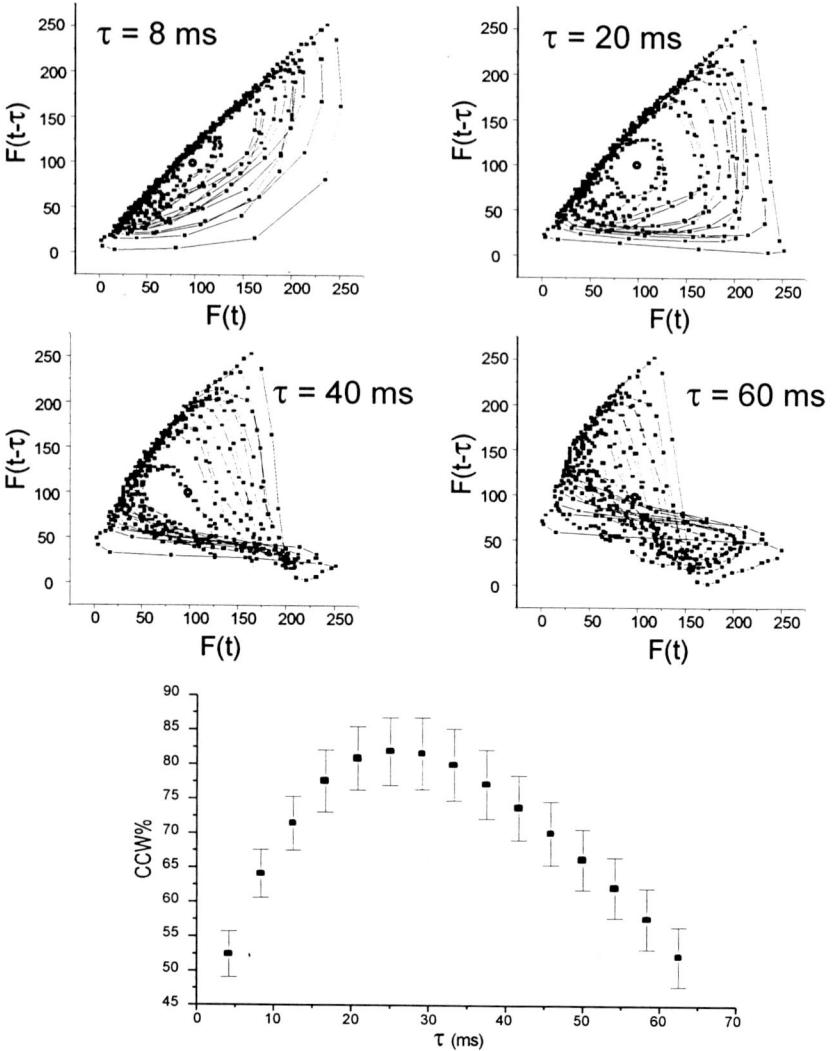

Figure 8. Phase space plots during atrial fibrillation. *Top:* Reconstructed state space via the time-delay embedding method for various values of τ. *Bottom:* The percentage of trajectories in phase space rotating counterclockwise for various values of τ.

record simultaneously from the endocardial and epicardial surfaces of the isolated, perfused right atrial preparation (see Fig. 2).[37] The preparations were always placed as shown, i.e., such that the crista terminalis was approximately aligned with the vertical axis, the pectinate muscles were to the left of the crista terminalis, and the sinoatrial node and smooth muscle region of the atrium were to the right of the crista terminalis as viewed from the endocardium. All epicardial images are presented as mirror images to allow direct comparison of epicardial and endocardial views. As shown in Figure 2, structures that are clearly distinguished in these epi-

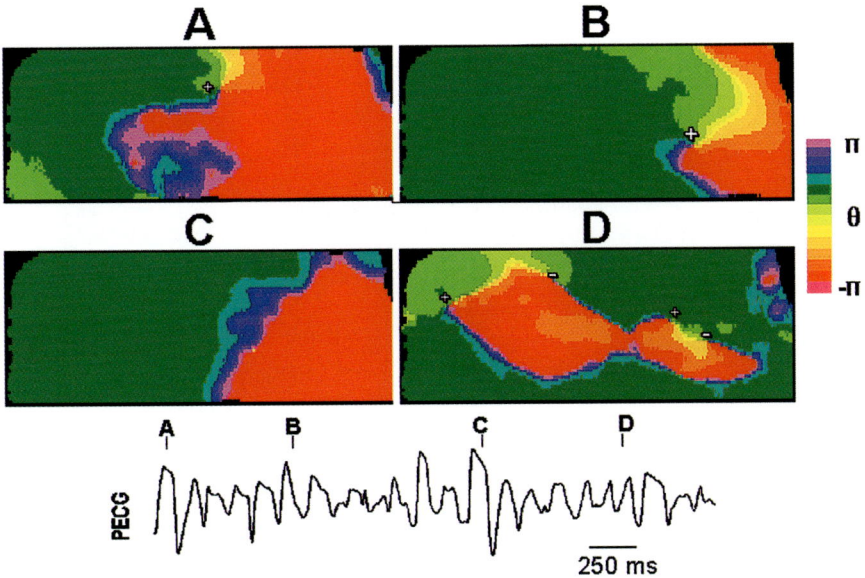

Figure 9. Phase singularities during atrial fibrillation (AF). **A** through **D.** Phase maps during sustained atrial fibrillation calculated for $\tau = 8$ ms. Clockwise phase singularities are denoted by $+$ and counterclockwise phase singularities are denoted by $-$. *Bottom:* Pseudo electrocardiogram of episode illustrating irregular, nonrepeating patterns characteristic of AF. The time of the phase "snapshots" are indicated. Images (240×50 pixels) were acquired at 240 fps with $>\Delta x = 0.160$ mm.

cardial images are the sulcus terminalis and the right atrial appendage, with the right ventricle in the background. For clarity, we present isochrones in multiples of 4 ms, even though the sampling interval was 120 or 240 fps. For example, an isochrone labeled as 80 ms is really the location of the wave front at time = 83.333 ms. For clarity, not all isochrones are displayed.

We found that activation patterns were highly dependent on the site of stimulation, and we observed preferential pathways for transmural wave propagation.[37] Activation patterns were highly dependent on the direction of muscle bundles and the excitation rate; waves blocked across the crista terminalis and pectinate muscles at fast rates. Pacing from the pectinate muscles was carried out in nine experiments at a variety of cycle lengths ranging from 500 to 160 ms. As shown by the isochrone maps in Figure 10, the excitation waves propagated away from the stimulation site in a roughly elliptical pattern, with the major hemiaxis oriented along the major pectinate muscle bundles. On the endocardium, the wave front was irregular and related to the underlying structure of the individual pectinate muscles. At the relatively low stimulation frequency used here (BCL = 500 ms), the pattern of wave propagation on the epicardium (Fig. 10) was similar to that observed on the endocardium. When we paced at faster rates, the activation patterns became more complex, with conduction block occurring at cycle lengths between 160 and 250 ms; no block

ENDO   EPI

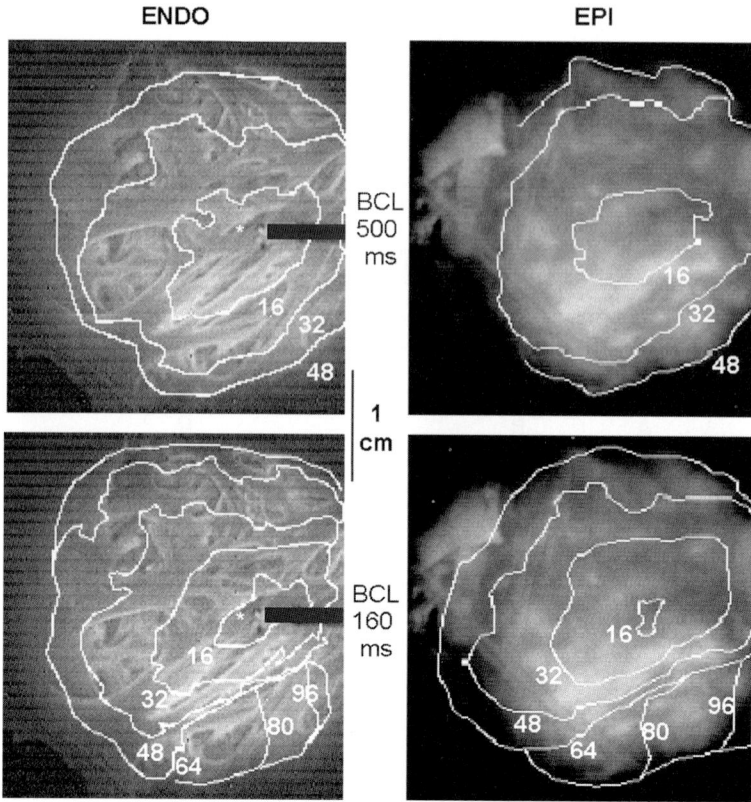

Figure 10. Activation of pectinate muscles. *Top:* Isochrone maps of endocardial (*left*) and epicardial (*right*) during pacing at a cycle length of 500 ms. Pacing at 500 ms resulted in fairly elliptical wave propagation on both surfaces. *Bottom:* Isochrone maps of endocardial (*left*) and epicardial (*right*) during pacing at a cycle length of 160 ms. Pacing at 160 ms caused the propagating wave to block across muscle bundles. Endocardial images were 256×110 pixels ($\Delta x = 0.133$ mm) and epicardial images were 258x118 pixels ($\Delta x = 0.132$ mm) acquired at 120 frames per second.

was observed at cycle lengths above 250 ms. An example of conduction block at a pectinate muscle during stimulation at a cycle length of 160 ms is shown in Figure 10 (bottom). The excitation wave propagated away from the stimulation site along a muscle bundle, but propagation in all directions was slower than at BCL = 500 ms. At BCL = 160 ms, the wave blocked below the stimulation site when attempting to cross a pectinate muscle, and propagated around a thin line of block corresponding to the border of that muscle. The time it took the wave to excite the pectinate muscle at BCL = 160 ms was twice as long as at BCL = 500 ms because of the slower propagation velocity and the block of the wave front at the faster rate. The patterns on the epicardium are similar to those in the pectinate muscle.

Under control conditions (no acetylcholine), sustained reentry could be induced in only 30% of the preparations (3 of 10). The reentrant waves propagated along thin lines of block at the junction of the crista terminalis and the smooth muscle. Reentry, as observed on the endocardium, was either clockwise or counterclockwise, and the average cycle length was 267 ± 51 ms. After the addition of acetylcholine (10^{-4} to 10^{-5} mol/L), stable reentrant waves could be initiated in 88% of the preparations (7 of 8). These waves rotated around lines of block along the crista terminalis and pectinate muscles with a cycle length of 150 ± 66 ms ($P < 0.05$ compared with control). Both the cycle length and the length of the line of block during reentry decreased after the addition of acetylcholine. In fact, a linear relationship between cycle length and line of block was observed.[37]

In two preparations, sustained reentry was localized in the pectinate muscle region after the addition of acetylcholine. The isochrone maps of endocardial and epicardial recordings from one example are shown in Figure 11, in which the reentrant wave rotated clockwise with a period of 81 ms. In this episode we adjusted the optics to zoom in on an area of the pectinate muscle, and recorded at 240 fps. The isochrones converged at the organizing center of the reentrant wave; however, we could not identify activation times at the center. The isochrones on the epicardium are similar to those observed on the endocardium except for a phase shift (see phase maps). The wave on the epicardium seems to be leading the endocardium by approximately 90°. One possible interpretation for this interesting observation is that, as a result of the 3-dimensional nature of the preparation, the activity in fact corresponds to a complex 3-dimensional reentrant wave[46] whose organizing center ("filament") is twisted.[47]

Discussion

Here we present evidence of the existence of phase singularities during AF (Fig. 9). However, these phase singularities did not survive for more than one complete rotation, and thus did not form rotors (sustained reentrant waves). Therefore, AF in the isolated sheep heart in the absence of acetylcholine was not sustained by the events in the right atrial free wall. The addition of acetylcholine shortens the wavelength and can result in rotor formation in isolated, arterially perfused right atrial preparations (Fig. 11) where the cut boundaries may influence the dynamics. Unlike the results presented here, during VF in isolated rabbit and sheep hearts, approximately 20% of phase singularities form rotors.[36] The atrial geometry is much more complex than the ventricular geometry, and hence the underlying mechanisms of AF and VF may differ.[17] In the ventricles, fibrillation appears to be maintained by rotors (i.e., functional reentry), while in the atria, fibrillation is probably maintained by both functional and anatomical reentry,[17,48–50] possibly localized in the left atrium.[49,50]

The optimal method to obtain the phase variable θ is still not clear. For the 2-dimensional representation of state space, dF/dt or F(t-τ) can be used to represent the second state variable. Here, for AF recorded at 240 fps, the choice of τ that maximized the number of trajectories that encircled the center (F_{mean}, F_{mean}) was 25 ms (Fig. 8). According to our hypothesis that a low dimensional attractor exists during fibrillation, and that we have chosen the center point appropriately, trajectories that circumvent

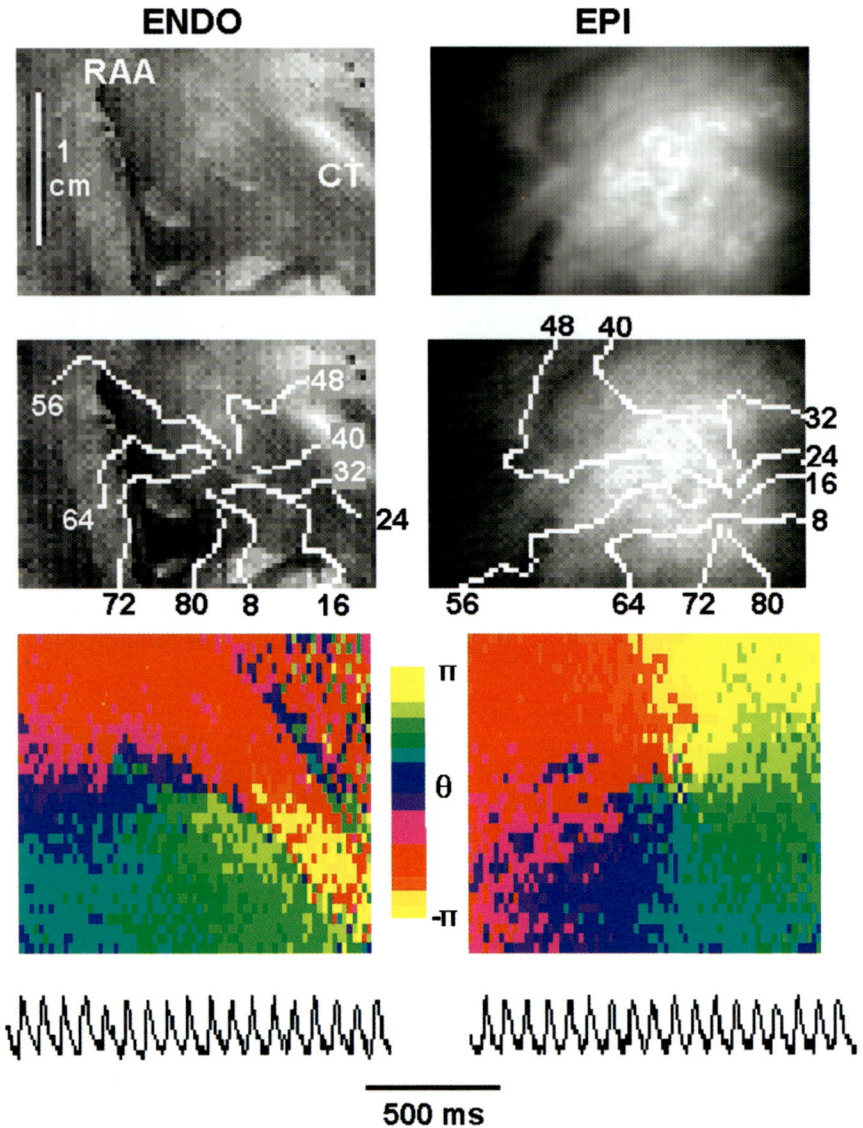

Figure 11. Reentry in the pectinate muscle region. *Top:* Images of endocardial (*left*) and epicardial (*right*) surfaces. *Middle:* Isochrone maps during one beat of a stable reentry with a period of 81 ms located in the pectinate muscle region. *Bottom:* Phase maps constructed with $\tau = 8$ ms from data with no spatial filtering and 3-point boxcar temporal filter. Endocardial images were 144×50 pixels ($\Delta x = 0.153$ mm) and epicardial images were 152×50 pixels ($\Delta x = 0.153$ mm) acquired at 240 frames per second. Individual site recordings are shown at the very bottom of the figure. Ensemble averaging of every two beats (39 frames) was accomplished ($P = 25$).

the center are suprathreshold activations and those that do not are sub-threshold,[36] as shown in Figure 12. For AF, approximately 70% to 80% of activations were suprathreshold (Fig. 8) compared to 90% in VF.[36] Furthermore, we speculate that an unstable fixed point exists in local state space that corresponds to the state at the site where a spatial phase singularity is located. Essentially, we believe that there exists an unstable fixed point in local state space resulting from the kinetics of the cardiac cell membrane during fibrillation. For example, the unstable fixed point might reside at $V_{threshold}$ where dV/dt diverges rapidly for nearby trajectories ($dV/dt > 0$ at $V = V_{threshold} + \epsilon$ and $dV/dt < 0$ at $V = V_{threshold} - \epsilon$, where ϵ is some small positive number) as shown schematically in Figure 12.

One limitation of using large values of τ is that this restricts the ability to localize the phase values in time. For example, using a value of $\tau = 25$ ms means that images four frames apart are used to calculate θ while dF/dt can be calculated using two consecutive frames. Alternatively, a smaller value of τ can be chosen and appears to work fine (Figs. 9 and 11). Although the value chosen for τ affected the number of spatial phase singularities, the spatiotemporal dynamics of the phase variable were always consistent with theoretical predictions.[38] The specific effects of the spatial and temporal integration of the CCD as well as the filters on the localization of spatial phase singularities are not known at this time. However, Figure 11 shows a spatial phase singularity from data acquired at 240 fps with no spatial filtering, a 3-point (12-ms) temporal filter, and $\tau = 8$ ms. Further theoretical development relating local kinetics to spatial phase singularities is required to determine the appropriate method to calculate θ.

The unique features of video imaging have allowed us to improve our understanding of the mechanisms of fibrillation[36] as well as the role of the structure of the heart.[14,37] With video imaging technology, correlation of the electrical activity in the heart with its structure is straight forward due its high spatial resolution and the fact that no electrodes are in contact with the sometimes highly convoluted surfaces of the heart (Figs. 10 and

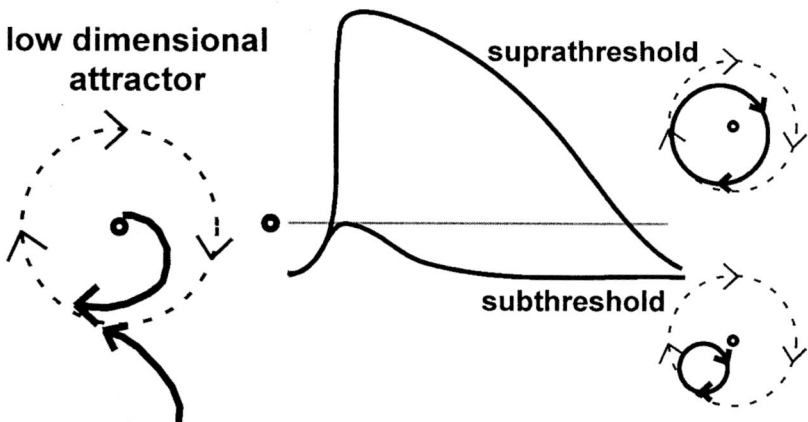

Figure 12. Low dimensional attractor during fibrillation. *Left:* Schema of phase space trajectories for a 2-dimensional limit cycle attractor. *Right:* Suprathreshold and sub-threshold activations represented in phase space.

11). In addition, the ability to record activity from a large number of sites allows a means to study electrical activity from a large portion of the heart surface with high spatial resolution (Figs. 2, 5, 6, 9, 10, and 11).[7,24,36] Finally, the ability to record transmembrane activity allowed us to construct a new phase variable, which has been essential for elucidating the mechanisms of fibrillation.[36]

References

1. Robles de Medina EO, Bernard R, Coumel P, et al. Definition of terms related to cardiac rhythm, WHO/ISFC Task Force. *Eur J Cardiol* 1978;8:127–144.
2. Myerburg RJ, Kessler KM, Interian A, et al. Clinical and experimental pathophysiology of sudden cardiac death. In Zipes DP, Jalife J (eds): *Cardiac Electrophysiology: From Cell to Bedside.* Philadelphia: W.B. Saunders Co.; 1990:666–678.
3. Wolf PA, Dawber TR, Thomas E Jr, Kannel WB. Epidemiologic assessment of chronic atrial fibrillation and risk of stroke: The Framingham study. *Neurology* 1978;28:973–977.
4. Scherf D. The atrial arrhythmias. *N Engl J Med* 1955;252:928.
5. Lewis T. *The Mechanism and Graphic Registration of the Heart Beat..* 3rd ed. London: Shaw & Sons; 1925:319–374.
6. Schuessler RB, Grayson TM, Bromberg BI, et al. Cholinergically mediated tachyarrhythmias induced by a single extrastimulus in the isolated canine right atrium. *Circ Res* 1992;71:1254–1267.
7. Gray RA, Jalife J, Panfilov AV, et al. Mechanisms of cardiac fibrillation: Drifting rotors as a mechanism of cardiac fibrillation. *Science* 1995;270:1222–1223.
8. Moe GK, Abildskov JA. Atrial fibrillation as a self-sustaining arrhythmia independent of focal discharge. *Am Heart J* 1959;58:59–70.
9. Allessie MA, Lammers WJEP, Bonke FIM, Hollen J. Experimental evaluation of Moe's multiple wavelet hypothesis of atrial fibrillation. In Zipes DP, Jalife J (eds): *Cardiac Electrophysiology and Arrhythmias.* Orlando: Grune & Stratton; 1985:265–275.
10. Janse MJ. Vulnerability to ventricular fibrillation. *CHAOS* 1998;8(1):149–156.
11. Fenton F, Karma A. Vortex dynamics in three-dimensional continuous myocardium with fiber rotation: Filament instability and fibrillation. *CHAOS* 1998;8(1):20–47.
12. Winfree AT. Electrical turbulence in three-dimensional heart muscle. *Science* 1994;266:1003–1006.
13. Janse MJ, Kléber AG, Capucci A, et al. Electrophysiological basis for arrhythmias caused by acute ischemia: Role of the subendocardium. *J Moll Cell Cardiol* 1986;18:339.
14. Gray RA, Pertsov AM, Jalife J. Incomplete reentry and epicardial breakthrough patterns during atrial fibrillation in the sheep heart. *Circulation* 1996; 94:2649–2661.
15. Mines GR. On circulating excitation on heart muscles and their possible relation to tachycardia and fibrillation. *Trans R Soc Can* 1914;4:43–53.
16. Garrey WE. Auricular fibrillation. *Physiol Rev* 1924;4:215–239.
17. Gray RA, Jalife J. Ventricular fibrillation and atrial fibrillation are two different beasts. *CHAOS* 1998;8(1):65–78.
18. Ideker RE, Klein GJ, Harrison L, et al. The transition to ventricular fibrillation induced by reperfusion following acute ischemia in the dog: A period of organized epicardial activation. *Circulation* 1981;63:1371–1379.
19. Smith WM, Wharton JM, Blanchard SM, et al. Direct cardiac mapping. In Zipes

DP, Jalife J (eds): *Cardiac Electrophysiology: From Cell to Bedside*. Philadelphia: W.B. Saunders Co.; 1993:849–858.

20. Allessie MA, Bonke FIM, Schopman FJC. Circus movement in rabbit atrial muscle as a mechanism of tachycardia. *Circ Res* 1973;33:54–77.

21. Davidenko JM, Pertsov AM, Salomonsz R, et al. Stationary and drifting spiral waves of excitation in isolated cardiac muscle. *Nature* 1991;355:349–351.

22. Pertsov AM, Davidenko JM, Salomonsz R, et al. Spiral waves of excitation underlie reentrant activity in isolated cardiac muscle. *Circ Res* 1993;72:631–650.

23. Cabo C, Pertsov AM, Baxter WT, et al. Wavefront curvature as a cause of slow conduction and block in isolated cardiac muscle. *Circ Res* 1994;75:1014–1028.

24. Gray RA, Jalife J, Panfilov AV, et al. Non-stationary vortex-like reentry as a mechanism of polymorphic ventricular tachycardia in the isolated rabbit heart. *Circulation* 1995;91:2454–2469.

25. Davidenko J. Spiral wave activity: A possible common mechanism for polymorphic and monomorphic ventricular tachycardias. *J Cardiovasc Electrophysiol* 1993;4:730–746.

26. Gray RA, Jalife J. Self-organized drifting spiral waves as a mechanism for ventricular fibrillation. *Circulation* 1996;94:I48.

27. Salama G, Morad M. Merocyanine 540 as an optical probe of transmembrane electrical activity in the heart. *Science* 1976;191:485–487.

28. Rosenbaum DS, Kaplan DT, Kanai A, et al. Repolarization inhomogeneities in ventricular myocardium change dynamically with abrupt cycle length shortening. *Circulation* 1991;84:1333–1345.

29. Gray RA, Ayers G, Jalife J. Video imaging of atrial defibrillation in the sheep heart. *Circulation* 1997;95:1038–1047.

30. Baxter WT, Davidenko JM, Loew LM, et al. Technical features of a CCD video camera system to record cardiac fluorescence data. *Ann Biomed Eng* 1997;25:713–725.

31. Efimov IR, Huang DT, Rendt JM, Salama G. Optical mapping of repolarization and refractoriness from intact hearts. *Circulation* 1994;90:1469–1480.

32. Gray RA, Ayers G, Jalife J. Video imaging of atrial defibrillation in the sheep heart. *Circulation* 1997;95:1038–1047.

33. Kanai A, Salama G. Optical mapping reveals that repolarization spreads anisotropically and is guided by fiber orientation in guinea pig hearts. *Circ Res* 1995;77:784–802.

34. Dorian P, Penkoske PA, Witkowski FX. Order in disorder: Effect of barium on ventricular fibrillation. *Can J Cardiol* 1996;12(4):399–406.

35. Takens F. Detecting strange attractors in turbulence. In Rand DA, Young LS (eds): *Dynamical Systems and Turbulence*. Lecture Notes in Mathematics. Vol. 898. Berlin: Springer-Verlag; 1981:366–381.

36. Gray RA, Pertsov AM, Jalife J. Spatial and temporal organization during cardiac fibrillation. *Nature* 1998;392:675–678.

37. Gray RA, Takkellapati K, Jalife J. Dynamics and anatomical correlates of atrial flutter and fibrillation. In Zipes DP, Jalife J (eds): *Cardiac Electrophysiology: From Cell to Bedside*. Philadelphia: W.B. Saunders Co.; 2000:432–439.

38. Winfree AT. *When Time Breaks Down*. Princeton: Princeton University Press; 1987.

39. Glass L, Mackay MC. *From Clocks to Chaos*. Princeton: Princeton University Press; 1988.

40. Elharrar V, Surawicz B. Cycle length effect on restitution of action potential duration in dog cardiac fibers. *Am J Physiol* 1983;244:H782-H792.

41. Gray RA, Jalife J. Spiral waves and the heart. *Int J Bifurc Chaos* 1996;6:415–435.

42. Kirchhof C, Chorro F, Scheffer GJ, et al. Regional entrainment of atrial fibrillation studied by high resolution mapping in open-chest dogs. *Circulation* 1993;88:736–749.

43. Spach MS, Miller WT 3d, Dolber PC, et al. The functional role of structural complexities in the propagation of depolarization in the atrium of the dog. *Circ Res* 1982;50:175–191.

44. Janse MJ. Anisotropic conduction in the atrium: Its role in arrhythmogenesis. In Attuel P, Coumel P, Janse MJ (eds): *The Atrium in Health and Disease.* Mt. Kisco, NY: Futura Publishing Co.; 1989:15–26.

45. Schuessler RB, Boineau JP, Bromberg BI, et al. Normal and abnormal activation of the atrium. In Zipes DP, Jalife J (eds): *Cardiac Electrophysiology: From Cell to Bedside.* Philadelphia: W.B. Saunders Co.; 1995:543–562.

46. Pertsov AM, Jalife J. Three-dimensional vortex-like reentry. In Zipes DP, Jalife J (eds): *Cardiac Electrophysiology: From Cell to Bedside.* Philadelphia: W.B. Saunders Co.; 1995:403–410.

47. Pertsov AM, Aliev RR, Krinsky VI. Three-dimensional twisted vortices in an excitable chemical medium. *Nature* 1990;345:419–421.

48. Kumagai K, Khrestian C, Waldo AL. Simultaneous multisite mapping studies during induced atrial fibrillation in the sterile pericarditis model. *Circulation* 1997;95:511–521.

49. Skanes AC, Mandapati R, Berenfeld O, et al. Spatiotemporal periodicity during atrial fibrillation in the isolated sheep heart. *Circulation* 1998;98(12):1236–1248.

50. Mandapati R, Skanes A, Chen J, et al. Stable microreentrant sources as a mechanism of atrial fibrillation in the isolated sheep heart. *Circulation* 2000; 101:194–199.

Chapter 15

Video Mapping of Spiral Waves in the Heart

William T. Baxter and Jorge M. Davidenko

Introduction

In their attempts to understand the mechanisms of cardiac arrhythmias, scientists have been motivated to develop increasingly sophisticated technologies to monitor the electrical activity of the heart with high resolution in both space and time. Propagation abnormalities in the heart, such as reentrant activation, may occur at different spatial scales, ranging from microreentry to rotors encompassing the entire ventricle. In addition, reentrant loops may travel away from the site of origin. This makes it desirable to record from large areas with high spatial resolution. Furthermore, it has proven helpful to directly visualize the complex structure of the myocardium, which may offer obstacles to propagating waves. Electrode mapping systems have been developed to record activity from hundreds, or even thousands, of points simultaneously from the heart surface.[1-3] Optical methods using voltage-sensitive dyes were developed by Cohen and his colleagues[4,5] and have been used to study a variety of electrically active tissues. In cardiac tissue, simultaneous recordings from multiple sites have been made by arrays of photodiodes,[6,7] laser scanning,[8] and charged coupled device (CCD) cameras.[9-11] Video optical mapping with CCD cameras has proven an effective tool in the analysis of the complex spatial patterns of propagation in cardiac arrhythmias. This chapter is divided into two parts. The first part describes the technical aspects of CCD cameras and their use in cardiac optical mapping, and the second part reviews one of the main results obtained from video mapping studies, namely, that spiral waves in the heart can act as the source of both monomorphic and polymorphic ventricular arrhythmias.

CCD Cameras for Cardiac Optical Mapping

The first optical mapping of cardiac tissue with a CCD camera was carried out in a Langendorff-perfused rabbit heart by Nassif et al.[12] The group of José Jalife, in Syracuse, NY, took full advantage of the video camera to

From Rosenbaum DS, Jalife J (eds): *Optical Mapping of Cardiac Excitation and Arrhythmias.*
©Futura Publishing Co., Inc., Armonk, NY, 2001.

study cardiac propagation in many forms: spiral waves as a mechanism of reentry in thin tissue slices[9,13] as well as the role of rotors in polymorphic arrhythmias[14,15] and ventricular fibrillation (VF)[16–18] in whole hearts. Furthermore, optical movies of pacing-induced electrical waves under special conditions showed the details of wave front propagation that could result in conduction block and subsequent reentry.[19,20] Direct correlation of activation patterns with the image of the preparation demonstrated that atrial fibrillation is affected by underlying physical structures.[21–23] In other cardiac optical mapping laboratories, CCD cameras have been used to analyze the virtual electrode effect[10] and VF.[11]

CCD Technology

CCDs were initially developed at Bells Labs (Murray Hill, NJ) as a form of computer memory, but their image-forming capabilities soon became evident due to silicon's sensitivity to visible light. CCDs are solid-state image sensors that have become as ubiquitous as the consumer camcorder, essentially replacing the large photocathode tubes seen in older television cameras. They acquire movies consisting of a series of still images, or frames. The acquisition of each frame is a 2-step process: the first is a light-sensing phase in which charge is accumulated, the second a readout phase in which the charge at each point is read off the chip and converted to voltage. CCDs are monolithic silicon devices divided into arrays of picture elements (pixels) by a matrix of deposited electrodes.[24] The pixels may be conceived as buckets or potential wells where incident photons are converted to electrons and charge is accumulated. Each site is eventually depicted as a point in the resulting image, with the brightness proportional to the number of photons received over a given period. After the period of accumulation (called the integration time), the CCD elements act as a bucket brigade, with each pixel passing its charge to its neighbor along the row (Fig. 1). At the end of the row is a vertical shift register, which then

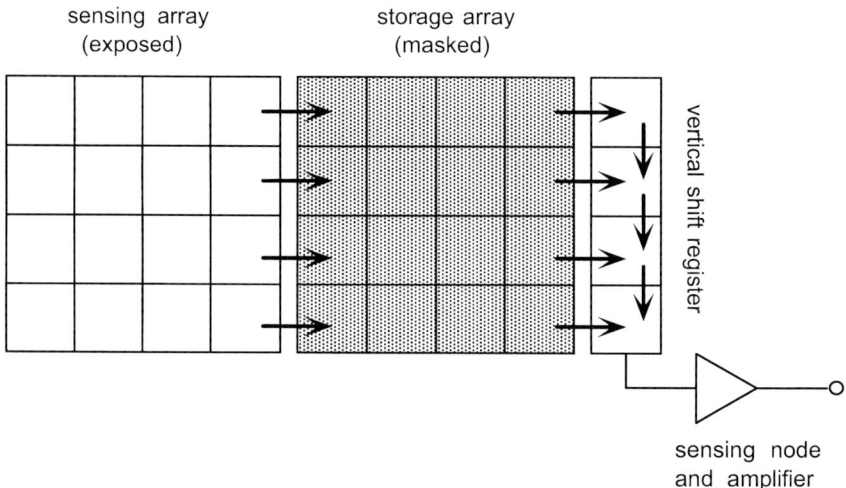

Figure 1. Schema of a frame-transfer charge coupled device.

shifts its column of charge packets to an amplifier that measures the charge from each pixel. Then another horizontal shift refills the vertical register, and so on until the entire array has been read out. At the end of the sequence, all pixels are reset to zero charge to begin the process anew—there is no carryover of charge from one frame to the next. Thus, while all pixels accumulate light simultaneously over the frame interval, each frame, or image, is converted to a serial analog signal of voltages. Compared to older photocathode tube technologies, CCDs have many advantages: they have high spatial resolution, good quantum efficiency, low noise, large dynamic range, and photometric accuracy. In addition, substrates may be manufactured with varying spectral sensitivities ranging from x-rays to the far infrared.[25] CCDs have been used extensively in astronomy and in the space program.[26,27] The charge-injection device (CID) is a variant of the CCD in which each cell has its own switch that senses charge rather than moving charge across the chip. While CIDs have some advantages, such as flexibility in readout, they suffer from several drawbacks, such as increased noise and lowered sensitivity.[28]

Technical Background

Here we define concisely some of the terms that are used in video imaging experiments and throughout this chapter. Additional definitions can be found in the Glossary at the end of the book. The amount of signal amplification, applied before digitization, is known as gain: high gain makes the image brighter but also increases noise. The black level, or offset, determines what brightness level will appear as black in the resulting image. It is useful to be able to manipulate the gain and offset; some cameras have nonadjustable factory-preset levels. Sensitivity indicates the lowest detectable light level. It may be expressed as the amount of voltage generated per unit of light intensity or, alternatively, as the least amount of light that will generate an image either at or just above the noise floor. Thus, camera makers express sensitivity in a variety of units, both photometric and electronic: lux, footcandles, $A/W/cm^2$, or $coulomb/J/cm^2$. Comparison of cameras is made even more difficult by the fact that manufacturers may report sensitivity without specifying whether the gain was off (equal to 1) or at maximum value. The term "saturation" is used for the overload point at which the pixel elements cannot convert any more photons. It is sometimes called well size (how deep the well or bucket is), and is measured in units of charge. On the other hand, the dynamic range expresses the span between the sensitivity and saturation levels, expressed as a ratio (e.g., the light intensity that produces saturation over the light intensity at the sensitivity level). Finally, the term "quantum efficiency" is used to indicate the likelihood that a photon reaching the sensor will be converted to an electron. Quantum efficiency of the entire optical system may be a more useful measure; this refers to the number of photons emitted by a light source that is eventually converted to electrons by the detector.

Sensitivity, saturation, and quantum efficiency are all sensitive to wavelength, and therefore should be expressed in terms of a given wavelength or spectrum. The voltage-dependent signal in optical mapping studies is typically quite small: approximately 5% of the background fluorescence for the dye di-4-ANEPPS.[29] Therefore, dynamic range is an important consideration for optical recording systems. Sensitivity is also required, especially at high frame rates, where brief exposure times will cause even intensely radiant objects to appear dark in the resulting images.

There are numerous sources of noise in optical detection systems, including dark signal, which is the output of a detector in the absence of illumination. The dark signal itself has several components: 1) dark current, or leakage current, is caused by electrons thermally generated within the CCD. It increases linearly with integration time, and increases by a factor of 2 for each 7°C. 2) Thermodynamic noise, or readout noise, is generated in the output amplifier. 3) Fixed-pattern noise refers to pixel-to-pixel variations that occur during chip fabrication. Both leakage current and thermodynamic noise may be reduced by cooling the sensor, an approach taken in many scientific grade CCDs. Fixed-pattern noise is eliminated when a background image is subtracted from all movie frames. Non-detector-related sources of noise include autofluorescence, nonspecific binding of the dye, mechanical vibration, 60 Hz pick-up noise, and shot noise. The last represents the ideal case and results from the statistical nature of photon emission from a light source.[5]

Varieties of CCD Cameras

The 2-step process of light integration and readout has implications for chip design. There are three basic CCD architectures: full-frame, frame-transfer, and interline.[30] Pixels still receive light even while the bucket brigade moves charge across the chip in the readout phase. Thus, an intense bright spot falling on one part of the array will appear as a smeared line in the resultant image. Full-frame cameras have a single light-sensitive area of pixels; therefore, a shutter must be closed to prevent light from reaching this area during the readout phase. Frame-transfer cameras have two equivalent areas of pixels, one covered by a mask (Fig. 1). An image is created in the exposed area during the integration phase and then rapidly shifted to the masked secondary storage area. Readout proceeds from the secondary area while the first area is accumulating the next image. The frame-to-frame transfer is very fast, typically a few microseconds. The time-limiting step is the readout phase; the on-chip amplifiers usually have speed limitations built into them to reduce internally generated noise.[31] Interline CCDs use the same approach as frame-transfer cameras, except that the masked array is interleaved with the accumulation array in the form of alternating columns. This makes them impervious to high-speed smearing, at the expense of reducing the horizontal spatial resolution by half.

The CCD chip itself must be incorporated into the electronics of the acquisition system, typically a camera. There are a wide variety of cameras but, for the purposes of cardiac optical mapping, we may distinguish several basic types: standard video, slow-scan, and high-speed cameras. Standard video cameras generate the standard Electronics Industries Association (EIA) broadcast video signal (RS-170 monochrome, and NTSC color in the United States and Japan; CCIR and PAL in Europe). Each frame in the television standard consists of two interlaced fields, one composed of odd lines, the other of even lines. Thus, at a standard readout time of 30 frames per second (fps), an effective frame rate of 60 fps may be obtained if each field is treated as one frame, at the expense of cutting the vertical resolution in half.[32]

The signal generated by a CCD chip may be acquired by a computer, in which case it must be digitized by a device called a frame grabber. Several megabytes of data may be written to the frame grabber's on-board video memory. Alternatively, newer frame grabbers act as simple digitizers that write directly to the computer's random access memory (RAM). In either case, the amount of memory determines the maximum length of the acquired movie, and the movie thus acquired must then be downloaded to the hard drive of the computer (or other peripheral device) before the next acquisition. Yet another alternative is to have the digitizing circuitry within the camera itself, which then outputs a digital signal (e.g., the RS-422 standard). Since this nonvideo signal does not need to adhere to television standards for image size and frame rate, the acquisition becomes significantly more flexible. Unfortunately, displaying a live image on a standard video monitor (useful for focusing, for example) may be a problem with such a system.

The term "scientific grade" usually applies to very sensitive slow-scan cameras used for recording low light level images, e.g., in biological microscopy[33] and astronomy.[27] Scientific grade CCDs typically have low noise, large dynamic range, high quantum efficiency, and high digital accuracy. They have frame readout rates on the order of seconds or even minutes, which limits their usefulness in the study of cardiac arrhythmias. Most of the scientific cameras are full-frame cameras, which means that they must be shuttered during the readout phase.

There are a number of high-speed image acquisition systems available at the time of this writing that are capable of acquiring data at hundreds, or even thousands, of frames per second. Because very fast exposure times are used, extremely high illumination is needed. These systems tend to use CCDs with approximately the same sensitivity as video-rate sensors. As a result, they have found a niche in applications that can supply all the light required, such as checking items on a moving assembly line.

CCDs Applied to Electrophysiology

In electrophysiological studies, video CCDs were not the initial photodetector of choice, primarily due to their low signal-to-noise (S/N) ratio and low temporal resolution (60 fps) compared with photodiodes (1 kHz). Temporal resolution may be effectively increased in a few ways: readout rates may be increased by decreasing the number of pixels used,[32,34] or repeatable sequences may be taken multiple times, slightly changing the start of the acquisition within the sequence each time.[10,35] As mentioned above, current high-speed cameras are not sensitive enough for optical mapping studies, while sensitive cameras are too slow. Nevertheless, the CCD camera's ability to deliver high-resolution images over a large recording area has furnished unique information about the propagation of the electrical impulse in cardiac tissue, and all three types of CCD camera have been used in cardiac optical mapping studies.

The Cohu 6500 Video Camera. Most of the video optical mapping at the Syracuse Health Science Center has been carried out with a Cohu 6500 video CCD camera (Cohu Inc., San Diego, CA; see reference 32 for details). This camera has a frame-transfer CCD array with 739×480 pixels (8.5×9.8 μ each) in a 6.4×4.8-mm exposed region. It has 56-dB S/N ratio, 0.4 lux sensitivity (no gain), 40% to 60% quantum efficiency in the range of the emission filter (640±50 nm), and external controls for gain and video offset. A TV zoom lens (f = 12.5 to 75 mm, f1.8, Navitar, Japan) focused the image onto the CCD array. Because the viewed area (approx. 20 mm) was larger than the sensor (6.4 mm), the lens system demagnified the image. This produced a depth of focus from 3 to 8 mm, depending on the magnification (see equation 1 in reference 7) A 250-W tungsten-halogen lamp was the light source. Camera output was digitized to 8 bits/pixel (256 gray levels) by the analog-to-digital (A/D) converter of a frame grabber board (model 12, Epix, Inc., Buffalo Grove, IL) with 16 Mb of memory. The 30-fps acquisition rate was increased to 60 fps noninterlaced (16.7-ms interframe interval), as described above, reducing the maximum number of lines from 480 to 240 lines of video. Even faster rates were obtained with use of external reset: in standard video, sensor integration is halted and frame readout is initiated by a vertical reset signal every 16.7 ms. The vertical reset may be sent at a faster rate, before the entire frame is read out, decreasing the number of video lines. The Epix frame grabber was programmed to provide the external vertical reset signal at 240, 120, and 60 Hz providing frame intervals of t = 4.2, 8.3, and 16.7 ms, with 60, 120, and 240 usable horizontal lines of video, respectively. This system has been remarkably flexible for studies in many different tissue preparations, including thin epicardial sheep muscle and whole Langendorff-perfused hearts from sheep, rabbits, and even mice.[35] Since most components are off the shelf and relatively inexpensive, the entire system could easily be duplicated; a dual-camera laboratory was set up for recording simultaneously from the epicardial and endocardial surfaces of isolated, perfused sheep right ventricle.[36]

Astromed Model 4100. John Wikswo and his colleagues[10] at Vanderbilt University employed a slow-scan cooled CCD camera (Model 4100, Astromed Ltd., Cambridge, UK) to examine the detailed geometry of potential changes around a stimulating electrode during the first few milliseconds of activation. The 12-bit resolution and high sensitivity of this camera enabled these investigators to acquire images at 0.5-ms exposure per frame, with light provided by a 2-W argon laser. Because of the limitations of this camera's frame rate, multiple pictures were taken of repeated stimulations at different temporal offsets, providing an effective temporal resolution of 2 ms. This approach requires highly repeatable activation sequences, but the resulting high-resolution images of a 6×6-mm area provide exquisite images of the virtual electrode effect.

The Dalsa 128 Camera. A high-speed system has been developed by Francis Witkowski et al.[11] based on a 128×128-pixel frame-transfer CCD with 12-bit resolution (model CA-D1–128S, Dalsa Inc., Waterloo, Ontario,

Canada). The pixels in this sensor are each 16×16 μ in a 2×2-mm array. The system is capable of running at 838 fps (1.2 ms per frame); its sensitivity was increased by using a 2-stage image-intensifier system and by cooling the camera to 15°C. The heart was illuminated by two 1-kW xenon arc lamps. Output was captured by a frame grabber (Dipix Technologies Inc., Ottawa, Ontario, Canada) with 256 Mb of memory, enabling nearly 10 seconds of continuous acquisition—a remarkable achievement considering the high frame rate.

Binning with the Dalsa Camera. The Dalsa line of area cameras also provides a binning option in which charge from four pixels (in a 2×2 square) may be summed into a single pixel. The number of elements is then decreased by a factor of 4, enabling faster readout, and the light-collecting ability is quadrupled. Lee et al.[37] used a Dalsa CA-DA-128S camera in this mode to study propagation abnormalities in transgenic mouse hearts. Images of 64×64 pixels were acquired at 1484 fps (0.67 ms per frame) by a digitizing frame grabber (Data Raptor-PCI, Bitflow, Inc., Woburn, MA), and written directly to the computer's RAM. With this approach acquisition time is limited by the amount of RAM, but similar systems may be configured to acquire directly to a small computer system interface (SCSI) device, permitting very long continuous acquisitions.

A Comparison of Photodetectors

At present, multisite optical imaging systems include photodiode arrays (PDAs), laser scanning systems, and CCD cameras. PDAs[6,7] have many excellent features: high S/N ratio (often >50), large dynamic range (12 or 16 bits), and fast acquisition rates (1 to 100 kHz). The number of elements in PDAs ranges from three to several hundred,[38] with the largest having more than 1000 elements.[39] Laser scanning systems[8,40] typically employ a single photodiode which monitors the entire field of view while acousto-optic deflectors rapidly shift the spot of illumination to different points on the tissue surface. Thus, they have many of the same operating characteristics of PDAs with the added advantage that the array of monitored points is not fixed, but can easily be programmed to any rectangular or even random configuration. CCD cameras have slower acquisition rates, although, as mentioned above, this has been pushed to the 1-kHz range. Most CCDs are less sensitive than photodiodes and have lower S/N ratios. The attraction of CCDs, however, lies in the great spatial resolution over a large area—ideal for analyzing complex wave patterns over several square centimeters. Activation of the tissue is visible on the monitor in real time, the field of view may be directed to the area of interest, and the magnification and frame rate may be quickly adjusted. The direct view of the tissue greatly simplifies problems of focusing and adjusting light levels. More importantly, the optical signal and the image of the preparation are acquired with the same detector at the same time so that there is a direct correlation between the signal and the image of the preparation.

The phenomenon of interest may dictate the best recording system. For instance, photodiode-based systems have high temporal resolution, high S/N ratio, but fewer recording elements, while CCDs have high spatial resolution, less temporal resolution, and variable S/N ratio. Girouard et al.[7] discuss the tradeoffs in S/N ratio incurred by varying temporal and spatial resolutions. CCD cameras are ideal for analyzing areas of slow conduction and block, which are precisely the areas of interest in many studies of arrhythmias,[2] and where extracellular electrograms are most difficult to interpret. For fine analysis of action potential characteristics such as the details of repolarization,[6] photodiode-based systems remain the best solution. For detailed analysis of wave front propagation, trends in technology indicate that CCD cameras will play an increasingly important role in the study of the complex activation patterns that accompany cardiac arrhythmias.

Video Mapping of Spiral Waves in the Heart:
A Common Mechanism for Monomorphic
and Polymorphic Ventricular Tachycardias

Reentrant activity in the heart has been classically envisioned as an electrical wave propagating over a 1-dimensional circuitous pathway and returning to its site of origin to reactivate that site. Such a model has clear application for many cardiac arrhythmias such as the reentrant activity observed in cases of Wolff-Parkinson-White syndrome. A "ring" formed by atrial tissue, AV nodal tissue, the His-Purkinje system, the muscle in the ventricle, and, finally, the accessory pathway may indeed be represented as a 1-dimensional system. Disconnecting the ring at any point will definitely interrupt the circulation of the impulse. However, reentrant arrhythmias may occur in the heart, where no distinct ring-like structure can be identified. In fact, reentry occurs in 2- and 3-dimensional structures with no evidence of anatomical circuits. Theoreticians have suggested that reentry in the absence of a circuit should not be approached with concepts derived from 1-dimensional models. Rather, 2- and 3-dimensional reentry should be analyzed using the concepts of wave propagation derived from models of generic excitable media.[41,42] Spiral waves are a property of 2-dimensional excitable media in which activation rotates around a center, thus providing a very general mechanism for reentrant activity.

Unfortunately, for cardiac electrophysiologists, the connection between spiral waves of activation occurring in excitable media (biological, chemical, or simulated by computer models) and cardiac reentrant activity, such as that observed during monomorphic ventricular tachycardia, was less than apparent. Aware of this lack of communication between scientists and cardiologists, our laboratory focused efforts on the development of models and techniques to improve our understanding of the mechanisms of reentrant arrhythmias in the heart. The high spatial resolution afforded by optical mapping with a CCD video camera provided the first convincing evidence of spiral wave activity in cardiac tissue.[9] Relatively long movies (several seconds) of self-sustaining spiral waves were recorded from the epicardial surface of the sheep ventricle. Both the center of rotation (the so-called core of the spiral wave) and the expanding peripheral arm were clearly monitored. Later, similar techniques were used to study spiral waves occurring in the isolated whole heart preparations.[14,16] In the following sections of this chapter we summarize the main features of spiral wave activation and how they may be applied to the understanding of reentry in the heart.

Once spiral waves of excitation were clearly recognized in cardiac tissue, the next step was to determine the extent to which other predictions derived from the studies of wave propagation in excitable media might be applied to reentry in the heart. Analogous to patterns observed in other systems, spiral waves in the heart may be separated into three types: stationary, drifting, and anchoring (that is, following a period of drift, the spiral wave becomes stationary by rotating around a small obstacle found in its path).

Stationary Spiral Waves and Monomorphic Arrhythmias

When the core of the spiral wave remains in the same position for many rotations (possibly indefinitely), the activity is called stationary. Stationary spiral waves offer a unique opportunity for the detailed analysis of the voltage (i.e., fluorescence) structure of the core. We have taken advantage of the high spatial resolution of the video images to study the characteristics of the core. Figure 2A shows an isochronal map of a clockwise spiral wave rotating over the surface of a thin slice of sheep epicardial muscle. The isochrones are 16.7 ms apart, the rotation period is 150 ms, the core is delineated by the gray region near the center. The core is an area that is excitable, but not excited, during rotation of the wave. Within the core, at the point marked by the asterisk, there is very low amplitude activation (below). Figure 2B shows the same tissue stimulated from the left at a cy-

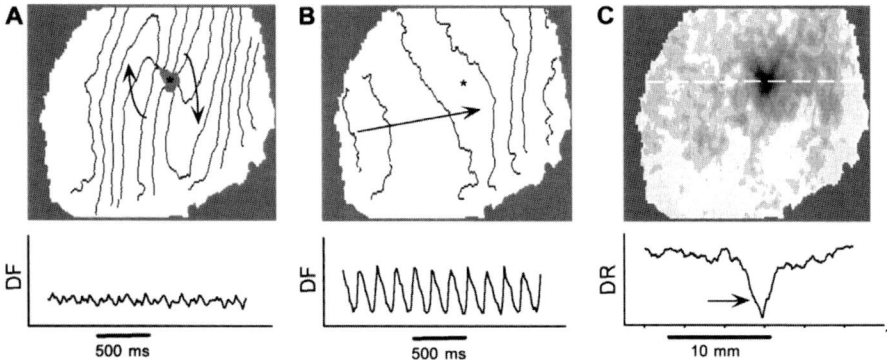

Figure 2. A. Self-sustained stationary spiral waves in sheep epicardial muscle. Isochrones show position of wave front every 17 ms, rotating around core (gray region near center). *Below:* Fluorescence changes over time at one location (asterisk in core). B. 17-ms isochrones of planar wave, stimulated from linear electrode along left edge. *Below:* Fluorescence changes at area that was previously the core (asterisk). C. Dynamic range map of activation in panel A. White corresponds to high-amplitude range over one cycle; dark equals low amplitude. *Below:* Profile of a horizontal line of pixels from the map (white dashed line). Arrow points to level of core in panel A.

cle length similar to the rotation period of the spiral, sending planar waves from left to right. In this case, the region of the former core is fully activated (below), indicating that the depolarized levels observed during this spiral wave are functionally determined (compare traces under panels A and B). In fact, the amplitude of the action potentials gradually decays toward the center of the core. A dynamic range map of the spiral episode was constructed by calculating the maximum minus the minimum amplitude over one rotation cycle for each spatial point. In Figure 2C, brightness corresponds to dynamic range, such that white regions have high dynamic range (high amplitude activations). The core shows up in this map as a dark region of decreased amplitude. A horizontal line of pixels through the core (shown at the bottom) displays the voltage profile of the core. The arrow shows the cut-off level used to outline the core in panel A. The dynamic range map of the planar wave (not shown) had high amplitudes throughout this region.

Spiral waves have also been observed in whole heart experiments.[14,16] Figure 3 shows one rotation from sustained counterclockwise rotating activity in a Langendorff-perfused rabbit heart, with a 133-ms rotation period. A pseudo-electrocardiogram (ECG) was computed by taking the difference between the left and right halves of each frame of the movie.[13] The resulting ECG (right) greatly resembles monomorphic ventricular tachycardia.

It should be noted that spiral waves may be extended into the third dimension. Three-dimensional spirals are called scroll waves,[41,43] and the core is thus extended into a linear structure called the filament. Scroll waves may take on extremely complex shapes within the mass of tissue. When we describe spiral waves on the surface of a 3-dimensional tissue preparation, the core is the point at which the filament intersects the surface.

Drifting Spiral Waves and Polymorphic Arrhythmias

One of the main contributions of the theory of spiral waves to cardiac electrophysiology was the idea that reentrant activity may persist even when the center of rotation is moving from beat to beat. Drifting spirals were consistently found in our preparations, initially in thin epicardial

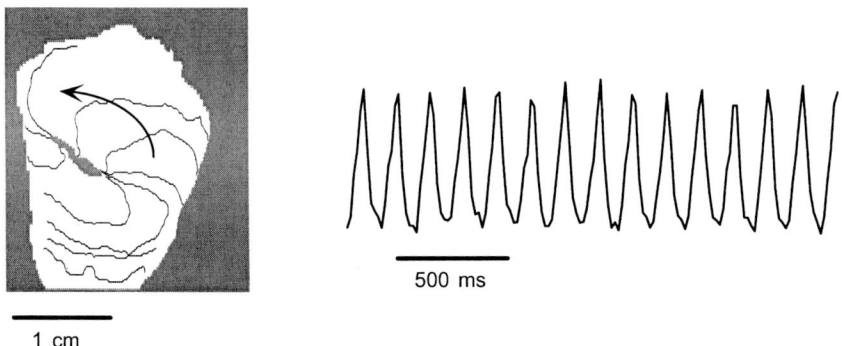

500 ms

1 cm

Figure 3. *Left:* Isochronal map of one rotation during ventricular tachycardia in the rabbit heart. *Right:* Pseudo-electrocardiogram of many rotations.

slices and later in whole hearts. Therefore, this phenomenon occurs in both 2- and 3-dimensional tissues. Drifting implies short circuiting of the wave front through the core of the spiral, which is compelling evidence that the core is indeed composed of excitable tissue.

The Doppler Effect and Torsade de Pointes. A drifting spiral behaves like any other moving source of waves and, as such, gives rise to spatial heterogeneities in the observed frequencies. Figure 4 is an illustration of a counterclockwise rotor drifting down and to the right. The spiral has two associated frequencies: the slow drift speed (large arrow), and the wave speed (small curved arrow), which is also the rotation period. Although these two velocities may be constant, the Doppler effect causes a point ahead of the core (B) to have a faster activation rate than a point behind the core (A). The coexistence of two frequencies that result from a single source represents an attractive model to explain the mechanism of some forms of ventricular tachycardias. In fact, one such form is the so-called torsade de pointes, in which the axis of the QRS complexes gradually changes the polarity in a sinusoidal manner. In the schematic recordings on the right side of Figure 4, arrows show the apparent direction of activation changing from B → A in the middle of the episode to A → B at the end. Earlier attempts to explain such a distinct transition of the QRS axis were based on the idea that the heart was activated by two separate foci with slightly different rates. It has been experimentally shown with dual electronic stimulation that in the presence of such an asynchronous activation of the ventricles, the axis of the QRS will vary in a predictable manner resembling the pattern observed during torsade de pointes. Although the model was able to reproduce the electrocardiographic pattern of the QRS, the idea that the real arrhythmia was the result of two separate foci that were activated simultaneously and had a slightly different firing rate was difficult to accept. Furthermore, because torsade de pointes usually manifests clinically as an episodic arrhythmia in which runs are quite reproducible in terms of electrocardiographic pattern, the "double focus" theory seems yet more unlikely. Alternatively, drifting spirals giving rise

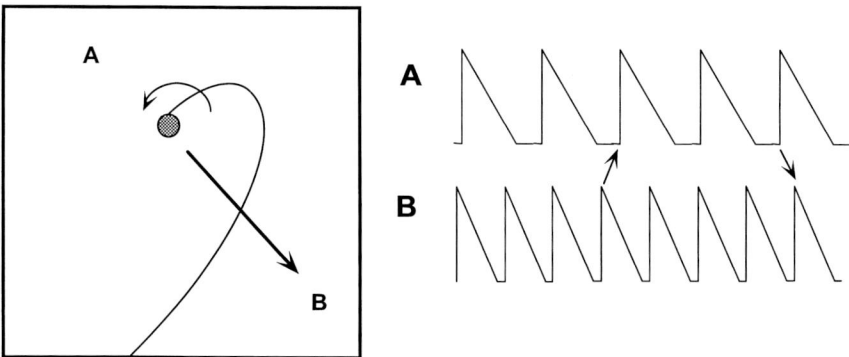

Figure 4. *Left:* Schema of Doppler effect in drifting spiral wave. Small curved arrow shows rotation, large straight arrow shows drift. *Right:* Activations have a slower frequency behind the spiral (A) than ahead of it (B). Arrows indicate apparent reversal of activation sequence at two different moments.

to more than one activation frequency from a single source is indeed a more attractive explanation.

Figure 5 shows isochronal maps of two rotations in a sequence of non-stationary ventricular tachycardia in the whole rabbit heart. In panel A, the core is in the upper left, near the base. Rotating waves drifted downward toward the apex with accompanying elongation of the core. Panel B, obtained about 500 ms later, shows the new position of the core, near the apex. When activation reached the apex, the center of rotation moved out of the field of view, then restarted again at the original location near the base. Panel C shows the typical pattern of shifting axis in the pseudo-ECG generated during the entire episode.

Mathematical and experimental models have shown that certain conditions of the medium (e.g., electrophysiological parameters) may induce the drift of spiral waves. For example, gradients in action potential duration or conduction velocity may induce spirals to drift into regions of longer action potential duration or slower conduction velocity. In recent publications, drifting spiral waves giving rise to patterns resembling torsade de pointes were observed in Langendorff-perfused rabbit hearts exposed to quinidine or the K channel blocker E-4031.[15]

Fibrillation. Torsadelike patterns are seen in the ECG, when drift velocities are approximately 10% of the propagation speed. If a spiral wave moves more rapidly, 30% or more of wave speed, it may give rise to fibrillatory ECG patterns.[16] Figure 6 shows three frames of a well-formed spiral during fibrillation in the rabbit heart. The spiral wave appeared out of the confluence of several wave fronts, meandered on the surface for five or six beats, then drifted out of the field of view. In this experiment, the heart was immersed in a beaker, with ECG leads on opposite sides. The ECGs recorded before, during, and after movie acquisition displayed irregular periodicity and morphology, resembling VF. Gray et al.[16] used the Doppler effect to relate the rotor's propagation speed and drift speed to the frequency spectrum of the ECG. Their prediction showed excellent correspondence with the recorded ECG. They concluded that a single rapidly drifting rotor in the heart may underlie VF.

Spiral waves have also been observed in fine-grained VF in sheep and rabbit whole hearts, but in this case there are many meandering "wavelets" moving across the heart surface. Spirals may last only one or two rotations

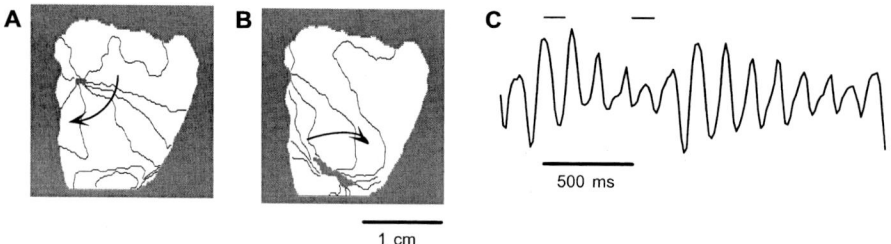

Figure 5. Isochrones of two rotations during unstable tachycardia in rabbit heart. **A.** Rotor near the base, initial isochrone at 333 ms. **B.** Same rotor has drifted toward apex 500 ms later. **C.** Pseudo-electrocardiogram. Small bars above represent times of the isochrone maps.

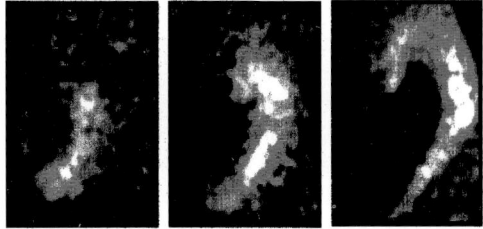

Figure 6. Three consecutive frames (17 ms apart) of a counterclockwise rotor during ventricular fibrillation in the rabbit heart. White = depolarized areas.

before disappearing, although sometimes they may persist for many rotations. Gray et al.[17] have devised a method of quantifying spatial and temporal order during cardiac fibrillation by labeling rotors as spatial phase singularities. These singularities may be tracked over time and have been found to obey several simple rules, such as forming or terminating with other singularities of opposite rotation. Their analysis reveals an unexpected amount of organization during fibrillation.

Anchoring Spiral Waves

Drifting spiral waves are usually short-lived. In most cases, the core finds boundaries of nonexcitable tissue and the activity is interrupted. However, in some episodes, the presence of very small heterogeneities may actually prevent the core from moving. In such cases, a drifting spiral becomes stationary. This sequence of events is responsible for an electrocardiographic pattern characterized by the presence of a polymorphic tachycardia with varying QRS axis as well as irregular cycle length, followed by a monomorphic tachycardia with uniform QRS morphology and cycle length. Such transitions have also been described during the spontaneous initiation of ventricular tachycardias in humans.[44]

In our experiments with thin epicardial slices, spiral waves were consistently initiated via cross-field stimulation.[13] The great majority of resulting rotors drifted to the boundary of the tissue and disappeared. However, in some cases the spiral attached to some heterogeneity and remained stable for extended periods. Experiments with whole hearts showed greater variety: initially, extra beats obtained by rapid pacing frequently appeared as complex, fibrillatory patterns. Then these patterns simplified with fewer wave fronts and longer wavelengths. Finally, one or two slow, high-amplitude activations would occur just before activity ceased. Unstable rotors were often observed during the second phase. These rotors could anchor and remain stable, but this has been extremely rare in whole rabbit and sheep hearts. The finding that stable tachycardias are rarely found in nonischemic whole animal hearts has been reported by other laboratories as well. The mechanism of anchoring is not fully understood, but both experiments and computer simulations have shown that rotating waves may anchor at points that are inexcitable. The cores of stationary spiral waves in thin tissue slices were often located at heterogeneities such as coronary vessels or small pieces of connective tissue. (In the extreme case, the core may be very large, as in the case of an infarct or an outflow tract.) In three dimensions, the mechanisms of anchoring are more complex. Simulation studies have shown that if only one end of the filament of a rotating scroll finds an anchor point while the other end is free to lash about, this may cause the anchored end to detach.[45] Therefore, the likelihood of anchoring is inversely proportional to the thickness of the tissues.[42] At one end of the spectrum, in thin, essentially 2-dimensional preparations, even small discontinuities offer a substrate for anchoring. As tissue thickness increases, the size of the obstacle must increase accordingly for anchoring to occur. Alternatively, the activity may be stabilized if both ends of the filament are anchored.

Conclusion

Video optical mapping techniques have significantly widened our knowledge of cardiac electrophysiology. In this chapter, we present results obtained with CCD video cameras. The high spatial resolution over a large recording area has permitted the analysis of complex spatiotemporal patterns. Spiral waves, a concept borrowed from theoretical and experimental studies of excitable media, have provided a useful description of reentrant activity in the heart. Spiral wave behavior provides a consistent mechanism underlying many tachyarrhythmias. Anchored, stationary spiral waves in cardiac tissue exhibit ECGs suggestive of monomorphic tachycardia. Sequences with drifting spiral waves manifest as polymorphic or fibrillatory episodes, depending on the speed of drift. High spatial resolution allows rotors to be tracked over time and space, permitting quantification of complex activation patterns.

References

1. Arisi G, Macchi E, Baruffi S, et al. Potential fields on the ventricular surface of the exposed dog heart during normal excitation. *Circ Res* 1983;52:706–715.
2. Dillon SM, Allessie MA, Ursell PC, Wit AL. Influence of anisotropic tissue on reentrant circuit in the epicardial border zone of subacute canine infarcts. *Circ Res* 1988;63:182–206.
3. Bayley PV, Johnson EE, Wolf PD, et al. A quantitative measurement of spatial order in ventricular fibrillation. *J Cardiovasc Electrophysiol* 1993;4:533–546.
4. Cohen LB, Salzberg BM, Davila HV, et al. Changes in axon fluorescence during activity: Molecular probes of membrane potential. *J Membr Biol* 1974;19:1–36.
5. Cohen LB, Lesher S. Optical monitoring of membrane potential: Methods of multisite optical measurement. In De Weer P, Salzberg BM (eds): *Optical Methods in Cell Physiology.* New York: Wiley-Interscience; 1986:71–99.
6. Efimov IR, Huang DT, Rendt JM, Salama G. Optical mapping of repolarization and refractoriness from intact hearts. *Circulation* 1994;90:1469–1480.
7. Girouard SD, Laurita KR, Rosenbaum DS. Unique properties of cardiac action potentials recorded with voltage-sensitive dyes. *J Cardiovasc Electrophysiol* 1996;7:1024–1038.
8. Dillon S, Morad M. A new laser scanning system for measuring action potential propagation in the heart. *Science* 1981;214:453–456.
9. Davidenko JM, Pertsov AV, Salomonsz R, et al. Stationary and drifting spiral waves of excitation in isolated cardiac muscle. *Nature* 1992;355:349–351.
10. Wikswo JP, Lin SF, Abbas RA. Virtual electrodes in cardiac tissue: A common mechanism for anodal and cathodal stimulation. *Biophys J* 1995;69:2195–2210.

11. Witkowski FX, Leon LJ, Penkoske PA, et al. Spatiotemporal evolution of ventricular fibrillation. *Nature* 1998;392:78–82.
12. Nassif GN, Dillon SM, Wit AL. Video mapping of cardiac activation. *J Mol Cell Cardiol* 1990;22(Suppl IV):S44.
13. Pertsov AM, Davidenko JM, Salomonsz R, et al. Spiral waves of excitation underlie reentrant activity in isolated cardiac muscle. *Circ Res* 1993;72(3):631–650.
14. Gray RA, Jalife J, Panfilov AV, et al. Nonstationary vortexlike reentrant activity as a mechanism of polymorphic ventricular tachycardia in the isolated rabbit heart. *Circulation* 1995;91:2454–2469.
15. Asano Y, Davidenko JM, Baxter WT, et al. Optical mapping of drug-induced polymorphic arrhythmias and torsade de pointes in the isolated rabbit heart. *J Am Coll Cardiol* 1997;29:831–842.
16. Gray RA, Jalife J, Panfilov AV, et al. Mechanisms of cardiac fibrillation. *Science* 1995;270:1222–1225.
17. Gray RA, Pertsov AM, Jalife J. Spatial and temporal organization during cardiac fibrillation. *Nature* 1998;392(5):75–78.
18. Vaidya D, Morley GE, Samie F, Jalife J. Reentry and fibrillation in the mouse heart: A challenge to the critical mass hypothesis. *Circ Res* 1999;85:174–181.
19. Cabo C, Pertsov AM, Baxter WT, et al. Wave-front curvature as a cause of slow conduction and block in isolated cardiac muscle. *Circ Res* 1994;75:1014–1028.
20. Cabo C, Pertsov AM, Davidenko JM, et al. Vortex shedding as a precursor of turbulent electrical activity in cardiac muscle. *Biophys J* 1996;70:1105–1111.
21. Gray RA, Pertsov AM, Jalife J. Incomplete reentry and epicardial breakthrough patterns during atrial fibrillation in the sheep heart. *Circulation* 1996;94:2649–2661.
22. Skanes AC, Mandapati R, Berenfeld O, et al. Spatiotemporal periodicity during atrial fibrillation in the isolated sheep heart. *Circulation* 1998;98:1236–1248.
23. Mandapati R, Skanes A, Chen J, et al. Stable microreentrant sources as a mechanism of atrial fibrillation in the isolated sheep heart. *Circulation* 2000;101:194–199.
24. Amelio GF. Charge-coupled devices. *Sci Am* 1974;Feb:22–31.
25. Janesick JR, Elliot T, Collins S, et al. Scientific charge-coupled devices. *Opt Eng* 1987;26(8):692–714.
26. Kristian J, Blouke M. Charge-coupled devices in astronomy. *Sci Am* 1982;Oct:66–74.
27. Janesick J, Blouke M. Sky on a chip: The fabulous CCD. *Sky Telescope* 1987;238–242.
28. Tseng HF, Ambrose JR, Fattahi M. Evolution of the solid-state image sensor. *J Imaging Sci* 1985;29:1–7.
29. Loew LM, Cohen LB, Dix J, et al. A naphthyl analog of the aminostyryl pyridinium class of potentiometric membrane dyes shows consistent sensitivity in a variety of tissue, cell, and model membrane preparations. *J Membr Biol* 1992;130:1–10.
30. Hooper CE, Ansorge RE, Browne HM, Tomkins P. CCD imaging of luciferase gene expression in single mammalian cells. *J Biolumin Chemilumin* 1990;5:123–130.
31. MacKay CD. Fast optical imaging techniques. In OS Wolfbeis (ed): *Fluorescence Spectroscopy: New Methods and Applications*. Berlin, New York: Springer-Verlag; 1993:25–30.
32. Baxter WT, Davidenko JM, Loew LM, et al. Technical features of a CCD video camera system to record cardiac fluorescence data. *Ann Biomed Eng* 1997;25:713–725.
33. Inoué S, Spring KR. *Video Microscopy*. 2nd ed. New York: Plenum Press; 1997.
34. Lasser-Ross N, Miyakawa H, Lev-Ram V, et al. High time resolution fluorescence imaging with a CCD camera. *J Neurosci Methods* 1991;36:253–261.
35. Morley GM, Vaidya DM, Samie FH, et al. A characterization of conduction in

the ventricles of normal and heterozygous Cx43 knockout mice using optical mapping. *J Cardiovasc Electrophysiol* 1999;10:1361–1375.

36. Mironov SF, Baxter WT, Zaitsev AV, Pertsov AM. Formation of ischemic border zone: An optical mapping study. *Circulation* 1997;96(8):I58.

37. Lee P, Morley GM, Huang Q, et al. Conditional lineage ablation to model human diseases. *Proc Natl Acad Sci U S A* 1998;95(19):11371-11376.

38. Falk CX, Wu JY, Cohen LB, Tang AK. Nonuniform expression of habituation in the activity of distinct classes of neurons in the Aplysia abdominal ganglion. *J Neurosci* 1993;13(9):4072–4081.

39. Hirota A, Sato K, Momose-Sato Y, et al. A new simultaneous 1020-site optical recording system for monitoring neural activity using voltage-sensitive dyes. *J Neurosci Methods* 1995;56:187–194.

40. Bove RT, Dillon SM. Optically imaging cardiac activation with a laser system. *IEEE Eng Med Biol* 1998;Jan/Feb:84–94.

41. Winfree AT. Scroll-shaped waves of chemical activity in three dimensions. *Science* 1973;181:937.

42. Winfree AT. Electrical turbulence in three-dimensional heart muscle. *Science* 1994;266:1003–1006.

43. Pertsov AM, Jalife J. Three-dimensional vortex-like reentry. In Zipes DP, Jalife J (eds): *Cardiac Electrophysiology: From Cell to Bedside.* 2nd ed. Philadelphia: W.B. Saunders Co.; 1995:403–410.

44. Bardy GH, Olson WH. Clinical characteristics of spontaneous-onset sustained ventricular tachycardia and ventricular fibrillation in survivors of cardiac arrest. In Zipes DP, Jalife J (eds): *Cardiac Electrophysiology: From Cell to Bedside.* Philadelphia: W.B. Saunders Co.; 1990:778–790.

45. Vinson M, Pertsov AM, Jalife J. Anchoring of vortex filaments in 3D excitable media. *Physica D* 1993;72:119–134.

Chapter 16

Video Imaging of Wave Propagation in a Transgenic Mouse Model of Cardiomyopathy

Faramarz Samie, Gregory E. Morley, Dhjananjay Vaidya, Karen L. Vikstrom, and José Jalife

Introduction

Familial hypertrophic cardiomyopathy (HCM) is a genetically transmitted disease with a dominant mode of inheritance.[1,2] Molecular genetic analyses have demonstrated that a myriad of mutations in the β-myosin heavy chain (MHC) and other sarcomeric proteins can cause HCM.[3] This disease has an estimated prevalence of 0.2% in the general population and is associated with disabling symptoms and life-threatening arrhythmias and, in fact, is the leading cause of sudden cardiac death in the young.[4] Unfortunately, however, the link between mutations in contractile proteins and their clinical manifestations such as arrhythmias is not well understood.

With the advent of technology to alter the mammalian genome, we have gained insight into the regulation and function of genes, the mechanisms of developmental and pathological processes, and the generation of animal models for human disorders. The mouse has proven to be the mammalian model system of choice for genetic analysis. Recently, several mouse models of familial HCM have been developed.[5,6]

We have chosen to study the effects of mutations in sarcomeric proteins on cardiac electrical function using a murine model of HCM.[6] This model is a transgenic mouse in which the coding region consists of a mutated rat α-MHC. Specifically, the first is a point mutation where glutamine has been replaced with arginine at position 403 in the MHC, and the second is a deletion of amino acids from positions 468–527 bridged by nine

This work was supported in part by grant PO1–39707. Faramarz Samie was supported by a Howard Hughes Medical Student Training Fellowship.
From Rosenbaum DS, Jalife J (eds): *Optical Mapping of Cardiac Excitation and Arrhythmias*. ©Futura Publishing Co., Inc., Armonk, NY, 2001.

281

nonmyosin amino acids. These mutations were predicted to interfere strongly with the interaction of actin and myosin. Phenotypically, this mouse exhibits the expected cardiac histopathology, including hypertrophy, myocellular disarray, fibrosis, and small vessel disease.

We initiated this study with the hope of understanding the mechanisms underlying arrhythmias and sudden cardiac death in this disease state. It is our hypothesis that, in the heart, structural alterations (e.g., fibrosis and myocellular disarray) of the appropriate size result in changes in the electrical activation sequence and therefore serve as an arrhythmogenic substrate.

To test this hypothesis we used a 9-lead mouse electrocardiogram (ECG) system[7] and a miniaturized optical recording system with high spatial and temporal resolution capable of imaging complex patterns of activation in the adult mouse heart.[7,8] We also developed a novel vector field technique to accurately quantify propagation velocity within the complex patterns of activation on the surface of the mouse heart. Finally, we developed analytical tools necessary to investigate the patterns of epicardial activation during sinus rhythm.

Methods and Results

Animal Husbandry

HCM transgenic mice, line 140,[3] were in the Department of Laboratory Animal Resources. Animals were maintained on a 12-hour light/dark cycle with free access to water and food. The Institutional Animal Use and Care Committee at the State University of New York Health Science Center at Syracuse approved all animal protocols.

Surface ECGs

Simultaneous body surface potentials were recorded from anesthetized animals (2.5% Avertin at 0.014 cc/g). Signals were amplified (200×; Biopack amplifier, Santa Barbara, CA), filtered (LP = 300 Hz, HP = 0.5 Hz), digitized (at 2751 Hz), stored in a computer, and displayed with commercially available software (AcqKnowledge, Biopack, Santa Barbara, CA). Recording electrodes were placed in the left and the right forlinks and the left hindlimb, and a reference electrode was placed in the right hindlimb (for details see references 7 and 8). Additionally, chest electrodes were placed along the left and right midaxillary line and a third electrode was placed on the sternum. With use of these electrode placements, the appropriate ECG leads were calculated.[9]

We measured several basic surface ECG parameters including heart rate, QRS duration, RR, PR, QT, and JT intervals with this system. Among the parameters measured, we found that both the QT and the JT intervals were prolonged in the transgenic mice, indicating an alteration in the ventricular repolarization. In Table 1, we report the results from 7 control and 7 HCM mice. Values are reported as mean±standard deviation. Figure 1 serves as a legend by demarcating the parameters of interest. A represen-

Table 1
Electrocardiographic Parameters in Control and HCM Mice

	HR (bpm)	RR (ms)	PR (ms)	QRS (ms)	QT (ms)	JT (ms)
Control	449.8±26.9	133.8±8.2	43.8±3.8	10.6±0.8	56.4±3.9	44.2±3.5
HCM	452.2±82.0	136.4±24.3	50.3±3.7	10.4±1.4	71.9±2.8	54.3±2.3

Mean±SD.
HCM = hypertrophic cardiomyopathy. HR (bpm) = heart rate in beats per minute.

tative 3-lead ECG tracing from one control and one HCM mouse also are displayed.

Perfusion System and Optical Mapping Set-Up

Langendorff Perfusion.　With the mice under deep anesthesia, the hearts were quickly removed through a sternotomy and rinsed in a Tyrode's so-

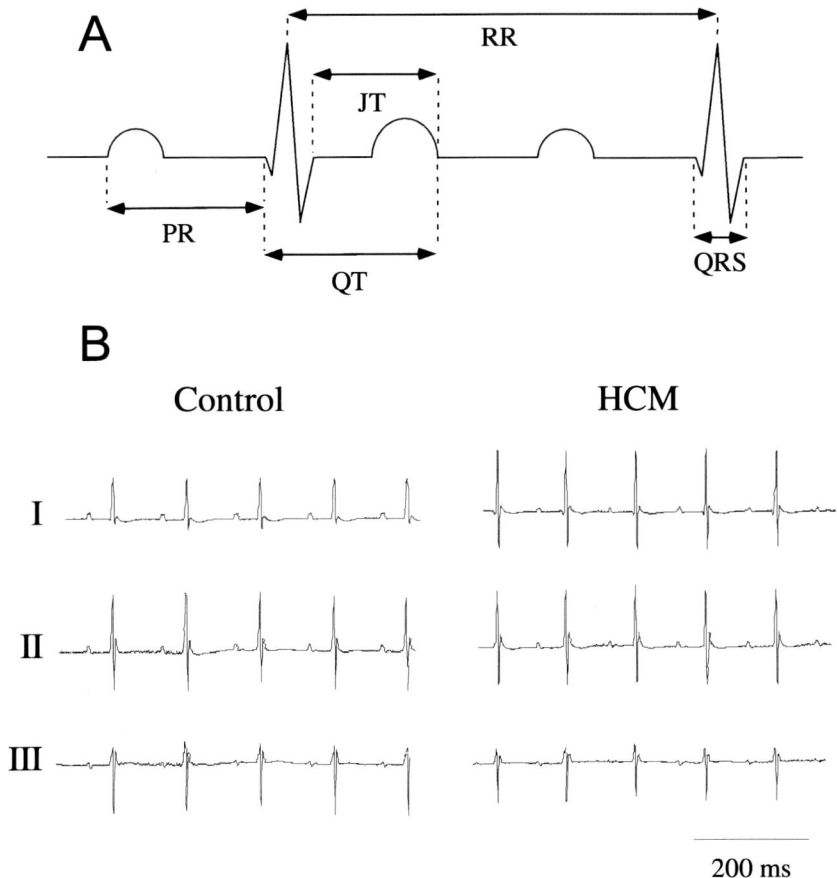

Figure 1. Electrocardiogram (ECG) traces. **A.** Schematic ECG trace demarcating the parameters of interest. **B.** Three representative ECG lead traces from a control and a hypertrophic cardiomyopathy (HCM) mouse.

lution equilibrated with a 95% O_2/5% CO_2 gas mixture. Hearts were then rapidly cannulated and perfused in a retrograde fashion via an aortic cannula with warm (37°C to 39°C) oxygenated Tyrode's solution (1.5 to 2.0 mL/min). Once connected to the Langendorff perfusion system, hearts were placed in a custom-built chamber where warm oxygenated Tyrode's solution was continuously superfused at 37°C to 39°C. This prevented the development of temperature gradients between the endocardium and the epicardium.

Stimulation Protocol. Bipolar pacing electrodes were placed near the center of the anterior and posterior left ventricle. Preparations were paced at cycle lengths from 80 to150 ms. The left ventricle was paced with use of pulses equivalent to 1.5× threshold amplitude at each cycle length with duration of 2 ms.

High-Resolution Mapping of the Mouse Heart. The hearts were stabilized against the glass front of the chamber for imaging. The mechanical movement of the heart was stopped by perfusion of the excitation-contraction uncoupler diacetyl monoxime (DAM, 15 mmol/L). To record optical signals, the voltage-sensitive fluorescent dye di-4-ANEPPS, an indicator of transmembrane voltage, was perfused.

The video imaging used was similar to that described previously.[10] Briefly, light from a 150-W xenon arc lamp (Opti Quip, Highland Mills, NY) was collimated and made quasimonochromatic by the use of an interference filter (520 nm) together with a heat filter. A fiberoptic cable delivered the excitation light to the epicardial surface of the heart. The emitted light was collected and passed through an emission filter (645 nm) and projected onto a charged coupled device (CCD) video camera (Dalsa Inc., Waterloo, Ontario, Canada) operating at a frame rate of approximately 1.5 kHz. Video images of the epicardial surface were acquired with an analog-to-digital frame grabber (Bitflow, Inc., Woburn, MA). To reveal the signal, the background fluorescence was subtracted from each frame. No temporal or spatial filtering was used in the data analysis. Hearts were optically mapped on both their anterior and posterior sides. Care was taken to position hearts so that similar anterior and posterior areas were mapped. We found that positioning the heart in these two orientations provided the largest viewing surface, with many readily defined anatomical landmarks.

Conduction Velocity Measurements

Figure 2 illustrates the method used to calculate conduction velocity (CV). Panel A shows the spatial distribution of the optical action potential signals, the high signal-to-noise ratio, and the high spatial resolution of the system. For illustrative purposes, only a few of the more than 1000 pixels that were in the viewing area of the heart are shown. Panel B shows the method that was used to calculate the activation time. The optical signal from each pixel was normalized to its maximal amplitude. A pixel was considered activated when the change in the fluorescence exceeded 50% of its maximal value. Activation times were calculated for each recorded pixel and an activation map was generated. Direction and magnitude of propagation were determined for each recorded site on the heart from the

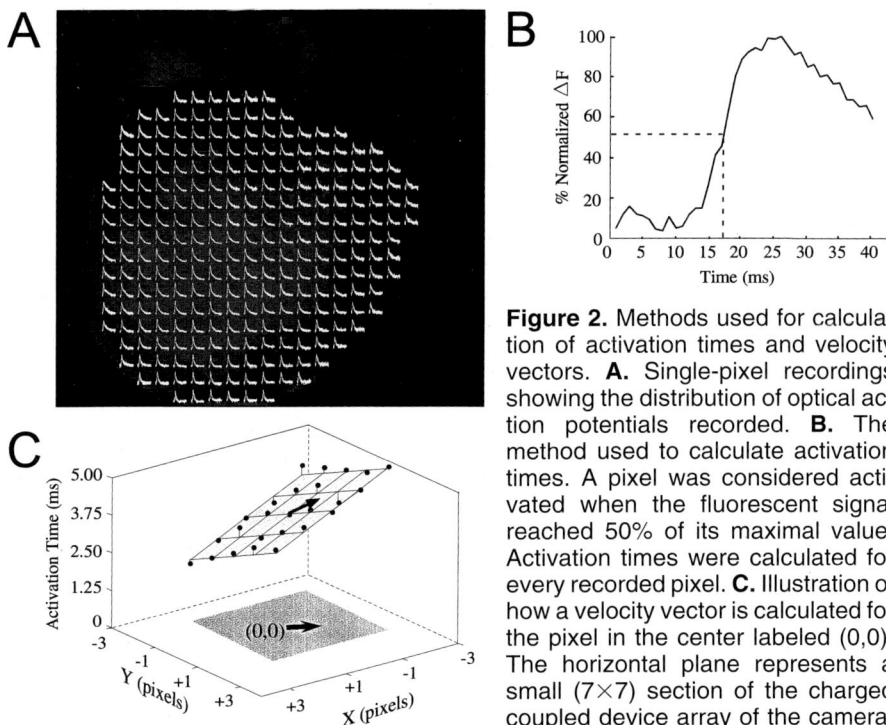

Figure 2. Methods used for calculation of activation times and velocity vectors. **A.** Single-pixel recordings showing the distribution of optical action potentials recorded. **B.** The method used to calculate activation times. A pixel was considered activated when the fluorescent signal reached 50% of its maximal value. Activation times were calculated for every recorded pixel. **C.** Illustration of how a velocity vector is calculated for the pixel in the center labeled (0,0). The horizontal plane represents a small (7×7) section of the charged coupled device array of the camera. The z-axis represents the activation time. To calculate a velocity vector, the activation times of a 5×5 array surrounding that pixel were fit to a plane using least-squares fit method. The direction on this plane that is increasing fastest represents the direction of perpendicular to wave front, and maximal slope represents the inverse of the speed of conduction in that direction.

activation times of neighboring pixels, in the following manner: The directional derivative of the activation time, t_a, at any point (x,y) represented the time taken by the wave front to travel a unit distance in a certain direction. The largest difference in activation times was found in the direction that was perpendicular to the wave front (i.e., in the direction in which the directional derivative was greatest). This maximal directional derivative can be calculated as the gradient of the t_a in space. The gradient represents the time taken by the activation front to travel a unit distance in the direction perpendicular to the wave front. The CV was defined as the distance traveled by the wave front per unit time. Hence, the magnitude of the CV in the direction perpendicular to the wave front was given by the inverse of the above gradient, whereas the direction of propagation was the same as the gradient.

The plot in Figure 2C shows the method used for calculation of a conduction vector. The horizontal plane (x-y) represents a small section of the recorded pixels and the vertical axis (z) represents the activation time for each given pixel. To calculate a velocity vector for the center pixel (0,0) the activation times for a 5×5 array were fit to a plane using least-squares fit. The direction on this plane where time was increasing fastest was found. This direction was perpendicular to the wave front and, along that path, the slope represented the inverse of the speed of propagation.

A comparison of conduction patterns and CVs obtained from a wild type and a transgenic mouse is shown in Figure 3. Panel A is a control isochrone map, and panel B is a similar map from an HCM mouse. In this color scheme, red indicates the initial site of activation, with each subsequent color band representing the position of the activation front every millisecond thereafter. Both maps were obtained by stimulating the epicardium using a pair of bipolar electrodes. The corresponding histograms of mean directional CV versus orientation are shown in panels C and D. The isochrone maps illustrate the patterns of epicardial conduction. The maps are similar in that they show nearly similar elliptical patterns of propagation. Moreover, no significant differences were found in the mean directional CV between wild type and transgenic mice. A summary of the CV_{max} and CV_{min} estimates from 5 control and 8 transgenic mice are shown

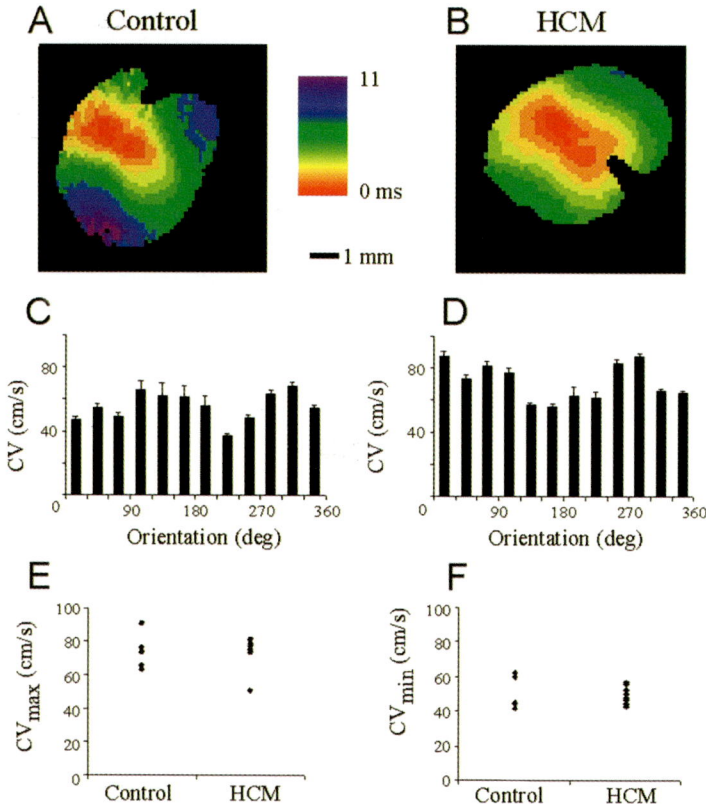

Figure 3. Conduction velocities and patterns of epicardial conduction in control and hypertrophic cardiomyopathy (HCM) mice. Isochrone maps and mean conduction velocity (CV) plots from a control (**A** and **C**) and an HCM (**B** and **D**) mouse show similar activation patterns. **E** and **F**. CV_{max} and CV_{min} estimates from 5 control and 8 transgenic mice. Each symbol represents a measurement from an individual mouse.

in panels E and F. They demonstrate a nearly identical distribution of velocities. On average, control mice showed a CV_{max} of 73.6 ± 4.8 cm/s and a CV_{min} of 50.9 ± 4.4 cm/s. These data were not statistically different from data in HCM mice, in which mean CV_{max} was 73.3 ± 3.9 cm/s and mean CV_{min} was 49.47 ± 1.8 cm/s.

Histology and 3-Dimensional Reconstructions

To better understand the distribution of the pathology in this model, we reconstructed a portion of the ventricular free wall from histological sections. To this end, following clcctrophysiological studies, the hearts were fixed in 10% formalin and embedded in paraffin. Serial 4-μm sections were cut transverse to the long axis of the heart and stained with Masson's trichrome. For 3-dimensional reconstructions, the region of interest was selected and every fourth section in that segment was projected onto a wall from a fixed distance. The outlines of the relevant structures (e.g., fibrosis, blood vessels, papillary muscle, and ventricles) were traced. The line drawings were then scanned into a computer and tagged image file format (TIFF) images were generated. With use of IP Lab Spectrum (Scientific Image Processing, Vienna, VA), the TIFF images were rotated with respect to one another and the correct alignment was calculated. With the software Canvas version 3.5 (Deneb Software, Miami, FL), the sections were digitally stained for contrast enhancement, and these images were used to generate the 3-dimensional volume of interest in another commercially available software, Spyglass Slicer (Spyglass Inc., Savoy, IL).

Figure 4 is an example of such a reconstruction. Panel A shows the entire width of the myocardium where the muscle is shown in orange and the areas of fibrosis are shown in yellow. Panel B shows a different perspective of the same reconstruction allowing for clear visualization of the extent of fibrosis as seen through the epicardial surface. From these reconstructions, it is clear that the majority of the fibrosis was located

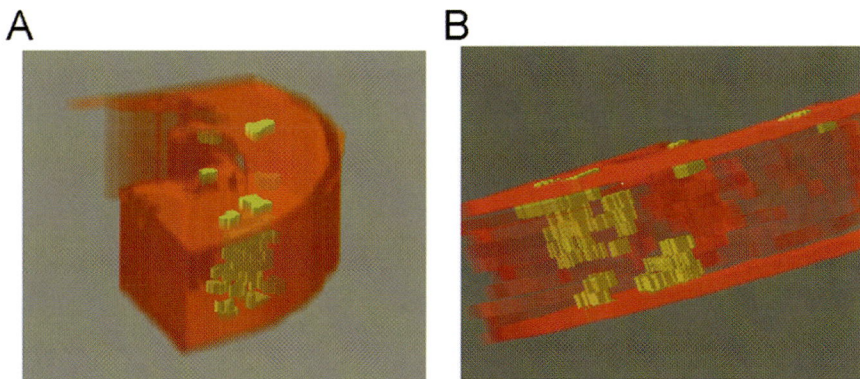

Figure 4. Three-dimensional reconstruction of a ventricular slab. Panels **A** and **B** are different views of the same region, and illustrate that fibrosis (yellow) is limited to the midmyocardium (orange).

within the midmyocardium, which may explain why neither the pattern of activation nor the conduction velocity of the transgenic hearts is altered upon epicardial stimulation. The likeliest explanation being that the effect of midmyocardial structures on epicardial conduction velocity was minimal when a bipolar electrode located on the epicardial surface applied stimulation.

Sinus Rhythm Analysis

To determine what effect, if any, midmyocardial structural changes have on ventricular propagation in the HCM mouse heart, we developed a technique to analyze the optical patterns of epicardial activation during sinus rhythm. To this end, activation maps of sinus rhythm in control and transgenic mice were generated. Subsequently, the activation maps were aligned with respect to one another, the time of activation was normalized in each map, and every pixel was then averaged with the corresponding pixels in the other maps. Finally, composite control and transgenic activation maps were generated and compared with each other.

The excitatory signal for a normal heartbeat begins in the sinus node then spreads to the AV node and bundle of His, and then to the bundle branches and Purkinje fibers. Finally, excitation spreads from the endocardium to the epicardium. On the surface, this process is seen as breakthroughs or sites of initial activation that appear at specific locations. From these regions, waves of excitation then emanate and activate the remainder of the ventricle. Figure 5 shows two composite activation maps obtained during sinus rhythm. Panel A is an average activation sequence ob-

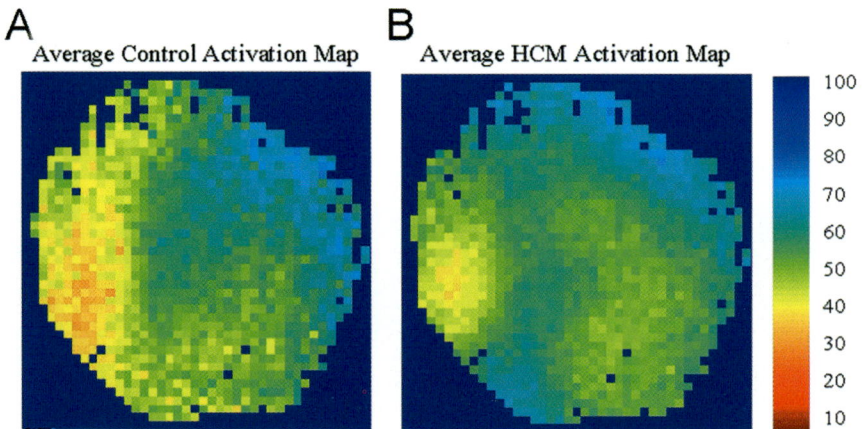

Figure 5. Composite activation maps obtained during sinus rhythm. **A.** An average activation map obtained during sinus rhythm from five control mice. In this color scheme, red represents the earliest site of activation and blue is the latest. **B.** A similar map obtained from eight hypertrophic cardiomyopathy (HCM) mice. From the comparison of the two maps, it is evident that the apex of the HCM mice is activated later. Presumably, this difference is due to the interaction of the wave front with the underlying structures in the midmyocardium.

tained from five control hearts. It demonstrates that there is one focused site of initial activation (red) located near the apex of the right ventricle and a second more diffuse site located in the left ventricle. These sites appear to be connected across the apex of the heart. Waves of excitation emanate from these regions and move toward the base, thus activating the remainder of the ventricle. Panel B is a composite activation map from eight HCM mice. A similar breakthrough pattern is seen. However, the two sites of initial activation are no longer connected across the apex. Consequently, waves of excitation move medially as well as toward the base. This interesting difference in the pattern of activation results in the delayed activation of the apex of the transgenic hearts, suggesting that the underlying obstacles imposed by areas of fibrosis (see Fig. 4) interfere with the propagating wave front. To quantify the variations in the patterns of activity, we calculated the standard error of the normalized activation time for each pixel on the average activation maps. It is known from statistics that in 95% of normal cases the activation time of any given pixel will occur within two standard errors of the average time of activation. Those pixels where the difference between mean activation time of control and HCM maps were greater than two standard errors were considered areas with significantly different activation pattern. However, it should be noted that up to 5% of isolated scattered pixels with spuriously significant differences may be found. In Figure 6, our map shows that more than 5% of pixels are significantly different; in addition, the clustering of differences also suggests a real difference in the pattern of activation.

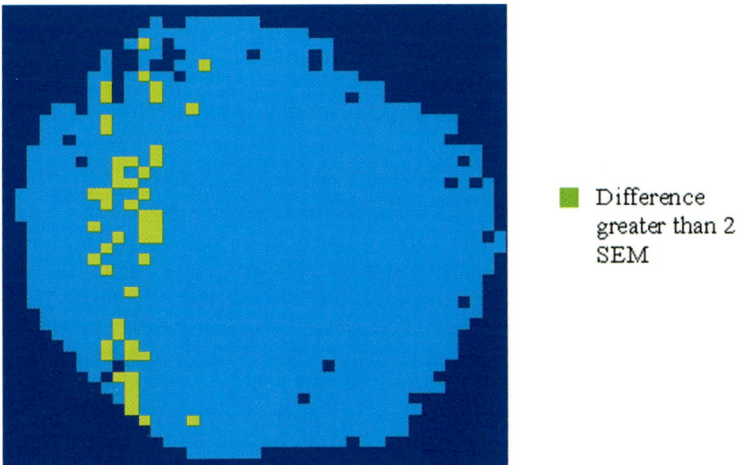

■ Difference greater than 2 SEM

Figure 6. Statistical comparison of activation maps obtained during sinus rhythm of 5 control and 8 transgenic hearts. The composite map illustrates the regions near the apex and septum (yellow) where a difference in the normalized time of activation was found between the control and the hypertrophic cardiomyopathy mice. This difference is greater than twice the standard error of the mean (SEM), suggesting that the visual observation of delayed activation in those regions is statistically significant. In addition, in histological sections of these regions we find the presence of fibrosis suggestive of the fact that the statistical difference found is indeed real.

Discussion

A Quantitative Method for the Study of Mouse Cardiac Electrophysiology

We have adapted established techniques in high-speed video optical mapping, using voltage-sensitive dyes, and electrocardiography to study electrical wave propagation in the mouse heart. We quantitatively measured epicardial conduction patterns and velocities in wild type and transgenic hearts from video movies by determining local conduction vectors, where we calculated the velocity and direction of propagation for 2500 individual recording sites. In addition, we developed optical means for studying the patterns of electrical excitation during sinus rhythm. We have found that, during epicardial stimulation, neither the pattern of activation nor the local conduction velocity in the transgenic mice is different from that observed and measured in the wild type mice. However, the sequence of excitation during sinus rhythm is different in the transgenic mice, which exhibit fibrotic changes in their hearts.

We have also measured several ECG parameters of anesthetized HCM and control mice. Our results are similar in conclusion to those reported previously by Berul et al.[11] In general, the ECG parameters reported for the mouse are variable and appear to be highly dependent on the anesthetic agent used.[12,13] The heart rate of the adult mouse has been reported to be between 200 and 636 bpm, with PR intervals ranging from 38 to 54 ms. Similarly, the QRS duration in the mouse range from 10 to 30 ms and the QT intervals range from 56 to 109 ms. Nevertheless, we have found, similar to that reported by Berul et al.,[11] that the QT and JT intervals are prolonged by approximately 16 ms and 10 ms, respectively, in the HCM mouse hearts as compared to control mice. This finding is indicative of an abnormality in the ventricular repolarization possibly due to the histopathology seen in these mice.

How do Obstacles Alter Wave Propagation?

Normally, the excitatory impulse for contraction begins in the sinus node and propagates through the atria to the ventricles. This process occurs without any difficulty in the presence of anatomical obstacles (e.g., blood vessels) under normal conditions. However, under certain critical conditions (e.g., reduced excitability) obstacles have been demonstrated to destabilize propagation, causing the formation of self-sustained vortices that result in uncontrolled excitation of cardiac tissue.[14] The formation of such vortices visually resembles vortex shedding in hydrodynamic systems.[15] But, why do such vortices form?

During the propagation of a wave initiated by a point source or a linear source, a repolarizing tail of finite dimensions always follows the wave front. Under these conditions, the wave front and wave tail never meet, and the distance that separates them corresponds to the wavelength of excitation.[16] In contrast, rotating waves show a unique phenomenon whereby the wave front and wave tail touch one another at a specific point, the wavebreak.[17,18] In such a case, the wave front velocity decreases toward the wavebreak, at which point the velocity is zero. A pronounced curvature is established close to the wavebreak so that the wave fails to activate the tissue ahead and instead rotates around a small region or pivoting point (i.e., the core); and although the core is excitable, it remains unexcited. Therefore, a self-sustained rotating wave may be initiated simply by inducing a wavebreak. This concept has utility for the understanding of reentry initiation, but it also explains the interaction of the wave fronts with anatomical and functional obstacles.[14,19,20]

It has been shown in in vitro experiments with the Belousov-Zhabotinsky (BZ) reaction,[19] as well as in cardiac muscle,[14] that under certain conditions, the broken ends of the wave fronts do not curve to form rotors but they maintain their elongated shape and contract. Eventually, as the result of continued shrinking of the broken ends, the excitation wave collapses, exhibiting decremental propagation. Using a generic model of an excitable medium Pertsov et al.[21] studied the conditions in which a propagating wave breaks after colliding with an obstacle. They demonstrated that a wavebreak leads to lateral instabilities and that the onset of such instabilities is associated with the existence of a critical curvature for propagation in the medium. The wave expands when the curvature of the wave front is lower than a critical value. However, when the obstacle is large enough or the expansion sufficiently slow, the broken wavefront could curve and give rise to a rotorlike activity. Inhomogeneities in cardiac muscle (e.g., fibrosis) may cause a break in a propagating wave, leading to lateral instabilities, and, depending on other parameters (e.g., excitability of the medium), the broken wave could contract and vanish or result in vortexlike activity. This was demonstrated experimentally by Cabo et al.,[14] who showed that excitability could control the fate or the ultimate outcome of a wave front when that wave front interacted with an anatomical obstacle, in the following way: Under conditions of reduced excitability they demonstrated that a broken wave could contract (i.e., conduction block); however, at an intermediate level of excitability, a broken wave could either continue onward, unaffected, or curve and expand, leading to rotor initiation. Therefore, the dynamics of lateral instabilities are determined not only by curvature but also by the excitability of the medium and the frequency of wave propagation, which, if fast, would also decrease excitability.

The characteristics of the obstacle, such as its shape and size, also play an important role in determining the formation of wavebreaks and vortexlike activity. For example, in the BZ reaction, in order for rotors to be initiated in the presence of an unexcitable obstacle, the barrier must have sharp corners; otherwise a wavebreak will not detach from a slowly curving barrier. Agladze et al.[19] also showed that if the obstacle is too small or the stimulation period is too long, then a planar wave initiated proximally to the obstacle will split at the obstacle into two waves with free ends, each circumnavigating the obstacle and eventually meeting again to form a single wave. On the other hand, if the size of the obstacle is sufficiently large (>1 mm), then the wave splits and the ends remain separated from the obstacle and from each other. However, as discussed earlier, the fate of the waves will ultimately depend on the conditions of excitability.

The concepts introduced here help to elucidate the mechanisms involved in the alterations seen in the pattern of excitation during sinus rhythm in the HCM mice. Simultaneously, they help to explain why more severe changes (e.g., arrhythmias) were not observed. As discussed above, the curvature, the state of excitability, the frequency of stimulation, and the nature of the obstacle all play an important role in determining the outcome of the wavebreaks. In this particular model of HCM, the histopathology observed is reminiscent of the human disease. However, the expressed phenotype (e.g., sclerotic patches) is not of a severe enough magnitude to result in dramatic changes in the electrophysiological properties of the heart (i.e., to induce arrhythmias).

Limitations of the Technique

All of our recordings were from the epicardial surface of the heart. It has been calculated that the signal recorded during epifluorescence recordings is from a layer of cells 0.3 mm thick.[22] This is certainly thinner than the mouse ventricular wall. Therefore, the epicardial recordings mostly reveal surface phenomenon. This is an important limitation, because the majority of the structural alterations are in the midmyocardium and during transmural activation (e.g., sinus rhythm) their true impact on the wave front may be diminished at the surface. Another limitation of our study is that we used DAM to remove the electrical-mechanical interaction in the cardiac cells. DAM has been shown to abbreviate action potential duration in sheep ventricular muscle[23]; however, its effects on mouse ventricle have been less studied.

Acknowledgments: We would like to thank Dr. Steven Landas and Dr. Robert Schelper for their guidance and assistance with the histology and 3-dimensional reconstructions. We also thank Dr. Sergey Minorov for his assistance with the 3-dimensional computer reconstructions. Finally, we thank Ms. Fan Yang and Mr. Jiang Jiang for their technical assistance.

References

1. Clark CE, Henry WL, Epstein SE. Familial prevalence and genetic transmission of idiopathic hypertrophic subaortic stenosis. *N Engl J Med* 1973;289:709–714.
2. Maron BJ, Bonow RO, Cannon RO, et al. Hypertrophic cardiomyopathy. Interrelations of clinical manifestations, pathology, and therapy. Part one. *N Engl J Med* 1987;316:780–789.
3. Vikstrom KL, Factor SM, Leinwand LA. Mice expressing mutant myosin heavy chains are a model for familial hypertrophic cardiomyopathy. *Mol Med* 1996;2:556–567.
4. Fananapazir L, McAreavey D, Epstein ND. Hypertrophic cardiomyopathy. In Zipes DP, Jalife J (eds): *Cardiac Electrophysiology: From Cell to Bedside.* 2nd ed. Philadelphia: W.B. Saunders Co.; 1995:769–779.
5. Geisterfer-Lowrance AAT, Christer M, Conner D, et al. A mouse model of familial hypertrophic cardiomyopathy. *Science* 1996;272:731–734.
6. Vikstrom KL, Leinwand LA. Contractile protein mutations and heart disease. *Curr Opin Cell Biol* 1996;8:97–105.
7. Morley GM, Vaidya DM, Samie FH, et al. A characterization of conduction in the ventricles of normal and heterozygous Cx43 knockout mice using optical mapping. *J Cardiovasc Electrophysiol* 1999;10:1361–1375.

8. Vaidya D, Morley GE, Samie F, Jalife J. Reentry and fibrillation in the mouse heart: A challenge to the critical mass hypothesis. *Circ Res* 1999;85:174–181.
9. Neuman MR. Biopotential amplifiers. In Webster JG (ed): *Medical Instrumentation: Application and Design.* Boston: Houghton Mifflin Co.; 1978:273–335.
10. Gray RA, Jalife J, Panfilov A, et al. Nonstationary vortex like reentrant activity as a mechanism of polymorphic ventricular tachycardia in the isolated rabbit heart. *Circulation* 1995;91:2454–2469.
11. Berul CI, Christe ME, Aronovitz MJ, et al. Electrophysiological abnormalities and arrhythmias in alpha MHC mutant familial hypertrophic cardiomyopathy mice. *J Clin Invest* 1997;99:570–576.
12. Christensen G, Wang Y, Chien KR. Physiological assessment of complex cardiac phenotypes in genetically engineered mice. *Am J Physiol* 1997; 272:H2513–H2524.
13. James JF, Hewett TE, Robbins J. Cardiac physiology in transgenic mice. *Circ Res* 1998;82:407–415.
14. Cabo C, Pertsov AM, Davidenko JM, et al. Vortex shedding as a precursor of turbulent electrical activity in cardiac muscle. *Biophys J* 1996;70:1105–1111.
15. Tritton DJ. *Physical Fluid Dynamics.* Berkshire, England: Van Nostrand Reinhold; 1977:21–27.
16. Jalife J, Gray RA, Morley GE, Davidenko JM. Self-organization and dynamical nature of ventricular fibrillation. *Chaos* 1998;8:79–93.
17. Krinsky VI. Mathematical models of cardiac arrhythmias (spiral waves). *Pharmacol Ther* 1978;B3:539–555.
18. Nagy-Ungvarai Z, Pertsov AM, Hess B, Müller SC. Lateral instabilities of a wave front in the Ce-catalyzed Belousov-Zhabotinsky reaction. *Physica D* 1992;61:205–212.
19. Agladze K, Keener JP, Müller SC, Panfilov A. Rotating spiral waves created by geometry. *Science* 1994;264:1746–1748.
20. Starobin JM, Zilbeter YI, Rusnak EM, Starmer CF. Wavelet formation in excitable cardiac tissue: The role of wave front-obstacle interactions in initiating high-frequency fibrillatory-like arrhythmias. *Biophys J* 1996;70:581–594.
21. Pertsov AM, Panfilov AV, Medvedeva FU. Instability of autowaves in excitable media associated with the phenomenon of critical curvature. *Biofizica* 1983;28:100–102.
22. Knisley SB. Transmembrane voltage changes during unipolar stimulation of rabbit ventricle. *Circ Res* 1995;77:1229–1239.
23. Liu Y, Cabo C, Salomonsz R, et al. Effects of diacetyl monoxime on the electrical properties of sheep and guinea pig ventricular muscle. *Cardiovasc Res* 1993;27:1991–1997.

Chapter 17

Optical Mapping of Cardiac Arrhythmias:
Clinical Insights and Applications

Douglas L. Packer

Evolution of Activation Mapping

During the 1970s and 1980s, substantial progress was made in the development of activation mapping techniques. As a result, the general principles of reentry, expounded by Mines[1] and others,[2] and the concept of macroreentrant circuits, suggested by early evaluations of the Wolff-Parkinson-White Syndrome,[3] were confirmed. Subsequent studies by Moe,[4] Durrer and Roos,[5] Wellens et al.,[6] Gallagher et al.,[7] and others extended these observations into the clinical arena. While much of this early work demonstrated that anatomical obstacles such as cardiac valves or vein orifices and scars were critical for the occurrence of reentry, the subsequent studies of Allessie et al.[8] and others clearly elucidated the relevance of reentry around an area of functional block as an alternative mechanism of arrhythmogenesis (Fig. 1). Those studies further validated the concept of the wavelength and its dependence on conduction velocity and tissue refractoriness, ideas already proposed in the work of Mines.[1]

The subsequent technological revolution of solid state electronics, embodied within high-speed computers, has further enabled simultaneous mapping from hundreds of tissue sites, thus allowing a further resolution of the mechanisms underlying both reentrant and point source arrhythmias.[9–12] Among other things, these advancing technologies have demonstrated the relationship between underlying pathology and electrical components of reentrant circuits. For example, the facilitating role of a critical central slow zone of conduction in serious ventricular tachycardias[12–15] has been illuminated.

A variety of in vitro studies have also provided evidence for triggered automaticity in the form of both early and late afterdepolarizations[16–18] and enhanced automaticity as alternative, nonreentrant mechanisms of arrhythmias. In many studies, these rhythm abnormalities were related to underlying pathology, while in others pharmacological agents produced the abnormal automaticity. Subsequently, these observations generated

From Rosenbaum DS, Jalife J (eds): *Optical Mapping of Cardiac Excitation and Arrhythmias.*
©Futura Publishing Co., Inc., Armonk, NY, 2001.

Anatomic obstacle   Scarred myocardium   Functional block

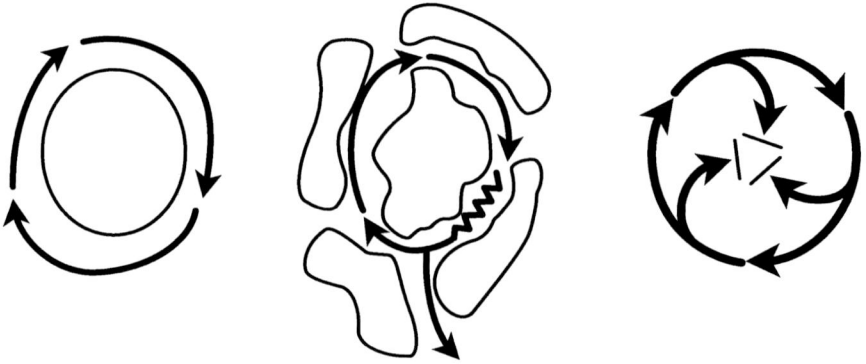

Figure 1. Candidate mechanisms of reentrant arrhythmias deduced from activation mapping. *Left:* Reentry around an anatomical obstacle. *Center:* Reentry around infarcted, scarred myocardium. *Right:* Reentry around a functional area of block.

from cellular and tissue level investigations have been extended to the intact heart, where in vivo and clinical investigations provided solid evidence for analogous electrophysiological processes. These techniques, however, have had several important limitations. First, even with multisite mapping, the quest for the additional understanding of arrhythmias was impeded by the limited number of available recording channels. This adversely limited recording site density and, therefore, the ability to spatially resolve a cardiac arrhythmia. Furthermore, multisite mapping techniques provided only indirect descriptions of repolarization of cardiac tissue. While the introduction of extrastimuli into sinus rhythm or various arrhythmias has revealed much about tissue refractoriness, this has fallen short of optimal analysis of the recovery of membrane potential, shown in a myriad of cellular studies to be critical for the understanding of that refractoriness and the occurrence of early or late afterdepolarizations. The interdependence of conduction and repolarization has thereby remained difficult to characterize. These limitations were responsible, in part, for the earlier notion that the properties of reentrant circuits were largely uniform,[19] even though recent studies have clearly demonstrated a dependence of impulse propagation on fiber orientation.[19–21] Despite these limitations, a substantial number of critical observations were, and continue to be, made with these methods.

Looking at the Cardiac Action Potential

In contrast to these approaches, the use of microelectrode techniques has been required for obtaining information about cellular recovery. Through this means of recording intracellular membrane potentials, the general voltage transitions occurring over the course of electrical activation and recovery have been chronicled. The nature of depolarization and its dependence on inward sodium current,[22] the restitution of excitability and its relationship to repolarization,[23] the interaction between ingoing

Na$^+$ currents and conduction velocity,[24–26] and the correlation of extra-cellular electrograms and the upstroke of the action potential seen on microelectrode recordings[27] have been established. The fundamental relationships between activation, recovery, and constituent intracellular and extracellular ion concentrations, as well as the modulation of transmembrane current by antiarrhythmic agents, have also been well studied.

While much information has been generated through these studies, microelectrode techniques have but a limited role in examining corresponding activation and recovery in the intact, beating heart. Maintaining an impalement during the cardiac cycle is difficult at best. Alternatively, means of generating surrogate monophasic action potentials in vivo[28] have been developed. Important correlations between electrical events and observations from single cell recording have been made in diverse areas from mechanoelectrical feedback[28–30] to the rate dependence of repolarization and remodeling of cellular electrophysiology in disease states. Unfortunately, the number of recordings that can be made simultaneously with this approach has been logistically constrained.

Development of Optical Mapping Techniques

At a time when electrophysiology had gazed nearly as far into the heart as available tools allowed, additional technologies have emerged that enable a substantially higher resolution look into the core of cardiac arrhythmias. Among the foremost is that of optical mapping techniques, which combine the strengths of activation and recovery mapping in a single, cohesive tool. The use of voltage-sensitive dyes, as originally developed by Cohen and coworkers,[31,32] has been further refined in the form of three fundamental imaging approaches using photodiodes,[33,34] laser scanning,[35] and the charged coupled device camera.[36–39] Each of these is founded on the principle that cardiac transmembrane potentials are reflected by the activity of the voltage-sensitive dye and its consistent response to a well-controlled, highly filtered light source. These techniques have been applied to examine membrane potentials as described in the chapters by Girouard and Rosenbaum (chapter 13),[40] Gray and Jalife (chapter 14),[41] and Baxter and Davidenko (chapter 15).[42] The relative merits of each of these approaches are also reviewed. This optical fingerprint can be recorded and analyzed in the form of effective action potentials from 100 to more than 100,000 epicardial sites. With this has come a substantial improvement in both spatial and temporal resolution of cardiac activation and recovery, as well as a straightforward analysis of the influences of recovery on the genesis and maintenance of cardiac arrhythmias. Once again, the advancement in techniques and technologies has allowed us to look further into the mechanisms responsible for arrhythmias.

What Do We Get for the Price of Technology?

Each of the chapters of this section reveals slightly different facets of optical mapping and the accompanying relevance to the clinician. As with the emergence of any other technology, it is important to take a step back for a critical look at its real utility in the clinical arena.

Understanding of Cardiac Electrophysiology

Theoretical and intact heart studies undertaken with these techniques more clearly elucidate underlying tachycardia mechanisms, and therefore provide an enhanced conceptual framework for considering arrhythmias in humans. For example, optical mapping studies have disclosed additional characteristics of reentrant wave fronts, "invisible" to the eye of activation mapping. Girouard and Rosenbaum,[40] using an essentially 2-dimensional guinea pig ventricle model of arrhythmias, elucidated the "dynamics" of reentry around an anatomical barrier. Specifically, their activation/recovery studies indicate that the wavelength is highly dependent on stimulation rate and propagation direction relative to cardiac fiber orientation. Moreover, these investigators show a substantial variance in the wavelength of a reentrant impulse as it transverses a reentrant pathway.

This is best understood in terms of excitability and "source-sink" relationships. The "source" can be viewed as the charge available in an advancing wave front that may contribute to activation of downstream tissue. The "sink" is the amount of charge or current required by a critical area of tissue to bring it to its propagation threshold. When "source" and "sink" currents are appropriately matched, impulse propagation continues. Girouard and Rosenbaum[40] further demonstrate that a source-sink mismatch occurs when a wave front advances across a transition from transverse to longitudinal orientation. In the setting of a limited available current at this pivot point, current spreads into parallel fibers with low longitudinal resistance (i.e., increased sink) (Fig. 2). The limited incoming current may be inadequate in the face of this rapid current drain, so conduction slows or stops. This process is reversed at points of transition from

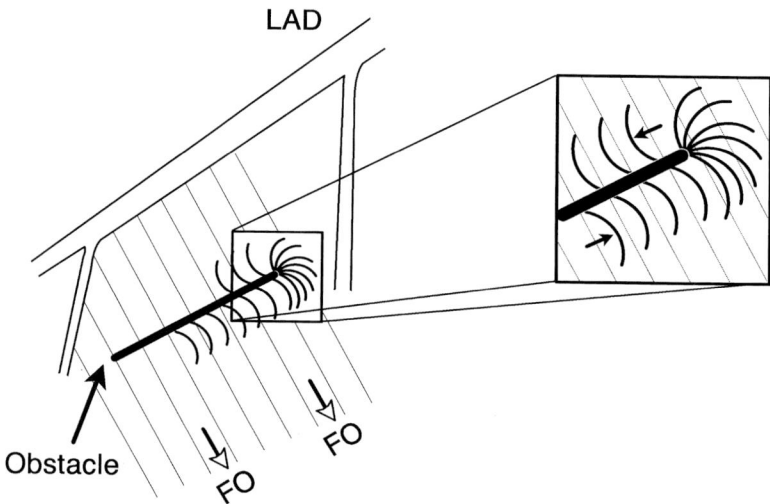

Figure 2. Impact of fiber orientation on occurrence of source-sink mismatches. *Left:* Consistent propagation transverse to fiber orientation with slowing at the pivot point. *Inset:* Increased curvature and increased sink as the wave front turns in the direction of fiber orientation, thus slowing or stopping conduction.

parallel to transverse fiber orientation and explains, in part, the marked variability of the wavelength during the course of one rotation around a reentrant pathway. The impact of fiber orientation on the excitable gap in a reentrant circuit is similarly explained. Furthermore, optical mapping studies help clarify the mechanism of initiation of some arrhythmias. For example, these findings indicate that the wavelength in an epicardial tissue zone increases substantially during slower sinus rhythm as a result of increases in recovery time. Since this precludes it from "fitting" into available tissue circuit dimensions, reentrant arrhythmias may not occur. The ability to record dynamic membrane potentials during the course of the cardiac cycle also provides a better understanding of the impact of action potential accommodation that occurs with changes in rate in the intact heart. An example of this is found in the modifications of recovery and conduction velocity that occur with an atrial or ventricular premature discharge. Here, a decrease in pacing or drive cycle length shortens tissue repolarization time and refractoriness, while premature stimuli introduced at progressively shorter coupling intervals result in greater conduction slowing (Fig. 3). Both lead to shorter possible induction wavelengths accompanied by higher arrhythmogenic propensity.[11,40]

Antiarrhythmic Drug Action

Optical mapping studies also demonstrate favorable mechanisms of action of antiarrhythmic drugs as they reverse wavelength adaptation or shortening during premature stimulation. Data from optical mapping studies show that the wavelength prolonging effect of sotalol is more than 3 times greater at the onset of tachycardia compared with that observed under steady-state tachycardia.[40] This exceptional manifestation of reverse use dependence in the intact heart provides a more solid mechanistic explanation

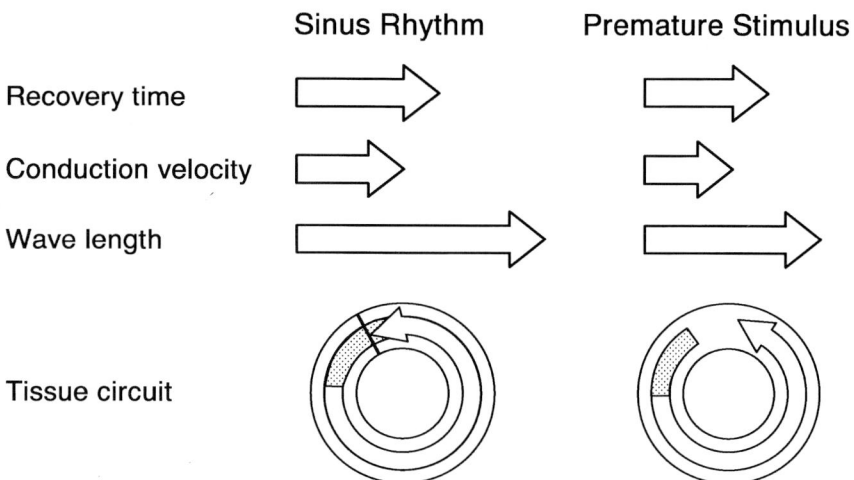

Figure 3. Alteration of tissue electrical properties with premature stimulation; the recovery time shortens as the conduction velocity slows. Together, these reduce the effective wavelength, allowing a candidate impulse to "fit" in a circuit tract.

for the preeminence of Class III drugs in general and of sotalol in specific in preventing ventricular tachycardia as seen in recent clinical trials.[43]

The enhanced resolution of optical mapping techniques presented in the chapters in this section also facilitates additional understanding of the nature of wave fronts in reentrant arrhythmia. As shown, a typical advancing wave front is curved, particularly toward the center or core around which that wave propagates.[37,41,42,44,45,46] This has several important implications. First, the "shape" of a resulting wave on the epicardial surface is that of a spiral rather than a flat leading edge. In three dimensions, the wave front takes on the appearance of a scroll. Furthermore, optical mapping studies demonstrate that the propagation velocity of such a spiral wave front is specifically related to its curvature.[41,42,46,47] Here, the greater the curvature of the wave front, the slower its propagation. Conversely, with more broad wave fronts, conduction velocity increases.

In the setting of a highly convex wave front,[47] however, an advancing source current may be so focused that available charge is insufficient for activating tissue both ahead and to the immediate sides of that convex wave front (Fig. 4). In contrast, a broad wave front has substantial more source current to bring to bear on activation in front of it. Since any area along the wave front is responsible for only a relatively small area of depolarization ahead of it, propagation continues.[47] Under certain circumstances, the source of current available during wave front propagation through a narrow neck of tissue and a resulting convex wave front may be inadequate to bring downstream tissue to threshold, and conduction may stop. This explanation can be invoked to explain anterograde block during sinus rhythm or decremental pacing in some accessory pathways.[47-49]

Insight into Clinical Arrhythmias

Optical mapping studies provide additional insight into the occurrence of clinically relevant arrhythmias. Although recent data clearly suggest that the cellular mechanism underlying torsade de pointes is the occurrence of early afterdepolarizations, this may only explain the initiation

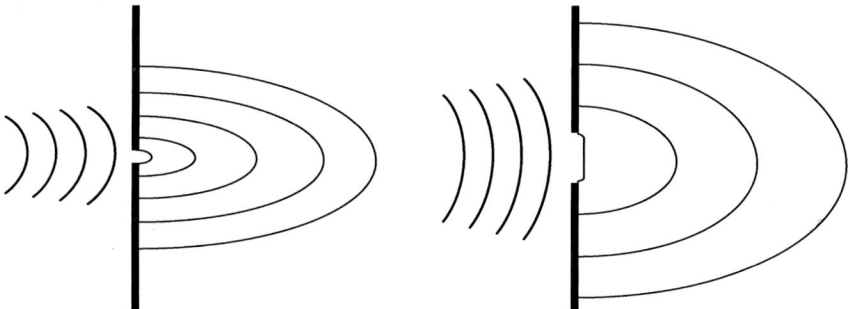

Figure 4. Impact of wave front curvature on tissue activation and conduction velocity. *Left:* Conduction through a narrow isthmus of tissue producing a convex wave front with resulting forward and side activation and conduction slowing. *Right:* Wide isthmus and broader wave front, adequate for continued wave conduction. Adapted from Cabo C, Pertsov AM, Baxter WT, et al. Wave-front curvature as a cause of slow conduction and block in isolated cardiac muscle. *Circ Res* 1994;75:1014-1028.

of this arrhythmia. Mechanisms of tachycardia *maintenance* and the actual twisting of the points have been unclear. Early studies[50] suggested that dueling focal trigger sites accounted for the polymorphic tachycardias seen in this arrhythmia. More recent work,[51,52] however, provides evidence that one or more drifting spiral waves may be a much more plausible explanation for the arrhythmia appearance, regardless of whether it occurs as a manifestation of drug-related proarrhythmia or as a spontaneously occurring event in a patient with a long QT syndrome.

Samie et al.[45] also provide evidence that underlying tissue pathology may be responsible, in part, for the multiplication of wave fronts and, thus, for polymorphic tachycardias seen in the setting of hypertrophic cardiomyopathies. In this case, advancing wave fronts may be broken up by structural abnormalities in the underlying tissue, again providing a clinically relevant explanation for the disproportionate member of variable ventricular tachycardias induced with programmed stimulation in this setting.[53] The concept of multiple or wandering rotors can also be extended to explain the activation patterns of ventricular fibrillation.[43,44] In contrast, the elucidation of spiral wave fronts through optical mapping further provides an explanation for the presence of clinical monomorphic tachycardias.[42] When rotating spirals occur singly, are stationary, or become anchored to an anatomical obstacle or to tissue sections, the ventricular arrhythmia appears monomorphic, as expected for epicardial breakthroughs from a specific, fixed location (Fig. 5).

In a somewhat analogous fashion, optical mapping studies have not only demonstrated the presence of multiple spiral wave fronts in the fibrillating atria, but have also extended previous observations generated with standard activation mapping[8] to provide reasons for the inherent frac-

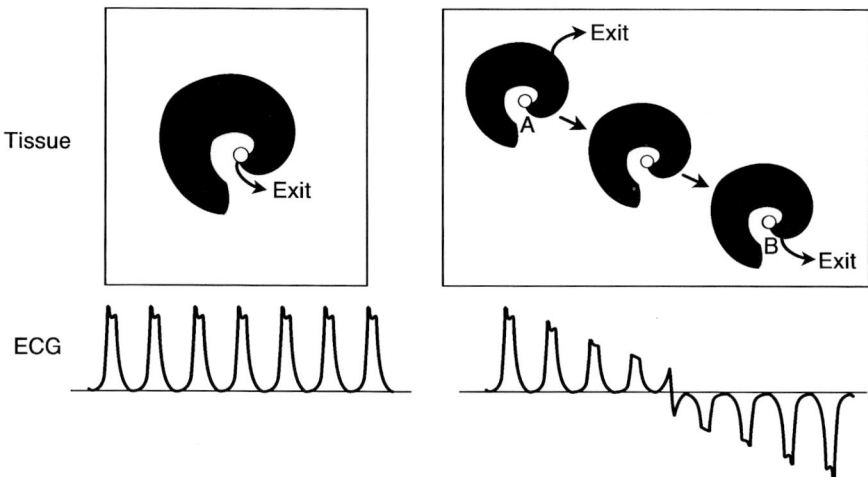

Figure 5. Result of an anchoring or wandering core on underlying arrhythmia morphology. *Left:* Fixed or anchored spiral core with constant QRS morphology on an electrocardiogram. *Right:* Core that wanders from site A to site B. The resulting shift in exit could result in a shift from one QRS morphology through a transition zone to an alternate QRS waveform.

tionation of propagation. Studies by several investigators[54,55] have shown the dependence of conduction, block, and refractoriness on the direction of propagation via pectinate muscle bundles originating near the crista terminalis. This is, once again, an elucidation of the structure/activity dependence of atrial fibrillation.[56] Finally, optical mapping studies have also provided insight into the mechanism of maintenance of atrial fibrillation by a single high-frequency source localized in the left atrium.[57,58]

Limitations

Importantly, there are limitations of these techniques that preclude their clinical application. The greatest of these is the absence of clear-cut "optical windows" through which voltage-sensitive events can be visualized in the beating heart. Motion artifact and accompanying noise, which also affect optical recording, must be resolved. Furthermore, given their potential cardiotoxicity, it is not possible to use the same voltage-sensitive dyes in the living organism as are used in experimental studies. Until recently, most optical recordings were also limited to those obtained at the epicardial surface. Several investigators have since developed tissue wedge recording methods that allow a "full thickness" look at myocardial activation and repolarization. Obviously, this approach is not possible in humans. Additional technological developments will therefore be required before this technique will provide direct mechanistic insight in patients. Until then, alternative methodologies will be required for a more direct examination of full thickness, multisite repolarization in the intact heart.

Fortunately, other mapping modalities have already provided new insights into the dynamics of membrane potentials on the endocardial surface. Noncontact mapping systems[59,60] can now generate isopotential maps of activation and recovery throughout the cardiac cycle. While the majority of resulting data are generated from electrical activation, by manipulating the recording threshold, a beginning glimpse into recovery may also be possible. It is likely that in the future alternative methodologies might enable an "optical" approach in patients. Other inherent fluorescent activities or voltage-dependent tissue changes might someday be visible with alternative scanning technologies such as ultrasound. For example, as described by Witkowski et al.,[44] the recent demonstration of naturally occurring fluorescence has already been harnessed to facilitate an optical evaluation of the process of gene expression in living cells.

Given the potential wealth of information available through such investigations, additional work in this general area will hopefully unleash other potent mapping capabilities in humans. Until then, we will continue to benefit from the advanced insights from in vitro and in vivo efforts such as those described in this section.

References

1. Mines GR. On circulation excitation on heart muscles and their possible relation to tachycardia and fibrillation. *Trans R Soc Can* 1914;3:43.
2. Mayer AG. *Rhythmical Pulsation in Scyphomedusae.* Washington, DC: Carnegie Institution of Washington, Publication 47. 1906.

3. Wolferth CC, Wood FC. The mechanism of production of short P-R intervals and prolonged QRS complexes in patients with presumably undamaged hearts: Hypothesis of an accessory pathway of auriculo-ventricular conduction (bundle of Kent). *Am Heart J* 1933;8:297–311.
4. Moe GK. On the multiple wavelet hypothesis of atrial fibrillation. *Arch Int Pharmacodyn Ther* 1962;140:183–188.
5. Durrer D, Roos JP. Epicardial excitation of the ventricles in a patient with W-P-W syndrome (type B). *Circulation* 1967;35:15–21.
6. Wellens HJJ, Schuilenberg RM, Durrer D. Electrical stimulation of the heart in patients with W-P-W syndrome, type A. *Circulation* 1971;43:99–114.
7. Gallagher JJ, Prichett ELC, Sealy WC, et al. The preexcitation syndromes. *Prog Cardiovasc Dis* 1978;20(4):285–327.
8. Allessie MA, Bonke FIM, Schopman FJG. Circus movement in rabbit atrial muscle as a mechanism of tachycardia. III. The "Leading Circle" Concept: A new model of circus movement in cardiac tissue without the involvement of an anatomical obstacle. *Circulation* 1977;41:9–18.
9. Frazier DW, Wolf PD, Wharton JM, et al. Stimulus-induced critical point: Mechanism for electrical initiation of reentry in the normal canine myocardium. *J Clin Invest* 1989;83:1039–1052.
10. Chen PS, Wolf PD, Dixon EG, et al. Mechanism of ventricular vulnerability to single premature stimuli in open-chest dogs. *Circ Res* 1988;62:1191–1209.
11. Smeets JL, Allessie MA, Lammers WJ, et al. The wavelength of the cardiac impulse and reentrant arrhythmias in isolated rabbit atrium. The role of heart rate, autonomic transmitters, temperature, and potassium. *Circ Res* 1986;58:96–108.
12. El-Sherif N, Smith RA, Evans K. Canine ventricular arrhythmias in the late myocardial infarction. 8. Epicardial mapping of reentrant circuits. *Circ Res* 1981;49:255–265.
13. Mehra R, Zieler RH, Gough WB, El-Sherif N. Reentrant ventricular arrhythmias in the late myocardial infarction. 9. Electrophysiologic-anatomic correlation of reentrant circuits. *Circulation* 1983;67:11–24.
14. Kienzle MG, Miller J, Falcone RA, et al. Intraoperative endocardial mapping during sinus rhythm: Relationship to site of origin of ventricular tachycardia. *Circulation* 1984;70:957–965.
15. Stevenson WG, Khan H, Sager P, et al. Identification of reentry circuit sites during catheter mapping and radiofrequency ablation of ventricular tachycardia late after myocardial infarction. *Circulation* 1993;88:1647–1670.
16. Jackman WM, Friday KJ, Anderson JL, et al. The long QT syndromes: A critical review, new clinical observations and a unifying hypothesis. *Prog Cardiovasc Dis* 1988;31;115–172.
17. Rosen MR. Cellular electrophysiology of digitalis toxicity. *J Am Coll Cardiol* 1985;5:22A-34A.
18. January CT, Riddel JM. Early after depolarizations. Mechanisms of induction and block. A role for L-type Ca^{++} current. *Circ Res* 1989;64:977–990.
19. Spach MS, Miller WT Jr, Geselowitz DB, et al. The discontinuous nature of propagation in normal canine cardiac muscle: Evidence for recurrent discontinuities of intracellular resistance that affect the membrane currents. *Circ Res* 1981;48:39–54.
20. Kadish AH, Spear JF, Levine JH, Moore EN. The effects of procainamide on conduction in anisotropic canine ventricular myocardium. *Circulation* 1986;74:616–625.
21. Girouard SD, Pastore JM, Laurita KR, et al. Optical mapping in a new guinea pig model of ventricular tachycardia reveals mechanisms for multiple wavelengths in a single reentrant circuit. *Circulation* 1993;93:603–913.
22. Weidmann S. Effects of calcium ions and local anesthetics on electrical properties of Purkinje fibers. *J Physiol (Lond)* 1955;129:568–582.

23. Boyett MR, Jewell BR. A study of the factors responsible for rate-dependent shortening of the action potential in mammalian ventricular muscle. *J Physiol (Lond)* 1978;285:359–380.

24. Hodgkin AL, Rushton WAH. The electrical constants of a crustacean nerve fiber. *Proc R Soc Lond B Biol Sci* 1946;133:444–479.

25. Walton MK, Fozzard HA. The conducted action potential: Models and comparison to experiments. *Biophys J* 1983;44:9–26.

26. Packer DL, Grant AO, Strauss HC, Starmer FC. Characterization of concentration- and use-dependent effects of quinidine from conduction delay and declining conduction velocity in canine Purkinje fibers. *J Clin Invest* 1989;83:2109–2119.

27. Spach MS, Miller WT, Miller-Jones E, et al. Extracellular potentials related to intracellular action potentials during impulse conduction in anisotropic canine cardiac muscle. *Circ Res* 1979;45:188–204.

28. Franz MR, Cima R, Wang D, et al. Electrophysiological effects of myocardial stretch and mechanism determinants of stretch-activated arrhythmias. *Circulation* 1992;86:968–978.

29. Lab MJ. Mechanoelectric feedback (transduction) in heart: Concepts and implications. *Cardiovasc Res* 1996;32:3–14.

30. Hansen DE, Craig CS, Hondeghem LM. Stretch-induced arrhythmias in the isolated canine ventricle: Evidence for the importance of mechanoelectrical feedback. *Circulation* 1990;81(3):1094–1105.

31. Cohen LB, Salzberg BM, Davila HV, et al. Changes in axon fluorescence during activity: Molecular probes of membrane potential. *J Membr Biol* 1974;19:1–36.

32. Cohen LB, Lesher S. Optical monitoring of membrane potential: Methods of multi-site optical measurement. In De Weer P, Salzberg MB (eds): *Optical Methods in Cell Physiology*. New York: Wiley-Interscience; 1986:71–99.

33. Efimov IR, Huang DT, Rendt JM, Salama G. Optical mapping of repolarization and refractionist from intact hearts. *Circulation* 1994;90:1469–1480.

34. Laurita KR, Girouard SD, Rosenbaum DS. Modulation of ventricular repolarization by a premature stimulus. Role of epicardial dispersion of repolarization kinetics demonstrated by optical mapping of the intact guinea pig heart. *Circ Res* 1996;79:493–503.

35. Dillon S, Morad M. A new laser scanning system for measuring action potential propagation in the heart. *Science* 1981;214:453–456.

36. Davidenko J, Pertsov A, Salomonsz R, et al. Stationary and drifting spiral waves of excitation in isolated cardiac muscle. *Nature* 1992;355:349–351.

37. Wikswo J, Lin S, Abbas R. Virtual electrodes in cardiac tissue. A common mechanism for anodal and cathodal stimulation. *Biophys J* 1995;69:2195–2210.

38. Witkowski F, Leon L, Penkoske P, et al. Spatiotemporal evolution of ventricular fibrillation. *Nature* 1998;392:78–82.

39. Nassif G, Dillon S, Wit A. Video mapping of cardiac activation. *J Mol Cell Cardiol* 1990;22(suppl IV):S44.

40. Girouard S, Rosenbaum DS. Mapping arrhythmia substrates related to repolarization: 2. Cardiac wavelength. In Rosenbaum DS, Jalife J (eds): *Optical Mapping of Cardiac Excitation and Arrhythmias.*. Armonk, NY: Futura Publishing Co., Inc.; 2001:227–243.

41. Gray RA, Jalife J. Video imaging of cardiac fibrillation. In Rosenbaum DS, Jalife J (eds): *Optical Mapping of Cardiac Excitation and Arrhythmias*. Armonk, NY: Futura Publishing Co., Inc.; 2001:245–264.

42. Baxter WT, Davidenko JM. Video mapping of spiral waves in the heart. In Rosenbaum DS, Jalife J (eds): *Optical Mapping of Cardiac Excitation and Arrhythmias*. Armonk, NY: Futura Publishing Co., Inc.; 2001:265–280.

43. Mason JW. A comparison of electrophysiologic testing with Holter monitoring

to predict antiarrhythmic-drug efficacy for ventricular tachyarrhythmias. *N Engl J Med* 1993;329:445–451.

44. Witkowski FX, Penkoske PA, Leon LJ. Optimization of temporal filtering for optical transmembrane potential signals. In Rosenbaum DS, Jalife J (eds): *Optical Mapping of Cardiac Excitation and Arrhythmias.* Armonk, NY: Futura Publishing Co., Inc.; 2001:79–92.

45. Samie F, Morley GE, Vaidya D, et al. Video imaging of wave propagation in a transgenic mouse model of cardiomyopathy. In Rosenbaum DS, Jalife J (eds): *Optical Mapping of Cardiac Excitation and Arrhythmias.* Armonk, NY: Futura Publishing Co., Inc.; 2001:281–293.

46. Pertsov A, Davidenko JM, Salomonsz R, et al. Spiral waves of excitation underlie reentrant activity in isolated cardiac muscle. *Circ Res* 1993;72:631–650.

47. Cabo C, Pertsov AM, Baxter WT, et al. Wave-front curvature as a cause of slow conduction and block in isolated cardiac muscle. *Circ Res* 1994;75:1014–1028.

48. De La Fuente D, Sasyniuk B, Mol GK. Conduction through a narrow isthmus in isolated canine atrial tissue: Model of the W-P-W syndrome. *Circulation* 1991;44:803–809.

49. Inoue H, Zipes DP. Conduction over an isthmus over an atrial myocardium in vivo: A possible model of W-P-W syndrome. *Circulation* 1987;76:637–647.

50. Bardy GH, Ungerleider RM, Smith WM, Ideker RE. A mechanism of torsades de pointes in a canine model. *Circulation* 1983;67:52–59.

51. Asano Y, Davidenko JM, Baxter WT, et al. Optical mapping of drug-induced polymorphic arrhythmias and torsade de pointes in the isolated rabbit heart. *J Am Coll Cardiol* 1997;29:831–842.

52. El-Sherif N, Chinushi M, Caref EB, Restivo M. Electrophysiological mechanism of the characteristic electrocardiographic morphology of torsades de pointes tachyarrhythmias in the long-QT syndrome: Detailed analysis of ventricular tridimensional activation patterns. *Circulation* 1997;96:4392–4399.

53. Fananapazir L, Chang AC, Epstein SE, McAreavey D. Prognostic determinates in hypertrophic cardiomyopathy. Prospective evaluation of a therapeutic strategy based on clinical, Holter, hemodynamic, and electrophysiologic findings. *Circulation* 1992;86:730–740.

54. Wu TJ, Yashima M, Xie F, et al. Role of pectinate muscle bundles in the generation and maintenance of intra-atrial reentry: Potential implications for the mechanism of conversion between atrial fibrillation and atrial flutter. *Circ Res* 1998;83:448–462.

55. Gray RA, Pertsov AM, Jalife J. Incomplete reentry and epicardial breakthrough patterns in the sheep heart. *Circulation* 1996;94:2649–2661.

56. Jalife J, Berenfeld O, Skanes A, Mandapati R. Mechanisms of atrial fibrillation: Mother rotors or multiple daughter wavelets, or both? *J Cardiovasc Electrophysiol* 1998;9:S2-S12.

57. Skanes AC, Mandapati R, Berenfeld O, et al. Spatiotemporal periodicity during atrial fibrillation in the isolated sheep heart. *Circulation* 1998;98:1236–1248.

58. Mandapati R, Skanes A, Chen J, et al. Stable microreentrant sources as a mechanism of atrial fibrillation in the isolated sheep heart. *Circulation* 2000; 101:194–199.

59. Schilling RJ, Peters NS, Davies DW. Simultaneous endocardial mapping in the human left ventricle using a non-contact catheter: Comparison of contact and reconstructed electrograms during sinus rhythm. *Circulation* 1998;98:887–898.

60. Peters NS, Jackman WM, Schilling RJ, et al. Images in cardiovascular medicine. Human left ventricular endocardial activation mapping using the novel non-contact catheter. *Circulation* 1997;95:1658–1660.

Section IV

Cardiac Defibrillation

Introduction:

Unique Role of Optical Mapping in the Study of Cardiac Defibrillation

José Jalife

Sudden cardiac death continues to occur at a perturbing rate in the United States. Recent estimates indicate that as many as 400,000 individuals die each year as victims of sudden cardiac death.[1] Studies on out-of-hospital collapse suggest that the initial rhythm observed in a victim of sudden cardiac death depends on the time elapsed from loss of consciousness to the first electrocardiogram (ECG). If that time is less than 4 minutes, ventricular fibrillation (VF) accounts for 95% of cases.[2] In these cases, early electrical defibrillation may be life saving. Defibrillation is the application of high-energy electrical shocks to stop hemodynamically dangerous ventricular arrhythmias, thereby allowing restoration of a cardiac rhythm that enables adequate ventricular contraction and, thus, perfusion of vital organs. Although the mechanism underlying defibrillation remains unclear, it is clear that effective VF termination by an electrical shock requires stimulation of myocytes by passing an adequate amount of current through them for an adequate period of time.[3] The relationship between the extracellular potential gradient distribution and the transmembrane potential has been the subject of much research for a number of years and recently optical techniques have come to occupy a central role in the quantitative study of that relationship.

Section IV of this text deals with the understanding, from the cellular to the organ level, of the manner in which high-energy shocks defibrillate or fail to defibrillate the heart. In chapter 18, Tung provides a detailed description of the use of voltage-sensitive dyes and a variety of optical detection systems to quantify the transmembrane potential response to externally applied electrical fields in single cardiac myocytes and cellular networks. In multicellular preparations, he demonstrates how the response differs depending on whether it is measured close to or far from the stimulating electrode. He illustrates also how virtual electrode effects arising from the underlying fiber structure of the tissue near the electrode lead to responses of opposite polarities. On the other hand, virtual sources may form far from the electrode at borders of strands or bundles of myocytes, or around cleft spaces. His experiments in single cells show that the transmembrane response has two components: one is fast and linear and the other, which is much slower, is nonlinear and dictated by changes in the active membrane currents. In chapter 19, Lin and Wikswo delineate for the reader their extensive theoretical and experimental results demonstrating the relevance of the bidomain model to the understanding of the response of cardiac tissues to large shocks. They also summarize far-reaching theoretical work using the bidomain model to make quantitative predictions that were later confirmed experimentally, and argue in favor of the use of that model as a realistic approach to link the molecular spatial scale associated with ion channel behavior to the macroscopic scale of the electrical behavior of the intact heart. In this regard, they demonstrate how epifluorescence imaging of the transmembrane potential has allowed wide recognition of the role of virtual cathodes and virtual anodes, and hence the importance of the complexity introduced by the unequal anisotropies of intra- and extracellular spaces to cardiac defibrillation, as well as the validation of the theoretical prediction of the formation of that unique pattern of quatrefoil reentry.[4]

In chapter 20, Knisley presents a study on the application of photodiode array (PDA) technology to the understanding of the mechanisms of cardiac defibrillation. He summarizes work accomplished in his laboratory during the last 10 years, using optical methods to test conjectures related to transmembrane voltage changes induced by electrical fields in isolated cardiac cells and whole hearts. With regard to the latter, he pays particular attention to the influence of fiber structure on the tissue response to electrical stimulation using unipolar point and line stimulation. His results and those from other laboratories lead him to propose that line stimulation may be more advantageous for defibrillation or other electrical antiarrhythmic therapy than point stimulation. On the one hand, previous results demonstrate that much more current can be delivered from a line electrode than from a point electrode. In addition, he argues, the change in membrane potential sign in the epicardium on either side of a line electrode can be made more uniform by orienting the electrode parallel to fibers, which might reduce the heterogeneous response of the ion channels to defibrillation shocks. Finally, he speculates that line stimulation may help to block activation fronts of fibrillation by producing a region of absolutely refractoriness and, thus, effectively stopping fibrillation. These ideas are interesting and deserve future experimentation. In chapter 21 Dillon also addresses the mechanisms of defibrillation as viewed by a series of laser scanning experiments, in which he mapped the spread of propagated electrical activation before, during, and after shocks applied to a fibrillating rabbit heart. He dedicates the first half of his chapter to describing why laser scanning was developed and how it works. He then looks at defibrillation as a reentrant rather than focal arrhythmia analyzed in terms of the "critical mass" hypothesis[5,6] or his more recently postulated "progressive depolarization" hypothesis,[7] as an extension of the "upper limit of vulnerability" hypothesis of defibrillation.[8] In fact, based on his optical mapping results, he postulates that the experimental data supporting the latter hypothesis could instead be interpreted in a manner consistent with the critical mass hypothesis. His progressive depolarization hypothesis uses traditional defibrillation concepts and takes advantage of what has been learned from optical mapping studies of defibrillation to explain defibrillation and shock-induced fibrillation.

Optical mapping has opened new windows of opportunity to answer a number of questions regarding the mechanisms of cardiac defibrillation. It is helping to address a number of fundamental questions regarding the effect of the extracellular electrical field produced by a shock on the transmembrane potential and what is the basis for the different effectiveness of shocks having different waveforms. In chapter 22, Efimov and Cheng present results derived from PDA experiments analyzing the role of virtual electrode-induced wave fronts and phase singularities in the mechanisms of success and failure of internal defibrillation. They nicely illustrate the manner in which monophasic shocks produce virtual electrode polarizations consisting of complex spatially and temporally distributed transmembrane potential changes, with large areas of positive and negative polarization. They show also that the second phase of a biphasic shock can lead to nonlinear reversal of virtual electrode polarization produced by the first phase. Importantly, they demonstrate that optimal biphasic defibrillation wave forms produce the most homogeneous polarization in the absence of virtual electrode formation, which is strongly influenced by the electrical and structural characteristics of the myocardium and the interface between the heart and other elements of the tissue bath in which the heart is immersed. They then focus on the role of spatial virtual electrode polarization gradients in the initiation of new activation wave fronts and the manner in which virtual electrodes may result in phase singularities, with consequent initiation of reentrant arrhythmias and failure to defibrillate.

In the closing chapter, chapter 24, Zipes wears his clinician's hat to discuss in his characteristic articulate way the reasons why we apply electricity to the heart as well as future clinical implications of cardiac defibrillation. He eloquently argues in favor of radiofrequency ablation as a revolution in the "cure" of patients suffering a wide variety of supraventricular tachyarrhythmias, and sees ablation as the next frontier in the treatment of atrial fibrillation. He reminds us that while pacing is an effective treatment for bradyarrhythmias, no major breakthroughs have occurred since the first ventricular pacemaker was introduced 50 years ago. Similarly, external defibrillation has seen important technical improvements over the last 25 years but no major scientific changes since it was first successfully applied in the clinic. On the other hand, Zipes sees the implantable defibrillator as truly revolutionary because of its unprecedented impact on patient survival and on the practice medicine. In his view, to develop new generation implantable defibrillator systems that are smaller, more reliable, longer lasting, and less painful for the patient, it will be essential to gain knowledge of mechanisms of fibrillation and defibrillation. Yet Zipes wonders what the ultimate gain will be, given the fact that less than 1% of patients with an implantable cardioverter defibrillator die suddenly every year.

After reviewing the three major ventricular defibrillation hypotheses (i.e., critical mass; upper limit of vulnerability, and progressive depolarization), as well as the mechanisms of defibrillation and how the bidomain model and the concept of virtual electrode have enhanced our understanding of how the heart responds to external electrical fields, Zipes reminds us that, in the final analysis, the most clinically relevant issue today is what causes fibrillation to start. He hypothesizes that sudden cardiac death results from an interaction between a transient trigger, often provided by the autonomic nervous system, and a remodeled, receptive myocardial substrate. Under the right conditions, that interaction may lead to reentry, abnormal automaticity, or triggered activity, to result in a ventricular tachyarrhythmia and ultimately sudden cardiac death. Thus, he recommends that major research initiatives over the next 10 years should be directed toward the understanding of the mechanisms of spontaneous initiation of arrhythmias.

References

1. Zipes DP, Wellens HJ. Sudden cardiac death. *Circulation* 1998;98:2334–2351.
2. Poole JE, Bardy GH. Sudden cardiac death. In Zipes DP, Jalife J (eds): *Cardiac Electrophysiology. From Cell to Bedside.* 3rd ed. Philadelphia: W.B. Saunders Co.; 2000:615–640.
3. Ideker RE, Wolf PD, Tang ASL. Mechanisms of defibrillation. In Tacker WA Jr. (ed): *Defibrillation of the Heart.* St Louis: Mosby; 1994:15–45.
4. Lin S-F, Roth BJ, Wikswo JP. Quatrefoil reentry in myocardium: An optical imaging study of the induction mechanism. *J Cardiovasc Electrophysiol* 1999;10:574–586.
5. Garrey WE. The nature of fibrillatory contraction of the heart. Its relation to tissue mass and form. *Am J Physiol* 1914;33:397–414.
6. Zipes DP, Fischer J, King RM, et al. Termination of ventricular fibrillation in dogs by depolarizing a critical amount of myocardium. *Am J Cardiol* 1975;36:37–44.
7. Chen PS, Shibata N, Dixon EG, et al. Comparison of the defibrillation threshold and the upper limit of ventricular vulnerability. *Circulation* 1986;73:1022–1028.
8. Dillon SM, Kwaku KF. Progressive depolarization: A unified hypothesis for defibrillation and fibrillation induction by shocks. *J Cardiovasc Electrophysiol* 1998;9:529–552.

Chapter 18

Response of Cardiac Myocytes to Electrical Fields

Leslie Tung

Introduction

Electrical fields and their associated currents are applied to the heart for therapeutic purposes in the clinical setting of pacemaking, cardioversion, defibrillation, and ablation.[1] The region of tissue targeted by the current may in some cases be highly localized (e.g., with pacemaking or electrical ablation) or in other cases global in extent (e.g., with defibrillation). The interaction of the local electrical field with the cardiac cell membrane is a fundamental link in the biophysical mechanisms underlying each of the therapeutic modalities. The interaction may be of many types, since in some cases cells respond to high-intensity nonuniform fields that are near the electrodes, while in other cases cells respond to low-intensity uniform fields in the bulk of the myocardium. Not only may the fields invoke direct (passive) electrical responses in the cell membranes, but other biophysical mechanisms may be triggered as well, such as the activation of active membrane ionic currents or massive changes in membrane permeability such as electroporation. In this chapter, we review the use of voltage-sensitive dyes to quantify the effect of externally applied electrical fields on the transmembrane potential of cardiac cells, both in isolation and as components of a cellular network in tissue.

Numerous questions arise in the context of the coupling between applied electrical field and cellular transmembrane potential, including: 1) Is the coupling process the same close to and far from the electrodes? 2) What role, if any, does the hierarchical arrangement of cells in the tissue structure play in the response of the cell membrane voltage? 3) Does the field invoke linear responses in the cell membrane? 4) How does the presence of active membrane currents through ionic channels and transporters in the cell membrane modify the transmembrane response? Insights into the answers to these questions can be gained from theoretical studies, which are detailed in large part in other chapters of this book, and some of which are briefly summarized below.

This work was supported by NIH grant HL48266.
From Rosenbaum DS, Jalife J (eds): *Optical Mapping of Cardiac Excitation and Arrhythmias.*
©Futura Publishing Co., Inc., Armonk, NY, 2001.

Passive tissue models are highly specific in their predictions of certain behavior. First, large amplitude changes in transmembrane potential are expected to occur in regions near the electrodes and at tissue boundaries as a result of the redistribution of current from the extracellular space into parallel extracellular and intracellular pathways for current flow.[2] Second, the diffusion of charge in the tissue away from the electrode should result in a time-dependent behavior of the transmembrane potential response.[3] Third, complex polarization patterns can arise owing to unequal anisotropy of the intracellular and extracellular domains of the tissue[4–6] or to discontinuities in intracellular resistance at gap junctions.[7,8] Fourth, the responses of transmembrane potential should be symmetric and should reverse symmetrically in polarity with reversals in field direction. Finally, active cellular[9–11] and tissue models[12] have shown that, following the initial polarization of the tissue produced by the applied field, ionic currents become activated or inactivated, resulting in further time-dependent behavior during the field pulse.

The many predictions of the theoretical work cited above concerning the coupling between applied electrical field and cellular transmembrane potential can be tested experimentally through the use of voltage-sensitive indicator dyes, which act as linear sensors of transmembrane potential in cardiac cells.[13] Unlike microelectrode recordings, which are sensitive to electrical artifacts during a stimulus pulse,[14] optical recordings of transmembrane potential (the electro-optical signal) are immune to these artifacts.[15] Furthermore, spatial variations in transmembrane potential can occur at subcellular length scales, which microelectrodes are unable to detect. Hence, the use of voltage-sensitive dyes is essential for the accurate recording of transmembrane potential responses during the application of electrical fields. The insensitivity of optoelectrical recordings to electrical interference has been exploited further in studies of cellular transmembrane potential responses to radiofrequency fields during electrical ablation.[16] The disadvantage in the usage of these dyes is that absolute potentials cannot be measured, so to circumvent this difficulty, the change in the optical signal for a known or estimated change in transmembrane potential (such as the amplitude of the action potential) is often used as a calibration signal.

Examples of electro-optical recordings of cellular responses to field stimulation are presented in this chapter. The discussion is divided into two parts: those for cells as members of a tissue or cellular network, and those for cells in isolation. These data provide important information regarding the coupling processes that are involved, and lend insight into the basic mechanisms of cellular responses to electrical fields that have been delineated by theoretical studies. The recordings are obtained by a variety of optical detection systems, which are described as encountered throughout this chapter.

Tissue Responses of Cells

The responses of cells within their tissue matrix to applied electrical fields are determined not only by their intrinsic responses to the fields as described in the next section, but also by cell-to-cell coupling via gap-junctional channels and the underlying tissue structure. Investigators interested in the mechanisms of cardiac responses to applied electrical fields have tended to partition the effects of electrical stimuli into sets of asymptotic behaviors. Examples include the "global" and "local" length scales of tissue responses,[17] "continuous" and "discrete" mechanisms for stimulation,[18] "near-field" and "far-field" responses in terms of distance from the stimulating electrode,[19] "primary" and "secondary" sources of transmembrane current,[7,20] and "surface" and "bulk" polarizations of the tissue.[21] Sobie and coworkers[22] have defined a "generalized activating function" that helps to unify much of the previous work under a single formalism by which the effects of a stimulus can be determined. The consequences of this function are discussed in the next section of this chapter.

Virtual Electrodes

The concept of virtual electrodes can be found in the work of Hoshi and Matsuda.[23] More recently it has been shown, based on the concept of the generalized activating function, that the transmembrane potential V_m responds to applied fields in two ways, one from the strength of the local electrical field E and the other from the spatial gradient of the local electrical field ∇E[22]:

$$\Delta V_m \sim aE + b\nabla E \qquad (1)$$

The notation ΔV_m is used here to indicate the change in V_m that occurs in response to the applied field. aE represents a virtual (Type I) source with strength equal to E, weighted by a, which is a function of the gradient in intracellular conductivity. $b\nabla E$ represents a virtual (Type II) source with strength proportional to ∇E, weighted by b, which is a function of the magnitude of intracellular conductivity. Therefore, the weighting functions a and b depend on the local tissue architecture. It should be noted that the description of equation 1 for virtual sources assumes that cardiac tissue behaves with the unique electrical properties of the so-called bidomain.[24]

Various aspects of the magnitude and polarity of tissue responses to virtual electrodes have been documented experimentally, as described in the following sections of this chapter.

The "Optrode"

To measure electro-optical responses in tissue, investigators have used a variety of methods, including photodiode arrays (PDAs), fiberoptic bundles, laser scanning systems, and charge coupled device (CCD) cameras. A different approach consisting of an "optrode"[25] is illustrated in Figure 1A. In brief, the optrode (a term borrowed from chemical sensors) consists of a single glass optical fiber, the tip of which acts as an exploring optoelectrode and which can be positioned with a micromanipulator. The other end of the optical fiber is coupled via a wavelength-dependent

A

Upper view

Beamsplitter

Green HeNe Laser

Interference filter

Multimode optical fiber

Light tight box

Optical fiber coupler

Dichroic mirror

Long pass filter

Photodetector

To signal data acquisition and processing

Front view

Micropositioner

Metal slab

Inner tube

Table

Heart

Micropositioner for optical fiber

Suction

Bath of Ringer's solution

B

electrolyte

current

optical fiber

glass tube

HEART SURFACE

C

d e f g h

c b a i

j

D

Hypodermic Needle

Optical Fiber

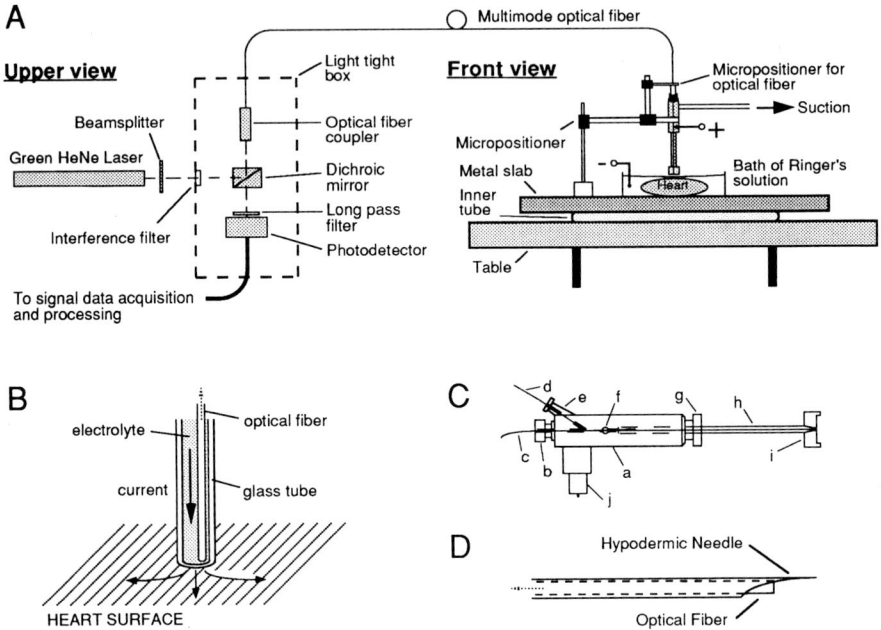

Figure 1. Optrode set-up. **A.** Schematic diagram. The output of a green He-Ne laser is reflected by a 580-nm dichroic mirror and coupled via a 20×, 0.4 numerical aperture fiberoptic coupler to the opposite end of the optical fiber. The power emitted from the fiber tip is 0.44 mW. The red fluorescence emitted by the dye is collected by the same fiber and routed back through the dichroic mirror and through a pair of 570-nm long-pass filters to a low-noise photodiode and transimpedance amplifier. The overall bandwidth of the electro-optical signal is 3 kHz. Modified from reference 25. **B.** Placement of optrode within an electrolyte-filled glass capillary tube used as an electrode. **C.** Suction cap added to tip of optrode to allow for mechanical stabilization of the optical fiber against the tissue and reduction of motion artifacts. The diagram shows a modified microelectrode holder (a) with a BNC mount (j). The airtight holes (b, e, g) are used to introduce the optical fiber (c), the stimulating Ag-AgCl electrode (d), and the glass pipette (h), respectively. A fourth hole (f) permits suction to be applied to the glass pipette. To the end of the glass pipette is glued a machined Plexiglas cap (i). The external diameter of the cap varies between 1 and 2.5 mm. The cavity in the cap has an internal diameter of 300 μm and a depth between 100 and 500 μm. Reproduced from reference 25. **D.** Placement of optrode within a hypodermic needle, such that the optrode tip is positioned at approximately the midpoint of the taper of the needle tip.

(dichroic) mirror to a 1.5-mW green He-Ne laser that acts as an excitation light source. The fiber transmits the excitation light to heart tissue that has been stained with a voltage-sensitive fluorescent dye such as di-4-ANEPPS (Molecular Probes Inc., Eugene, OR). The fluorescence emitted by the dye is collected by the same fiber and routed back through the dichroic mirror and an optical filter to a low-noise photodiode and amplifier. The coupling optics, filters, and photodetector are enclosed in a Faraday shielded light-proof box that allows experiments to be conducted under lowered, ambient light conditions without the necessity of a dark room.

The optrode design, while limited to single point measurements, allows for great flexibility in its usage. For example, the optrode can be used to measure changes in transmembrane potentials in tissue directly underneath a stimulating pipette electrode (Fig. 1B). Addition of a cap with suction allows for stabilization against motion artifacts (MAs), a problem that commonly plagues optoelectrical measurements. Unlike PDA or video imaging systems that require a clear "line of sight" between the tissue and the photodetector, the optrode is extremely flexible in terms of its accessibility to tissue locations, and can record transmembrane potentials remotely over distances at least 30 feet away with little degradation in signal. Measurements of transmembrane potentials can even be obtained from within the myocardial wall, by inserting the optrode down the bore of a hypodermic needle, which allows easy penetration into the midmyocardium (Fig. 1D).

Figure 2 shows illustrative optoelectrical recordings obtained from the ventricles of hearts from different species. Panels A through D were obtained as surface recordings from the epicardium, while panel E was obtained from the midmyocardium, using a 140-μm diameter glass optical fiber placed within a 30-gauge hypodermic needle.

Cellular Responses Near a Point Electrode

The optrode has been used to characterize the cellular transmembrane responses on the surface of tissue in the vicinity of a unipolar stimulating electrode. In this scenario, the stimulation current densities and electrical fields are expected to be relatively high and nonuniform and fall off exponentially or even more rapidly with distance from the electrode. Several key experimental findings are described below.

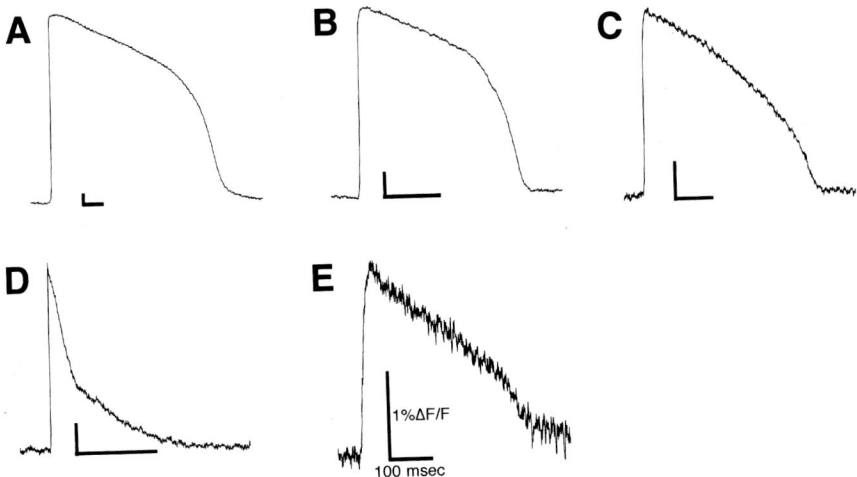

Figure 2. Optical recordings of action potentials from epicardial surfaces of **A**) bullfrog ventricular epicardium; **B**) guinea pig ventricular epicardium; **C**) rabbit ventricular epicardium; **D**) rat ventricular epicardium; and **E**) rabbit ventricular midmyocardium. An optical fiber with 100-μm core diameter was used. Scale bars are 100 ms horizontal and 1% fluorescence change vertical. Unpublished data, from S. Lu and L. Tung.

Regions of Oppositely Polarized Responses and the "Virtual Electrode" Effect. It has been increasingly recognized from theoretical work that the orientation of the cardiac fibers and the tissue architecture are important factors governing the tissue response.[22,26] Bullfrog atrium was used because the fibers are relatively parallel and present a well-defined directional axis. Experiments were conducted with a 0.3-mm diameter, stimulating point electrode placed on the endocardial surface, with the return electrode placed in the bath solution. The heart was stained by 20 to 30 μmol/L of the voltage-sensitive dye di-4-ANEPPS, as previously described.[25] With 10-ms duration square stimulus pulses, V_m near the electrode decays monotonically to zero when measured in a direction transverse to the fiber axis (Fig. 3, lower row). However, if V_m is measured along the fiber axis, regions of *opposite* polarity can be observed (Fig. 3, upper row), as predicted by car-

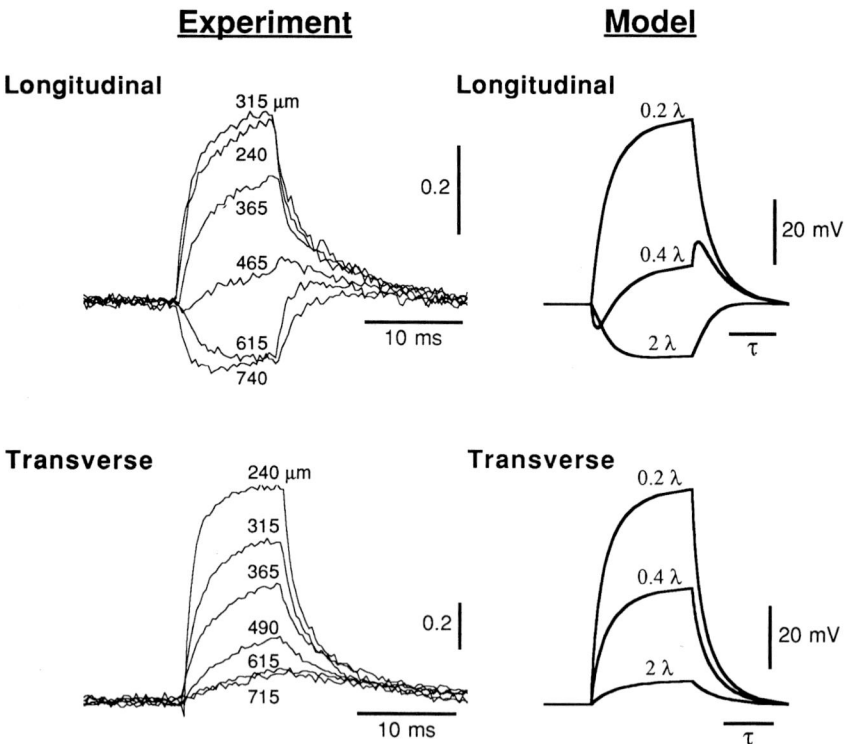

Figure 3. Experimental data showing the virtual electrode effects around a stimulating cathodal electrode. *Left column:* Experimental data. Numbers refer to distance from the stimulating electrode, in μm. *Right column:* Computer simulations using a passive membrane model. Data are presented in units of λ (space constant) and τ (time constant). *Upper row:* Data along the longitudinal fiber axis. At sites closest to the electrode, the membrane undergoes maximum depolarization. At increasing distances, the membrane potential becomes less positive and eventually hyperpolarizes. Model and data show a relatively good fit. *Lower row:* Data along the transverse fiber axis. At sites closest to the electrode, the membrane undergoes maximum depolarization. Unlike the longitudinal direction, the membrane potential decreases monotonically with distance, always exhibiting a depolarizing behavior. Adapted from reference 34.

diac bidomain tissue models.[4,26,28] These coexisting regions of *opposite* polarity are a consequence of the anisotropic characteristics of the intra-cellular and extracellular conductances that couple together adjacent cells along the longitudinal and transverse axes. The results of a simple computational model of an anisotropic tissue are also shown in Figure 3 (right column), and reproduce the qualitative aspects of the measured ΔV_m (left column).

Other investigators have made similar observations of virtual electrode effects near stimulus point electrodes,[29,30] as well as with other electrode configurations,[31,32] as described in other chapters of this text.

Response of Transmembrane Potential V_m Directly Underneath a Stimulating Electrode. The design of the optrode makes feasible the unique ability to record cellular transmembrane potentials directly *underneath* the stimulating electrode. This can be accomplished by using a hollow glass capillary tube that is filled with conductive solution so that it can be used as a stimulating electrode. The optrode is then placed down the bore of the pipette as shown previously in Figure 1B. In this study, an isolated flap of frog ventricle was stimulated while at rest, and V_m was recorded directly on the epicardial surface underneath the stimulating electrode.[33,34] For a given stimulus amplitude, the responses were found to be asymmetrical with respect to stimulus polarity, with larger changes occurring in the positive, depolarizing direction (Fig. 4A). These observations may be explained by the nonlinear electrical behavior of the membrane, which has a passive current-voltage relation that rectifies in the inward direction (i.e., has a higher resistance in the depolarizing direction). This condition is known to be the case from independent experiments on single cells using the whole cell voltage-clamp technique.[35] Because the stimulus acts like a current source near the electrode, a larger voltage change results in the depolarizing direction.

Another point to note is that with these diastolic stimuli, activation of the action potential can occur, either with depolarizing polarities (shown here as "make excitation" at 1 and 9.2 times the excitation threshold) or as "break excitation" (at −9.2 excitation threshold). This active response is superimposed on the passive membrane response to the stimulus pulse and therefore poses as a confounding factor in the study of field-induced responses. For that reason, investigators often apply the test stimulus during the early plateau (absolute refractory period) of the action potential, when the inward sodium channel is inactivated.[31,32,34,36–39] We see that the tissue response changes dramatically when the stimulus is applied during the action potential plateau (Fig. 4B). First, the excitatory response is completely eliminated. Second, the voltage response is again asymmetrical but now larger in the negative, hyperpolarizing direction. These observations suggest that the current-voltage relation of the membrane exhibits outward rectification during the plateau, a condition substantiated in this tissue by experiments using the voltage-clamp technique.[40] Similar observations regarding the asymmetry of ΔV_m and the polarity of the asymmetry have been made in the vicinity of cleft spaces in monolayers of cultured cardiac cells[38,39] and in single cells, as discussed in a later section.

The optrode has also been used to monitor ΔV_m in response to high-intensity shocks with current density in the range of several hundred

A

B

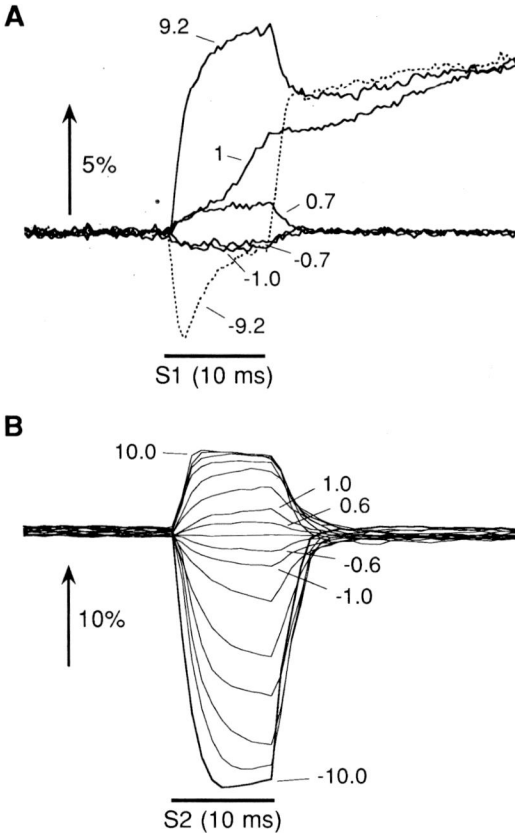

Figure 4. Transmembrane potential responses of cells underneath a stimulating pipette electrode (0.3 mm in diameter) in the epicardial surface of a flap of frog ventricle stained with 25 μmol/L of the voltage-sensitive dye di-4-ANEPPS. **A.** Responses for 10-ms rectangular stimuli applied during rest. Three current pulses with differing amplitudes (0.7, 1, and 9.2 times excitation threshold) were applied, with positive and negative polarities. The heavy bar indicates the on time of the stimulus pulse (S). For the positive responses, stimuli with intensities of 1 and 9.2 were excitatory and resulted in an action potential. For the negative responses, an intensity of −9.2 resulted in break excitation. **B.** Responses for 10-ms rectangular stimuli applied during the action potential plateau. Current pulses with amplitudes of 0.6, 1.0, 2.0, 3.6, 5.4, 6.9, 8.3, and 10.0 times excitation threshold were applied, with positive and negative polarities. Adapted from reference 27.

mA/cm².⁴¹ Ten-millisecond shock pulses of varying intensity and polarity were applied to frog ventricle in diastole, and ΔV_m was quantified directly under the stimulating electrode by an optrode. Both the shock-induced action potential amplitude (Fig. 5) and resting potential amplitude decreased sigmoidally with shock intensities exceeding 10 to 20 times diastolic threshold. The half-maximum points for the shock-induced action potential amplitude were 185 and 238 mA/cm², with the smaller value for the anodal pulses ($P = 0.02$). These values of current density may conceivably be attained in parts of the heart for certain electrode shapes, configurations, and shock intensities. Finally, ΔV_m was observed to increase with shock amplitude, and to reach a maximum of about −2 times the amplitude of the preshock action potential (APA_c) for anodal shocks and about 1.25 times APA_c for cathodal shocks, relative to the resting membrane potential (not shown). The observations in the hyperpolarizing direction, in which the ΔV_m increases, reaches a limit of nearly 3 times APA_c, and then declines during the shock pulse, are consistent with the process known as electroporation. Electroporation is a field-induced reorientation of the molecular structure of the lipid bilayer of the cell membrane that occurs when the transmembrane potential exceeds a threshold voltage of several hundred

A **B**

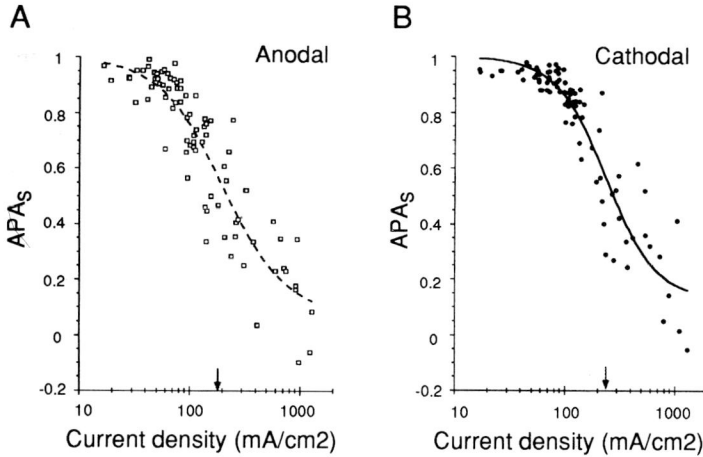

Figure 5. Action potential amplitude induced by the shock (APA_s) as a function of the shock intensity for anodal and cathodal pulses. **A.** Anodal shock data. The data were fit by a sigmoidal function, which reached an asymptote of 0.08 of the control action potential amplitude (APA_c). The half-maximum point of the curve fit (ED_{50}) is indicated by the arrow and was estimated by analysis of covariance to be 185 mA/cm². **B.** Cathodal shock data. The data were fit by a sigmoidal function, which reached an asymptote of 0.03 of APA_c. ED_{50} was 238 mA/cm². Reproduced from reference 41.

millivolts.[42] The reorientation results in the formation of aqueous-filled pores that allow the nonspecific exchange of ions and macromolecules across the membrane, and at the same time limits the ΔV_m that can develop.

Cellular Responses Remote from the Electrode

It is generally accepted that what constitutes remote in an electrical sense is a distance much greater than the length of tissue over which passive electrical activity can spread, i.e., the length constant for linear, passive electrical cables. The length constant is typically several hundred microns at rest but can vary in size over the time course of an action potential, becoming smaller during the upstroke and larger during the plateau, owing to changes in membrane resistance. At locations remote from the stimulating electrodes, current densities and electrical fields are expected to be relatively uniform spatially, but to be at their lowermost values compared with the remainder of the heart. Yet somehow, electrical fields are able to induce responses in cellular transmembrane potentials even in these remote regions. To verify whether cells in the "far-field" can be stimulated directly rather than as the result of propagated electrical activity originating from tissue stimulated near the electrodes, the following experiment was performed.

Latency Delay Decreases with Increasing Stimulus Strength. An exploring optrode was used to measure the latency delay for excitation by field stimulation. In the experiment shown in Figure 6A, an optrode was placed at the center of an isolated flap of bullfrog atrium. Stimulation was provided by two parallel wire electrodes. The measured ΔV_m at the center of

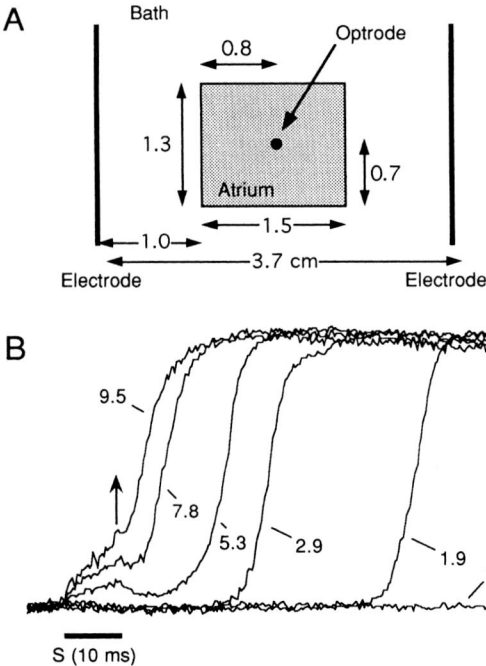

Figure 6. Far-field responses. **A.** A flap of bullfrog atrium approximately 1.3×1.5 cm in dimension was placed between a pair of stimulating wire electrodes. **B.** Electro-optical potentials measured with an exploring optrode positioned at the center of the flap, for varying stimulus strengths. Each of the optical recordings was normalized to its maximum intensity. The timing of the rectangular stimulus pulse is indicated by the heavy bar. Stimuli intensities ranged from 1 to 9.5 times excitation threshold (ET). Latency delay from the end of the stimulus pulse to the midpoint of the upstroke of the action potential varied from 90 ms for the stimulus of intensity 1× ET to 5 ms for the stimulus of intensity 9.5× ET. An optical fiber with 100-μm core diameter was used. Unpublished data from E. Sobie and L. Tung.

the flap to a 10-ms rectangular stimulus pulse are shown in Figure 6B for pulse strengths ranging from 1 to 9.5 times the excitation threshold. It is clear that with increasing pulse strength, the latency delay measured from the end of the pulse to the upstroke of the action potential decreases from 90 ms to 4 ms. At the lowest stimulus intensity, the delay is consistent with the lag time for propagation of electrical activity from the border of the tissue (where excitation presumably occurred as a near-field effect). However, at the highest stimulus intensity, the latency delay is much shorter than can be accounted for by the time required for electrical propagation, and hence one can infer that excitation is virtually instantaneous at the center of the flap. These data support the idea that the cell membranes respond directly to the applied electrical field. While these results might not be applicable to stimulation of the heart as a whole, they do suggest that direct excitation may be possible in structures up to a centimeter in dimension (such as the heart wall), for field strengths about an order of magnitude larger than the minimal levels required for tissue excitation. From equation 1, we see that in a region of tissue where the field is relatively uniform, the responses may be the result of Type I virtual sources provided that the cardiac fibers have a spatially varying direction or conductivity. Recent studies that substantiate the presence of virtual electrodes in the tissue bulk are reviewed in the next few sections of this chapter.

Virtual Sources Form Around Tissue Clefts. In a study of monolayers of cultured rat myocytes stimulated by electrical fields, polarization patterns were observed in the tissue regions surrounding cleft spaces, such that the side closer to the anode was depolarized and the side closer to the cathode was hyperpolarized.[38] In a follow-up study, the magnitude of the polarizations was found to vary monotonically with the cleft size.[39] These experimental findings of the spatial distribution and polarities of ΔV_m around the cleft are consistent with results obtained from computer simulations based on equation 1.[22] However, a result not predicted by the simulations was that the responses tended to be asymmetrical, being larger in the hyperpolarizing direction than in the depolarizing direction. This finding is discussed later in this chapter.

Virtual Sources Form at Tissue Borders. Polarization patterns at the borders of linear strands of cultured cardiac cells can be measured using the PDA mapping system developed by Fast.[43,44] A 100-μm-width linear strand of neonatal rat myocytes was stimulated transversely by a uniform electrical field (Fig. 7). Like the case of the tissue cleft, the two sides of the strand

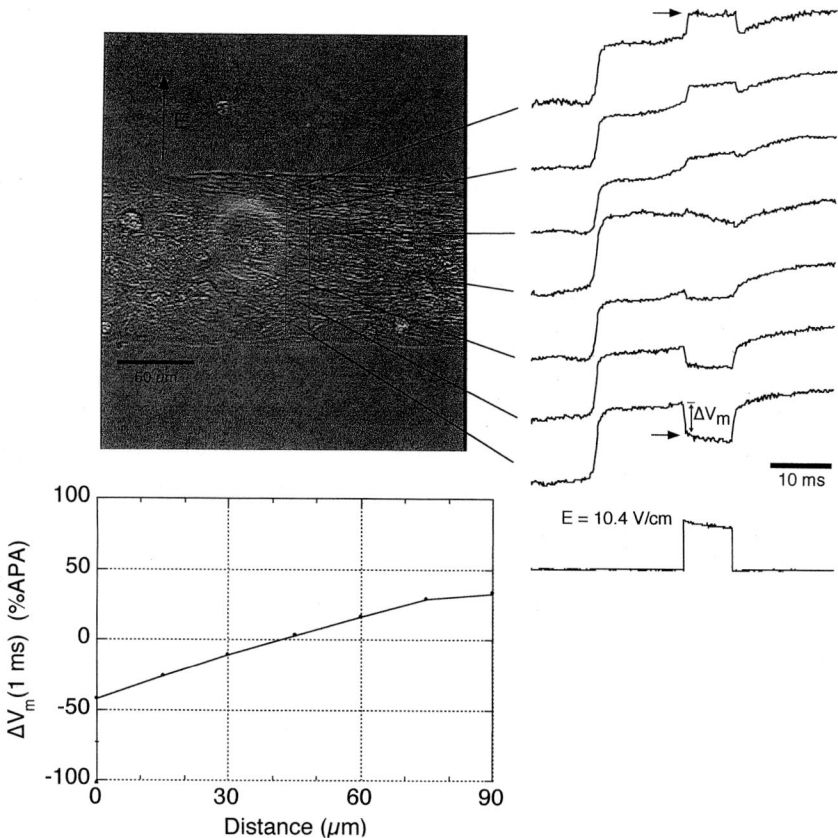

Figure 7. Transmembrane potential responses (ΔV_m) in a 100-μm-wide linear strand during transverse field stimulation. A 10-ms S2 field pulse was applied in the transverse direction to a linear strand of cultured neonatal rat heart cells during the plateau of their action potentials. The cells were stained with 2 μmol/L RH237. A nonuniform polarization pattern resulted, with maximum hyperpolarization on the edge facing the anode and maximum depolarization on the edge facing the cathode. The distribution of ΔV_m was approximately linear across the cross-section of the strand as shown in the lower graph. Unpublished data from L. Tung and A. Kléber.

polarize in opposite directions, although the signs are reversed so that the side facing the anode hyperpolarizes while the side facing the cathode depolarizes. The initial part of ΔV_m, measured 1 ms after the onset of the S2 pulse, varies linearly with position across the strand width. Such a result is as expected from passive cable theory for finite length fibers in which the fiber length is small compared with the space constant.[45]

Single Cell Responses

The theory of single cell responses to field stimulation was developed to describe the general, steady-state responses of spheroidal cells to uniform fields,[46] and also responses in the context of ellipsoidal cells in alternating electrical fields,[47] electroporation of spherical or ellipsoidal particles,[48,49] electrophotoluminescence of chloroplast vesicular membranes,[50] and cells stained with voltage-sensitive dyes[51] to cite but a few examples. In the cardiac literature, the analysis of single cell responses can also be found in numerous studies.[9–11,52–54] From these works, it is well known that with field stimulation, the cell surface membrane will polarize nonuniformly, with the side facing the cathode having a depolarizing response, and the side facing the anode having a hyperpolarizing response. In the simplest case of a spherical cell in a uniform field under static conditions, ΔV_m has an often-cited sinusoidal dependence around the perimeter of the cell:

$$\Delta V_m = 1.5 E_o\, a \sin \theta \qquad (2)$$

where E_o is the field strength, a the cell radius, and θ the circumferential angle. In general, however, the precise cell shape, orientation of the cell with respect to the field direction, and spatial uniformity of the field all will influence the exact profile of transmembrane potential that develops. For the case of a spheroidal cell with a passive membrane in a uniform electrical field, the maximum transmembrane potential that will develop follows the function KE_og, where K is a shape form factor and g a generalized conductivity parameter that is a function of the cell dimensions.[46] The importance of the orientation of the cell with respect to the electrical field,[55,56] as well as a possible asymmetry in excitation threshold with reversals in field direction owing to cell shape,[57] have been documented in nonoptical experiments.

For step changes in field intensity that occur during the onset of a field stimulus pulse, ΔV_m will charge in a time interval much shorter than the membrane time constant. For example, for spherical cells with passive membranes, equation 2 can be rewritten as,

$$\Delta V_m = 1.5 E_o\, a \sin \theta \left[1 - e^{-t/\tau} \right] \qquad (3)$$

where the reciprocal of the time constant is $\dfrac{1}{\tau}$

$$\frac{1}{\tau} = \frac{1}{R_m C_m} + \frac{1}{0.5(R_i + 2R_e)C_m} \qquad (4)$$

R_m is the area-specific membrane resistance, C_m the area-specific membrane capacitance, R_i the access resistance to the membrane through the intracellular conductive pathways, and R_e the access resistance through the extracellular conductive pathways. In general, the second term of equation 4 dominates over the first.

For cells with active membranes, a second but slower time-dependent behavior emerges after the rapid component of the membrane response.[9] This behavior is determined by the active currents in the cell membrane that are activated or inactivated to varying degrees, depending on their location along the cell length.

Single Cell Optical Recordings

To test the model predictions, two different photodetector systems were developed for single cell measurements, as shown schematically in Figures 8 and 9. The first, shown in Figure 8, used a mechanically steered laser beam focused to a 15-μm spot on different parts of the cell.[58] The beam from a 0.2-mW green He-Ne laser (543 nm) passed through a mechanical shutter (model 846HP, Newport Corp, Irvine, CA), reflected off a 2-dimensional motorized mirror (model 6800, Cambridge Tech, Watertown, MA), and was focused by a set of relay lenses into the epi-illumination port of an inverted microscope (Diaphot, Nikon Instruments, Tokyo, Japan). The beam passed through a 546-nm excitation filter, reflected off a 580-nm dichroic filter and up onto the specimen plane in which cells were placed and stained with voltage-sensitive dye. The fluorescent light was collected by the same microscope objective and passed back through the

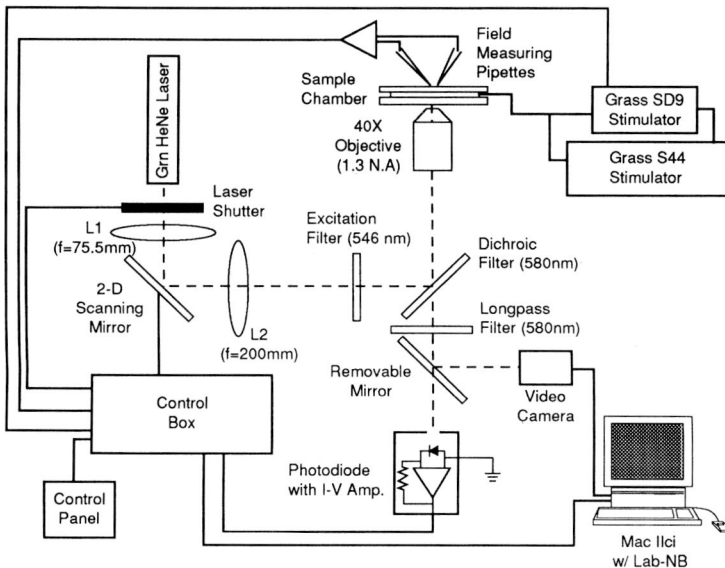

Figure 8. Set-up for measurements of single cell fluorescence, using a steerable laser excitation light source and a single photodetector. See text for details of the system.

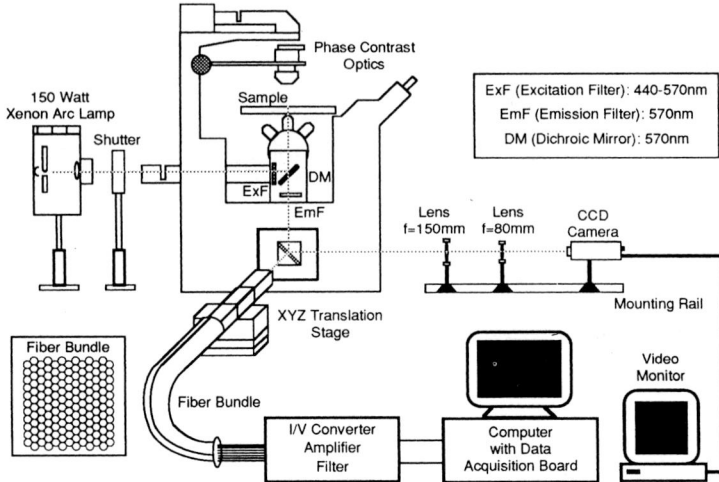

Figure 9. Set-up for measurements of single cell fluorescence, using a broadband xenon arc light source and a photodiode array coupled to the microscope via an optical fiber bundle. See text for details of the system.

dichroic mirror and a 580-nm long-pass filter and focused onto a photodiode (model S2386–5K, Hamamatsu Photonics Corp., Bridgewater, NJ) and current-to-voltage converter (OPA111, Burr-Brown Corp., Tucson, AZ) with a 1-GΩ feedback resistor. By the nature of its design, this system was limited to single point measurements at any one instant of time.

A second photodetector system (Fig. 9) was developed to perform optical mapping of many sites in parallel, based on the approach of Rohr and Kucera.[59] Light from a 150-W xenon arc lamp (Optiquip, Highland Mills, NY) was gated through a mechanical shutter (Vincent Associates, Rochester, NY) and coupled to the epi-illumination port of an inverted microscope (Diaphot, Nikon Instruments). A 149-element fiberoptic bundle consisting of an ordered hexagonal array of 1-mm-diameter plastic fibers (Boston Optical Fibers, Westboro, MA) was constructed and positioned with one end at the video port of the microscope. Between five and seven adjacent elements of the bundle were coupled at their other ends to individual photodiodes and current-to-voltage amplifiers. The signals were then routed to a 64-channel-capacity data acquisition board (Sheldon Instruments, Provo, UT) running on a 200-MHz industrial computer (ANT Computers, Walnut, CA). Images of the cell were captured by a video camera (Cohu, San Diego, CA).

Dual Components of the Field Response

In this section, only results using the optical mapping system (Fig. 9) are presented. Readers interested in the results of the mechanically steered laser system are referred to reference 58. Single rat ventricular cells were obtained by standard enzymatic dissociation techniques and stained with 135-μmol/L di-8-ANEPPS for 5 minutes. The results of one experiment are shown in Figure 10.

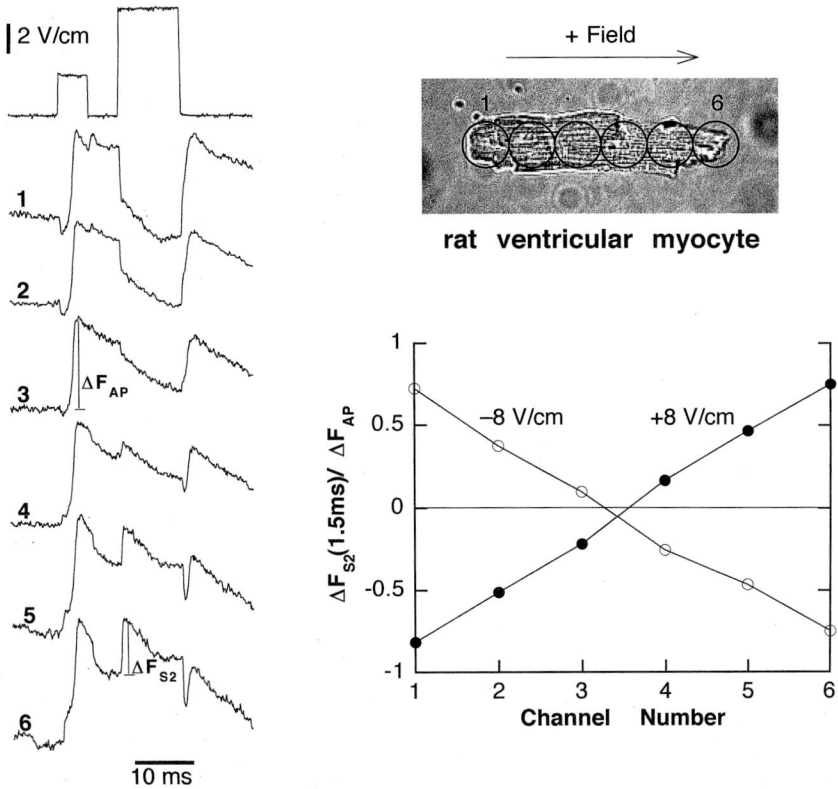

Figure 10. Single cell response to uniform field stimulation. A 14.5-V/cm field was applied along the long axis of an adult rat ventricular cell. Fluorescence from the cell was imaged via six optical fibers running to six photodetectors. The optical field of each of the fibers is shown with a circle overlaying the cell image, which was obtained by a video camera. The transmembrane responses were nonuniform along the length of the cell, and were maximum in the depolarizing direction at the end of the cell facing the cathode and maximum in the hyperpolarizing direction at the other end of the cell. The change in fluorescence (open circles) was measured 1.5 ms after the onset of the S2 pulse, and showed completely linear responses along the length of the cell. The responses were symmetric around zero when the field was reversed (filled circles). Unpublished data from V. Sharma, S. Lu, and L. Tung.

Here, a uniform electrical field was applied along the long axis of a single cell. Six optical fibers were positioned to collect portions of the cell fluorescence as shown in the image on the upper right. The optoelectrical responses (left column) show very clearly the reciprocal polarization of the cell membrane along the cell length, typical of cell responses to field stimulation. The initial component of the S2 response measured 1.5 ms after the onset of the S2 pulse is plotted against position along the cell (graph on the lower right). A linear behavior was observed that changed polarity and remained linear in a symmetric way with a reversal in field polarity. The magnitude of the response at the hyperpolarized end of the cell was approximately the same as the response at the depolarized end, regardless of the field direction.

Other investigators have measured the responses of single cardiac cells to field stimulation applied either at rest[13,60] or as in the experiment of Figure 10 during the action potential plateau.[36,58] Regardless of when the shock is applied, the response consists of an initial rapid component that occurs at the temporal resolution of their measurement systems (as fast as 70 μs[13]), followed by a slower, smaller, time-dependent component. In general, the initial rapid component has opposite signs at the two ends of the cell and varies linearly in amplitude with field strength, while the time-dependent component is nearly the same all along the cell length.

In contrast, responses of cardiac tissue to field stimulation are presented in Figures 3, 4, and 6, and show only the slow time-dependent component, without an initial rapid component. The different behavior might be due to the difference in the size of the recording spots in the tissue and cell experiments (100 μm versus 15 μm), which, for the tissue, would be sufficiently large to allow averaging of the subcellular responses to occur. Since the rapid component of the cellular response is symmetrically distributed in polarity around the center of the cell (Fig. 10), its spatial average would be zero, and hence might remain undetected when averaged.

It has been suggested that discontinuities in intracellular resistance at gap junctions may act as localized virtual sources that are separated by distances equal to the cell length.[7,61] If these effects were indeed to occur in tissue during field stimulation, one would expect that both depolarizing and hyperpolarizing responses (the so-called "sawtooth" effect) could be observed if the spatial resolution of the measurement system were sufficiently fine (i.e., finer than the cell length). Indeed, the "sawtooth" would be the tissue-level correlate to the rapid component of the single cell response. Neither optical recordings nor microelectrode recordings obtained at high spatial resolution have yet successfully documented such changes, at least in tissue with normally coupled cells.[38,60,62] This finding may be the result of the staggered arrangement of cells in the lateral direction,[63] such that the sawtooth pattern may be smoothed out owing to electrotonic interactions between sources of opposite polarities.[64]

On the other hand, it is clear that the rapid component response exists for certain geometries of cellular networks, such as monolayers of cultured neonatal heart cells that possess clefts[38,39] or narrow strands of cultured neonatal heart cells that are transversely stimulated (Fig. 7). These two cases may have tissue correlates in the form of cell bundles and laminar sheets,[65,66] and the bending of fibers around capillaries,[39] respectively. More generally, the dual rapid and slow components of the membrane response may be a general characteristic of cellular networks in which oppositely polarized virtual sources exist in pairs and are closely spaced on a length scale less than a space constant.[67]

Asymmetry in the Responses Having Opposite Polarity

For either field polarity, the transmembrane potential responses in Figure 10 are nearly symmetric around zero at the onset of the stimulus pulse. However, with time, all of the pulses exhibit a similar slow hyperpolarization time course, so that by the end of the pulse there is an asymmetry in the magnitude of the responses that is biased in the hyperpolarizing direction (not plotted). The amount of asymmetry may not be so clear in the recordings in Figure 10, in which some of the hyperpolarization arises naturally as part of the normal repolarization sequence of the cell, but in cells with much longer action potentials and slower rates of repolarization, the hyperpolarizing behavior during the stimulus pulse becomes more evident. Similar asymmetries between hyperpolarized and depolarized ΔV_m for field stimuli applied during the action potential plateau have been noted previously, with responses under a stimulating electrode (Fig. 4), around cleft spaces,[38,39] in intact tissue,[37] and at the borders of narrow strands (Fig. 7). These observations suggest that an intrinsic property of the cell membrane (some ionic current, for example) is responsible for the common behavior seen in these diverse settings.

Saturating Behavior at High Shock Intensities

As discussed earlier for tissue experiments (Fig. 5), ΔV_m for high-intensity fields can exhibit additional, complex behavior. With field intensities in excess of 50 V/cm, ΔV_m at both ends of the single cell acquires a slope that decays toward 0 mV.[68] This behavior is consistent with that expected from electroporation of the cell membrane, in which the conductance of the membrane rises by several orders of magnitude[69] and therefore acts to short circuit the transmembrane voltage. Electroporation is also expected to result in a limit in the maximum transmembrane potential that can develop, as was shown in sea urchin eggs using voltage-sensitive dyes and pulsed laser fluorescence microscopy.[49]

Summary

Electro-optical recordings of cardiac cells and tissue allow the testing and validation of the theoretical basis for the coupling between applied electrical fields and the cellular transmembrane potential during electrical stimulation. It is now known that the coupling process differs close to and far from the electrodes. Underneath the electrode, the transmembrane potential responds in a manner that likely reflects the nonlinear impedance properties of the cell membrane. Near the electrode, virtual electrode effects arising from the organized fiber structure of the tissue may be prominent, leading to regions of oppositely polarized responses. Far from the electrode, virtual sources may form at the borders of strands or bundles of cardiac cells, or around cleft spaces. Recordings from single cells show that the field response consists of two components. The first is complete in less than 1 ms, has opposite signs at the two ends of the cell, and varies linearly with field intensity. The second is much slower in time course, is governed by changes in the active membrane currents, and is relatively homogeneous across the cell. Finally, the field responses of certain but not all geometries of cellular networks can mimic the qualitative behavior of the single cell response.

Acknowledgments: I especially wish to acknowledge the contributions of current and past students in the Cardiac Bioelectric Systems Laboratory at the Johns Hopkins University, including Michel Neunlist, Vinod Sharma, Steven Lu, and Eric Sobie.

References

1. Tacker WAJ. *Defibrillation of the Heart.* St. Louis: Mosby-Year Book; 1994.
2. Weidmann S. Electrical constants of trabecular muscle from mammalian heart. *J Physiol* 1970;210:1041–1054.
3. Jack JJB, Noble D, Tsien RW. *Electric Current Flow in Excitable Cells.* Oxford: Oxford University Press; 1976.
4. Sepulveda NG, Roth BJ, Wikswo JP Jr. Current injection into a two-dimensional anisotropic bidomain. *Biophys J* 1989;55:987–999.
5. Trayanova N, Eason J, Henriquez CS. Electrode polarity effects on the shock-induced transmembrane potential distribution in the canine heart. *Proc Ann Int Conf IEEE Eng Med Biol Soc* 1995;17:317–318.
6. Roth BJ, Wikswo JP Jr. The effect of externally applied electrical fields on myocardial tissue. *Proc IEEE* 1996;84:379–391.
7. Plonsey R, Barr RC. Effect of microscopic and macroscopic discontinuities on the response of cardiac tissue to defibrillating (stimulating) currents. *Med Biol Eng Comput* 1986;24:130–136.
8. Krassowska W, Frazier DW, Pilkington TC, Ideker RE. Potential distribution in three-dimensional periodic myocardium—Part II: Application to extracellular stimulation. *IEEE Trans Biomed Eng* 1990;37:267–284.
9. Tung L, Borderies J-R. Analysis of electrical excitation of cardiac muscle cells. *Biophys J* 1992;63:371–386.
10. Leon LJ, Roberge FA. A model study of extracellular stimulation of cardiac cells. *IEEE Trans Biomed Eng* 1993;40:1307–1319.
11. Krassowska W, Neu JC. Response of a single cell to an external electric field. *Biophys J* 1994;66:1768–1776.
12. Roth BJ, Wikswo JP Jr. Electrical stimulation of cardiac tissue: A bidomain model with active membrane properties. *IEEE Trans Biomed Eng* 1994;41:232–240.
13. Windisch H, Ahammer H, Schaffer P, et al. Optical multisite monitoring of cell excitation phenomena in isolated cardiomyocytes. *Pflugers Arch* 1995;430:508–518.
14. Jones JL, Jones RE, Balasky G. Improved cardiac cell excitation with symmetrical biphasic defibrillator waveforms. *Am J Physiol* 1987;235:H1418–H1424.
15. Salama G, Lombardi R, Elson J. Maps of optical action potentials and NADH fluorescence in intact working hearts. *Am J Physiol* 1987;252:H384–H394.
16. Wu C-C, Fasciano RW, Calkins H, Tung L. Sequential changes in action potential of rabbit epicardium during and following radiofrequency ablation. *Pacing Clin Electrophysiol* 1996;19:580.
17. Krassowska W, Pilkington TC. Two-scale asymptotic analysis for modeling activation of periodic cardiac strand. *Math Comput Model* 1992;16:121–130.
18. Trayanova N, Roth BJ. Mechanisms for cardiac stimulation. *Proc Ann Int Conf IEEE Eng Med Biol Soc* 1993;15:817–818.
19. Fishler MG, Sobie EA, Tung L, Thakor NV. Modeling the interaction between propagating cardiac waves and monophasic and biphasic field stimuli—the importance of the induced spatial excitatory response. *J Cardiovasc Electrophysiol* 1996;7:1183–1196.
20. Plonsey R, Barr RC. Inclusion of junction elements in a linear cardiac model through secondary sources: Application to defibrillation. *Med Biol Eng Comput* 1986;24:137–144.
21. Trayanova NA, Roth BJ, Malden LJ. The response of a spherical heart to a uni-

form electric field: A bidomain analysis of cardiac stimulation. *IEEE Trans Biomed Eng* 1993;40:899–908.

22. Sobie EA, Susil RC, Tung L. A generalized activating function for predicting virtual electrodes in cardiac tissue. *Biophys J* 1997;73:1410–1423.

23. Hoshi T, Matsuda K. Excitability cycle of cardiac muscle examined by intracellular stimulation. *Jpn J Physiol* 1962;12:433–446.

24. Henriquez CS. Simulating the electrical behavior of cardiac tissue using the bidomain model. *Crit Rev Biomed Eng* 1993;21:1–77.

25. Neunlist M, Zou SZ, Tung L. Design and use of an "optrode" for optical recordings of cardiac action potentials. *Pflugers Arch* 1992;420:611–617.

26. Roth BJ. How the anisotropy of the intracellular and extracellular conductivities influences stimulation of cardiac muscle. *J Math Biol* 1992;30:633–646.

27. Tung L, Neunlist M, Sobie EA. Near-field and far-field stimulation of cardiac muscle. In *Clinical Applications of Modern Imaging Technology II*. Bellingham, WA: SPIE Press; 1994:367–374.

28. Wikswo JP. Tissue anisotropy, the cardiac bidomain, and the virtual cathode effect. In Zipes DP, Jalife J (eds): *Cardiac Electrophysiology: From Cell to Bedside*. 2nd ed. Philadelphia: W.B. Saunders Co.; 1995:348–361.

29. Knisley SB. Transmembrane voltage changes during unipolar stimulation of rabbit ventricle. *Circ Res* 1995;77:1229–1239.

30. Wikswo JP Jr, Lin SF, Abbas RA. Virtual electrodes in cardiac tissue: A common mechanism for anodal and cathodal stimulation. *Biophys J* 1995;69:2195–2210.

31. Efimov IR, Cheng YN, Biermann M, et al. Transmembrane voltage changes produced by real and virtual electrodes during monophasic defibrillation shock delivered by an implantable electrode. *J Cardiovasc Electrophysiol* 1997;8:1031–1045.

32. Knisley SB, Baynham TC. Line stimulation parallel to myofibers enhances regional uniformity of transmembrane voltage changes in rabbit hearts. *Circ Res* 1997;81:229–241.

33. Neunlist M, Tung L. Optical recordings of ventricular excitability of frog heart by an extracellular stimulating point electrode. *Pacing Clin Electrophysiol* 1994;17:1641–1654.

34. Neunlist M, Tung L. Spatial distribution of cardiac transmembrane potentials around an extracellular electrode. Dependence on fiber orientation. *Biophys J* 1995;68:2310–2322.

35. Tung L, Morad M. A comparative electrophysiological study of enzymatically isolated single cells and strips of frog ventricle. *Pflugers Arch* 1985;405:274–284.

36. Knisley SB, Blitchington TF, Hill BC, et al. Optical measurements of transmembrane potential changes during electric field stimulation of ventricular cells. *Circ Res* 1993;72:255–270.

37. Zhou X, Ideker RE, Blitchington TF, et al. Optical transmembrane potential measurements during defibrillation-strength shocks in perfused rabbit hearts. *Circ Res* 1995;77:593–602.

38. Gillis AM, Fast VG, Rohr S, Kléber AG. Spatial changes in transmembrane potential during extracellular electrical shocks in cultured monolayers of neonatal rat ventricular myocytes. *Circ Res* 1996;79:676–690.

39. Fast VG, Rohr S, Gillis AM, Kléber AG. Activation of cardiac tissue by extracellular electrical shocks. *Circ Res* 1998;82:375–385.

40. Goldman Y, Morad M. Ionic conductances during the time course of the cardiac action potential. *J Physiol* 1977;268:655–695.

41. Neunlist M, Tung L. Dose-dependent reduction of cardiac transmembrane potential by high intensity electrical shocks. *Am J Physiol* 1997;273:H2817-H2825.

42. Neumann E, Sowers AE, Jordan CA. *Electroporation and Electrofusion in Cell Biology.* New York: Plenum Press; 1989.
43. Fast VG, Darrow BJ, Saffitz JE, Kléber AG. Anisotropic activation spread in heart cell monolayers assessed by high-resolution optical mapping—role of tissue discontinuities. *Circ Res* 1996;79:115–127.
44. Tung L, Kléber AG. Virtual sources associated with linear and curved strands of cardiac cells. *Am J Physiol Heart Circ Physiol* 2000;279:H1579-H1590.
45. Gaylor DC, Prakah-Asante K, Lee RC. Significance of cell size and tissue structure in electrical trauma. *J Theor Biol* 1988;133:233–237.
46. Klee M, Plonsey R. Stimulation of spheroidal cells—the role of cell shape. *IEEE Trans Biomed Eng* 1976;23:347–354.
47. Bernhardt J, Pauly H. On the generation of potential differences across the membranes of ellipsoidal cells in an alternative electrical field. *Biophysik* 1973;10:89–98.
48. Jeltsch E, Zimmerman U. Particles in a homogeneous field: A model for the electrical breakdown of living cells in a Coulter counter. *Bioelectrochem Bioenerg* 1979;6:349–384.
49. Hibino M, Shigemori M, Itoh H, et al. Membrane conductance of an electroporated cell analyzed by submicrosecond imaging of transmembrane potential. *Biophys J* 1991;59:209–220.
50. Farkas DL, Korenstein R, Malkin S. Electrophotoluminescence and the electrical properties of the photosynthetic membrane. *Biophys J* 1984;45:363–373.
51. Gross D, Loew LM, Webb WW. Optical imaging of cell membrane potential changes induced by applied electric fields. *Biophys J* 1986;50:339–348.
52. Platzer D, Windisch H. Modeling the complex behavior of single cardiomyocytes during and after field stimulation. *Proc Ann Int Conf IEEE Eng Med Biol Soc* 1993;15:823.
53. Quan W, Cohen TJ. Field stimulation of single cardiac cell—the dependency of membrane excitation on waveform shape and cellular refractoriness. *Proc Ann Int Conf IEEE Eng Med Biol Soc* 1993;15:869–870.
54. Fishler MG, Sobie EA, Thakor NV, Tung L. Mechanisms of cardiac cell excitation with premature monophasic and biphasic field stimuli—a model study. *Biophys J* 1996;70:1347–1362.
55. Bardou AL, Chesnais JM, Birkui PJ, et al. Directional variability of stimulation threshold measurements in isolated guinea pig cardiomyocytes: Relationship with orthogonal sequential defibrillating pulses. *Pacing Clin Electrophysiol* 1990;13:1590–1595.
56. Tung L, Sliz N, Mulligan MR. Influence of electrical axis of stimulation on excitation of cardiac muscle cells. *Circ Res* 1991;69:722–730.
57. Ranjan R, Thakor NV. Electrical stimulation of cardiac myocytes. *Ann Biomed Eng* 1996;23:812–821.
58. Cheng DK, Tung L, Sobie EA. Nonuniform responses of transmembrane potential during electric field stimulation of single cardiac cells. *Am J Physiol* 1999;277(1 Pt. 2):H351-H362.
59. Rohr S, Kucera JP. Optical recording system based on a fiber optic image conduit: Assessment of microscopic activation patterns in cardiac tissue. *Biophys J* 1998;75:1062–1075.
60. Windisch H, Müller W, Ahammer H, et al. Optical potential mapping helps to reveal discrete-natural-phenomena in cardiac muscle. *Int J Bifurcation Chaos* 1996;6:1925–1933.
61. Roth BJ, Krassowska W. The induction of reentry in cardiac tissue. The missing link: How electric fields alter transmembrane potential. *Chaos* 1998;8:204–220.
62. Zhou X, Rollins DL, Smith WM, Ideker RE. Responses of the transmembrane

potential of myocardial cells during a shock. *J Cardiovasc Electrophysiol* 1995;6:252–263.

63. Spach MS, Heidlage JF. A multidimensional model of cellular effects on the spread of electrotonic currents and on propagating action potentials. *Crit Rev Biomed Eng* 1992;20:141–169.

64. Juhlin SP, Promann JB. Dimensional comparison of the sawtooth pattern in transmembrane potential. In *Computers in Cardiology*. Washington, DC: IEEE Press; 1994:413–416.

65. Sommer JR, Scherer B. Geometry of cell and bundle appositions in cardiac muscle: Light microscopy. *Am J Physiol* 1985;248:H792-II803.

66. LeGrice IJ, Smaill BH, Chai LZ, et al. Laminar structure of the heart: Ventricular myocyte arrangement and connective tissue architecture in the dog. *Am J Physiol* 1995;269:H571–H582.

67. Susil RC, Sobie EA, Tung L. Separation between virtual sources modifies the response of cardiac tissue to field stimulation. *J Cardiovasc Electrophysiol* 1999;10:715–727.

68. Knisley SB, Grant AO. Asymmetrical electrically induced injury of rabbit ventricular myocytes. *J Mol Cell Cardiol* 1995;27:1111–1122.

69. Tovar O, Tung L. Electroporation and recovery of the cardiac cell membrane with rectangular voltage pulses. *Am J Physiol* 1992;263:H1128–H1136.

Chapter 19

New Perspectives in Electrophysiology from the Cardiac Bidomain

Shien-Fong Lin and John P. Wikswo, Jr.

Introduction

For many years, the uniform double layer model was widely accepted and used to describe the macroscopic electrical behavior of cardiac tissue. It predicted that outside a closed wave front, there should be no extracellular potential. In 1977, Corbin and Scher[1] measured the extracellular potential outside an expanding wave front and found a positive potential parallel to the fibers and a negative potential perpendicular to them. This observation was inconsistent with the uniform double layer model, and implied that a new and more general model was required to accurately relate the extracellular and transmembrane potentials. Corbin and Scher explained their results in terms of nonuniform dipole strength within the wave front, with the individual dipoles aligned with the fiber axis. Colli-Franzone and colleagues[2] developed an oblique dipole model to explain the experimental data.

An alternative model, with few ad-hoc assumptions, is the bidomain model, in which a 3-dimensional electrical cable represents the cardiac syncytium with distinct intracellular and extra cellular spaces separated by cell membrane.[3–11] The bidomain model treats the macroscopic heart as a continuous, nonlinear, 3-dimensional cable, with the effects of intercellular junctions incorporated into the anisotropic intracellular conductivities. As shown in Figure 1, this view is supported by the fact that the intracellular spaces of all cardiac cells are connected together sufficiently tightly through the gap junctions in the intercalated disks to form a 3-dimensional syncytium that can carry currents and support voltage gradients in all directions. Similarly, the cells share a common extracellular space that also forms a 3-dimensional conductor. Because of the tissue architecture, the electrical conductivities of the intracellular and extracellular spaces are directionally dependent, i.e., anisotropic, such that each domain in the model has its own anisotropic electrical resistivity. This also leads to the well-known anisotropic conduction velocity. At present,

From Rosenbaum DS, Jalife J (eds): *Optical Mapping of Cardiac Excitation and Arrhythmias.* ©Futura Publishing Co., Inc., Armonk, NY, 2001.

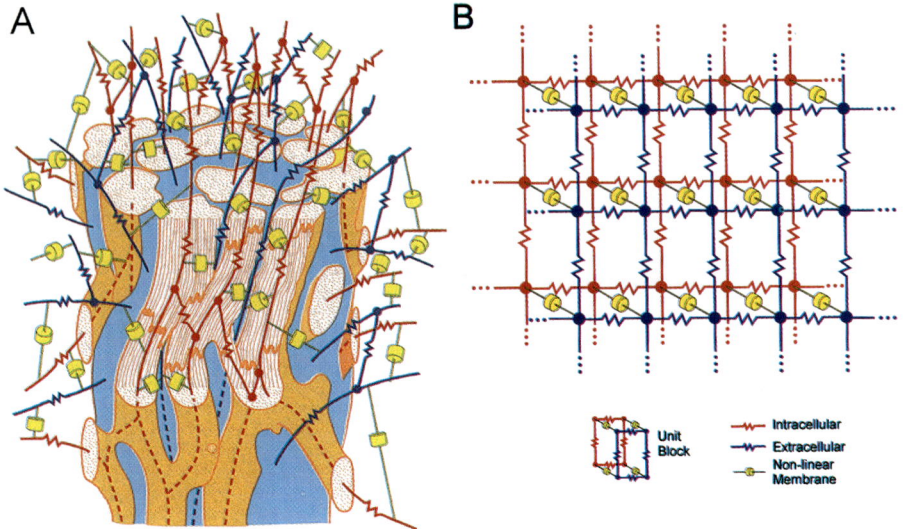

Figure 1. Schematic representation showing how the syncytial nature of cardiac tissue can be represented by a 3-dimensional coaxial cable. Intracellular (red) and extracellular spaces (blue) are represented by a pair of superimposed, 3-dimensional resistor arrays that are interconnected by the nonlinear membrane, represented by the yellow cylindrical elements. **A.** Irregular bidomain reflecting actual cardiac cellular structure. *Bottom:* Cardiac cells (red) are surrounded by the extracellular space (blue). *Middle:* Equivalent resistor network is superimposed on the cell structure, with the intracellular resistor network in red and the extracellular network in blue. The two are connected by the yellow nonlinear membrane elements. *Top third:* The resistor and membrane network is shown alone. Such cellular-scale bidomain models have yet to be implemented. **B.** A regular, 2-dimensional bidomain suitable for numerical calculations; the entire pattern can be translated out of the page to create a 3-dimensional bidomain. The choice of the resistors would define the fiber direction, in that the intracellular resistance would be 10 times greater across the fibers than along them for a 10:1 intracellular anisotropy ratio; the extracellular anisotropy would be 4:1. Typically, one element of a 3-dimensional bidomain mesh would be 100 μm to 1 mm on a side and, as such, would represent a large number of individual cardiac cells.

the complicated heterogeneous geometry in Figure 1A is homogenized to form the idealized, locally homogeneous, and highly regular bidomain seen in Figure 1B.

Mathematically, the bidomain model accounts fully for the syncytial nature of cardiac tissue, including the effects of tissue anisotropy, using a pair of coupled, partial differential equations governing the intracellular, V_i, and extracellular, V_e, potentials

$$\nabla \cdot \sigma_i \nabla V_i = \beta(C_m \partial V_m / \partial t + J_{ion}) - I_i$$

$$\nabla \cdot \sigma_e \nabla V_e = -\beta(C_m \partial V_m / \partial t + J_{ion}) - I_e$$

where σ_i and σ_e are the anisotropic electrical conductivity tensors of the two spaces (S/m), C_m is membrane capacitance per unit area (F/m²), β is the ratio of cell membrane area to tissue volume (m^{-1}), J_{ion} is the membrane ionic current per unit area (A/m^2), and I_i and I_e are the intracellularly and extracellularly applied external current sources per unit volume (A/m^3).

While these equations are easier to solve if the anisotropies of the intracellular and extracellular space are assumed to be the same, the physiologically realistic values for the tissue resistivities show the intracellular resistivity transverse to the fiber direction to be 10 times that of the resistivity along the fibers, for an intracellular anisotropy ratio of 10 to 1, while the ratio for the extracellular space is 4 to 1.[8,12,13] When the bidomain model has equal anisotropy ratios for the intracellular and extracellular spaces, it predicts zero extracellular potential outside a closed wave front, just as does the uniform double layer. However, if the two spaces are assigned the physiologically realistic, differing anisotropy ratios, the model predicts a variety of unexpected and interesting effects. In 1987, we showed that for a model with unequal anisotropy ratios, the extracellular potential is qualitatively similar to that observed by Corbin and Scher, with a region of positive extracellular potential leading the wave front in the direction along the fibers.[12]

Another implication of the bidomain model, first reported by Plonsey and Barr,[8] is that the intracellu lar and extracellular action currents associated with an expanding wave front are not equal and opposite. Rather, they form closed loops of net current with a fourfold (quatrefoil) symmetry. We realized that these current loops produce a magnetic field, whose quatrefoil pattern provides a unique signature of wave front propagation,[12] and that current injection produces a similar but quantitatively different pattern.[10] We have measured this magnetic field pattern using a high spatial resolution superconducting quantum interference device (SQUID) magnetometer scanned over a tissue slice from a dog heart.[14] Measurement of the magnetic field is a particu larly sensitive test of the bidomain model and unequal anisotropy ratios, because in the limit of equal anisotropy ratios, the magnetic field vanishes.

The doubly anisotropic bidomain model was rarely used to study electrical stimulation of cardiac tissue prior to 1989, when we calculated the transmembrane potential induced in a 2-dimensional bidomain stimulated with a unipolar electrode.[10] For strong stimuli, the boundary of the depolarized tissue under the cathode (the virtual cathode) has a complex, "dog-bone" shape that results in the wave front originating farther from the cathode in the direction perpendicular to the fibers than in the direction parallel to them. Concurrent with this theoretical study, we measured the virtual cathode size and shape in a dog by back-extrapolating the extracellular action potential wave front measurements to their site of origin.[15] We found a dog-bone-shaped virtual cathode that increased in size as the stimulus strength increased and was similar in shape to that predicted by the bidomain model.[16] The observed virtual cathode shape is sensitive to the tissue and membrane electrical properties and may provide a way to assess the effects of different drugs on cardiac tissue.[17] However, it was not until the widespread use of epifluorescence imaging of the transmembrane potential that the role of virtual cathodes and virtual anodes, and hence the importance of the complexity introduced by the unequal anisotropy ratios, became widely recognized.

As experience was gained with the doubly anisotropic bidomain model, it became clear that the model might be able to explain several long-standing puzzles in cardiac electrophysiology, including the mechanisms for cathodal and anodal make and break excitation,[11] as well as predict specific details of not-yet-observed phenomena, such as how a long premature pulse from a point source could induce a quatrefoil reentry pattern due to unequal dual anisotropies in myocardium.[18–22] As we see when these two predictions and their confirmation are discussed later in this chapter, there is now unequivocal evidence, at least macroscopically, that the traditional model of cardiac tissue as a nonlinear monodomain should be replaced by a nonlinear bidomain with dual anisotropies.

The peculiar distribution of tissue depolarization and hyperpolarization, as described by virtual cathodes and anodes, during and immediately after tissue excitation, raises an important question as to how these patterns interact with wave front propagation. Because these patterns are more pronounced when the intensity of the stimuli approximates that required for defibrillation, their interaction with dynamic wave fronts should have important implications in defibrillation research. Thus, there is increasing evidence that tissue anisotropy, as described by the unequal anisotropy bidomain model, determines the spread of stimulus and action currents in a manner that affects the initiation and propagation of action potentials in both the normal and the abnormal heart. It is from this perspective that we describe the evolution of our imaging system and discuss how the bidomain model and epifluorescence imaging of the cardiac transmembrane potential support new perspectives in cardiac electrophysiology.

Optical Imaging Approach

Because the bidomain responses in cardiac tissue are manifested more clearly in the transmembrane potential rather than in the extracellular potential, the optical recording technique is ideally suited to allow high-resolution observation of bidomain behavior. During the past few years, we have developed several imaging systems with different configurations specifically designed for a variety of bidomain research projects. The first system, shown in Figure 2, was a small-field, synchronous-capture epifluorescence cardiac imaging technique with wide dynamic range and high temporal and spatial resolution to image point activation patterns.[23,24] The wide dynamic range and precise timing control of the system provided us with the capability to capture synchronously a small, fractional change in the laser-induced epifluorescence proportional to transmembrane potential change. Boxcar averaging techniques in which the stimulus timing was sequentially shifted with respect to the stroboscopic illumination of the heart allowed us to achieve frame exposure times of only 0.5 ms and interframe intervals of a millisecond with a camera that had an intrinsic speed of only 7 frames per second (fps).

Subsequently, the camera system was upgraded to allow asynchronous imaging of aperiodic events such as fibrillation. The image sensor (a charged couple device [CCD] camera) was replaced by a frame-transfer CCD, which employs a double buffer technique to shorten the data trans-

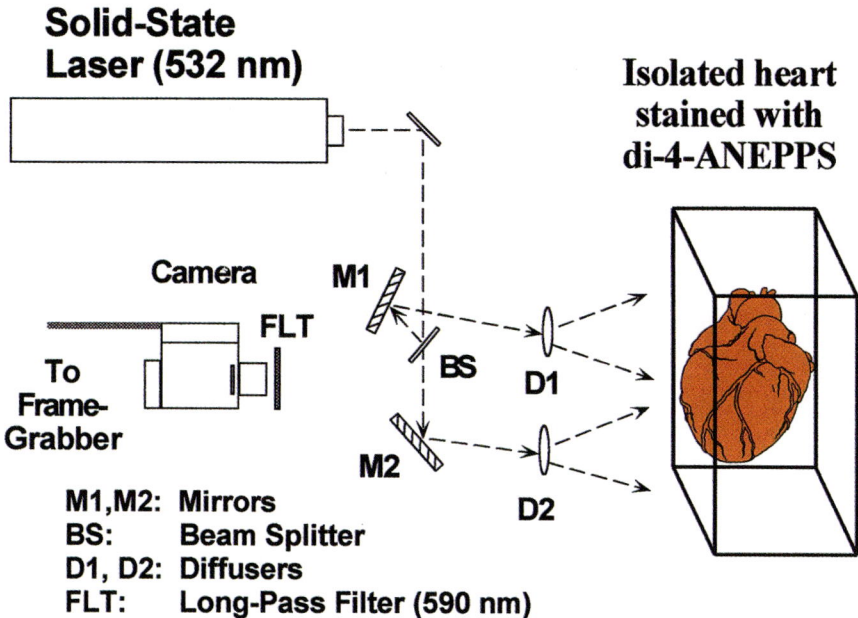

Figure 2. The first-generation synchronous imaging system developed at Vanderbilt to study cathodal and anodal make and break excitation. An acousto-optic modulator (not shown) in the laser beam allowed modulation of the laser intensity to provide submillisecond exposures of the heart to the laser illumination. Boxcar averaging techniques that involved stepwise adjustment of the interval between sequential stimuli and the laser illumination made it possible to record a sequence of 0.5-ms images separated by 1 ms with a camera that could record only 7 frames per second. Reprinted, with permission, from reference 24.

fer time. The fast frame speed led to the discovery of a quatrefoil reentry pattern[25] that had only been inferred by theoretical analyses but had never been observed in real tissue. In the meantime, a panoramic imaging technique was successfully developed to allow visualization of wave fronts on the entire heart surface,[26] as shown in Figures 3 and 4. It is now possible to measure with unprecedented detail wave front propagation on the entire heart surface. Such a capability is especially favorable for fibrillation and defibrillation studies, because the formation, maintenance, and dynamics of the reentrant patterns can be traced and measured realistically in whole heart models, not restricted to either small local areas or to only one view of the heart. We are currently completing the development of an interactive 3-dimensional wave front visualization procedure,[26,27] as well as automated, geometrical measurement of wave fronts. These are best accomplished by digitizing the 3-dimensional heart geometry using noncontact methods. The interactive visualization will allow free tilting and rotation of the computerized heart model with the animated wave fronts attached to it as texture. Such a capability will greatly facilitate geometrical tracing and measurement of the wave fronts.

The imaging system was upgraded in 1997 to a higher speed of 267 to 330 fps, with a frame resolution of 128×64 pixels.[27] This was achieved by

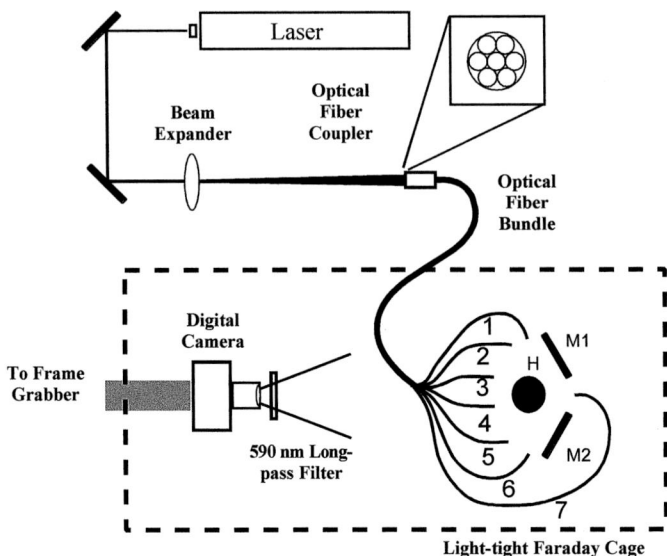

Figure 3. Schematic layout of the panoramic imaging system developed at Vanderbilt. The mirrors M1 and M2 not only allowed the camera to view the front of the heart, but also provided two other simultaneous views that included lateral and posterior portions of the heart. The seven optical fibers could be adjusted to provide uniform illumination over the entire heart.

replacing the cooled CCD camera with a faster room temperature camera, and by increasing the speed of the frame grabber and the computer. In addition, a graphic user interface panel was designed to allow fast playback of the acquired image sequences with simplified processing algorithms. More advanced image processing, including temporal/spatial filtering and analysis of electrodynamics, is performed after the experiment to improve the image quality and to extract important wave front information. Movies are produced to allow visualization of the dynamics of wave front propagation. These movies were found to be superior to frame-by-frame inspection in revealing the dynamic information due to the involvement of human visual perception. Recently, we have completed the design of camera-control software to obtain a maximum imaging speed of 1200 fps at 64×64 pixels with a 12-bit digitization.

The Role of Virtual Electrodes in Cardiac Stimulation

A surprising and unexpected result of our early bidomain simulations[10] was that during unipolar cathodal stimulation, cardiac tissue is depolarized in a dog-bone-shaped region (the virtual cathode) that lies underneath and adjacent to the cathodal electrode, and that a pair of hyperpolarized regions (virtual anodes) exist adjacent to the cathode along the directions parallel to the myocardial fibers. Until the application of high-resolution optical imaging, the complete dog-bone-shaped activation patterns had not been observed directly, despite numerous predictions from

A .

B .

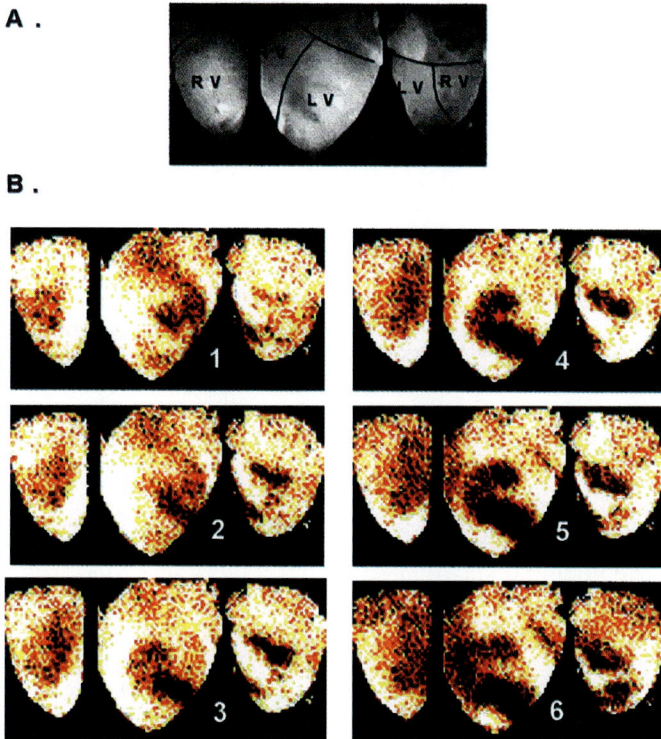

Figure 4. Panoramic imaging of spiral reentry. **A.** A frame of unprocessed fluorescence image showing the three views of the heart obtained simultaneously with the camera. The central image is the frontal view of the heart, predominantly the anterior left ventricle. The side images are obtained simultaneously using two mirrors. These side mirror images were flipped left to right to provide contiguous anatomical features. Lines have been added to indicate the left ventricle (LV) and the right ventricle (RV). **B.** Six successive frames of the processed images containing the information about V_m distribution at different times during fibrillation. The black patterns represent fully depolarized tissue. Note the evolution of the spiral wave front in the central panels and an independent reentrant pattern on the rightmost images. These frames are out of a set of 100 recorded at 67 frames per second with a 2-ms laser exposure time.

model calculations and electrode experiments that inferred its existence.[15] In 1995, three laboratories, including ours, published experimental results[23,28,29] that provided unequivocal evidence in support of the prediction that stimulation with a point electrode creates perpendicularly positioned virtual cathodes and virtual anodes, with the orientation of the patterns determined by the local muscle fiber orientation.[10] The shape of the virtual cathode and anodes was most clearly shown in our images recorded from refractory epicardial tissue of an isolated rabbit heart, as shown in Figure 5A.

We considered stimulation not only with a cathode, but also with an anode. In this case, the tissue is hyperpolarized under the anode but depolarized at regions along the fiber direction (virtual cathodes), as can be seen in Figure 5B.

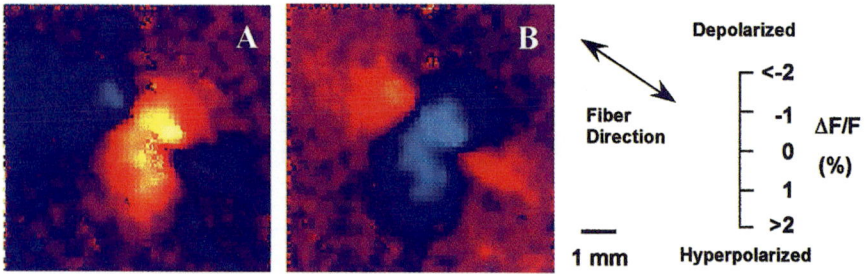

Figure 5. False-color images of the transmembrane potential associated with injection of current into refractory cardiac tissue. **A.** Image for a −10-mA, 2-ms cathodal S2 stimulus applied at a point electrode. Note the dog-bone-shaped virtual cathode (orange) and the pair of adjacent virtual anodes (blue). The fiber orientation is from lower right to upper left. The range in colors corresponds to a total fluorescence change of greater than 4%. **B.** Complementary image for a +10-mA, 2-ms anodal S2 stimulus at the same location on the heart. Note that the dog bone is now the virtual anode (blue), whereas the adjacent areas are the virtual cathodes (orange). Reprinted from reference 23, with permission from *Biophys J.*

While the virtual electrodes in Figure 5 were recorded from refractory tissue, for which there would be no propagating response, the same effects would be expected for application of a stimulus to resting cardiac tissue. Most importantly, the simultaneous existence of virtual cathodes and anodes for either a cathodal or anodal stimulus provides a mechanism for anodal stimulation: if the depolarization is strong enough, a wave front can be excited that propagates outward from the pair of virtual cathodes that are adjacent to the central, anodal dog-bone. This mechanism for anodal stimulation is called anodal make, because it occurs after the start (or make) of the stimulating pulse. The role of virtual cathodes and anodes for cathodal make and anodal make stimulation is shown schematically in Figure 6.

Theoretical models also showed that virtual electrodes play an important role in anodal break and cathodal break stimulation.[11] Anodal break and cathodal break stimulation of cardiac tissue have both been observed for decades,[30–34] but no adequate mechanism appropriate to cardiac tissue had been proposed until the bidomain studies. Break stimulation is defined as excitation that occurs upon the termination (or break) of a long stimulus pulse. With the doubly anisotropic bidomain model, the predicted mechanism of cathodal break stimulation is as follows: The strong hyperpolarization within the virtual anode removes any inactivation of the sodium channels resulting from the prolonged depolarization, and thereby renders the tissue excitable, but during the stimulus, there is no charge available by which this tissue could be stimulated. The tissue within the virtual cathode is depolarized throughout the duration of the pulse and remains unexcitable after the end of the stimulus for an interval approximately equal to the refractory period. However, upon the break of the stimulus, the positive charge that has been localized inside the cells within the depolarized virtual cathode can now diffuse into the hyperpolarized tissue within the virtual anode and excite it. Figure 6D shows how the activation wave fronts (yellow lines) will propagate away from the pair of virtual anodes adjacent

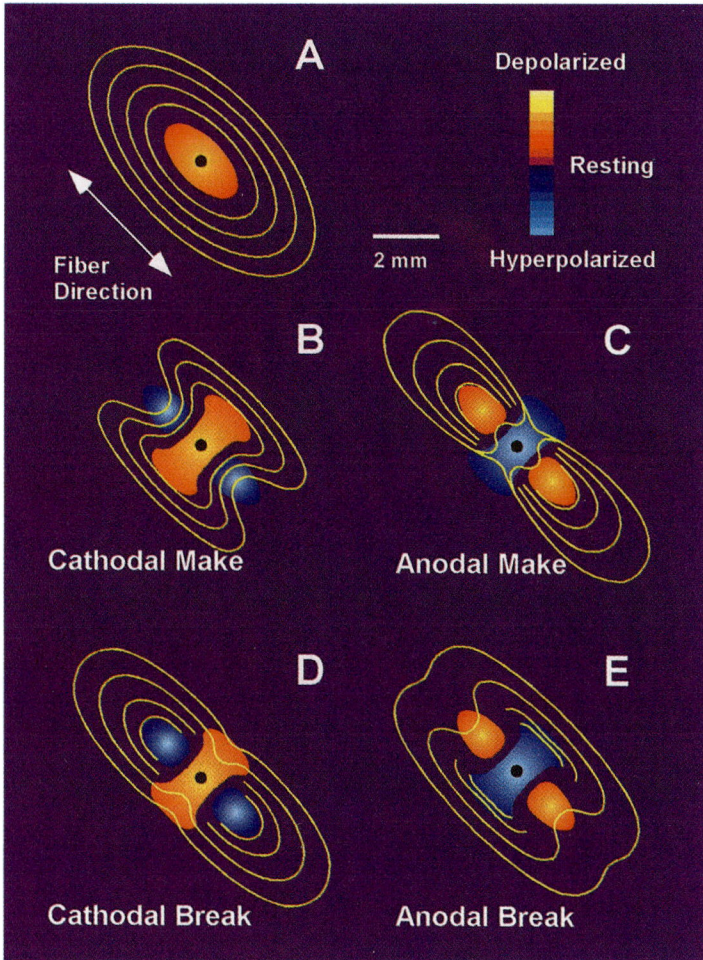

Figure 6. Schematic representation of the theoretical predictions of action potential propagation for point stimulation of cardiac tissue (based on references 9 through 11). **A.** Cathodal make stimulation in an equal anisotropy model. An elliptical region of tissue would be directly depolarized (orange) by a strong point stimulus (black dot) and would act as a virtual cathode. An elliptical action potential wave front (yellow lines separated by 2 ms) would propagate away from the edge of the virtual cathode. **B.** Cathodal make stimulation in a model with differing anisotropic conductivities for the intracellular and extracellular spaces. The virtual cathode is yellow to orange and the virtual anode is blue. The resulting propagating wave front would initially have the transverse dog-bone shape, but because of the greater longitudinal conduction velocity, the wave front would become elliptical by the time it was 5 mm from the stimulus electrode. **C.** The same model as in B, but for anodal make stimulation. A pair of action potential wave fronts propagating outwardly from the virtual cathodes (orange) merge and form an elliptical wave front within 1 cm of the stimulus electrode. **D.** The same model for cathodal break stimulation. Early activation occurs from the virtual anodes (blue) along the fiber direction. **E.** Anodal break stimulation, in which initial activation progresses transverse to the fibers from the dog-bone-shaped virtual anode (blue). Reprinted from reference 23, with permission from *Biophys J.*

to the dog-bone-shaped virtual cathode, but will be blocked initially from propagating through the refractory virtual cathode.

A similar mechanism was predicted to underlie anodal break stimulation, with the exception that a smaller amount of charge is stored within the pair of virtual cathodes and the nonlinearity of the membrane conductance may play a larger role in the stimulation process. This process is shown in Figure 6E, wherein the anodal break activation again propagates away from the virtual anode, which in this case is dog-bone shaped, and is delayed by the pair of adjacent virtual anodes.

Using our synchronous fluorescence imaging system, we verified all four mechanisms of unipolar stimulation: cathodal make, anodal make, cathodal break, and anodal break.[11] As shown in the leftmost column of Figure 7, we were able to observe the initial activation patterns of all four

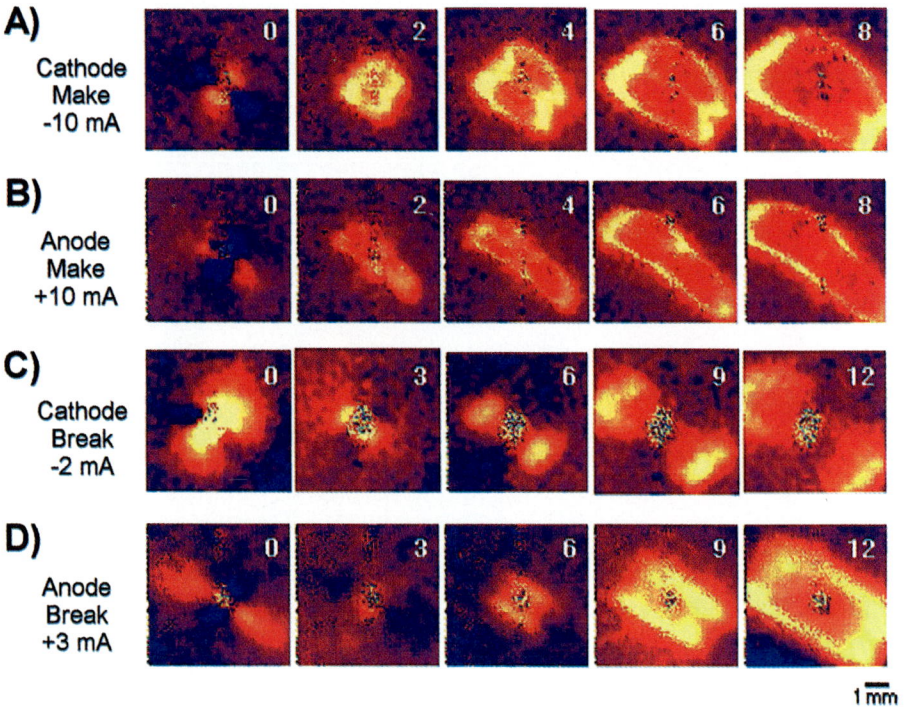

Figure 7. Virtual electrodes and the four modes of excitation of cardiac muscle. Each frame is a false-color image of the transmembrane potential associated with injection of current into fully repolarized, excitable cardiac tissue. The number in each frame is the time in ms. **A.** Cathodal make stimulation with 1-ms, −10-mA stimulus current; **B.** 1-ms, +10-mA anodal make stimulation of the same heart; **C.** 180-ms −2-mA cathodal break stimula tion of another heart; and **D.** 150-ms +3-mA anodal break stimulation of a third heart. For each row, the leftmost images are at the end of the stimulus (0 ms) and the other images are at 2-ms intervals (A and B) or 3-ms intervals (C and D) thereafter. The direction of the epicardial fibers is from lower right to upper left. Note that in both cathodal make and anodal make excitation, the early propagating wave fronts in the 2-ms and 4-ms frames are seen to originate from the orange virtual cathodes in the 0-ms frame; in break excitation, the early propagating activity in the 3-ms and 6-ms frames originates from the hyperpolarized virtual anodes in the 0-ms frame. Reprinted from reference 23, with permission from *Biophys J.*

different modes of cardiac stimulation, as well as the subsequent outwardly propagating wave fronts. The agreement with the theoretical predictions (Fig. 6) is remarkable.

The experimental observation of these phenomena would have been difficult using electrical mapping techniques that record the extracellular signals, because the early activation patterns appear only in the transmembrane potential distribution,[10] and these activation patterns are essentially embedded in the electrical stimulus artifact. Thus, optical techniques provided, for the first time, the ability to image directly and with submillimeter spatial resolution both the virtual anodes and cathodes during activation and the subsequent propagating wave fronts. Our results clearly demonstrated that current injection into the extracellular space of tissue with unequal anisotropies simultaneously produces distinct depolarized and hyperpolarized regions of transmembrane potential that are the mechanism by which anodal make and anodal break excitation occurs. This study also demonstrated that the differing anisotropic conductivities of the intra- and extracellular spaces are not just a biophysical curiosity but play a significant role in the stimulation of the heart with strong electrical current.

Discovery of Quatrefoil Reentry

Single spiral wave rotors with circular movement, and two opposing rotors with a figure-of-8 reentrant pathway are basic patterns of electrically induced reentry in normal cardiac muscle that provide the fundamental elements for understanding and treatment planning of many cardiac arrhythmias. In contrast to anatomical reentry that arises from an anatomical obstacle or inhomogeneity about which the reentrant excitation propagates, both of these functional reentry patterns can be produced in anatomically homogenous tissue solely by the interaction between a spatial gradient in stimulus strength and another spatial gradient in excitability. As a result, the reentrant activation propagates around a phase singularity, i.e., a region of tissue whose electrical phase is indeterminate, with the spiral wave exhibiting a single singularity and a wave front that extends from this singularity to the edge of the active tissue, and figure-of-8 reentry having a pair of singularities that define the ends of a wave front.

Theoretical studies based on the dual anisotropies in cardiac tissue suggested the existence of an unusual 4-loop reentry.[18–22] Using numerical simulations, Roth and Saypol[20–22] found that when the pacing (S1) and the premature (S2) stimuli were delivered at the same site on the tissue, the hyperpolarization at the virtual anode shortened the refractory period of the S1 wave front parallel to the fibers, and the depolarization at the virtual cathode lengthened the refractory period of the S1 wave front perpendicular to the fibers. Thus, a wave front initiated by the S2 stimulus could propagate parallel to the fibers, but was blocked perpendicular to them. This "arc of functional conduction block" would lead to a fourfold symmetrical reentrant pattern in their computer model, shown in Figure 8.

Similar to other functional reentry patterns, the reentry is established by the interaction of a spatial gradient in excitability following the S1 stimulus with a differing spatial gradient in the strength of the S2 stimulus.

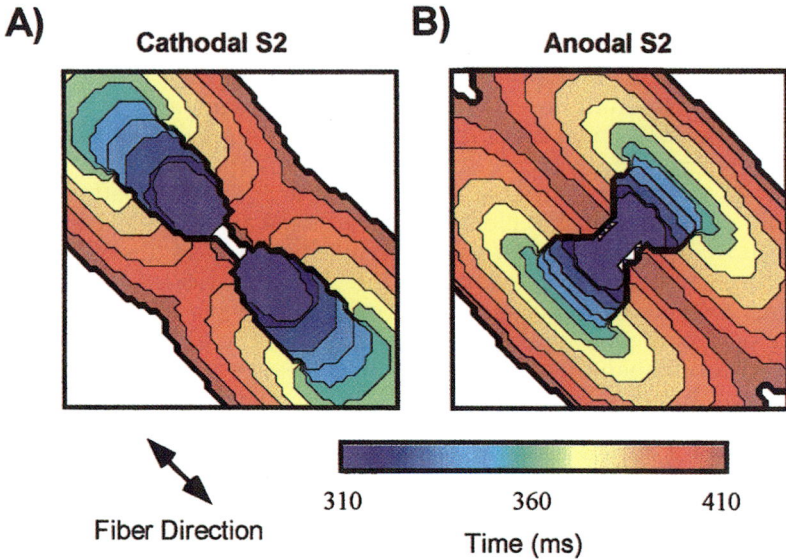

Figure 8. The predicted sequence of quatrefoil reentry in cardiac tissue. **A.** The isochrones (10 ms separation) following a strong cathodal S2 break stimulus applied to refractory tissue as predicted by the bidomain model of cardiac tissue. The strong S2 stimulus was delivered to tissue that was still refractory from the earlier, twice-threshold S1. Because of the tissue anisotropy, the cathodal S2 produces a dog-bone-shaped virtual cathode region that maintains the tissue depolarization and refractoriness. The adjacent anodal regions on either side of the dog-bone are hyperpolarized by S2, which returns the tissue to excitability. At the end of S2, charge flows from the cathodal region into the anodal ones, so that activation propagates along the fiber axis but is blocked from spreading transversely. Subsequently, the wave front propagates around the region that was directly polarized during the S2 stimulus, so that the S2 wave fronts finally reenter toward the electrode from both sides, collide near the electrode, and then launch another wave front that again moves along the fiber direction. **B.** The isochrones predicted for an anodal break S2. Courtesy of Bradley Roth.

Winfree[19] has described this in terms of the critical point hypothesis, in which phase singularities, about which the reentrant wave front propagates, are created at the intersection of the excitability contour T* and the stimulus threshold contour S*. In spiral wave reentry, crossed-field stimulation by a pair of orthogonal line electrodes produces orthogonal T* and S* that cross at the point that defines the fixed end of a spiral wave; figure-of-8 reentry occurs when the T* generated by a planar S1 wave front crosses a circular S* from a point stimulus, producing a pair of singularities that define the ends of a single wave front. Quatrefoil reentry is unique in that it can be produced by sequential stimulation by a single electrode: a nearly elliptical T* from S1 is cut four times by the dog-bone-shaped S* of a strong S2 delivered at the same stimulus site. Consequently, there are four phase singularities that define the ends of a pair of synchronized wave fronts.

Using our frame-transfer CCD camera system, we performed high-speed imaging to investigate the induction mechanism of such a peculiar reentrant pattern. In 16 isolated, Langendorff-perfused rabbit hearts, high-speed optical imaging at 133 or 267 fps allowed us to observe the induced response with a unipolar point electrode. Delivering long stimuli during the vulnerable phase created the novel quatrefoil-shaped reentry pattern consisting of two pairs of opposing rotors. Successful induction occurred in a narrow range of coupling intervals. A dog-bone pattern of virtual electrodes was established during the premature stimulus (Fig. 9A). Wave fronts that were launched began to propagate from the virtual anodes immediately after the termination of S2. The alternating blocking and conducting effects of the virtual electrodes, as well as the boundary between virtual cathode and virtual anode, provided the necessary substrate for quatrefoil reentry. As predicted by the theory, the direction of propagation of the reentrant spiral wave fronts reversed with a reversal in S2 polarity (not shown). Because of interference by secondary wave fronts propagat-

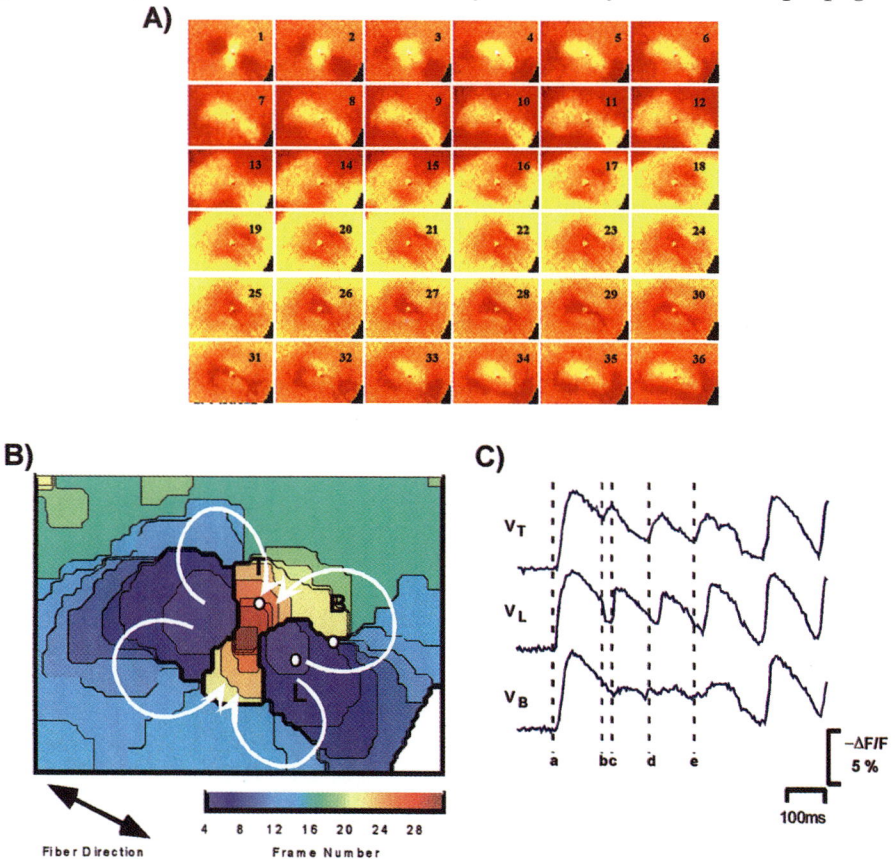

Figure 9. A. Dye-fluorescence images of the transmembrane potential of an isolated rabbit heart as a function of space and time during cathodally induced quatrefoil reentry. A cathodal S2 stimulus (-20 mA, 20 ms) is applied at the center of the tissue; the stimulus ends after frame 1. Adjacent frames are separated in time by 3.8 ms, and show a 20×13.5-mm^2 area of tissue. The arrow indicates the fiber direction. **B.** Pseudo-color isochronal map showing the position of the activation wave front at subsequent times after the end of the S2 stimulus. **C.** The transmembrane potential as a function of time, at the three different locations marked T, L, and B. The vertical dotted line a is the time of the last S1 stimulus, b and c are the start and end of the S2 stimulus, and d and e are start times of subsequent depolarizations in the VT trace. The V_B trace shows that the B recording site in panel B is within or near the region of functional block.

ing back into the region of the reentrant pattern, quatrefoil reentries were not sustained and lasted between one and four complete cycles.

One of the key findings of our studies of quatrefoil reentry is that for strong shocks we can clearly distinguish between cathodal make or anodal make activation, for which the wave front propagates away from the depolarized virtual cathode, and cathodal break or anodal break activation, for which activation propagates from the hyperpolarized virtual anode. Activation of cardiac tissue by the break mode of stimulation may prove to be an additional new mechanism for defibrillation.

Tissue-Medium Interface

The role of the tissue surrounding the heart is important in transthoracic defibrillation, in that the distribution of defibrillation currents and the fraction of currents that actually enter the heart are determined by the conductivity of the skin, the thoracic muscles and ribs, the lungs, the mediastinum, and the great vessels. The effects of the extracardiac tissues and great vessels on intracardiac defibrillation, such as with an implantable defibrillator, is not well known. Studies of internal defibrillation are conducted on intact humans either during transthoracic surgery or in the catheterization lab, on intact dogs or dogs with exposed hearts supported in a pericardial cradle, and on isolated rabbit or dog hearts in air or in a conducting bath. In each of these preparations, the heart is located in a different conducting environment, and if the surrounding environment has any effect on cardiac defibrillation, then there could be substantial differences between studies conducted with different conductor configurations. An example of the effect of extracardiac conductivity is shown in Figure 10,[35] which demonstrates the modeling results of tissue response from an endocardial shock. Although the endocardial response appears to be the same, the epicardium shows different activation patterns due to different tissue-medium interface conditions.

In a monodomain model of the heart, the heart-tissue interface serves as a boundary between two regions of differing conductivity, and the primary effect of the interface is to alter the direction of the electrical field and thereby bend the lines followed by the electrical current. In the bidomain model, the situation is substantially more complex. For example, current flowing in a passive monodomain, such as the blood, crosses into the bidomain by the extracellular space, and then proceeds to redistribute itself between the intra- and extracellular spaces in accordance with the length constant of the tissue. The transmembrane potential reflects this redistribution of current and shows the effect predominately within a length constant of the surface.

Although the bidomain boundary effects have been the subjects of some theoretical debate,[36] there have been few direct observations of boundary effects. One of the clearest demonstrations involves comparison of the epicardial transmembrane potential during application of intracardiac defibrillation-strength shocks. Figure 11A shows tissue response from an endocardial anodal shock with an isolated, Langendorff-perfused rabbit heart pressed against the frontal glass window of the bath. The activation

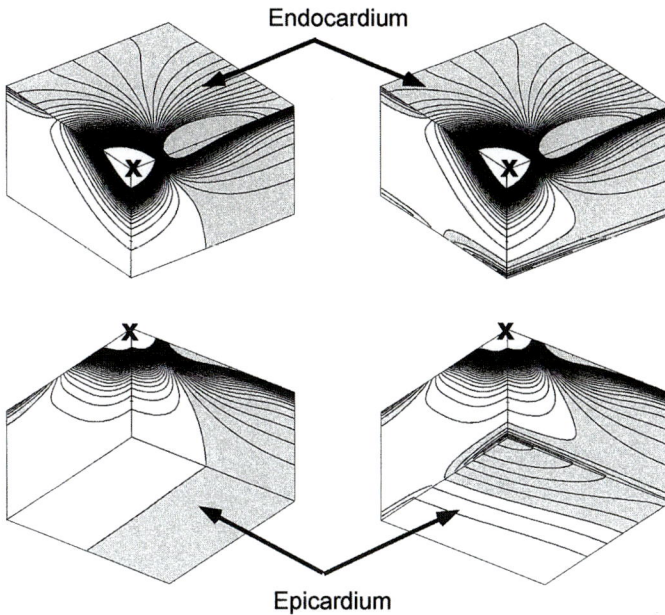

Figure 10. Model predictions of the transmembrane potential during intracardiac defibrillation in a slab of cardiac tissue that is 5 mm × 5 mm × 3 mm thick. Only one quarter of the tissue is shown. *Left:* Endocardial (upper) and epicardial (lower) views of the potential distribution when the epicardial surface is bounded by an insulator. The shaded regions have a negative transmembrane potential change due to the shock. Contours are every 300 mV; contours above 20 V and below −7 V have been omitted. *Right:* The same views when the epicardial surface is bounded by a conducting bath. Note the two endocardial distributions are similar but there is a pronounced rotation of the potential distribution and the zero-volt line between the two boundary conditions. Reprinted from reference 35, with permission of *IEEE Trans Biomed Eng.*

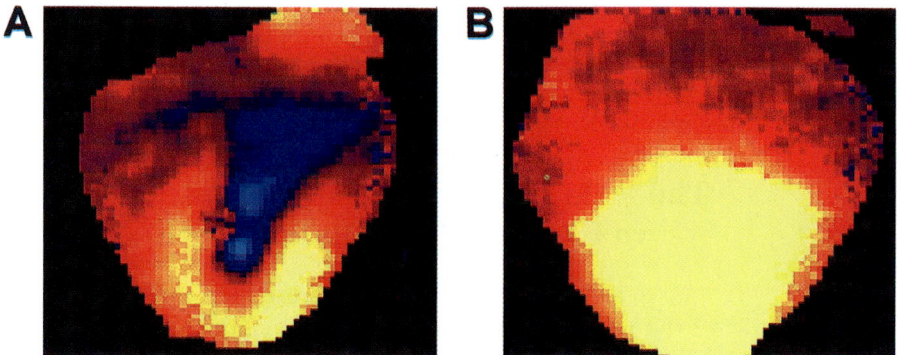

Figure 11. The dye fluorescence image of the epicardial surface of an isolated rabbit heart during an intracardiac defibrillation-strength anodal shock. **A.** The heart is pressed against a glass plate to produce a horseshoe-shaped depolarized region (yellow) surrounding a hyperpolarized one (blue). **B.** The heart is suspended freely in the bath, and only depolarization is evident on the epicardium.

pattern shows a horseshoe-shaped depolarized region surrounding a negatively polarized region. Such an epicardial observation of bipolar response from endocardial shocks is consistent with the result obtained in the right ventricle by Efimov et al.[37] However, when the heart was suspended in the bath without being pressed against the frontal window, the tissue response did not show such a horseshoe pattern (Fig. 11B), and the negative polarization cannot be observed from optical recordings on the epicardium.

The difference between these two epicardial responses could be the result of 1) changes in the propagation of direct activation during the shock, or 2) differences between the heart-medium interface through the action of pressing the heart against the frontal window. Using high-speed imaging at 1200 fps with a frame interval of 0.8 ms, we observed the progression of tissue response during the shock. The results showed that the negative polarization was not detectable with our instrumentation when the heart was freely suspended in the bath. Therefore, we conclude that the high impedance created by the heart-plate interface is responsible for the bipolar response as shown in Figure 11A, in that the plate serves as a no-current boundary and prevents current from leaving the bidomain at the epicardium and from producing a large transmembrane potential change at the monodomain/bidomain interface.

For the first time, the ability to observe regions of depolarization and hyperpolarization during the shock and to identify these in terms of virtual anodes and cathodes had made possible the detailed examination of the mechanisms by which a defibrillation shock alters the state of cardiac tissue over large regions of the heart. Studies by the group of Efimov[37,38] as well as those studies reported in this chapter demonstrate that the transmembrane potential distribution on the epicardial surface depends upon whether the heart is hanging free in a bath or pressed up against an insulating window. Mathematical modeling by Latimer and Roth[35] confirms that the epicardial potential distribution is altered significantly between a surrounding material of air or saline. All of these observations suggest that interpretations of transmembrane potentials on the epicardial surface during defibrillation are strongly affected by the surrounding environment. We conclude from these studies that investigators studying defibrillation mechanisms must be aware that the transmembrane potential distributions on the epicardial surface depend upon the electrical conductivity of the surrounding medium.

The Role of the Bidomain Model in Cardiac Defibrillation

In the past few decades, a trend in defibrillation research has been established toward the understanding of mechanistic shock action. Chronologically, the proposed defibrillation mechanisms include total extinction,[39] critical mass,[40,41] upper limit of vulnerability (ULV),[42] and synchronization of repolarization.[43] Other defibrillation mechanisms, including more speculative ones such as perturbation of chaotic systems,[44] generated a lot of interest, and experimental results have been gathered to support the chaotic nature of ventricular fibrillation.[45,46]

The relationship between defibrillation energy or voltage or current and the likelihood of success has been found experimentally to be well described by a sigmoid-shaped curve, reflecting a probabilistic function.[47] Actual defibrillation thresholds (DFTs) must be determined experimentally, and even mathematical models of defibrillation current distributions require empirical calibration.[48] Surprisingly, there is no theory or mathematical model that provides a first-principles connection between the vast knowledge of cellular cardiac electrophysiolo gy and the growing understanding of fibrillation and defibrillation. Today, there are no models that can predict, from a description of ion channel kinetics, the response of a fibrillating heart to a defibrillation shock. The role of tissue anisotropy in the distribution of defibrillation currents is unknown.

It is no coincidence that the progress in defibrillation research is tightly coupled to the capability of the research instrumentation, especially the exponential increase over the years in the number of recording sites on the heart. It is through the advances in instrumentation that many different levels of defibrillation mechanisms can be pursued.[49] By recording simultaneously from a large number of sites, more global information, such as reentrant conduction pathways, location of the ectopic focus, or wave front curvature, can be investigated. The hypotheses of total extinction and critical mass were proposed when only a small number of recording sites were available. Such views have led to the argument over continued versus regenerated fibrillation wave fronts.[50,51] In contrast, the ULV hypothesis has been studied extensively by the group of Ideker and Chen,[42,49,50] with an electrical mapping system of more than 200 recording sites. This hypothesis has significant clinical implications because a correlation between ULV and DFT has been suggested.[42] However, the ULV hypothesis has been reevaluated recently, in theory and in experiment,[52,53] as a result of rare experimental observations of critical point formation resulting from delivered shocks, and also due to the dynamic variation of isocontours during the shock. The ability to record the transmembrane potential using optical recording techniques has led to a recent hypothesis of synchronization of repolarization.[43]

Of all of the questions presented by cardiac defibrillation, the most fundamental relates to the interaction between the electrical field of the shock and the transmembrane potential of individual cardiac cells. It is well recognized that the myocardial syncytium has cablelike properties, including an exponential drop in transmembrane potential with distance from an extracellular electrode, described by a length constant of 1 or 2 mm. Hence, during a defibrillation shock, one might expect that cells only within a few length constants of the electrodes would experience appreciable changes to their transmembrane potential, and that the bulk of the heart would be unaffected. However, it is clear that a sufficiently strong defibrillation shock, delivered by some combination of transthoracic, epicardial, or intracavitary electrodes, can render virtually all of the heart transiently unexcitable.

Obviously, changes in transmembrane potential are required to render cardiac tissue unexcitable, but a uniform cable can carry large amounts of current, appropriately distributed between the intracellular and extracellular spaces, without requiring transmembrane potential differences beyond several length constants from the electrodes. One hypothesis to address this problem was advanced 10 years ago: with the sawtooth mechanism, the discrete cell-to-cell resistance at the gap junctions causes each cell to be depolarized and hyperpolarized on opposite ends.[54,55] If the sawtooth has sufficient amplitude, one end of each cell would be depolarized above threshold, and the resulting sodium influx would then depolarize the entire cell. This could provide a possible explanation of how a shock can activate a large volume of tissue. Despite its theoretical plausibility and observation of the phenomena in a single, isolated myocyte[56,57] and a single strand of myocytes,[58] the search in real tissue or in wider cultured strands for this specific sawtooth excitation has been unsuccessful,[59,60] apparently because the staggering of adjacent myocardial cells provides shunt pathways across the high-resistance cell junctions, thereby attenuating the sawtooth amplitude.

An alternative bidomain mechanism for the interaction of defibrillation shocks with bulk myocardium was suggested by Trayanova and colleagues[61]: the curvature of the cardiac fibers and the un equal anisotropy ratios cause depolarization and hyperpolarization throughout the heart, in that as the applied stimulating currents transverse the heart, they encounter fibers at different orientations, which would induce a redistribution of current between the intracellular and extracellular spaces and a concomitant change in the transmembrane potential. Their analysis also predicted that the transmembrane potential at the heart surface is quite different from the transmembrane potential below the surface. The differences may be so large that the surface may be depolarized while the bulk of the tissue is hyperpolarized.

Another bidomain mechanism has been proposed to explain the defibrillation of bulk myocardium. Under the syncytial heterogeneity hypothesis,[62] localized heterogeneities in the cellular volume fraction (the ratio of intracellular to extracellular space in a given element of myocardial tissue) at the level of a few percent could lead to current redistributions that are sufficient to depolarize the tissue. This hypothesis can be generalized to include localized heterogeneities of any number of bidomain parameters, or even millimeter-scale changes in tissue connectivity or conductivity. Thus, it appears that the bidomain model and the underlying tissue anisotropy may hold the answer to the fundamental questions of how strong shocks can inactivate most of the heart.

As a first step toward quantifying shock-tissue interactions during defibrillation, we have used optical imaging of the epicardial transmembrane potential V_m during far-field stimulation.[63] Langendorff-perfused, di-4-ANEPPS-stained, isolated rabbit hearts with atria excised were immersed in a $10 \times 10 \times 15$ cm^3 bath of Tyrode's solution. Following 20 right ventricular pacing pulses at a constant cycle length of 500 ms, a diastolic 1-ms S2 was delivered to plate electrodes at the ends of the bath to produce horizontal shock fields of ± 3.3, ± 6.7, or ± 10 V/cm. High-speed optical imaging at 322 fps measured V_m changes during and after S2. The heart axis was at either $0°$, $45°$, or $90°$ to the vertical. The prompt response of V_m was recorded in the frame taken during S2. To detect shock-induced asymmetries in V_m, we calculated the x and y components (p_x and p_y) of the dipole moment of the V_m image by integrating the prompt-response image intensity weighted by the x or y distance from the center of a pre-S2 image. Figure 12 shows the

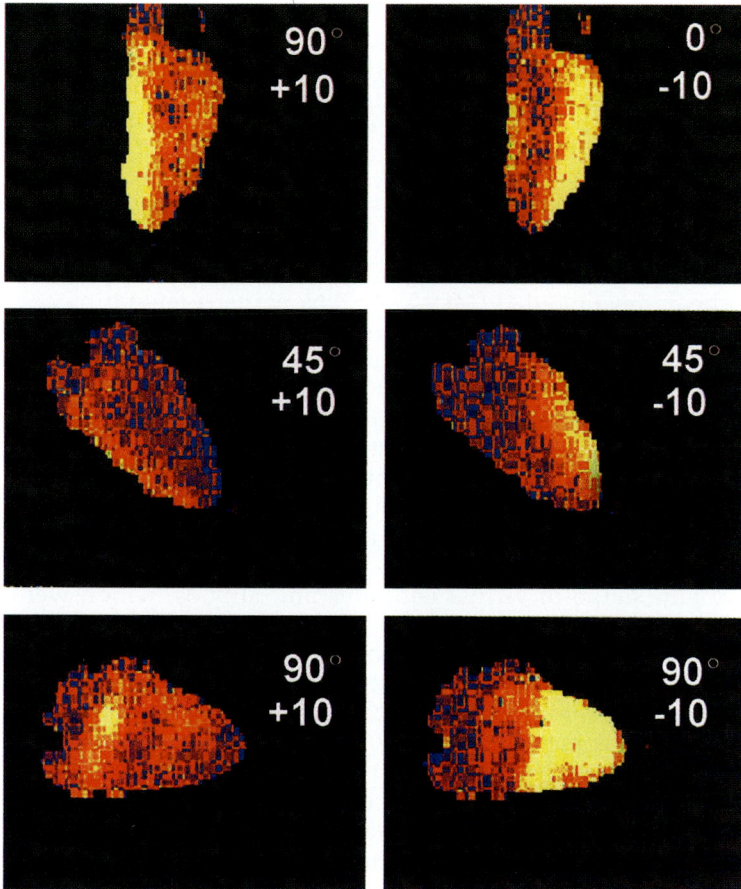

Figure 12. The prompt response of an isolated rabbit heart to field stimulation by a horizontal electrical field at three different angles and shock polarities (±10 V/cm). Red/yellow is depolarization. For 90°, +10 V/cm, the valve ring may block the field. Otherwise, the pattern is clearly determined by the orientation and sign of the field and not the orientation of the heart, consistent with the monodomain/bidomain boundary between the surrounding bath and the heart.

prompt responses of shocks delivered horizontally with the heart at three angles. Spherical and ellipsoidal models of cardiac shock response using a bidomain with unequal intracellular and extracellular anisotropy ratios and fiber curvature predict that the dominant epicardial effect arises from the monodomain/bidomain interface, which to first order is independent of the orientation of the underlying fibers. As a result, the cardiac surface facing the cathodal electrode would exhibit depolarization while the surface facing the anode would hyperpolarize.[61,64] If macroscopic or cellular conductivity discontinuities play the dominant role in defibrillation, prompt depolarization would be expected on both sides of the heart. Our data show that p_x is determined by shock strength and polarity; our data are not yet adequate to ascertain whether we can detect secondary, fiber orientation effects, in the form of a p_y dipole moment or curvature of the isopotential line between the depolarized and hyperpolarized regions of the epicardium. We are continuing with these experiments, and are devising experimental configurations for which the boundary effects should be smaller than those due to bidomain anisotropies or heterogeneities.

Conclusions

Over the past decade, a variety of linear and nonlinear bidomain models have been developed.[11,12,14–17,23,65,66] New instrumentation and experimental techniques have been devised to test quantitative predictions by these models, and we have conducted a series of in vitro experiments to provide qualitative and quantitative tests of most of the specific predictions of the bidomain model. The results present convincing evidence that at the spatial scale of 1 mm and larger the bidomain model accurately describes the electrical behavior of cardiac tissue, particularly its response to strong electrical shocks. The bidomain model with unequal electrical anisotropies has been used to make a number of surprising and nonintuitive predictions that were not anticipated by earlier models, such as the existence and shape of virtual cathodes and anodes, which were subsequently confirmed experimentally. The unequal anisotropy bidomain model provides the first explanation of how cathodal and anodal make and break stimuli induce propagating activation. The experimental confirmation of quatrefoil reentry is the capstone of these predictions.

The bidomain model has led to the replacement, during excitation from a point source of strong currents, of the traditional concept of an elliptical excitation wave front with a cloverleaf, or dog-bone, excitation pattern.[11,23] Furthermore, the shock effects from either far-field shock electrodes, epicardial patches, or internal coil electrodes have been shown to be consistent with bidomain predictions.[37,63,67–69] It is important to emphasize that the phenomena that validate the bidomain model all result from differences in the electrical anisotropy of the electrical conductivities of the intracellular and extracellular spaces. Because of these differences, the spatial distribution of stimulus currents will differ between the two spaces, which in turn leads to previously unexpected transmembrane potential distributions. These phenomena in turn have led to the revision of several historical concepts in cardiac electrophysiology, including defibrillation mechanisms. A representative case is the reevaluation of the critical point hypothesis,[18,70] which was based on simple excitation and repolarization gradients to determine the intersecting singularity points. The complex rather than simple pattern of excitation gradients will make it necessary to review this important hypothesis in fibrillation and defibrillation theory.[52]

Given the recent demonstrations of the cardiac bidomain response and the growing acceptance of the bidomain concept in the cardiac electrophysiology community, it is worthwhile to contemplate the future contributions that such a model may offer. Historically, the electrical behavior of the membrane of isolated cardiac myocytes has been studied using patch-clamp recordings and carefully designed current and voltage protocols. The immediate response of cardiac tissue to electrical stimulation, as occurs during pacing and defibrillation, has been studied with micropipettes that measure the transmembrane potential, V_m, of a single cardiac cell, or with dye/fluorescence techniques that record from a number of adjacent cells, or with macroscopic electrodes that are placed within the myocardium or on the epicardial, endocardial, or torso surfaces. The models used to explain the resulting data have a similar span in spatial scales and describe, for example, the kinetics of single ion channels or the movement of activation wave fronts through the heart. The challenge facing defibrillation research is to couple channel-scale and cellular-scale observations to those of the whole heart, recognizing that in fibrillation all scales are active: from the single channel to the macroscopic geometry of the reentry pathways.

Thus, a detailed understanding of the propagation of electrical activity through ventricular myocardium requires a knowledge of both the electrical behavior of an individual cardiac cell and the role of the cardiac syncytium that couples together the 4 billion cells that form the ventricles. A similar range of scales occurs in atrial fibrillation. Over the past decade, patch-clamp techniques, coupled with molecular biology, have been providing an increasingly clear picture of ion channel structure and the role of specific ion channels in the cardiac action potential. Progress has been slower in combining this knowledge with models of myocardial tissue, primarily because of the formidable computational challenge imposed by the requirements for 10-μm spatial discretiza tion and 5-μs time steps in a simulated block of myocardium, no less the entire heart. At present, models that support active propagation of wave fronts are discretized at the scale of a millimeter, and hence cannot include cellular level effects such as the explicit role of intercellular discontinuities and intracellular gradients in voltage or channel density. Although the spatial resolution and geometric and physiological complexity of models is continually increasing, it is unlikely that a single model will be able to span between the ion channel and the whole heart. Given the present impossibility of such a calculation, *the bidomain model offers great promise as a physiologically realistic intermediate step to link the submicron spatial scale associated with molecular electrophysiology to the 10-cm spatial scale of macroscopic electrical behavior of the intact heart.* Toward this end, the bidomain model has already far exceeded the ability of other models to make quantitative predictions regarding cardiac electrical activity that subsequently have been verified experimentally. The coupling of realistic bidomain models of the entire heart with detailed electrophysiological models of the cardiac membrane promises to be a fruitful area of cardiac research.

From this perspective, there are a number of questions that remain to be answered, about the bidomain model and about cardiac electrophysiology. At issue are concerns such as how best to describe the actual cardiac syncytium at all spatial scales, how spatial variations in electrical anisotropies, other bidomain parameters, and tissue macrostructure affect propagation of depolarization and the spread of repolarization, and how myocardium responds to external electri cal stimuli of differing time courses. The clinical cardiac literature is replete with observations of electrophysiological phenomena that have defied theoretical explanation, such as the strength-interval characteristics of two sequential stimuli and the differences in threshold for monophasic and biphasic stimuli. Other areas of interest include the exact angular dependence upon conduction velocity, wave front curvature during collisions, and the effect of the conductivity of the medium surrounding the heart on both propagating action potentials and defibrillation shock distributions. Some phenomena, such as the directional dependence of the rate of rise of V_m, have been addressed with models that may be unnecessarily complicated or whose wider impli cations are not fully understood, such as cardiac models with large numbers of discrete cells. As the role of individual ion channels is described in finer and finer detail, the severity of the gap between our understanding of the molecular electrophysiology of the heart and our knowledge of how the $\approx 10^9$ cardiac cells interact to form the heart is becoming more pronounced. Reentrant phenomena that exist at spatial scales of 1 mm to 1 cm will undoubtedly be governed by both ion channel kinetics and the nature of the 3-dimensional cardiac cable, which in some cases must include local heterogeneities. Addressing these questions and others will require further refinement of the advanced optical, electrical, and magnetic recording techniques developed so far, and may require extension of the bidomain model to include the effects of regional heterogeneities and discontinuities in tissue conductivity.

References

1. Corbin LV, Scher AM. The canine heart as an electrocardiographic generator. Dependence on cardiac cell orientation. *Circ Res* 1977;41:58–67.
2. Colli-Franzone P, Guerri L, Viganotti C, et al. Potential fields generated by oblique dipole layers modeling excitation wavefronts in the anisotropic myocardium. Comparison with potential fields elicited by paced dog hearts in a volume conductor. *Circ Res* 1982;51:330–346.
3. Muler AL, Markin VS. Electrical properties of anisotropic neuromuscular syncytia. I. Distribution of the electrotonic potential. *Biofizika* 1977;22:307–312.
4. Muler AL, Markin VS. Electrical properties of anisotropic neuromuscular syncytia. II. Distribution of a flat front of excitation. *Biofizika* 1977;22:518–522.
5. Muler AL, Markin VS. Electrical properties of anisotropic neuromuscular syncytia. III. Steady state of the front of excitation. *Biofizika* 1977;22:671–675.
6. Tung L. *A Bidomain Model for Describing Ischemic Myocardial DC Potentials* [PhD dissertation]. Cambridge, MA: MIT; 1978.
7. Geselowitz D, Miller W. A bidomain model for anisotropic cardiac muscle. *J Biomed Eng* 1983;11:191–206.
8. Plonsey R, Barr RC. Current flow patterns in two-dimensional anisotropic bisyncytia with normal and extreme conductivities. *Biophys J* 1984;45:557–571.
9. Roth B, Wikswo J Jr. A bidomain model for the extracellular potential and magnetic field of cardiac tissue. *IEEE Trans Biomed Eng* 1986;33:467–469.
10. Sepulveda NG, Roth BJ, Wikswo JP Jr. Current injection into a two-dimensional anisotropic bidomain. *Biophys J* 1989;55:987–999.
11. Roth BJ. A mathematical model of make and break electrical stimulation of cardiac tissue by a unipolar anode or cathode. *IEEE Trans Biomed Eng* 1995;42:1174–1184.
12. Sepulveda NG, Wikswo JP Jr. Electric and magnetic fields from two-dimensional anisotropic bisyncytia. *Biophys J* 1987;51:557–568.
13. Roth BJ. Electrical conductivity values used with the bidomain model of cardiac tissue. *IEEE Trans Biomed Eng* 1997;44:326–328.

14. Staton DJ, Friedman RN, Wikswo JP Jr. High resolution SQUID imaging of octupolar currents in anisotropic cardiac tissue. *IEEE Trans Appl Superconduct* 1993;3:1934–1936.

15. Wikswo JP Jr, Wisialowski TA, Altemeier WA, et al. Virtual cathode effects during stimulation of cardiac muscle: Two-dimensional in vivo experiments. *Circ Res* 1991;68:513–530.

16. Roth BJ, Wikswo JP Jr. Electrical stimulation of cardiac tissue: A bidomain model with active membrane properties. *IEEE Trans Biomed Eng* 1994;41:232–240.

17. Turgeon J, Wisialowski TA, Wong W, et al. Suppression of longitudinal versus transverse conduction by sodium channel block. Effects of sodium bolus. *Circulation* 1992;85:2221–2226.

18. Winfree AT. Electrical instability in cardiac muscle: Phase singularities and rotors. *J Theor Biol* 1989;138:353–405.

19. Winfree AT. Ventricular reentry in three dimensions. In Zipes DP, Jalife J (eds): *Cardiac Electrophysiology: From Cell to Bedside.* Philadelphia: W.B. Saunders Co.; 1990:224–234.

20. Roth BJ, Saypol JM. The formation of a reentrant action potential wave front in tissue with unequal anisotropy ratios. *Int J Bifur Chaos* 1991;1:927–928.

21. Saypol JM, Roth BJ. A mechanism for anisotropic reentry in cardiac muscle. *J Cardiovasc Electrophysiol* 1992;3:558–566.

22. Roth BJ. Nonsustained reentry following successive stimulation of cardiac tissue through a unipolar electrode. *J Cardiovasc Electrophysiol* 1997;8:768–778.

23. Wikswo JP Jr, Lin S-F, Abbas RA. Virtual electrodes in cardiac tissue: A common mechanism for anodal and cathodal stimulation. *Biophys J* 1995;69:2195–2210.

24. Lin S-F, Abbas RA, Wikswo JP Jr. High-resolution high-speed synchronous epifluorescence imaging of cardiac activation. *Rev Sci Instrum* 1997; 68:213–217.

25. Lin S-F, Roth BJ, Echt DS, Wikswo JP Jr. Complex dynamics following unipolar stimulation during the vulnerable phase. *Circulation* 1996;94:I714.

26. Lin S-F, Echt DS, Wikswo JP Jr. Panoramic whole-heart optical mapping of ventricular fibrillation. *Circulation* 1996;94:I48.

27. Lin S-F, Wikswo JP Jr. Panoramic optical imaging of transmembrane potential propagation in isolated heart. *J Biomed Opt* 1999;4:200–207.

28. Neunlist M, Tung L. Spatial distribution of cardiac transmembrane potentials around an extracellular electrode: Dependence on fiber orientation. *Biophys J* 1995;68:2310–2322.

29. Knisley SB. Transmembrane voltage changes during unipolar stimulation of rabbit ventricle. *Circ Res* 1995;77:1229–1239.

30. Brooks C, Hoffman BF, Suckling EE. *Excitability of the Heart.* New York: Grune and Stratton; 1955.

31. Dekker E. Direct current make and break thresholds for pacemaker electrodes on the canine ventricle. *Circ Res* 1970;27:811–823.

32. Goto M, Brooks C. Membrane excitability of the frog ventricle examined by long pulses. *Am J Physiol* 1969;217:1236–1245.

33. Lindemans FW, Heethaar RM, van der Gon JJ, Zimmerman AN. Site of initial excitation and current threshold as a function of electrode radius in heart muscle. *Cardiovasc Res* 1975;9:95–104.

34. Ehara T. Rectifier properties of canine papillary muscle. *Jpn J Physiol* 1971; 21:49–69.

35. Latimer DC, Roth BJ. Electrical stimulation of cardiac tissue by a bipolar electrode in a conductive bath. *IEEE Trans Biomed Eng* 1998;45:1449–1458.

36. Roth BJ. Effect of a perfusing bath on the rate of rise of an action potential propagating through a slab of cardiac tissue. *Ann Biomed Eng* 1996;24:639–46.

37. Efimov IR, Cheng YN, Biermann M, et al. Transmembrane voltage changes produced by real and virtual electrodes during monophasic defibrillation shock

delivered by an implantable electrode. *J Cardiovasc Electrophysiol* 1997; 8:1031–1045.

38. Entcheva E, Eason J, Efimov IR, et al. Virtual electrode effects in transvenous defibrillation-modulation by structure and interface: Evidence from bidomain simulations and optical mapping. *J Cardiovasc Electrophysiol* 1998;9:949–961.

39. Wiggers CJ. The mechanism and nature of ventricular defibrillation. *Am Heart J* 1940;20:399.

40. Mower MM, Mirowski M, Spear JF, Moore EN. Patterns of ventricular activity during catheter defibrillation. *Circulation* 1974;49:858–861.

41. Zipes DP, Fischer J, King RM, et al. Termination of ventricular fibrillation in dogs by depolarizing a critical amount of myocardium. *Am J Cardiol* 1975;36:37–44.

42. Chen P-S, Shibata N, Dixon EG, et al. Comparison of the defibrillation threshold and the upper limit of ventricular vulnerability. *Circulation* 1986;73:1022–1028.

43. Dillon DM. Synchronized repolarization after defibrillation shocks. A possible component of the defibrillation process demonstrated by optical recording in rabbit heart. *Circulation* 1992;85:1865–1878.

44. Garfinkel A, Spano ML, Ditto WL, Weiss JN. Controlling cardiac chaos. *Science* 1992;257:1230–1235.

45. Garfinkel A, Chen PS, Walter DO, et al. Quasiperiodicity and chaos in cardiac fibrillation. *J Clin Invest* 1997;99:305–314.

46. Chen PS, Garfinkel A, Weiss JN, Karagueuzian HS. Spirals, chaos, and new mechanisms of wave propagation. *Pacing Clin Electrophysiol* 1997;20:414–421.

47. Davy JM, Fain ES, Dorian P, Winkle RA. The relationship between successful defibrillation and delivered energy in open-chest dogs: Reappraisal of the "defibrillation threshold" concept. *Am Heart J* 1987;113:77–84.

48. Sepulveda NG, Wikswo JP Jr, Echt DS. Finite element analysis of cardiac defibrillation current distributions. *IEEE Trans Biomed Eng* 1990;37:354–365.

49. Walcott GP, Knisley SB, Zhou X, et al. On the mechanism of ventricular defibrillation. *Pacing Clin Electrophysiol* 1997;20:422–431.

50. Chen P-S, Wolf PD, Ideker RE. Mechanism of cardiac defibrillation: A different point of view. *Circulation* 1991;84:913–919.

51. Witkowske FX, Penkoske PA, Plonsey R. Mechanism of cardiac defibrillation in open-chest dogs using unipolar DC-coupled simultaneous activation and shock potential recordings. *Circulation* 1990;82:244–260.

52. Roth BJ. The pinwheel experiment revisited. *J Theor Biol* 1998;190:389–393.

53. Kwaku KF, Dillon SM. Shock-induced depolarization of refractory myocardium prevents wave-front propagation in defibrillation. *Circ Res* 1996;79:957–973.

54. Plonsey R, Barr RC. Effect of microscopic and macroscopic discontinuities on the response of cardiac tissue to defibrillating (stimulating) currents. *Med Biol Eng Comput* 1986;24:130–136.

55. Krassowska W, Pilkington TC, Ideker RE. Periodic conductivity as a mechanism for cardiac stimulation and defibrillation. *IEEE Trans Biomed Eng* 1987;34:555–560.

56. Knisley SB, Blitchington TF, Hill BC, et al. Optical measurements of transmembrane potential changes during electric field stimulation of ventricular cells. *Circ Res* 1993;72:255–270.

57. Tung L, Sliz N, Mulligan MR. Influence of electrical axis of stimulation on excitation of cardiac muscle cells. *Circ Res* 1991;69:722–730.

58. Fast VG, Kléber AG. Cardiac tissue geometry as a determinant of unidirectional conduction block: Assessment of microscopic excitation spread by optical mapping in patterned cell cultures and in a computer model. *Cardiovasc Res* 1995;29:697–707.

59. Zhou X, Rollins DL, Smith WM, Ideker RE. Responses of the transmembrane potential of myocardial cells during a shock. *J Cardiovasc Electrophysiol* 1995;6:252–263.

60. Gillis AM, Fast VG, Rohr S, Kléber AG. Spatial changes in transmembrane potential during extracellular electrical shocks in cultured monolayers of neonatal rat ventricular myocytes. *Circ Res* 1996;79:676–690.

61. Trayanova NA, Roth BJ, Malden LJ. The response of a spherical heart to a uniform electric field: A bidomain analysis of cardiac stimulation. *IEEE Trans Biomed Eng* 1993;40:899–908.

62. Fishler MG. Syncytial heterogeneity as a mechanism underlying cardiac far-field stimulation during defibrillation-level shocks. *J Cardiovasc Electrophysiol* 1998;9:384–394.

63. Wikswo JP Jr, Lin S-F. The prompt response of the transmembrane potential distribution of rabbit epicardium to defibrillation-strength field stimulation. *Pacing Clin Electrophysiol* 1998;21:940.

64. Entcheva E. *Cardiac Tissue Structure-Electric Field Interactions in Polarizing the Heart: 3D Computer Models and Applications* [PhD dissertation]. Memphis, TN: University of Memphis; 1998.

65. Wikswo JP Jr. Tissue anisotropy, the cardiac bidomain, and the virtual cathode effect. In Zipes DP, Jalife J (eds): *Cardiac Electrophysiology: From Cell to Bedside.* Philadelphia: W.B. Saunders Co.; 1995:348–361.

66. Sepulveda NG, Wikswo JP Jr. Bipolar stimulation of cardiac tissue using an anisotropic bidomain model. *J Cardiovasc Electrophysiol* 1994;5:258–267.

67. Zhou X, Ideker RE, Blitchington TF, et al. Optical transmembrane potential measurements during defibrillation-strength shocks in perfused rabbit hearts. *Circ Res* 1995;77:593–602.

68. Lin S-F, Wikswo JP Jr. Endocardial defibrillation-strength stimulus produces bipolar responses and charge diffusion in rabbit left ventricle. *J Am Coll Cardiol* 1998;31:36A.

69. Trayanova NA, Roth BJ, Malden LJ. The response of a spherical heart to a uniform electric field: A bidomain analysis of cardiac stimulation. *IEEE Trans Biomed Eng* 1993;40:899–908.

70. Frazier DW, Wolf PD, Wharton JM, et al. Stimulus-induced critical point: Mechanism for electrical initiation of reentry in normal canine myocardium. *J Clin Invest* 1989;83:1039–1052.

Chapter 20

Mechanisms of Defibrillation:
1. Influence of Fiber Structure on Tissue Response to Electrical Stimulation

Stephen B. Knisley

Introduction

Electrical stimulation of biological tissue has been used in experimental or therapeutic settings ranging from cellular drug delivery or gene transfer via electroporation to life-saving electrical defibrillation of the heart.[1-3] Optimizing the effects of electrical stimulation requires an understanding of the mechanism of stimulation. The mechanism may be considered to have various steps, including: 1) the stimulation pulse changes the transmembrane voltage during or soon after the onset of the pulse; 2) the change in transmembrane voltage alters states of transmembrane voltage-dependent ion channels in the cell membrane (or creates electropores); and 3) the altered channels introduce effects such as the production or alteration of action potentials, arrhythmias, or defibrillation. The research described in this chapter was undertaken to gain insight into the first step mentioned, i.e., the transmembrane voltage change that occurs during the pulse (ΔV_m).

We hypothesized that the ΔV_m in the heart during a current pulse that is given when the membrane is highly refractory will depend on the current strength and the passive electrical properties of the heart. Early concepts of passive properties of tissue were determined by applying electrical current to nerve axons or cardiac fibers.[4-6] These properties were thought of in terms of physical or mathematical models, e.g., the transmembrane potential in nerve after a brief shock developed as would potential on a capacitor charged through a resistor,[4] and the ΔV_m during current application in a nerve or cardiac Purkinje fiber was fit to a space constant defined for a continuous linear core conductor.[5-7] The ideas of

This work was supported by National Institutes of Health Grant HL52003, and American Heart Association Grants AL 950032 and 9740173N. Dr. Knisley is an Established Investigator Awardee of the American Heart Association.

From Rosenbaum DS, Jalife J (eds): *Optical Mapping of Cardiac Excitation and Arrhythmias.*
©Futura Publishing Co., Inc., Armonk, NY, 2001.

the membrane time constant and 1-dimensional fiber space constant are still useful in limited cases. However, insights from more recent mathematical models of 2- or 3-dimensional myocardium[8–10] indicate that results from 1-dimensional theory cannot be simply applied to multidimensional hearts. In the 2- or 3-dimensional cases, ΔV_m during stimulation is predicted to have a complex spatial pattern instead of a simple exponential decay with a space constant as occurs in a 1-dimensional model.[11]

A mathematical model,[9] and not actual measurements of the ΔV_m, was the first to indicate the complex ΔV_m that occurs in the heart during unipolar stimulation. That a model showed the ΔV_m first is partly due to the fact that for decades it has been difficult or impossible to measure the ΔV_m in hearts. Previously, the only experimental technique for measuring transmembrane voltage had used glass microelectrodes with the tip inserted into the intracellular space.[12] With use of microelectrode methods, the voltage can be recorded differentially between the microelectrode tip inside a cell and another electrode located somewhere in the extracellular space. Such recordings can indicate absolute transmembrane voltages during most of an action potential. However, the microelectrode method cannot generally measure ΔV_m when extracellular current exists in the preparation. Even the local currents that are generated near the leading edge of a propagating action potential (which are much smaller than currents applied during a defibrillation shock) can produce noticeable errors in microelectrode measurements of transmembrane voltage such as dV/dt of the action potential phase zero depolarization and the time constant of the action potential foot.[13] During a strong externally applied shock, a prominent spike generally occurs in microelectrode recordings. The spike can be produced by the potential difference between the extracellular electrode and the point in the extracellular or interstitial space just outside of the membrane impaled by the intracellular microelectrode. The spike obscures transmembrane voltage during the shock. This problem can be lessened in multicellular tissue in vitro by subtracting sequential measurements for repeated events with the microelectrode tip outside and then inside of a cell or by adjusting relative positions of electrode tips.[13–15] Such tip positioning techniques are complicated because the tip is normally too small to see with a light microscope. Even if the spike can be overcome, a second limitation of microelectrodes for measurement of ΔV_m is the small number of sites that can be explored simultaneously. This limitation arises because space for micromanipulators that hold the microelectrodes is limited, and the probability exists that an intracellular tip will spontaneously come out of the cell.

The optical methods with transmembrane voltage-sensitive fluorescent dyes have overcome the limitations described for ΔV_m measurement with microelectrodes. With optical methods, light is measured that follows changes in transmembrane voltage and is not directly affected by extracellular current.[16–18] Also, optical methods can measure the light at many sites simultaneously, allowing spatial distributions of ΔV_m to be mapped during a single stimulation pulse. Thus, optical methods are advantageous for studies of the distribution of ΔV_m in the heart.

During the last 10 years, my research has employed optical methods to test hypotheses concerning transmembrane voltage changes in isolated cardiac cells and whole hearts. Some of the studies have focused on the ΔV_m produced during application of electrical stimulation and whether the ΔV_m depends on the fiber orientation. This chapter describes three studies that revealed the ΔV_m during unipolar point and line stimulation in isolated hearts and the role of the fiber structure of the hearts.

Experimental Preparation

Hearts from anesthetized New Zealand White rabbits were quickly isolated and arterially perfused with saline containing (in mmol/L) 129 NaCl, 4.5 KCl, 1.8 $CaCl_2$, 1.1 $MgCl_2$, 26 $NaHCO_3$, 1 Na_2HPO_4, 11 glucose, 0.04 g/L bovine serum albumin bubbled with a gas mixture of 95% O_2 and 5% CO_2, at a pH of 7.3 to 7.4 and a temperature of 35°C to 37°C. Some of the hearts were endocardially prefrozen with liquid nitrogen to produce a 1-mm layer of surviving epicardium.[19,20]

Cellular contraction that develops mostly during repolarization[18,21] can introduce heart motion that affects optical signals during the cardiac cycle. The motion was lessened by placing a transparent plate in contact with the recording region and by adding the electromechanical uncoupler diacetyl monoxime at a concentration of 15 to 20 mmol/L.[22] Diacetyl monoxime did not noticeably affect ΔV_m in single cells or hearts.[18,23] In some experiments, fluorescence emission ratiometry was used to lessen the effect of heart motion on optical signals.[24,25] With the ratiometry, an electromechanical uncoupling drug was not necessary.

Fluorescence Recording with Laser Scanner

Optical action potentials were recorded with transmembrane voltage-sensitive fluorescent dye, blue or green excitation light, and a detector that sensed red fluorescence. Hearts were usually stained by adding a concentrated stock solution of di-4-ANEPPS (Molecular Probes Inc., Eugene OR), dissolved in ethanol or dimethyl sulfoxide, to 100 to 500 mL of the perfusing solution at a final dye concentration of 0.01 mg/mL for 2 to 15 minutes.[26] In some experiments the dye WW781 was used at a final concentration of 0.005 mg/mL.

A laser scanner[27–29] excited fluorescence by scanning an array of spots with an argon ion laser beam having a wavelength of 488 or 514 nm. Acousto-optic deflectors were used to steer the beam. Although the array could contain 128 spots, it usually contained 63 spots. The focused excitation beam had a nominal diameter of 100 μm. The size of the scanned region of the heart was determined by software that controlled the angle of laser deflection. The size also depended on the distance from the acousto-optic deflectors to the heart, which was typically 60 cm. A fluorescence sample was taken while the beam dwelled at each spot just before jumping to the next spot. During each millisecond of recording, the beam completed a scan of all spots and one sample was taken of a voltage signal proportional to the stimulation current. Thus, the stimulation pulse strength and times of the beginning and end of the pulse were recorded in the same data stream that contained the fluorescence data.

For any one spot, fluorescence excited by the laser represented the group of cells at the spot. When the laser then jumped to a second spot, fluorescence represented cells at the second spot because fluorescence from the previous spot died quickly (fluorescence lifetimes of standard fluorophores are 1 to 10 ns, i.e., orders of magnitude shorter than the time for the laser to jump[30]). Since the scan order was prescribed, knowledge of which spot corresponds to each sample was contained in the order of samples. With this method, there was no need to focus a fluorescence image of the heart onto an image plane containing charged coupled device (CCD) or photodiode array detectors, which are described in other chapters of this text.

Fluorescence light intensity could be sufficiently weak that shot noise was noticeable. Fluorescence light could be increased and noise reduced by 1) increasing the laser power (the power of laser light that passed to the heart was typically 2 to 20 mW); 2) increasing the amount of dye in the heart by increasing dye perfusion time or dye concentration in perfusate; and 3) increasing the fraction of the fluorescence light that was collected. Fluorescence light emanated from the heart in essentially all directions, and hence much of the fluorescence light did not reach the light collector. In experiments with the transmembrane voltage-sensitive dye di-4-ANEPPS, collection was adequate when a 2″ photocathode window of a photomultiplier tube was placed as close as possible (e.g., 5 to 8 cm) to the recording region without blocking the laser light. In experiments with the calcium-sensitive fluorescent dye Fluo-3, which had fluorescence intensity in hearts much lower than that of di-4-ANEPPS, it was necessary to increase the fraction of fluorescence light collected. A convex reflector was positioned in front of the recording region. The laser light was passed to the heart through a hole in the center of the reflector. A photomultiplier tube then collected fluorescence that was concentrated behind the heart.[31] This increased the intensity of collected fluorescence by a factor of 18 compared with the intensity when the photomultiplier tube was in front of the heart.

A red glass filter covered the photocathode to block reflected laser light and to allow fluorescence light containing desired wavelengths to pass onto the photocathode. In different studies using di-4-ANEPPS, the filter passed fluorescence containing wavelengths longer than 570 to 645 nm.

The photocurrent was converted to a voltage signal with a gain of 10^5 V/A. The signal was then electrically filtered with a pass-band of direct current (DC) to 80,000 Hz. This wide pass-band allowed the signal to settle quickly each time the laser beam moved to the next spot. The signal was digitized at a sampling rate of 64,000 Hz. This produced a sampling interval of 1 ms for each spot.[23,29]

The fiber direction was typically estimated from the fast axis of optically measured activation isochrones produced by pacing. Activation times at the recording spots were determined as the time of the midpoint of the fast rising phase of the action potential.[20,32] The array of laser spots could be quickly rotated by recalculating grid coordinates to orient the array at a desired angle relative to the fast axis. In some hearts the fiber direction was determined by microscopically examining 5-μm myocardial sections that were prepared after heart fixation, or by identifying minute tissue striations after staining the surface with Evans blue dye and transilluminating with an optical fiber placed on the opposite side of the ventricular wall.[33]

Transmembrane Voltage During Stimulation

Stimulation electrodes were usually fabricated from chlorided Ag or stainless steel. Since the metallic electrodes block or reflect light, the ΔV_m was not measured directly under an electrode. Optical measurement directly under an electrode is possible with an "optrode" consisting of an optical fiber inside of a glass pipette[34] or with a transparent indium-tin-oxide electrode.[35] With metallic electrodes, care was required to avoid blocking laser beams when electrodes were inside the laser array. Typically, the electrodes were positioned on the heart first. Then the laser array location on the heart was adjusted by micromanipulating the final mirror that passed laser light to the heart until electrodes and leads did not block laser light for any spots. During adjustments, the laser array was viewed with a magnifying loupe. Leads were covered with candle-black to prevent possible reflection of coherent laser light, which is a potential danger to the investigator. Provided that distance between laser spots was greater than 1 mm, up to 25 electrodes and leads could be placed in a 1-dimensional electrode array within the laser grid.[33,36]

A transparent plate gently contacted the heart to flatten the recording region, mechanically stabilize the heart, and hold the stimulation electrodes that were attached to the plate. Contact pressure was lower than perfusion pressure so as to avoid occlusion of epicardial vessels. In some experiments the heart was placed in a physiological saline bath and the stimulation electrode was positioned in the bath at various distances from the myocardial surface.[37] Hearts were usually paced at a strength 2 to 4 times threshold to produce action potentials at a rate of 3 to 4 Hz. A 5- to 20-ms test stimulation pulse, during which ΔV_m was to be measured, was given typically after the rising phase of an action potential and before cells had recovered excitability. The membrane's fast inward sodium channels are highly refractory at this time. Hence, the ΔV_m was not obscured by large regenerative inward sodium current or phase zero depolarization during the stimulation pulse.[18] Responses during the pulse were not strictly passive, since nonlinearities were observed, e.g., a negative ΔV_m that had larger magnitude than the positive ΔV_m after reversing stimulation polarity,[38] and a few spots that did not switch ΔV_m sign when shock polarity was reversed.[39,40]

The ΔV_m at each spot was determined as the difference in fluorescence during the test stimulation and fluorescence at the same time relative to the action potential phase zero depolarization in a preceding action potential that did not receive the test stimulation (control). Each ΔV_m was expressed as a fraction of the amplitude of the action potential phase zero depolarization from the same recording.[18]

Statistical analyses were performed using individual ΔV_m measurements. To help visualize spatial distributions, contour lines of a given ΔV_m were generated by Surfer (Golden Software Inc., Golden, CO) using the regional variable theory technique of Kriging[41] or by PV Wave.[42]

Results

Unipolar Point Stimulation

Fluorescence recordings were obtained from a rabbit heart placed under a laser epifluorescence microscope.[39] The microscope was previously used to measure from a 5-μm spot on single cells.[18] For experiments with hearts, spot size was increased to 60 μm by moving the heart closer to the objective lens. Figure 1 shows fluorescence recordings from one rabbit heart. The unipolar test stimulation electrode location on the epicardium and the stimulation current strength and polarity were constant in the three trials. However, the fluorescence recording location under the objective lens was changed between trials by moving the heart and test stimulation electrode that were attached to a single manipulator. Thus, we recorded at locations immediately adjacent to the electrode (0 mm), as well as 0.5 mm and 1 mm away from the electrode. The line containing the test

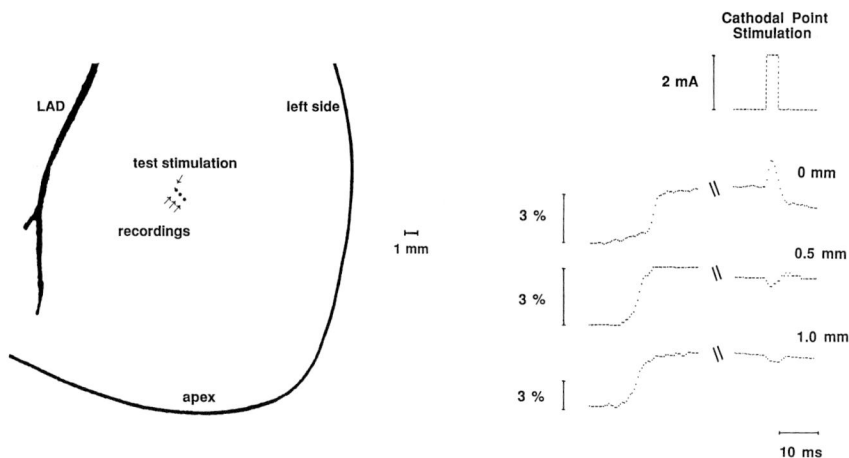

Figure 1. *Left:* Enlarged diagram of the anterior left ventricle showing the stimulation and recording region, and recordings obtained in experiments with an epifluorescence microscope. Test stimulation with strength of 2 mA was applied from a 25-μm-diameter wire electrode (see downward-oriented arrow pointing toward stimulation site). Fluorescence recordings were obtained from three 60-μm-diameter recording sites on epicardium (see spots with three parallel arrows pointing to them), which were immediately adjacent to (0 mm), 0.5 mm away from, and 1 mm away from the electrode in the direction along fibers. The left anterior descending artery (LAD) is shown at left. The outlines of the left side and apex of the heart are shown. *Right:* Recordings at different distances from a cathodal point stimulation electrode. Stimulation pulse is indicated in the top recording. Fluorescence recordings are interrupted where indicated by double slashes after the upstrokes, and then begin again 25 ms later. Myocardium adjacent to electrode (0 mm) underwent a positive transmembrane voltage change during the pulse (positive ΔV_m). At 0.5 mm and 1.0 mm away from the electrode, myocardium underwent negative ΔV_m. Calibration bars on left indicate the stimulation current and percent of total fluorescence. Effect of fluorescence decrease due to photobleaching of the fluorescent dye was eliminated by linear subtraction. From reference 39, with permission.

stimulation and recording locations was approximately parallel to the local fiber direction on the anterior left ventricle.[43,44] The action potential upstroke produced by a pacing pulse given elsewhere on the heart is shown in the left part of each recording. The test stimulation pulse was given 75 ms after the pacing pulse.

The myocardium adjacent to the cathodal electrode underwent positive ΔV_m during the test stimulation pulse. The peak of this ΔV_m was 55% of the action potential amplitude. At 0.5 mm away from the electrode, the myocardium underwent negative ΔV_m during the test pulse. The peak of this ΔV_m was -15% of the action potential amplitude. Also at 1.0 mm away from the electrode, the myocardium underwent negative ΔV_m during the pulse. The peak of the ΔV_m at 1.0 mm was -11% of the action potential amplitude. Other trials showed that the ΔV_m sign at a recording location could be reversed by reversing the S2 stimulation polarity. An unexpected finding was that ΔV_m signs at the spots 0.5 mm or 1 mm from the electrode in the direction along the fibers were negative for cathodal stimulation and positive for anodal stimulation, which are the opposite of signs that occur in a 1-dimensional cable.[45]

In other experiments, the ΔV_ms at spots in various directions from the point electrode were examined by using a laser scanner system to record from many spots simultaneously (Fig. 2).[23] An example of the recordings is shown in Figure 3 for cathodal test stimulation. The recordings are arranged to correspond to the locations of their laser spots. The stimulation produced negative ΔV_ms in regions away from the electrode on the axis from the upper left to lower right. The approximate locations of the regions are indicated by "-" signs. Since cathodal stimulation was known to produce positive ΔV_ms immediately under the electrode,[46] the regions of negative ΔV_ms were defined as reversed ΔV_m regions. The stimulation produced positive ΔV_ms in regions indicated by "+" signs on a perpendicular axis, indicating that ΔV_m was not the reverse of that which occurs under the electrode. A new action potential that may have begun elsewhere on the heart was observed at all laser spots after the membrane had nearly repolarized.

Figure 4 shows examples of contour maps of the ΔV_ms produced by the test stimulation. Stimulation and recording locations were the same for both maps. Test stimulation was given 24 ms after the phase zero depolarizations in the center of the recording region. Reversed ΔV_m regions existed in the upper left and lower right of each map in which cathodal stimulation produced negative ΔV_ms and anodal stimulation produced positive ΔV_ms. Centers of reversed ΔV_m regions were approximately 2.5 mm away from the stimulation electrode. On the axis perpendicular to the axis of reversed ΔV_m regions, stimulation either had no effect or cathodal stimulation produced positive ΔV_ms and anodal stimulation produced negative ΔV_ms.

Trials in which the test stimulation was given in diastole with no diacetyl monoxime added to the solution showed that fluorescence contained deflections consistent with those during stimulation in systole. However, unlike recordings of stimulation during the refractory period, the recordings for diastolic stimulation also contained large deflections that corresponded to excitation of the fast inward sodium current (Figs. 8 and 9 in reference 47). The stimulation-induced excitation began in re-

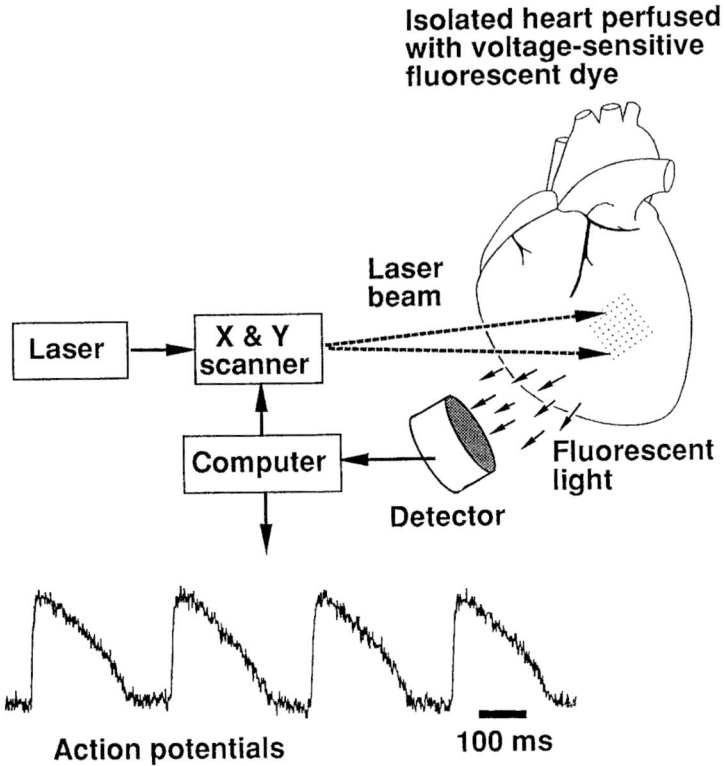

Isolated heart perfused with voltage-sensitive fluorescent dye

Laser beam

Laser → X & Y scanner

Computer

Detector

Fluorescent light

Action potentials

100 ms

Figure 2. Diagram of laser scanning method to record action potentials from epicardium of isolated, perfused hearts stained with transmembrane voltage-sensitive dye. Laser beam repeatedly scanned an array of 64 recording spots on the epicardium every millisecond. Fluorescence that followed changes in transmembrane voltage of cells at each recording spot was detected with a photomultiplier tube. Individual action potential recordings for each spot were obtained by collating fluorescence samples that had been taken during scanning. From reference 43, with permission (©1995 IEEE).

gions along or across the fibers where the ΔV_m was positive (Figs. 5 through 8 of reference 23). Excitation where ΔV_m was positive agrees with the fact that recovered transmembrane voltage-dependent sodium channels become activated when transmembrane voltage is changed in the positive direction by an electrical pulse.[48] Thus, our results support conclusions that fluorescence deflections during stimulation in systole indeed represent ΔV_ms, and that similar ΔV_ms exist during stimulation in diastole, though the stimulation in diastole also produces large deflections due to excitation of recovered sodium channels.

Unipolar Line Stimulation

We hypothesized that effects of line stimulation may be predicted by considering the line electrode to be a set of point electrodes that together produce the sum of the various ΔV_ms produced by each point electrode.

Cathodal stimulation

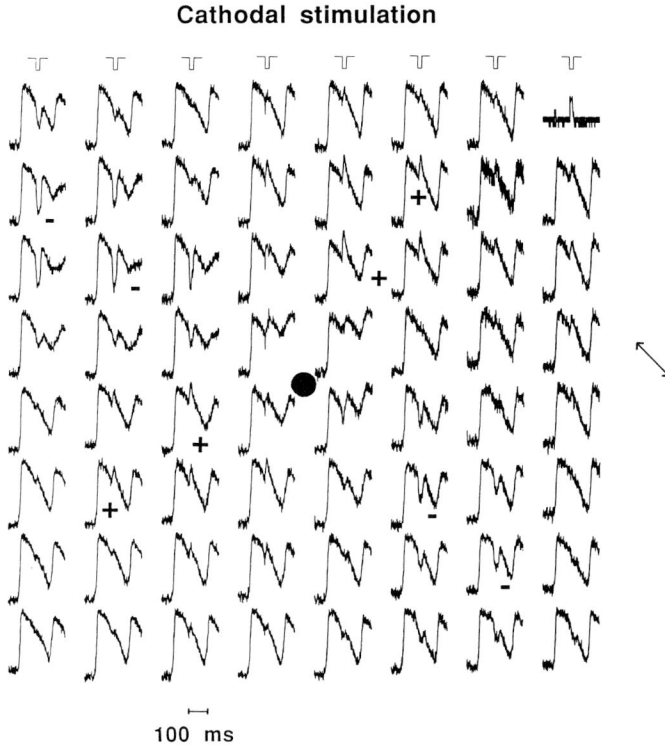

Figure 3. Effect of 40-mA unipolar cathodal test stimulation during an action potential produced by pacing. Test stimulation was applied in the center (filled circle). Timing of the last pacing pulse and test stimulation pulse is indicated in upper right recording. Timing of the test stimulation pulse is also indicated above columns. Cathodal test stimulation produced negative ΔV_ms in regions away from the electrode on one axis (−) and positive ΔV_ms in regions on a perpendicular axis (+). Distance between adjacent recording spots in a line or column was 1.14 mm. The perfusing solution contained 20 mmol/L diacetyl monoxime. Arrow indicates fast propagation axis. From reference 23, with permission.

One prediction is, for a finite-line electrode oriented parallel to fibers, the sign of ΔV_m does not reverse away from the electrode in the direction perpendicular to fibers. If true, then such stimulation would enhance uniformity of ΔV_m. To test this, measurements of ΔV_m were performed during line stimulation parallel and at other angles with respect to the fibers.[36]

Unlike a point electrode, in which current enters the heart at a small electrode area, a line electrode produces current entry into the heart that is distributed along the length of the electrode. The distribution is not necessarily uniform, e.g., a model of a disc electrode has greater current at electrode edges than in the center.[49] The distribution may affect ΔV_ms; e.g., points that have more current should contribute more to the ΔV_ms than points that have less current. This effect may occur in addition to any effect of orientation of the line electrode with respect to fibers. Thus, we sought to determine the distribution of current from a line electrode.

Cathodal stimulation   **Anodal stimulation**

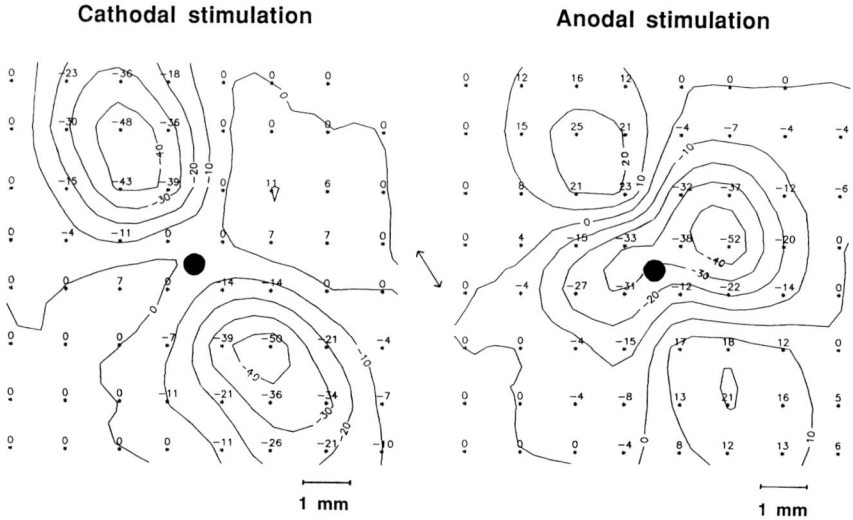

1 mm   1 mm

Figure 4. Contour maps of ΔV_ms produced by 15-mA unipolar test stimulation applied in the center (filled circle). ΔV_ms at each laser spot (asterisk) are indicated as a percentage of the pacing-induced action potential amplitude. Contour lines are shown for ΔV_ms of 10% to −40% for cathodal stimulation and 20% to −40% for anodal stimulation in increments of 10%. Regions of reversed ΔV_m occurred for either stimulation polarity (upper left and lower right of each map). The perfusing solution contained 20 mmol/L diacetyl monoxime. Arrow indicates fast propagation axis. From reference 23, with permission.

We tested a finite-element model of a line electrode in a 2-dimensional conductor, an Ag line electrode in which current distribution during stimulation was estimated from the darkening produced by electrically induced AgCl formation, and a line electrode composed of individual points in which current was measured for each point. The results for all three methods indicate that points near line electrode ends had greater current than points near the electrode center. Figure 5 shows the fraction of cur-

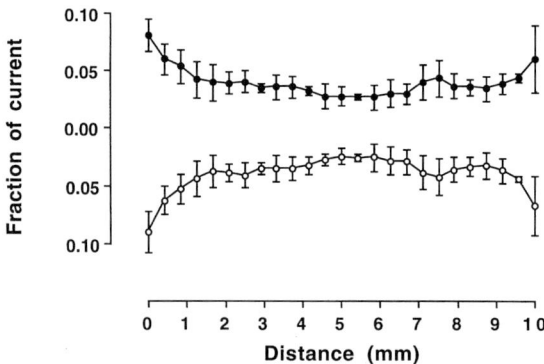

Figure 5. Distribution of current entering heart from line electrode consisting of 25 terminals positioned on left anterior epicardium of four rabbit hearts. Filled symbols represent anodal stimulation. Open symbols represent cathodal stimulation. Means and standard deviations of current from terminals are shown as fractions of total current from all terminals. The total current strength was 143 ± 66 mA. Current was greater at terminals near electrode ends compared with between ends. From reference 36, with permission.

rent that passed through each of the points. For anodal stimulation, current through points at electrode ends, i.e., 0 and 10 mm, was 10.4±6.9 mA while average current for all points was 5.7±2.6 mA ($P = 0.032$ for current at ends versus average current, n = 8 hearts x ends). For cathodal stimulation, current through points at electrode ends was -11.8±7.4 mA while average current for all points was $-5.7±2.7$ mA ($P = 0.012$ for current at ends versus average current, n = 8 hearts × ends).

Figure 6 shows measurements and contours of ΔV_m produced by stimulation with a line electrode parallel to fibers in a rabbit heart. The

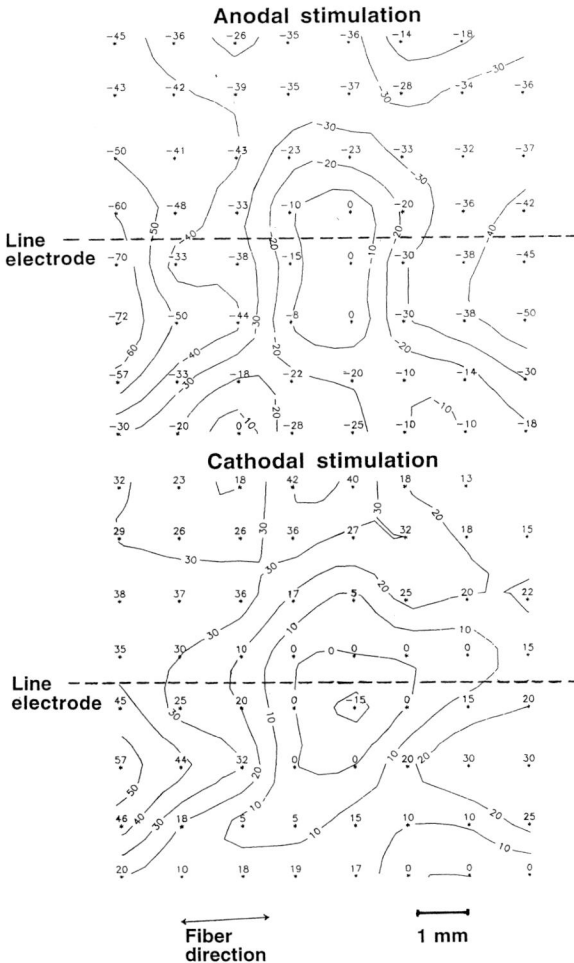

Figure 6. Measurements and contours of ΔV_ms during stimulation with a line electrode parallel to fibers. The stimulation current strength was 172 mA. The ΔV_ms at each laser spot (asterisk) are indicated as percentages of the pacing-induced action potential amplitude. Contour lines are shown for ΔV_m of -60% to -10% for anodal stimulation and -10% to 50% for cathodal stimulation in increments of 10%. Anodal stimulation produced negative ΔV_ms and cathodal stimulation produced positive ΔV_ms. Arrow indicates fast propagation axis. From reference 36, with permission

ΔV_ms having the largest magnitudes in the recording region occurred during anodal stimulation, had a negative sign, and were located near electrode ends. Anodal line stimulation produced negative ΔV_ms at most recording spots, including spots less than 1 mm from the stimulation electrode and spots as far as 3 to 4 mm from the electrode. A region existed near the center of the line electrode where small ΔV_ms occurred. None of the recording spots underwent a positive ΔV_m during the anodal line stimulation pulse.

Cathodal stimulation was tested after reversal of the line stimulation leads. The cathodal stimulation produced positive ΔV_ms at most recording spots. A region of small ΔV_ms existed near the center of the line electrode in which distinct negative ΔV_m occurred (e.g., recording at row 5 column 5).

Figure 7 shows measurements and contours of ΔV_m during stimulation from a line electrode oriented perpendicular to fibers. Anodal stimulation produced negative ΔV_ms at all 16 recording spots 0.5 mm from the line stimulation electrode. Some spots farther away from the electrode underwent positive ΔV_ms. Of the 31 recording spots in the leftmost two columns and the rightmost two columns, 23 underwent positive ΔV_ms. The ΔV_ms were negligible at some spots 4 mm to the left or right of the center of the line electrode. Cathodal stimulation from a line electrode perpendicular to fibers frequently produced positive ΔV_ms at spots near the line electrode. Many spots farther away from the line electrode underwent negative ΔV_ms. Of the 31 recording spots in the leftmost two columns and the rightmost two columns, 22 underwent negative ΔV_ms.

Tests of a line electrode oriented at various angles with respect to fibers showed that for electrode orientations parallel to fibers to within approximately 15° to 20°, many spots underwent ΔV_ms of one sign while few spots underwent ΔV_ms of the other sign. In contrast, when electrode orientations were nonparallel to fibers, the ΔV_ms had either sign.

The results described above for line stimulation apply only to regions of epicardium on either side of the electrode. Regions beyond the ends of a line electrode undergo complex distributions of ΔV_m that include ΔV_m of both signs when the line electrode is parallel to fibers.[36]

Discussion

Optical Method for the Study of Electrical Stimulation

Optical methods using transmembrane voltage-dependent fluorescent dye for the study of the distributions of ΔV_m overcome some limitations of microelectrode methods. Optical methods do not produce the electrical spike or artifact that can occur in microelectrode recordings. Also, optical methods can provide measurements from many spots, which has allowed mapping of spatial distributions of ΔV_m. In our experiments, localization of measurements at 64 individual spots was accomplished by controlling the locations of excitation of dye fluorescence with a scanned laser beam.[27,29] Alternatively, localization can be performed with optical fibers to direct the excitation light to, and to collect fluorescence from, a location on the tissue.[46,50] In other methods, dye can be excited with broad field

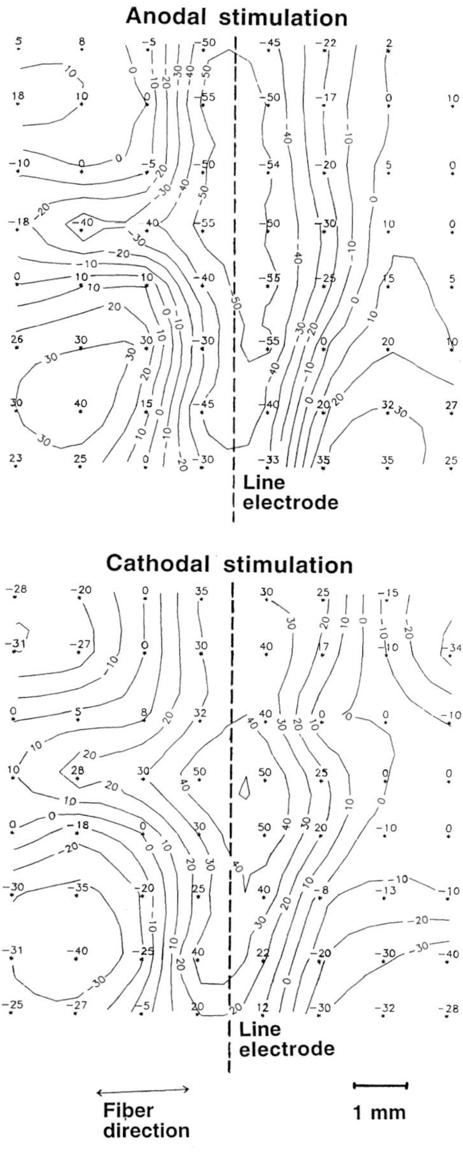

Anodal stimulation

Cathodal stimulation

Fiber direction

1 mm

Line electrode

Figure 7. Measurements and contours of ΔV_ms during stimulation with a line electrode perpendicular to fibers. The stimulation current strength was 172 mA. The ΔV_ms at each laser spot (asterisk) are indicated as percentages of the pacing-induced action potential amplitude. Contour lines are shown for ΔV_m of −50% to 30% of the pacing-induced action potential amplitude for anodal stimulation and −30% to 50% for cathodal stimulation in increments of 10%. Anodal stimulation produced negative ΔV_ms at spots near line electrode and positive ΔV_ms at many spots away from electrode. Cathodal stimulation produced positive ΔV_ms at spots near line electrode and negative ΔV_ms at many spots away from electrode. Arrow indicates fast propagation axis. From reference 36, with permission.

light. Then, localization at multiple sites can be accomplished via collection of fluorescence using a lens to project an image of the fluorescent tissue onto an array of light detectors.[51–56]

Technical challenges to optical mapping of the ΔV_m include shot noise resulting from measurement of a small amount of light, effects of tissue motion due to cardiac contraction, and the fact that the fluorescence does not indicate absolute transmembrane voltage. We have increased the fluorescence light as described in the "Methods" section of this chapter. We have lessened cardiac contraction with an electromechanical uncoupler, diacetyl monoxime. Studies of this drug have consistently found that it markedly decreases cardiac contraction. There is not full agreement on the extent to which diacetyl monoxime affects the fast inward sodium current or conduction velocity.[22,43,57,58] To avoid possible effects on the sodium current, we eliminated diacetyl monoxime during measurements of excitation produced by the test stimulation during diastole.[23] Diacetyl monoxime does not markedly change the myocardial diffusion constant,[43] which suggests that it does not change the intracellular resistances that are determinants of ΔV_m in hearts. Diacetyl monoxime does not alter action potential amplitude.[22,57,58] These results indicate that diacetyl monoxime does not influence our measurements in which ΔV_m was expressed as a fraction of action potential amplitude.[18,23,36,39,40,59–61] Recently, we found that by performing fluorescence emission ratiometry, we can lessen the effect of heart motion on the fluorescence recording without use of an electromechanical uncoupler. The ratiometry was performed with di-4-ANEPPS by division of a DC-coupled signal representing green fluorescence emission by a simultaneous and collocal DC-coupled signal representing red fluorescence emission.[24,25]

We hypothesized that ΔV_m as a fraction of action potential amplitude indicates the magnitude of transmembrane voltage change in millivolts, provided that we have an estimate of action potential amplitude under the experimental conditions.[18,60] We tested this with fluorescence measurements at ends of isolated single ventricular myocytes exposed to electrical field stimulation. In normal solution, magnitudes of ΔV_m in millivolts (estimated by assuming a normal action potential amplitude of 130 mV) approximately matched magnitudes that are expected theoretically in the cells (i.e., the product of electrical field strength and half of the cell length).[62,63] Also, when solution potassium was increased (which is known to decrease the action potential amplitude in cardiac tissue[64]) the ΔV_m as a fraction of action potential amplitude increased, supporting the hypothesis.

Regardless of quantitative uncertainty in the magnitude of ΔV_m measured optically, the sign of ΔV_m can be absolutely determined by optical methods. This follows from the fact that the fluorescence emitted from the membrane, given a constant excitation light intensity, changes monotonically (and linearly) with changes in transmembrane voltage.[16] However, artifacts that do not represent a change in transmembrane voltage are possible during shocks. For example, the intensities of excitation light that reaches the membrane and fluorescence that reaches the light collector may be altered by electrically induced gas bubbles. Also, an electrical spark can occur during a defibrillation shock that introduces light that does not represent a transmembrane voltage change (S. B. Knisley, PhD, unpublished data, April 1998). Light from indicator lamps on stimulation equipment can change during a shock pulse, which can introduce an artifact in fluorescence recordings if this light is not blocked. Thus, reasonable care is required in the performance and analysis of experiments that incorporate electrical shocks and optical methods.

Point and Line Stimulation

The ΔV_m in the region surrounding the electrode during unipolar stimulation in the rabbit ventricle is different from that in 1-dimensional myocardial preparations, in which ΔV_m decreases approximately exponentially in accordance with the fiber space constant. In rabbit ventricle, ΔV_m reverses sign just a few millimeters away from the electrode in the fiber direction, becoming negative for cathodal simulation and positive for anodal stimulation, i.e., the opposite of ΔV_m along a 1-dimensional fiber.[5] While our initial findings of virtual electrode effects along fibers were inconsistent with the established 1-dimensional theory,[39] several facts argued that our results were correct: 1) both positive and negative ΔV_m were found during a single stimulation pulse, which cannot be caused by a spark that could only increase light; 2) the results fit a 2-dimensional theory that explained the distribution of ΔV_m[9]; 3) for stimulation in diastole, early membrane excitation occurred where ΔV_m was positive, which indicated that membrane sodium channels responded to ΔV_m as expected from known transmembrane voltage dependence of sodium channels[23,39,47]; 4) the ΔV_m distribution accounts qualitatively for electrical recordings of excitation produced by cathodal stimulation[65]; and 5) the ΔV_m was highly reproducible in our laboratory and was found with point stimulation independently in other laboratories.[23,38,39,54]

The ΔV_m sign reversal along fibers in rabbit hearts is not simply explained by the activating function described for a fiber in 3-dimensional conductive saline.[66] This is partly because the reversal occurred even with an insulating plate that displaced saline on the epicardium.[23,36] The ΔV_m sign reversal can be explained by bidomain models of 2- or 3-dimensional anisotropic myocardium in which the ratio of transverse to longitudinal resistance in the intracellular domain differs from the ratio in the extracellular domain.[9] Indeed, measurements indicate that the ratios of transverse to longitudinal resistance are different in the intracellular domain (9.4) compared to the extracellular domain (2.7) in superfused calf trabecular muscles.[67]

We found that line stimulation produced ΔV_m having approximately uniform sign in the epicardium on either side of the electrode when the electrode was oriented parallel to the myocardial fibers and nonuniform sign when the electrode was perpendicular or at some intermediate angles to the fibers. This can be predicted qualitatively by the hypothesis that summation of the ΔV_m produced by each point within a line electrode determines the effect of the whole electrode. For a finite elongated electrode oriented perpendicular to fibers, summation of the ΔV_m produced by points in the line would result in regions of reversal of the sign of ΔV_m on either side of the line electrode. For an electrode parallel to fibers, summation of the ΔV_m produced by the points would result in no reversal of the sign of ΔV_m on either side of the electrode.

The findings that magnitudes of ΔV_m are large near ends of the line electrodes are consistent with the greater density of current that entered the heart near ends. Thus, ΔV_m contributions from points near electrode ends are larger than the contributions from points between ends.[36]

Possible Significance for Electrical Defibrillation

In order to defibrillate, a shock should not induce arrhythmias.[68] The ΔV_m produced by point stimulation may induce arrhythmias when the stimulation is given in the vulnerable period. A mathematical bidomain model of the myocardium has been used to demonstrate that positive ΔV_m of the tissue under a point cathodal electrode and away from the electrode in the direction perpendicular to the fibers, and negative ΔV_m in the direction parallel to the fibers, modify the refractory period differently in the two directions resulting in unidirectional block and stable reentry.[69] Optical mapping has shown quatrefoil reentry induction by a related mechanism.[70] These reports suggest that the nonuniformity of ΔV_m sign produced by point stimulation, in which ΔV_m has opposite signs on different axes, may be disadvantageous. Also, the small size of a point electrode limits the amount of current that can be applied.

We have speculated that line stimulation may be advantageous for defibrillation or other electrical antiarrhythmic therapy. We have found that much more current can be delivered from a line electrode than from a point electrode.[23,36] Line electrodes can be introduced into cardiac chambers by transvenous catheterization or onto the epicardium by an epidural needle.[71] Introduction techniques may allow implantation in various regions of the heart without requiring thoracotomy. The ΔV_m sign in the epicardium on either side of a line electrode can be made more uniform by orienting the electrode parallel to fibers, as described for positive ΔV_m during cathodal stimulation and negative ΔV_m during anodal stimulation. Such a line electrode might lessen the inhomogeneity of the ion channel responses to stimulation that is thought to be related to electrical induction of arrhythmias or defibrillation failure.[44,68-70,72-74]

Also, line stimulation may help to block activation fronts of fibrillation. Such block may halt fibrillation. When the electrode is anodal, the negative ΔV_m may cause inward sodium channels that are already inactivated to recover.[75] This may allow the region to become excitable, undergo a new action potential after the end of the stimulation pulse, and quickly become absolutely refractory. Also, in the case where the electrode is cathodal, the positive ΔV_m may excite any recovered sodium channels, causing an action potential and absolute refractoriness. Activation fronts of fibrillation are expected to block when they encounter a region that is absolutely refractory.[76] Future experimentation may indicate significance of line stimulation in arrhythmia induction and defibrillation.

References

1. Förster W, Neumann E. Gene transfer by electroporation: A practical guide. In Neumann E, Sowers AE, Jordan CA (eds): *Electroporation and Electrofusion in Cell Biology*. New York: Plenum Press; 1989:299–318.
2. Tung L. Electroporation of cell membranes. *Biophys J* 1991;60:297–306.
3. Geddes LA, Bourland JD. Tissue stimulation: Theoretical considerations and practical applications. *Med Biol Eng Comput* 1985;23:131–137.
4. Blair EA, Erlanger J. On excitation and depression in axons at the cathode of the constant current. *Am J Physiol* 1936;114:317–327.
5. Hodgkin AL, Rushton WAH. The electrical constants of a crustacean nerve fibre. *Proc R Soc B* 1946;133:444–479.
6. Weidmann S. The electrical constants of Purkinje fibres. *J Physiol* 1952; 118:348–360.

7. Jack JJB, Noble D, Tsien RW. Linear cable theory. In *Electric Current Flow in Excitable Cells*. Oxford: Clarendon Press; 1975:25–66.

8. Plonsey R, Barr RC. Current flow patterns in two-dimensional anisotropic bi-syncytia with normal and extreme conductivities. *Biophys J* 1984;45:557–571.

9. Sepulveda NG, Roth BJ, Wikswo JP Jr. Current injection into a two-dimensional anisotropic bidomain. *Biophys J* 1989;55:987–999.

10. Roth BJ, Wikswo JP Jr. Electrical stimulation of cardiac tissue: A bidomain model with active membrane properties. *IEEE Trans Biomed Eng* 1994;41:232–240.

11. Wikswo JP Jr. The complexities of cardiac cables: Virtual electrode effects. *Biophys J* 1994;66:551–553.

12. Ling G, Gerard RW. The normal membrane potential of frog sartorius fiber. *J Cell Comp Physiol* 1949;34:383–396.

13. Knisley SB, Maruyama T, Buchanan JW Jr. Interstitial potential during propagation in bathed ventricular muscle. *Biophys J* 1991;59:509–515.

14. Knisley SB, Smith WM, Ideker RE. Effect of intrastimulus polarity reversal on electric field stimulation thresholds in frog and rabbit myocardium. *J Cardiovasc Electrophysiol* 1992;3:239–254.

15. Zhou X, Smith W, Rollins D, et al. Transmembrane potential changes caused by shocks in guinea pig papillary muscle. *Am J Physiol* 1996;271:H2536-H2546.

16. Ehrenberg B, Farkas DL, Fluhler EN, et al. Membrane potential induced by external electric field pulses can be followed with a potentiometric dye. *Biophys J* 1987;51:833–837.

17. Windisch H, Ahammer H, Schaffer P, et al. Optical multisite detection of membrane potentials in single cardiomyocytes during voltage clamp. In Nagel JH, Smith WM (eds): *Proc Ann Int Conf IEEE Eng Med Biol Soc*. Piscataway, NJ: Institute of Electrical and Electronics Engineers, Inc.; 1991:0605–0606.

18. Knisley SB, Blitchington TF, Hill BC, et al. Optical measurements of transmembrane potential changes during electric field stimulation of ventricular cells. *Circ Res* 1993;72:255–270.

19. Allessie MA, Schalij MJ, Kirchhof CJHJ, et al. Experimental electrophysiology and arrhythmogenicity: Anisotropy and ventricular tachycardia. *Eur Heart J* 1989;10(Suppl E):2–8.

20. Hill BC, Hunt AJ, Courtney KR. Reentrant tachycardia in a thin layer of ventricular subepicardium: Effects of *d*-sotalol and lidocaine. *J Cardiovasc Pharmacol* 1990;16:871–880.

21. Knisley SB, Smith WM, Ideker RE. Prolongation and shortening of action potentials by electrical shocks in frog ventricular muscle. *Am J Physiol* 1994;35:H2348-H2358.

22. Li T, Sperelakis N, Teneick RE, et al. Effects of diacetyl monoxime on cardiac excitation-contraction coupling. *J Pharmacol Exp Ther* 1985;232:688–695.

23. Knisley SB. Transmembrane voltage changes during unipolar stimulation of rabbit ventricle. *Circ Res* 1995;77:1229–1239.

24. Kong W, Johnson PL, Knisley SB. Reduction of motion artifacts and photobleaching during multiwavelength ratiometric optical recording of action potentials and intracellular calcium transients in rabbit hearts. *Pacing Clin Electrophysiol* 2000;23:608. Abstract.

25. Knisley SB, Justice RK, Kong W, Johnson PL. Fluorescence emission ratiometry indicates cardiac repolarization and resting membrane potential changes without requiring pharmacological motion inhibition. *Pacing Clin Electrophysiol* 2000;23:616. Abstract.

26. Fluhler E, Burnham VG, Loew LM. Spectra, membrane binding, and potentiometric responses of new charge shift probes. *Biochemistry* 1985;24:5749–5755.

27. Dillon S, Morad M. A new laser scanning system for measuring action potential propagation in the heart. *Science* 1981;214:453–456.

28. Morad M, Dillon S, Weiss J. An acousto-optically steered laser scanning system for measurement of action potential spread in intact heart. In De Weer P, Salzberg BM (eds): *Optical Methods in Cell Physiology*. New York: Society of General Physiologists and Wiley-Interscience; 1986:211–226.

29. Hill BC, Courtney KR. Design of a multi-point laser scanned optical monitor of cardiac action potential propagation: Application to microreentry in guinea pig atrium. *Ann Biomed Eng* 1987;15:567–577.

30. Lakowicz JR, Szmacinski H, Nowaczyk K, et al. Fluorescence lifetime imaging. *Analytical Biochemistry* 1992;202:316–330.

31. Knisley SB. Mapping intracellular calcium in rabbit hearts with Fluo 3. In *17th Annual International Conference—Engineering in Medicine and Biology Society*. Montreal, Canada: IEEE, 1995: (electronic medium).

32. Spach MS, Kootsey JM. Relating the sodium current and conductance to the shape of transmembrane and extracellular potentials by simulation: Effects of propagation boundaries. *IEEE Trans Biomed Eng* 1985;32:743–755.

33. Knisley SB, Trayanova N, Aguel F. Roles of electric field and fiber structure in cardiac electric stimulation. *Biophys J* 1999;77:1404–1417.

34. Neunlist M, Zou S-Z, Tung L. Design and use of an "optrode" for optical recordings of cardiac action potentials. *Pflugers Arch* 1992;420:611–617.

35. Knisley SB. Evidence for roles of the activating function in electric stimulation. *IEEE Trans Biomed Eng* 2000;47:1114–1119.

36. Knisley SB, Baynham TC. Line stimulation parallel to myofibers enhances regional uniformity of transmembrane voltage changes in rabbit hearts. *Circ Res* 1997;81:229–241.

37. Knisley SB, Fast V, Pollard AE. Anisotropy of membrane polarization decreases when an electrode is separated from the myocardial surface. *Circulation* 1999;100:I786.

38. Neunlist M, Tung L. Spatial distribution of cardiac transmembrane potentials around an extracellular electrode: Dependence on fiber orientation. *Biophys J* 1995;68:2310–2322.

39. Knisley SB, Hill BC, Ideker RE. Virtual electrode effects in myocardial fibers. *Biophys J* 1994;66:719–728.

40. Knisley SB, Pollard AE, Ideker RE. Changing shock polarity causes a "no-switch" region where transmembrane voltage hyperpolarizes with either polarity. *Pacing Clin Electrophysiol* 1998;21:847.

41. Ripley BD. *Spatial Statistics*. New York: John Wiley & Sons; 1981:44–54.

42. Snyder WV. Algorithm 531 contour plotting. *ACM Trans Math Software* 1978;4:290–294.

43. Knisley SB, Hill BC. Effects of bipolar point and line stimulation in anisotropic rabbit epicardium: Assessment of the critical radius of curvature for longitudinal block. *IEEE Trans Biomed Eng* 1995;42:957–966.

44. Knisley SB, Hill BC. Optical recordings of the effect of electrical stimulation on action potential repolarization and the induction of reentry in two-dimensional perfused rabbit epicardium. *Circulation* 1993;88(Pt. I):2402–2414.

45. Weidmann S. Electrical constants of trabecular muscle from mammalian heart. *J Physiol* 1970;210:1041–1054.

46. Neunlist M, Tung L. Optical recordings of ventricular excitability of frog heart by an extracellular stimulating point electrode. *Pacing Clin Electrophysiol* 1994;17:1641–1654.

47. Knisley SB. Optical mapping of cardiac electrical stimulation. *J Electrocardiol* 1997;30(Suppl):11–18.

48. Hodgkin AL, Huxley AF. A quantitative description of membrane current and its application to conduction and excitation in nerve. *J Physiol* 1952;117:500–544.

49. Wiley JD, Webster JG. Analysis and control of the current distribution under circular dispersive electrodes. *IEEE Trans Biomed Eng* 1982;BME-29:381–389.

50. Krauthamer V, Davis CC, Gan E-T. Two-point electrical-fluorescence recording from heart with optical fibers. *IEEE Trans Biomed Eng* 1994;41:1191–1194.
51. Gray RA, Jalife J, Panfilov A, et al. Nonstationary vortexlike reentrant activity as a mechanism of polymorphic ventricular tachycardia in the isolated rabbit heart. *Circulation* 1995;91:2454–2469.
52. Girouard SD, Pastore JM, Laurita KR, et al. Optical mapping in a new guinea pig model of ventricular tachycardia reveals mechanisms for multiple wavelengths in a single reentrant circuit. *Circulation* 1996;93:603–613.
53. Windisch H, Müller W, Tritthart HA. Fluorescence monitoring of rapid changes in membrane potential in heart muscle. *Biophys J* 1985;48:877–884.
54. Wikswo JP Jr, Lin S-F, Abbas RA. Virtual electrodes in cardiac tissue: A common mechanism for anodal and cathodal stimulation. *Biophys J* 1995; 69:2195–2210.
55. Gillis AM, Fast VG, Rohr S, et al. Spatial changes in transmembrane potential during extracellular electrical shocks in cultured monolayers of neonatal rat ventricular myocytes. *Circ Res* 1996;79:676–690.
56. Fast VG, Rohr S, Gillis AM, et al. Activation of cardiac tissue by extracellular electrical shocks: Formation of "secondary sources" at intercellular clefts in monolayers of cultured myocytes. *Circ Res* 1998;82:375–385.
57. Liu Y, Cabo C, Salomonsz R, et al. Effects of diacetyl monoxime on the electrical properties of sheep and guinea pig ventricular muscle. *Cardiovasc Res* 1993;27:1991–1997.
58. Rubart M, Biermann M, Wu J, et al. Differential effects of cytochalasin D and 2,3-butanedione monoxime on cardiac excitation-contraction coupling. *Biophys J* 1998;74:A55.
59. Zhou X, Ideker RE, Blitchington TF, et al. Optical transmembrane potential measurements during defibrillation-strength shocks in perfused rabbit hearts. *Circ Res* 1995;77:593–602.
60. Knisley SB, Grant AO. Asymmetrical electrically induced injury of rabbit ventricular myocytes. *J Mol Cell Cardiol* 1995;27:1111–1122.
61. Holley LK, Knisley SB. Transmembrane potentials during high voltage shocks in ischemic cardiac tissue. *Pacing Clin Electrophysiol* 1997;20:146–152.
62. Tung L, Sliz N, Mulligan MR. Influence of electrical axis of stimulation on excitation of cardiac muscle cells. *Circ Res* 1991;69:722–730.
63. Klee M, Plonsey R. Stimulation of spheroidal cells—The role of cell shape. *IEEE Trans Biomed Eng* 1976;23:347–354.
64. Kishida H, Surawicz B, Fu LT. Effects of K^+ and K^+-induced polarization on $(dV/dt)_{max}$ threshold potential, and membrane input resistance in guinea pig and cat ventricular myocardium. *Circ Res* 1979;44:800–814.
65. Wikswo JP Jr, Wisialowski TA, Altemeier WA, et al. Virtual cathode effects during stimulation of cardiac muscle: Two-dimensional in vivo experiments. *Circ Res* 1991;68:513–530.
66. Rattay F. Analysis of models for extracellular fiber stimulation. *IEEE Trans Biomed Eng* 1989;36:676–682.
67. Clerc L. Directional differences of impulse spread in trabecular muscle from mammalian heart. *J Physiol* 1976;255:335–346.
68. Ideker RE, Tang ASL, Frazier DW, et al. Basic mechanisms of ventricular defibrillation. In Glass L, Hunter P, McColloch A (eds): *Theory of the Heart*. New York: Springer-Verlag; 1991:533–560.
69. Saypol JM, Roth BJ. A mechanism for anisotropic reentry in electrically active tissue. *J Cardiovasc Electrophysiol* 1992;3:558–566.
70. Lin S-F, Roth BJ, Wikswo JP Jr. Quatrefoil reentry in myocardium: An optical imaging study of the induction mechanism. *Pacing Clin Electrophysiol* 1998;21:854.
71. Sosa E, Scanavacca M, D'Avila A, et al. A new technique to perform epicardial

mapping in the electrophysiology laboratory. *J Cardiovasc Electrophysiol* 1996;7:531–536.

72. Frazier DW, Wolf PD, Wharton JM, et al. Stimulus-induced critical point: Mechanism for electrical initiation of reentry in normal canine myocardium. *J Clin Invest* 1989;83:1039–1052.

73. Knisley SB, Smith WM, Ideker RE. Effect of field stimulation on cellular repolarization in rabbit myocardium: Implications for reentry induction. *Circ Res* 1992;70:707–715.

74. Efimov IR, Cheng Y, Wagoner DRV, et al. Shock-induced critical points: A mechanism of defibrillation failure. *Pacing Clin Electrophysiol* 1998;21:962.

75. Swartz JF, Jones JL, Jones RE, et al. Conditioning prepulse of biphasic defibrillator waveforms enhances refractoriness to fibrillation wavefronts. *Circ Res* 1991;68:438–449.

76. Kwaku KF, Dillon SM. Shock-induced depolarization of refractory myocardium prevents wave-front propagation in defibrillation. *Circ Res* 1996;79:957–973.

Chapter 21

Mechanisms of Defibrillation:
2. Application of Laser Scanning Technology

Stephen M. Dillon and Kevin F. Kwaku

Electrical defibrillation is the only sure, safe, and immediate means of rescue from cardiac sudden death due to ventricular fibrillation (VF). It is the passage of an electrical shock through the heart to arrest the rapid, erratic activation of the ventricle and replace it with a slower, more organized rhythm capable of restoring the heart's ability to pump blood to itself and to the rest of the body. Though much of its technical refinement has occurred in the last few decades, the electrical defibrillation process itself was first recognized more than 100 years ago.[1] We are still faced with the question of understanding how this essential life-saving technique works. While much remains to be learned about a wide variety of cardiac arrhythmias and their therapies, defibrillation has been particularly obscure because of the highly complex nature of fibrillation itself and because of the incapacitation of electrical recording instrumentation by the shock. The last decade, however, saw a sharp increase in the investigation of defibrillation brought on primarily by the introduction of shock-resistant electrical mapping techniques[2,3] and, somewhat later, the introduction of optical recording methods.[4–9]

In past reviews, we[10] and others[11] have described defibrillation from a bottom-up mechanistic approach in which a connection between the magnitude and waveform of the shock is ultimately tied to the dynamics of wave front propagation. The importance of the latter is predicated on the assumption that VF is perpetuated by the reentry of such wave fronts. In this chapter I instead look at defibrillation from the standpoint of how what we know relates to a traditional view of defibrillation, such as the critical mass hypothesis[12,13] or our own progressive depolarization[14] hypothesis. This traditional view considers the presence of propagating wave fronts after the shock to be a risk factor for failed defibrillation. Accordingly, the key to defibrillation will be to understand how shocks terminate

Supported by the Sidney Kimmel Cardiovascular Research Center and grant R01 HL-49246 from the National Heart, Lung, and Blood Institute of the National Institutes of Health, Bethesda, MD.

From Rosenbaum DS, Jalife J (eds): *Optical Mapping of Cardiac Excitation and Arrhythmias.* ©Futura Publishing Co., Inc., Armonk, NY, 2001.

fibrillation wave fronts. Other factors, such as the ability of the shock to prolong[5,15,16] and synchronize[17] repolarization or to evoke ectopic activity, also enter into the defibrillation process but only when a shock fails to eliminate all wave fronts or when shock field strengths become pathologically excessive. Although the traditional viewpoint taken by this chapter differs from the upper limit of vulnerability[18] hypothesis of defibrillation, the processes it describes is nevertheless pertinent since fibrillation wave front termination is a necessary, albeit not a sufficient, condition for successful defibrillation in that scheme. Last, this chapter assumes that VF is in essence a reentrant rather than focal[19] arrhythmia, which despite ample supporting experimental evidence, remains an unproved conjecture.

The process of fibrillation wave front termination was directly addressed by a laser scanning study that mapped the spread of propagated electrical activation before, during, and after shocks applied to a fibrillating rabbit heart.[6] Since this technique is markedly different from other optical mapping methods detailed in this book (however, see references 9 and 20), the first half of this chapter describes why laser scanning was developed and how it works.

Laser Scanning Overview

One common approach to optical mapping involves projecting an image of the myocardium onto an array of photodetectors, either photodiodes[21–26] or a charged coupled device (CCD) imager,[27–30] a so-called multiple detector focal plane approach. Laser scanning by contrast is a nonimaging technique that employs a single photodetector.[31] It was developed in response to unique circumstances, the first of which was a desire for a high depth of field in order to accommodate intact hearts. It also arose from the need to alter flexibly the number and position of recording sites. This design also enabled us to work around the difficulty inherent in illuminating large areas of the heart using incandescent or arc lamp sources (see reference 30), a less pressing problem today with the availability of efficient dyes. Another advantage, specific to the author at that time, was having to construct only one as opposed to 100 or more photodetectors in order to perform optical mapping.

Mapping by laser scanning is performed simply by causing a spot of laser illumination to visit, rapidly and repeatedly, a series of sites on the heart. A high-speed laser beam deflector is used to move the laser spot around on the surface of the heart in a random access manner under the control of a computer. While the beam is scanned across the heart, a single high-speed photodetector records the fluorescence emitted from each of the sites as they are illuminated in turn. The computer that controls the laser spot position also digitizes the fluorescence signal from the photodetector. In this way it is possible to associate a particular fluorescence level with a particular site during successive scans. The optical recordings from each site are reconstructed by reassembling the time series of fluorescence values associated with each site. The number of sites that can be mapped and the temporal resolution for each recording site are dependent on how quickly the laser beam can be repositioned from site to site and on how rapidly the photodetector is able to respond to the change in fluorescence caused by the repositioning of the laser beam. If the laser scanning system can reposition the laser spot and record a new fluorescence value in S μs, then it would be possible to repeatedly sample each site in a scan of N sites every T = N*S/1000 ms. Therefore, the number of sites in a scan can be reduced to increase the temporal resolution of the measurements, or the sampling time can be increased in order to increase the number of recording sites, i.e., the spatial resolution.

Figure 1 shows a block diagram of the laser scanning system presently in use. As in the first scanning system, we use the voltage-sensitive dye WW781[32] to transduce membrane potential into a fluorescence signal. When excited by red light, the dye fluoresces at just longer than visible red wavelengths. The original scanning system used the 633-nm wavelength beam from a 20-mW He-Ne laser. However, even though the dye quantum efficiency declined at longer excitation wavelengths, in this present design we use the 647-nm wavelength beam from a 400-mW Krypton Laser (Innova 90K, Coherent, Palo Alto, CA), a power increase that more than offsets the decreased fluorescence emission. (In another scanning system[33] we have used the voltage-sensitive dye di-4-ANEPPS and so have incorporated an argon ion laser to provide the green excitation light needed for that dye.) The use of a more powerful laser raises the concern of photodynamic damage. However, only a fraction of this power reaches a particular site on the heart because the laser spot continuously moves. For example, after power losses through the deflection system and optics (see Fig.

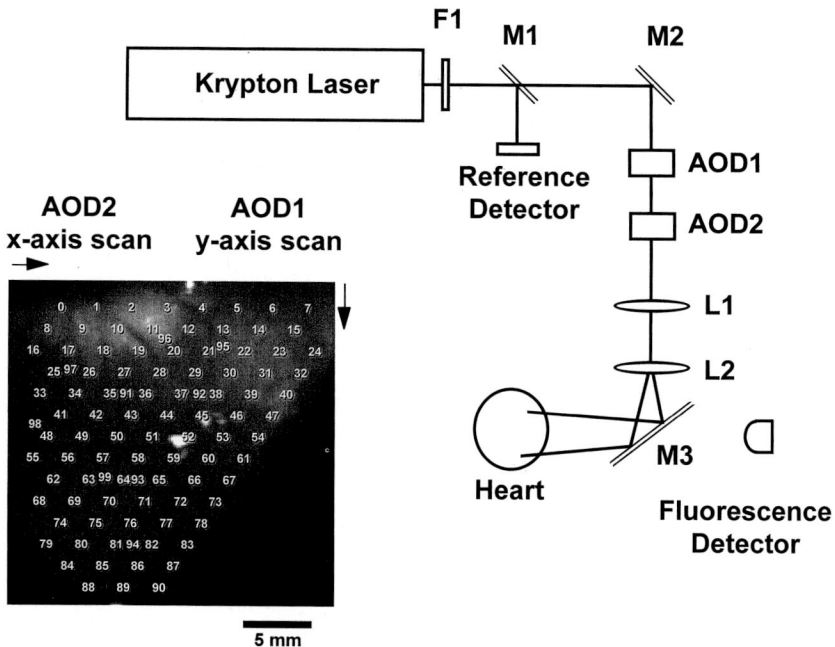

Figure 1. Schematic diagram of laser scanning system for optical mapping. AOD = acousto-optic deflector.

1) were accounted for, only 55 mW of laser power reached the heart. In the present configuration, it illuminates a 0.2-mm-diameter spot but does so only 1% of the time when there are 100 sites in a scan. This yields an average power density of 1.75 W/cm^2. By comparison, in some of our other studies of defibrillation[5,17,34] we used a fiber pick-up, which delivered 10 mW continuously to a 0.25-mm-diameter spot to yield a power density of 20 W/cm^2 and registered no damage.

The rapid positioning of the laser beam on the heart is accomplished by a pair of acousto-optic deflectors (AOD1 and AOD2). A portion of the laser beam entering an acousto-optic deflector emerges at an angle to the original beam. The exit angle of this deflected laser beam can be electronically controlled. To position a laser spot in two dimensions, a pair of these devices is used to first deflect the laser beam along the vertical axis and then, taking that vertically deflected beam, to deflect it along the horizontal axis. Two lenses (L1 and L2) convert these angular deflections of the laser beam into lateral translations on the surface of the preparation. In the present configuration theses acousto-optic deflectors can reposition the laser spot within 5.5 μs of a change in the command signal from the computer.

As the laser spot is moved from site to site, a portion of the emitted fluorescence is intercepted by a single fluorescence photodetector. Although we have not done so, a lens may be inserted between the detector and the heart in order to increase the light collection efficiency. However, there is no need to form an image of the heart on the detector because, since fluorescence can arise only from the illuminated spot, the spatial discrimination is achieved here by the size of the laser spot. The fluorescence detector does not respond instantaneously to changes in light level caused by repositioning the laser spot but requires a finite time to settle to a new fluorescence reading. Taking into account this delay and the time required for laser beam repositioning, a total of 10 μs is required to sample fluorescence at each site. Therefore, optical recordings from 100 sites can be obtained, each consisting of fluorescence values sampled at 1000 times per second (1 ms = 100 sites*10 μs/site/1000 μs/ms).

To increase the uniformity of light collection by the fluorescence detector, we used a dichroic mirror (M3) to align the axes of the illumination and detection optics. This mirror (530DRLP, Omega Optical, Inc., Brattleboro, VT) reflects the laser beam but permits passage of fluorescence light of a longer wavelength. Thus, the heart can be viewed face-on by the fluorescence detector and illuminated face-on by the laser. Care must be taken to use the dichroic mirror in correct orientation with respect to the linear polarization of the laser beam. In this set-up the light leaving the acousto-optic deflection system has a vertical polarization. This means that the dichroic mirror will work best when oriented as portrayed in the top view illustrated in Figure 1.

The krypton ion laser is used for both its high power and the collimation of its light beam. Since the acousto-optic deflectors move the laser beam through a small angle, a tightly collimated light beam is needed in order to resolve the maximum number of separate laser spots. However, use of this laser presents its own unique problems, the first of which is the glow from the electrical discharge within the laser tube that can be picked up as noise by the fluorescence detector. Insertion of an interference filter (F1) rejects this plasma glow by permitting passage of only the 647 laser emission line. This filter (647BP10, Omega Optical, Inc.), however, is not 100% efficient and so it reduces the power available to the scanning system. A more serious problem involves the fluctuations in the laser beam power caused by variations in the electrical discharge current and mode hopping. The latter is due to the fact that the laser cavity can accommodate more than one resonant mode. Each mode, however, may produce different amounts of light. Thus, the laser beam can spontaneously and unpredictably fluctuate in power as the distribution in cavity resonance modes shifts in time. To cure this problem we reduced the gain of the laser cavity by forcing the laser beam through an aperture within the resonator. Under these conditions only the most efficient resonant mode was sustained. Fortunately, it was also the one that produced the most highly collimated beam. The residual laser noise was reduced with use of an analog divider integrated circuit (MPY634, Burr-Brown Corp., Tucson, AZ) to modulate the signal from the fluorescence detector in inverse proportion to the laser power. The laser power was measured using a beam splitter (M1) to reflect 10% of the laser beam power onto reference detector. This detector had the same bandwidth characteristics as the fluorescence detector. The fluorescence signal was fed into the numerator input of the divider circuit while the reference detector signal was fed into the denominator. This reduced the noise from a 1% peak-to-peak noise envelope to 0.1%.

Acousto-optic Deflection

The acousto-optic deflection system relies on the interaction between the laser beam and ultrasound waves within glass or some other interaction medium.[35] This interaction can impart an angular deflection on the laser beam, a deflection that is then converted into a position change by a lens. In a recent description of a laser scanning-based imaging system,[33] we described in detail the basics of this acousto-optic interaction. Acousto-optic deflection can be briefly described by likening it to Bragg reflection of x-rays by the lattice arrangement of atoms in a crystal. The difference is that the "crystal" structure is created in an interaction medium by the ultrasound waves. These sound waves alternatively compress and expand the medium at the crest and troughs of the sound waves. These compressions and expansions in turn alter the optical index of the medium. These changes in optical index are spaced at the wavelength of the sound wave. For the ultrasound frequencies used, this can be as small as several microns. Therefore, the ultrasound wave creates what is in effect a diffraction grating consisting of changes in optical index in the medium. Just as an ordinary optical grating can diffract light, so can this index grating. Therefore, a laser beam entering the medium at the correct angle, defined as the Bragg angle, will be "reflected" (in actuality diffracted) back out at the same angle by the sound waves. The undiffracted portion of the laser beam passes through along the same path. Diffraction efficiencies of 50% to 75% are typical of most commercial acousto-optic deflectors. The exit angle of the reflected laser beam can be varied by changing the wavelength of the ultrasonic waves and the angle of the ultrasound wave fronts. The latter is needed because changing the acoustic wavelength also changes the Bragg angle needed for efficient diffraction of the light. Since the alignment of the entering laser beam is fixed, the Bragg angle condition is satisfied by simultaneously tilting the angle of the sound waves with respect to the entering laser beam. This occurs automatically because the ultrasound transducers are fabricated in the form of a "phased array." The ultrasound wavelength is changed by changing the frequency of the radiofrequency (RF) voltage driving the ultrasound transducers attached to the interaction medium. From the standpoint of the operator, the angle of the reflected laser beam changes when the frequency of the RF drive signal is changed, which, when it originates from a voltage-controlled oscillator, occurs when the command voltage signal originating in the computer changes. The change in laser beam exit angle is not instantaneous but instead occurs during the time it takes for the new ultrasound waves to propagate to the laser beam in the crystal and through it. These parameters are determined by the physical properties of the acousto-optic deflector and by the position and diameter of the laser beam.

Figure 2 is a block diagram of the acousto-optic deflector configuration. This scanning system uses a deflector (EFL D250, Inrad, Inc., Northvale, NJ) for each axis of laser beam movement. (This manufacturer no longer supplies acousto-optic deflectors but several others, including Isomet Corp., Springfield, VA; Brimrose Corp., Baltimore, MD; and In-

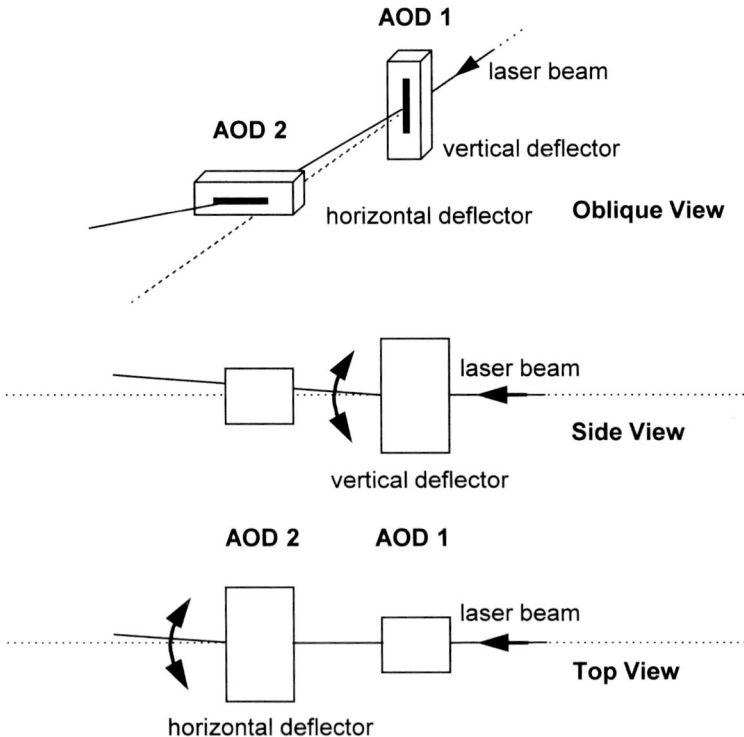

Figure 2. Alignment and orientation of acousto-optic deflectors (AODs).

traAction Corp., Bellwood, IL, sell similar devices). The upper part of the figure shows a face-on, oblique view of the deflection stage in which the laser beam enters from the rear of the diagram along the laser axis denoted by the dashed line. The vertical deflector (AOD1) is shown upright on the page but in reality it is rotated slightly backward in order to satisfy the baseline Bragg angle condition. This diagram shows only the deflected laser beam emerging from the vertical stage (first-order diffraction) and not the lower intensity nondeflected (0 order diffraction) and doubly deflected (higher order diffraction orders) beam. This vertically deflected beam then enters the horizontal deflection stage (AOD2). This stage is rotated 90° with respect to the vertical stage. This stage is also tilted backward at the minimum deflection angle so that the vertically deflected beam passes through the vertical aperture of the horizontal deflection device. Though not drawn this way, this stage is also rotated slightly clockwise in order to establish the minimum Bragg angle between the device and the vertically deflected laser beam. The double deflected laser beam thus exits the acousto-optic stages at a horizontal and vertical angle with respect to the laser tube axis. This figure also diagrams the relationships between the two deflection stages from two other views. Again, the devices are drawn without showing the small angular adjustments needed to satisfy the Bragg angle requirements just discussed.

High-efficiency acousto-optic devices that are presently available rely on interaction media that have birefringent optical characteristics as opposed to the glass acousto-optic deflectors we first used,[36] that have no optical activity. This means that the polarization properties of the laser light must be taken into account. The devices used in this present system require a vertically polarized laser beam. Fortunately, most laser beams are vertically polarized and so can be directly passed, as is, through the vertical acousto-optic deflection stage. In the course of vertically deflecting the laser beam, the device also rotates its polarization by 90°. This action makes it possible to send the laser beam directly into the horizontal deflector since it requires a horizontally polarized laser beam. If the horizontal and vertical deflection stages are interchanged, the system will operate very poorly because of the inappropriate polarization. Other acousto-optic deflectors convert a vertically polarized beam into a circularly polarized one and so a retardation plate is needed to bring the deflected beam back into linear polarization (e.g., the Isomet devices described in reference 33).

Optical Characteristics

A set of lenses is needed to transform the small angular deflections imposed on the laser beam by the acousto-optic deflectors into a linear translation of a laser spot on the surface of the heart. This is done by a pair of lenses: the first converts the angular deflection into a lateral translation (L1) and the second (L2) projects an image of the translated laser spot onto the surface of the heart. A positive focal length lens will bring light rays entering it to a point on the plane that is determined by the angle of the entering light ray. This plane is located at the lens focal length F from the lens. The change in spot position Δx caused by a change in the laser beam angle $\Delta\theta$ is described by the equation $\Delta x = F*\Delta\theta$, where $\Delta\theta$ is small, as is the case with acousto-optic deflection. This is illustrated on the right side of the diagrams in Figure 3, in which parallel light rays from a laser beam converge at various points in the focal plane of lens L1 (50-mm focal length plano-convex achromat) as a function of entry angle. For the purposes of illustration, this diagram considers only one axis of deflection. Descriptions given here simultaneously apply to deflections imparted to the laser beam along the other axis. This schematic diagram exaggerates the size of the laser beam relative to the lens and the angles of the light rays. The beam entering at $\theta = 0$ corresponds to the nondeflected laser light that passes through the deflection stage. These light rays come to focus at a point along the axis defined by the beam exiting the laser. Rays at angles θ_1 and θ_2 correspond to the minimum and maximum deflection angles of the laser beam. These beams are brought to focus at the corresponding points x_1 and x_2 in the L1 focal plane. Intermediate deflection angles fill out the range of laser spots along the line between x_1 and x_2.

The acousto-optic devices used in this set-up impose a maximum $\Delta\theta$ of 49 milliradians ($\sim 2.8°$). This means that the laser spot will traverse a Δx = 2.5 mm span in the focal plane of lens L1. A second lens (L2) is used to magnify this span approximately 10 times to a $\Delta x'$ of 24.7 mm at the position of the heart. This lens (100 ms focal length double convex achromat) is positioned at an object distance of approximately 110 mm from the focal point of L1. This will refocus the scanned laser beam at an image dis-

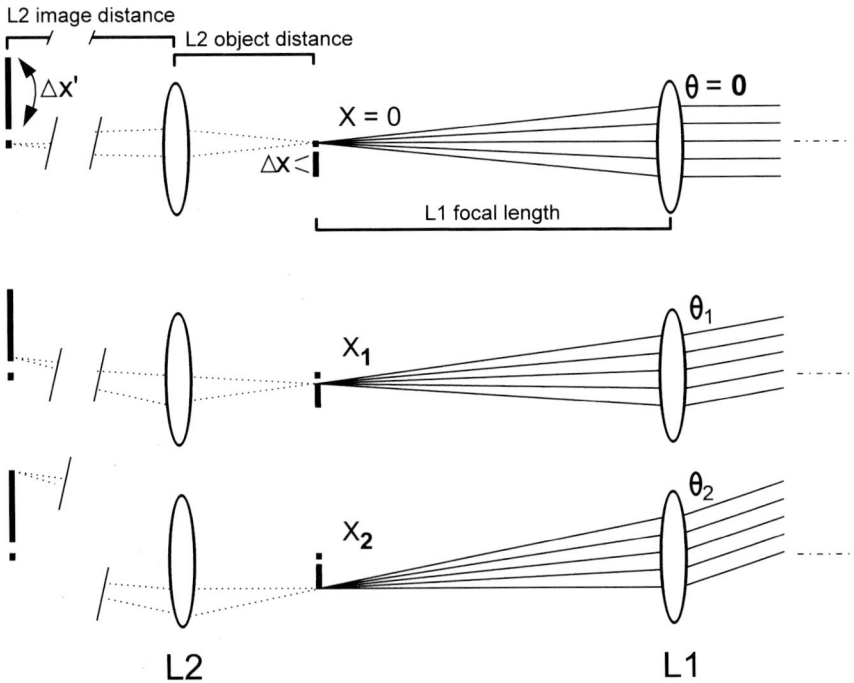

Figure 3. Ray diagram for the imaging optics of the laser scanning system.

tance of 1100 mm (~43″) from L2, a point at which the heart should be positioned. Such a long object distance, combined with the small width of the laser beam at L2, even after expanding outward after the first focal point, results in a very high effective F# (low aperture) for the imaging optics. This means that the deflected laser beam will remain in focus over several centimeters' distance on either side of the focal plane centered on the heart. This is illustrated by Figure 5 of reference 33, which shows a scanned image remaining in sharp focus at different points in front of and behind the prime focal plane centered on the heart's normal position.

By varying the position of L2 to change the magnification, or changing the focal length of L1 to change the size of the scan at the focal point of L1, it is possible to easily change the size of the scan pattern so that both large and small hearts can be optically mapped. Regardless of the changes in the scan pattern size, the spatial resolution of the scanner will remain fixed. The spatial resolution of the scanning system is defined as the number of laser spots that can be placed side by side across the span of the scan and still remain distinguishable. The maximum resolution of the present system is 137 spots along each axis. In practice, we calibrated the software to operate as if the maximum resolution was 128 spots per axis. One factor determining the spatial resolution is the fact that a laser beam, though highly collimated, is not perfectly parallel but diverges slightly. The number of resolvable spots, in turn, is determined by the ratio of the maximum angular sweep that the acousto-optic devices can impose divided by the self-divergence angle of the laser beam. Since the maximum angular sweep is effectively fixed by our choice of deflection hardware and laser wavelength, the only way to increase the spatial resolution is to reduce the laser beam self-divergence angle by expanding the beam diameter. This would have the effect of increasing the number of resolvable spots. This approach was taken in the first laser scanning system constructed,[36] and the result was that the acousto-optic deflection stage had to be several feet long in order to accommodate the beam-reshaping optics for each deflection stage. However the acousto-optic devices now used have a naturally higher maximum deflection angle and so in the present configuration the laser beam was not expanded. This permitted us to construct a compact deflection stage that was not unwieldy and did not suffer the light losses introduced by additional lenses. Another important reason for not expanding the laser beam to increase spatial resolution was that this would also increase the time required to reposition the laser beam. Movement of the laser from one spot to the other is not complete until the new acoustic wave fronts have enough time to propagate across the width of the laser beam. The 128 spot per axis resolution we currently employ is more than sufficient to map the heart since on average the scan sites are 2 mm apart, a separation corresponding to 10 spots.

Another limit on the spatial resolution is the stability of the laser spot position. Mechanical vibrations in the optical set-up or variability in the frequency of the RF driver or noise on the control voltage signal will cause uncertainties in the laser spot position and so reduce the effective spatial resolution. The position stability of the present system was measured by recording the output from a position-sensitive diode over a 1-second period. It showed that the spot position stability along either axis was within 5% of the laser spot diameter.

Fluorescence Photodetector

In addition to the acousto-optic deflector speed, the performance of the fluorescence photodetector plays an important role in determining how quickly the system can scan from spot to spot on the heart. Figure 4 shows tracings that illustrate how both of these parameters respond to a command to change the spot position. The beginning of these traces corresponds to the delivery of a new spot position command signal. The laser spot position trace does not respond at first, but after a delay it undergoes a transition signaling the disappearance of the spot at the old position at its appearance at the new position. The laser spot movement was complete within 5.5 μs of the change in command voltage. The initial delay (acoustic latency) was 2.6 μs and was in part due to the time required for the RF generators to respond to a new command voltage signal by delivering a new frequency of RF excitation to the ultrasonic transducers in the acousto-optic deflectors. It is important to minimize this delay, and in order to do so we chose RF drivers (DE-70M and DE-70BM, IntraAction Corp.) that were able to make the transition to a new RF frequency quicker than those drivers sold by the manufacturer of the acousto-optic deflector. Because of this mixing of manufacturers we had to carefully match the frequency range (50 to 100 MHz), maximum RF power (0.3 W), and impedance (50 Ω) of the acousto-optic deflectors to the capabilities of the drivers. The IntraAction drivers we used supplied in excess of 4 W RF power, and we were able to operate them beyond the specified bandwidth of 50 to 90 MHz. These drivers were able to respond to step change in command voltage within 0.5 μs. The remaining 2.1 μs of acoustic latency was due to the time required for the ultrasound wave fronts to propagate to the position of the laser beam. While this can be minimized by positioning the devices, in practice it is difficult to minimize it in both devices while retaining optimal alignment between AOD1 and AOD2. Care was taken, however, to ensure that both devices produced the same amount of propagation delay. The 2.9-μs aperture filling time corresponds to the time required by the ultrasound wave fronts to propagate across the width of the laser beam. As discussed above, this delay can be reduced, but at the cost of reducing the spatial resolution and adding more optical components.

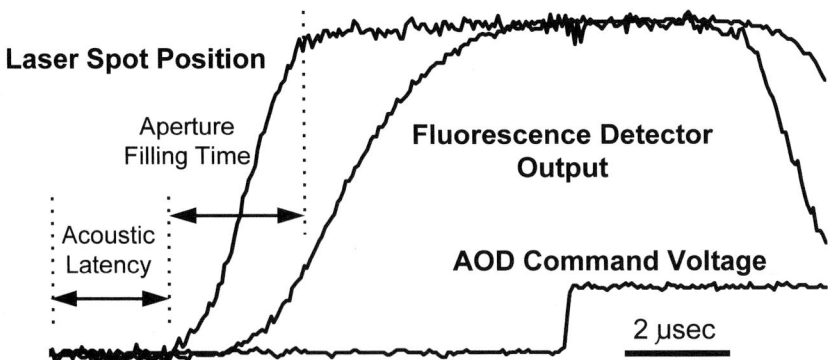

Figure 4. Response time for laser spot positioning and the fluorescence detector. AOD = acousto-optic deflector.

Figure 4 also shows that the fluorescence detector response lags the laser spot position signal. The photoamplifier does not settle to its final value until 10 μs after the step change in the acousto-optic deflector command voltage, at which time its output is sampled by the computer's analog-to-digital (A/D) converter. This reflects the limitations in the upper cut-off frequency of the photoamplifier-photodiode combination. One could reduce the sampling time a few microseconds by taking advantage of the fact that during the acoustic latency period no changes in signal occur; however, we have not done so. The response time of the photodetector is a function of the performance of the electronics and of the willingness to trade an increased noise level for faster operation. The latter is because the higher signal bandwidth required to speed the photodetector operation also admits a greater frequency range of noise components. There was an additional penalty owing to the nature of the photodiode-photoamplifier configuration. We used a single photodiode (600-PIN-RM, Quantrad Sensor, Santa Clara, CA) connected to an operational amplifier (OP-27, Precision Monolithics Inc., Santa Clara, CA) configured as a 1×10^5 volts per ampere transimpedance configuration. The capacitance of the photodiode causes the amplifier bandwidth for noise to extend out to the operational amplifier limiting bandwidth rather than to the lower bandwidth established for the signal. For this reason it is important to select an operational amplifier whose limiting bandwidth is just enough to handle the signal so that the additional bandwidth margin available for excess noise is limited. Another confounding factor is that photodiode capacitance increases as larger photodiodes are used in order to intercept more light. We desired a larger photodiode area so that it could be located further from the heart in order to increase the uniformity of signal pick up. Typically, we place the photodetector 4 to 7 cm from the heart. To reduce the photodiode capacitance we applied a 90-V reverse bias to the photodiode. This not only reduced the background noise but it also decreased the intrinsic time constant of the photodiode. A high reverse bias voltage also increased the leakage or "dark" current, but in our case it did not matter since the noise associated with a larger dark current was far less than the baseline photoamplifier noise. In order to reject the reflected laser light and selectively pass the fluorescence signal, a glass long-pass filter (RG665, 3 mm thickness, Schott Glass Technologies, Duryea, PA) was placed in front of the photodiode. The photoamplifier output underwent a subsequent stage of amplification resulting in a total system gain of 5×10^6 volts per ampere of photodiode current. At this second amplification stage, an adjustable offset current was introduced to subtract the background fluorescence so that the changes in fluorescence could be amplified and subsequently digitized. Following amplification, this signal then underwent compensation for laser noise according to the description given above.

After digitization, a 20-mV peak-to-peak noise level was recorded while the photodetector was kept in the dark. When the heart is illuminated, the photodetector noise can increase due to the residual laser noise that is carried on the background fluorescence. In most measurement applications involving a low light level, the limiting noise is determined by the quantum shot noise of the resting light level and the dark current. Our application differs in that the noise floor is set by either the photodetector background noise or, at higher background fluorescence levels, by the residual laser noise. It is normal practice to use a photomultiplier where high-speed responses are desired in low light level environments.[9,20] We instead chose to use a photodiode because it reduced the size of the photodetector, eliminated a high-voltage power supply, and removed the possibility of burning out the photomultiplier by inadvertent illumination.

One recurrent source of confusion with regard to the laser scanning approach is in regard to the Nyquist criterion and the generation of alias signals. Fourier analysis of optical signals of VF recorded continuously through the photodetector during single site illumination showed us that the main frequency component present in the data was always less than 20 Hz. This measurement agrees with data obtained by Girouard et al.[37] In some episodes there were harmonic peaks at higher frequencies, but these always reached insignificant power (<<1% of the main power peak) by 100 Hz, which was still considerably less than the 500 Hz required by the Nyquist theorem on the basis of the 1-kHz sampling rate of each site. Confusion arises because we use a photodetector whose bandwidth far exceeds the 1-kHz digitization rate of each channel and so, by standard application of the Nyquist criterion, signal aliasing would be predicted to occur. However, the criterion does not apply to the laser scanning system since it can be considered analogous to a multiplexed data acquisition system wherein the laser deflector comprises the analog multiplexor and the fluorescence detector the high-speed, high-bandwidth sample-and-hold amplifier. Such a data acquisition system can digitize multiple channels of low-bandwidth analog signals.

Computer System

A standard IBM-PC-compatible computer was used to control the laser beam movement and to digitize the fluorescence signals. Laser spot position control signals for each axis were generated by a pair of programmable waveform synthesizers (WSB-10, Qua Tech, Akron, OH). Data were acquired and digitized with 12-bit resolution (DT2821-G-16SE, Data Translation, Marlboro, MA). A timing signal was added to the A/D data stream to register the timing of events such as shocks and pacing stimuli. The optical recordings presented in this chapter had the baseline fluorescence signal component subtracted and have been filtered using a 5-ms boxcar algorithm. The system could scan a maximum area of 24.7×24.7 mm with this optical configuration, though the effective scan area was generally limited to 20×20 mm, because of the hearts' curvature at the far edges of the scan area. The typical inter-recording site distance was ≈2 mm. The area to be scanned is outlined by the experimenter. Software then automatically fills this area with 100 sites laid down in a regular pattern so that each site within the scan area had four or six equidistant nearest neighbors.

Optical Mapping of Defibrillation

We have long used the isolated, perfused rabbit heart as an experimental model for defibrillation studies, as have others. This model has demonstrated the crucial behaviors needed for such a study: it exhibits a classic dose-response defibrillation probability curve in response to shocks,[6,38] its electrocardiogram is rapid and erratic during VF,[6,39] and optical maps of epicardial activation[6] have demonstrated the expected picture of a shifting pattern of complete and partial reentry loops, isolated wavelets, and wave front collisions, mergers, and bifurcations. A Langendorff perfusion method was used to support the hearts physiologically after their removal from New Zealand White rabbits (~3 kg). The hearts were perfused with Tyrode's solution under a 40 cm of water pressure head, and the perfusate was gassed and warmed to maintain a ventricular temperature of ~36°C. The voltage-sensitive dye WW781 was added to the perfusate to a concentration of 4 mg/L (5.3 μmol/L) and remained in the perfusate throughout the experiment. The calcium channel blocker D600 (2 μmol/L) was also added to eliminate visible contractions. (Other experiments without D600 were able to reproduce the same basic phenomenon described below but by using coupling interval rather than optical membrane voltage to gauge refractoriness.) Test and rescue defibrillation shocks were generated by a pair of battery powered defibrillators (models 2384 and 2326, Medtronic Inc., Minneapolis, MN). They generated monophasic, truncated-exponential waveforms having a 5-ms duration with 58% average tilt (test shock), and a 4- to 6-ms duration with 63% tilt (rescue shock). The test shocks ranged in strength from those that never defibrillated to those that consistently defibrillated. The shocks were applied between stainless steel mesh electrodes in the form of a band encircling the ventricular apex and a cup underlying the ventricular apex. These electrodes were also used to pass 60-Hz current through the ventricle in order to induce VF.

The recording protocol was to induce VF and allow it to proceed, while perfusion continued, for 10 seconds before the initiation of a 1- to 1.3-second optical scanning sequence. During this time a test shock and a rescue shock were applied and, following the latter, the ventricle was paced in order to generate a control action potential for calibration purposes. Optical recordings were made primarily from the right ventricular free wall, though several recordings mapped activity on the left ventricle and the anterior border of the right and left ventricles. The primary means of analysis was the construction of activation maps depicting the propagation of depolarization prior to, during, and following the application of the test shocks. Activation times in each laser scan were initially marked by a computer algorithm, followed by manual correction of inappropriate marks. Activation times were taken as the temporal midpoint of depolarizing deflections, whether these were due to ongoing fibrillation activity or to shocks. Isochronal activation maps were constructed from activation times at all sites, plotted with respect to the time of the test shock. Impulse conduction block was judged to occur between adjacent sites if the activation times differed by at least 20 ms.

Shock-Induced VF Wave Front Reset

Figure 5 is an illustrative example of the results obtained in this study, the "reset" of fibrillation by depolarization evoked by the shock. A partic-

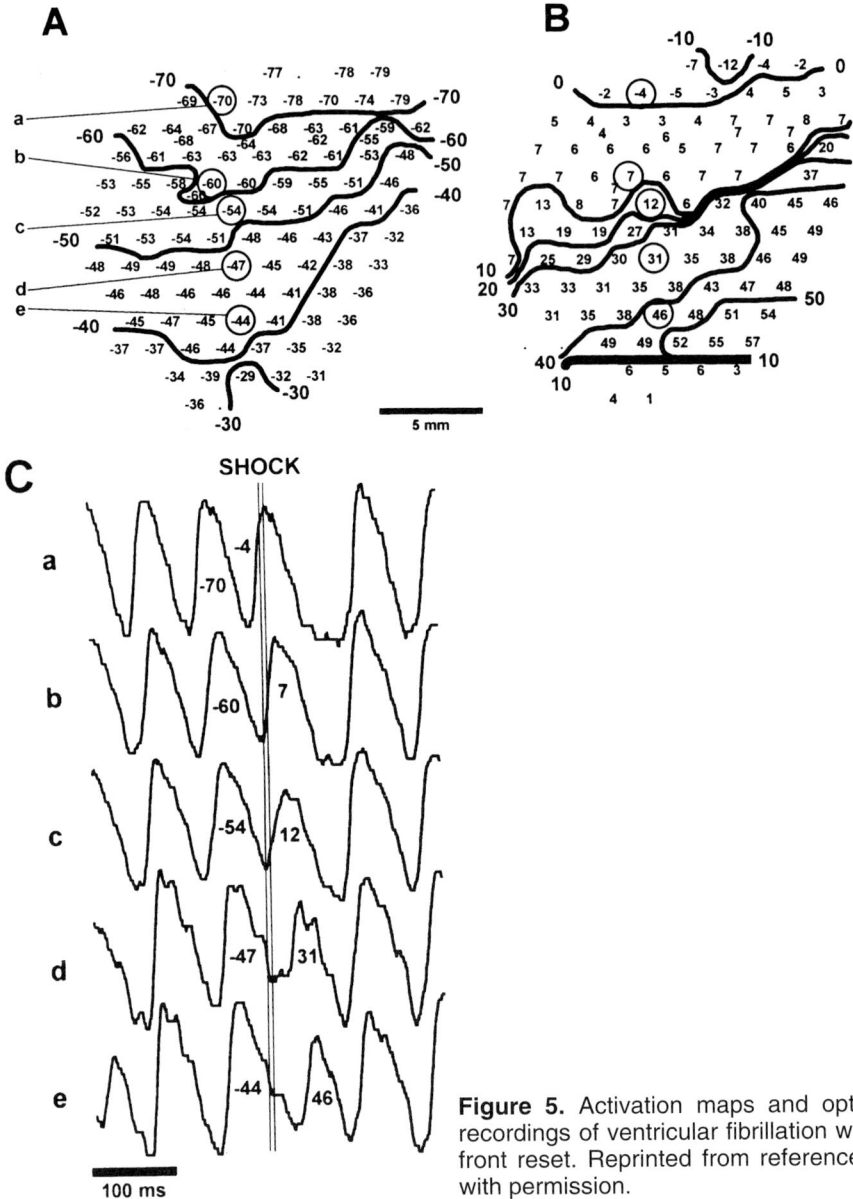

Figure 5. Activation maps and optical recordings of ventricular fibrillation wave front reset. Reprinted from reference 6, with permission.

ularly organized pattern of VF wave front propagation was selected in order to best illustrate this process. From time to time, fibrillation lost its complex appearance and demonstrated short runs of coherent activation wave fronts. (See Fig. 2 in reference 6 for an example of complex VF activation in the rabbit.) Panel A shows the downward progress of the last wave front to activate the recording area before delivery of a shock. This wave front was broad and coherent and could be expected to leave behind a similarly organized pattern of myocardial recovery. Panel B shows that the next sequence of activation began with the appearance of another wave front at the top of the map. This too propagated in a downward direction and, had the shock not been applied, would have probably completed activation of the recording area much as the prior wave front. However, coincident with the delivery of a shock at 0 ms, a broad area of isochronous activation (10-ms isochrone) is registered a third of the way down from the top of the map. Conduction was blocked along the right portion of the 10-ms isochrone but it continued in an initially downward direction along its left portion. Activation of the remainder of the recording area was completed by a rightward pivot of this downwardly moving wave front. The sample optical recordings in panel C indicate that the broad area of activation inside the 10-ms isochrone was due to the depolarizing actions of the shock. The downward progression of the preshock activation wave depicted in panel A is reflected in the latency of the preshock upstrokes labeled -70 to -44 ms in traces a through e. Because of the entry of the second wave front depicted in panel B, the upstroke at site a was already under way at -4 ms at the time of the shock. Sites b and c show simultaneous commencement of depolarization coincident with the application of the shock. Whereas in the preceding beat there was a latency in upstroke generation times, the simultaneous onset of depolarization at time 0 indicates that depolarization in and around isochrone 10 was elicited by the shock. Propagated activation resumes after the depolarizing actions of the shock as is evidenced by the latency in upstroke generation at sites d and e in subsequent isochrones. In summary, the events depicted in panel B can be described as instances wherein the shock pre-excited myocardium that was about to be depolarized by the preshock wave front. On the left side of the recording area this shock-induced depolarization continued propagation, i.e., activity was effectively "reset" forward in space. On the right side, by contrast, the depolarization remained stationary, i.e., it was blocked.

Based on this result and on many similar to it, it became apparent that postshock electrical activity did not arise from continuations of preshock wave fronts but rather from areas of depolarization evoked by the shock itself. This assumption neglects instances of trivial shock strengths too small to evoke depolarization. If the goal of a defibrillation shock is to eliminate postshock propagating activity, then the process should not be couched in terms of terminating existing wave fronts but should instead be in terms of preventing postshock wave fronts. If a wave front is identified as the leading edge of regenerative depolarization, then any shock that pre-excites myocardium in advance of a preshock wave front effectively terminates that wave front since regenerative activity mediated by that wave front ceases. However, propagating activity does not end with elimination of the preshock wave fronts but instead may be continued by wave fronts that arise at the leading edges of depolarization evoked by the shock.

At this point in the description of the experimental data, it is important to address a potentially confusing usage of the term "depolarization" in relation to the effects of a shock. As in our prior publications, the membrane effects of shocks are described as shock-induced depolarizations. However, this must not be taken to mean a literal elevation of the membrane potential due to the outward flow of current across the membrane.

Rather, depolarization here is used to connote excitation of the membrane, i.e., stimulation, a process in which the shock ultimately evokes a regenerative depolarizing response due to the ionic processes at work in the cellular membrane. Accordingly, even a shock that initially hyperpolarizes the myocardium before subsequently exciting a depolarizing response would be said to have caused shock-induced depolarization. It is extremely important to keep this distinction in mind because other investigators have described distinct roles for the explicit depolarization and hyperpolarization of separate areas of the ventricle that occur during the shock.[40] In the phenomena described in our studies,[5,6,17,34] the predominant effect of a shock was to induce a depolarizing response. While hyperpolarizing responses were observed, they usually occurred prior to ultimate regenerative membrane depolarization.

In order to understand the interactions between shocks and fibrillation wave fronts, it is useful to consider the process analogous to the resetting or circus movement reentry by a shock. Figure 6 illustrates such an analogy by depicting in panel A the reentry of an impulse in an anatomically defined circuit. Lying between the advancing depolarizing "head" of the wave front and its receding repolarizing "tail" is a stretch of myocardium not yet activated by it, the "excitable gap." An excitable gap, whether comprising myocardium that is partially or wholly excitable, is considered necessary for the maintenance of reentry since wave front head

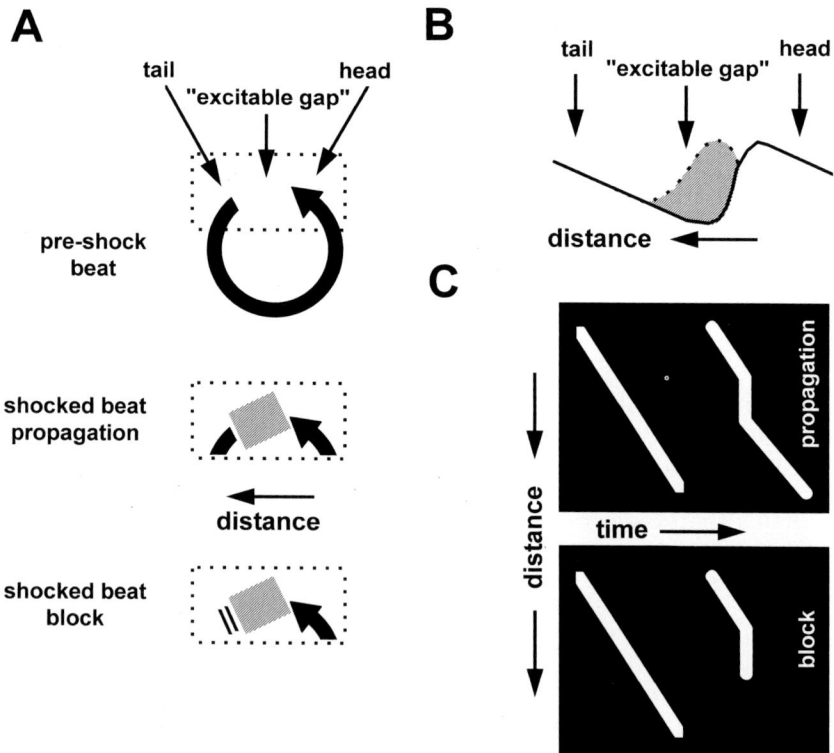

Figure 6. Schematic illustration of excitable gap-shock interactions.

would be unable to perpetuate itself through regenerative depolarization. There is evidence that not only do reentrant tachycardias possess an excitable gap[41] but that atrial fibrillation[42] and VF[43] do as well. The situation depicted at the top of panel A could be considered similar to those of a preshock fibrillation wave front. Application of a shock depolarizes myocardium (shading) in an area extending from the head of the wave front up to some point along the trailing wake of repolarization. Wave front propagation could then continue from the leading (left) edge of the shock-depolarized area (middle drawing) or it could remain stationary, i.e., blocked (bottom drawing). Panel B illustrates a hypothetical membrane voltage profile through the reentrant circuit before and immediately after the shock. The repolarizing wake of the wave front tail is represented by the negative sloping membrane voltage profile. The oncoming wave of depolarization causes a spatially abrupt increase in membrane potential. The excitable myocardium lies in the valley of membrane potential between the head and tail. Upon application of a shock, the membrane potential profile of this section is elevated through excitation by the shock. The level of shock-induced depolarization tapers off in the direction of the repolarizing tail as a result of the decreased ability of the shock to excite progressively less repolarized myocardium. Postshock wave front propagation could then arise at this leading (left) edge of the zone of shock-induced depolarization.

Panel C of Figure 6 illustrates the hypothetical process of VF wave front reset by a shock by using a modified time-space plot[44] of the membrane potential along a line projected across the ventricle. It is constructed by converting the membrane voltage profile illustrated in panel B into image intensity, i.e., a grayscale in which maximally depolarized myocardium is white and fully repolarized myocardium is black. A series of such shaded lines are then stacked next to each other in time sequence. The counterclockwise movement of the impulse in panel A is depicted as a downward movement of the depolarization front. For simplicity, no gray levels are shown in this example—only white for the peak of the action potential wave front. In both parts of panel C the preshock wave front sweeps out a rightward sloping diagonal from left to right and top to bottom. Entry of preshock wave front at the top of the image commences the next round of reentrant excitation. The shock depolarizes the myocardium ahead of the wave front and is depicted in the time-space plot as the vertical, downward segment. The success or failure of propagation away from the shock-depolarized area will give rise to two different patterns on the time-space plot. In the upper plot a wave front continued away from the vertical segment depicting the shock-depolarized zone. In the bottom plot propagation failed, i.e., was blocked, and so the vertical segment ended. In this case the shock terminated reentry because the shock-induced depolarization was somehow prevented from propagating. In the upper plot reentry continued after the shock, since a new wave front immediately commenced propagation around the circuit, i.e., a postshock wave front was not prevented. In both cases the preshock wave front was effectively terminated since it could no longer excite the myocardium ahead of it due to its premature activation by the shock. Therefore, it is most useful to describe shock outcome in terms of the ability of the shock-induced depolarization to propagate rather than as a description of the fate of the preshock wave front.

Figure 7 illustrates the effects of a shock on a fibrillation wave front by using the time-space plot approach shown in Figure 6. Panel A reproduces the isochronal map of activation immediately preceding and following application of the shock shown in Figure 5. Panel B is a grayscale image of the "optical membrane potential" distribution in this same area 1 ms before the shock was delivered. A bilinear interpolation was performed to estimate the optical membrane voltages at points between the measurement sites.[45] The resulting data were then converted to a grayscale image calibrated on the basis of the transition from fully repolarized (black) to fully depolarized (white) myocardium seen in the stimulated beat following defibrillation. This image shows that the depolarizing head of the incoming wave front had advanced to the position of the 0-ms isochrone in panel A. It also shows the trailing tail of repolarization due to the downward propagation of the preceding VF wave front whose movement was illustrated in panel A of Figure 5. Lying between these features is a zone of relatively repolarized myocardium, which is denoted as the excitable gap. The optical recordings in Figure 5 show that the myocardium in this area did not fully recover to the level of the resting potential. This was almost always the case for all recordings during fibrillation. The optical membrane potential profile in the direction of preshock wave front propagation was sampled along the two lines indicated by the white dashes. The left line runs through the section of the recording area where propagating activity continued after the shock. The right line samples the section in which postshock propagation

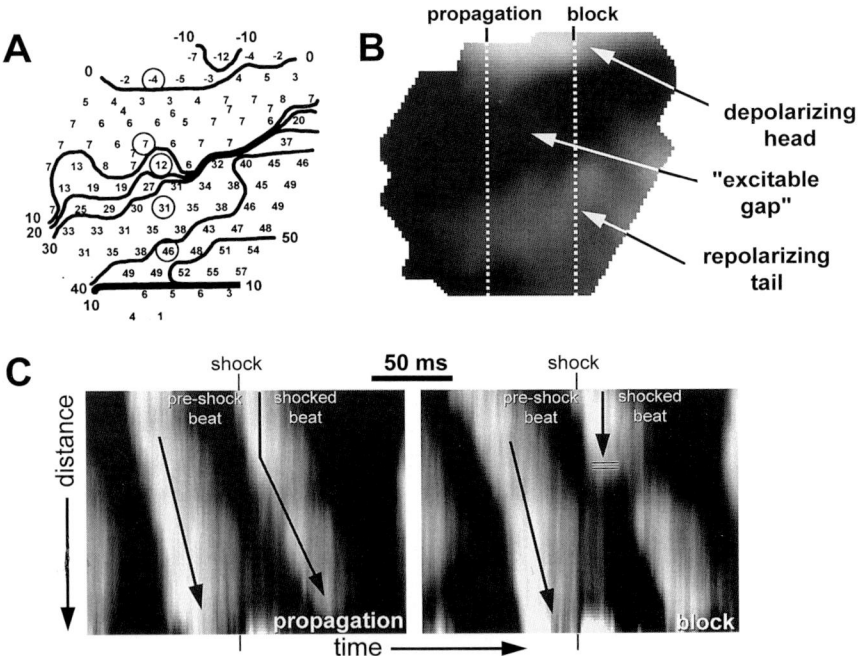

Figure 7. Space-time diagram of ventricular fibrillation wave front reset.

was blocked. The two time-space plots shown in panel C were then created using the potential distributions along these lines as a function of time.

In both images of panel C, conduction of the preshock wave front is indicated by the downward sloping, left-to-right track of depolarized myocardium. This pattern reflects the path of the preshock wave front depicted in panel A of Figure 5. The next wave front had just entered the top of the recording area immediately before the shock, as indicated by the short extent of depolarization down from the top of both plots. With application of the shock, this zone of depolarization extended straight downward in both images as a consequence of the shock stimulating the myocardium ahead of the wave front. Subsequent conduction differed because in the left plot the zone of depolarization continued its downward extension along a track parallel to the preshock wave front. Note that there was no interruption in propagation after the shock in this part of the recording area. The right plot shows that no conduction ensued from the leading edge of the downward segment elicited by the shock. Postshock depolarization reappeared in the right plot only after a delay (dashed arrow). Examination of the isochronal map in panel B of Figure 5 indicates that this later depolarization was due to conduction from the left side of the map where the shock-induced depolarization continued propagation. The depolarization patterns depicted in panel C of Figure 5 match those which would be expected to occur in a hypothetical instance of reentrant excitation reset by a shock as illustrated in Figure 6. Therefore, with the limitations that are discussed later in this chapter, it is useful to envision the interaction between a shock and VF wave fronts in terms of resetting process. Therefore, in order to eliminate VF wave fronts, the shock must reset them in a way as to prevent their continued propagation, such as in the right plot of panel C.

Figure 8 illustrates the hypothetical outcomes of the VF wave front reset process in response to shocks of increasing strength. Hypothetical membrane voltage profiles that would exist before and after shocks of increasing voltage, $V_3 > V_2 > V_1$, are shown in panel A. The shaded areas represent the area of myocardium between the advancing head of one VF wave front and the receding tail of another that is depolarized by the shock. The membrane voltage (V_m) at the leading edge of the shock-depolarized areas is denoted by $Vm_1 > Vm_2 > Vm_3$ (increasing less negative potentials). These are the potentials prevailing at the time of shock application, and they are drawn here to indicate an increasing level of depolarization with increasing shock strength. In each of the drawings, the membrane potential level corresponding to the onset of the effective refractory period (ERP) is indicated by Vm_{ERP}. Normally, the ERP denotes the longest coupling interval at which a premature stimulus of any amplitude is not able to evoke a propagating stimulus. In this context the Vm_{ERP} represents the most repolarized potential at which depolarization of the membrane, whatever its origin, is not able to evoke a propagating response. If the leading edge of depolarization is pushed sufficiently high up along the repolarizing tail of the preceding impulse, it will border myocardium whose excitability due to sodium channel inactivation is sufficiently reduced so as to be unable to support continued regenerative depolarizing activity, i.e., conduct an impulse. Thus, the shock-induced depolarizations evoked

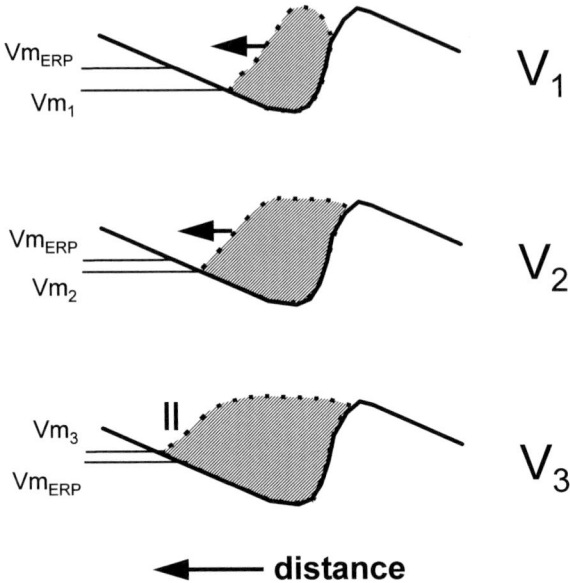

Figure 8. Schematic illustration of the excitable gap excitation.

by shocks of strengths V_1 and V_2 might still be able to propagate because the membrane voltage at the leading edge of the shock-depolarized area is more negative than the Vm_{ERP}. However, shock V_3 pushes the leading edge of depolarization into the zone of effective refractoriness and so it will not evoke a propagated depolarization. Therefore, even though sufficiently strong shocks are able to depolarize myocardium at almost any point during the action potential, propagated depolarization could only occur if the leading edge of depolarization is more negative than the membrane voltage corresponding to the onset of that which is the equivalent of the ERP for shock-induced depolarizations. The resetting analogy therefore predicts that the incidence of postshock propagation will fall to zero when the membrane voltage at the leading edge of the shock-depolarized area exceeds a certain value.

The above prediction was verified for test shocks applied to a fibrillating rabbit heart.[6] Figure 9 plots the incidence of postshock propagation away from the leading edge of the shock-depolarized area against the optical membrane potential prevailing there at the time of the shock. The optical V_m is given as the percentage of the full action potential amplitude (APA) of the postdefibrillation stimulated beat. A 0% V_m corresponds to resting potential and 100% to the control action potential amplitude. The filled circles plot the propagation incidence following test shocks of various voltages and the unfilled circles plot the propagation incidence of free-running VF action potentials. The latter data were obtained by analyzing the optical action potentials at one VF cycle length prior to the shock. The optical recordings and activation maps were analyzed as if a shock had occurred, a sham shock, at this fixed but arbitrary time. Both of these plots show that the likelihood of postshock wave front propagation is maximal when the leading edge of the depolarized area arises in the low end of the

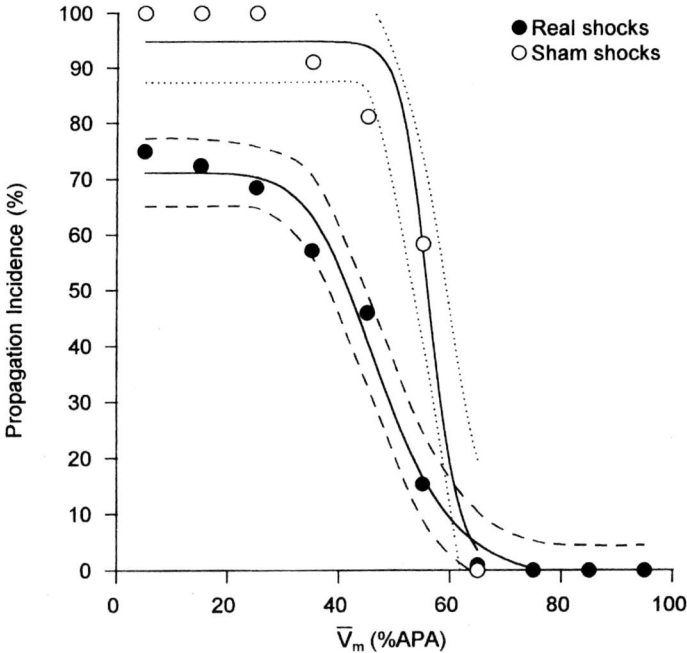

Figure 9. Plot of propagation incidence for shocked and unshocked ventricular fibrillation wave fronts. Reprinted from reference 6, with permission.

range of membrane potentials. Note that here the shock-evoked depolarizations are overall less likely to propagate. In this model the nascent shock-induced wave front would be adjacent to the least refractory and therefore most excitable regions of myocardium present during VF. Also, both curves show a steep decrease in propagation incidence as the leading edge of the area of shock-induced depolarization is pushed up into higher potentials. This is consistent with an increasing refractoriness and therefore decreasing excitability of the myocardium into which the shock-induced depolarization could propagate. At a certain point, here at 65% APA, the propagation incidence of both free-running VF wave fronts and those induced by a shock effectively disappears. In terms of the model, this value represents the onset of effective refractoriness of the fibrillating myocardium, Vm_{ERP}. The fact that Vm_{ERP} represents an upper limit on conduction for the sham shock as well as the real shock data points suggests the operation of a more general electrophysiological phenomenon rather than one particular to depolarizations evoked by shocks. That there were no data points for sham shocks above the Vm_{ERP} can be seen to reflect the reentrant nature of fibrillation since depolarizations could only arise as a result of wave front propagation. The Vm_{ERP} therefore represents the upper limit of membrane potential for which the myocardium is able to support regenerative depolarizations during VF. By contrast, the plot for real shocks shows data points for membrane voltages in excess of Vm_{ERP}. This is consistent with the phenomenon we first demonstrated,[5] that sufficiently strong shocks are able to evoke depolarizing responses from myocardium during nearly the entire duration of the action potential save just after upstroke generation. Therefore, while a shock is able to evoke depolarizing responses in membranes residing at potentials in excess of Vm_{ERP}, this depolarization could not propagate beyond the shock-depolarized region because the adjoining myocardium was unable to support regenerative sodium channel activation. To explain the ability of shocks to depolarize refractory myocardium it was hypothesized[5] that they evoke bipolar membrane voltage responses through microscale[46] or macroscale[47] virtual electrode effects. The excitability of inactivated sodium channels could be restored in the membranes hyperpolarized by the shock, and these membranes were subsequently excited by currents from the membranes depolarized by the shock.

Relationship of VF Wave Front Reset to Defibrillation

Given that VF is generally regarded as a reentrant process, it is clear that defibrillation must bring about the immediate or eventual cessation of propagating wave fronts. This is true whether one considers the critical mass[12,13] or our own progressive depolarization[14] hypotheses for defibrillation, in which defibrillation is thought to occur when all or most of the wave fronts are terminated. It is also true in the case of the upper limit of vulnerability[18] hypothesis but with a significant difference. In this hypothesis the shock must first halt all wave fronts in order to defibrillate, but more importantly it must fail to reinitiate VF. In both schemes the shock must first stop all propagating activity. What we describe here is an indication of how this process is most properly viewed. In stopping propagation, the emphasis is not on stopping the existing VF wave fronts but rather on preventing the shock from launching new ones. The data obtained by our laser scanning system indicate that a loose analogy may be drawn between the process of resetting a reentrant wave front and the interaction between shocks and fibrillating ventricle. A single reentrant circuit in the form of a spiral wave[48] or a leading circle[49] has been hypothesized to be able to effectively maintain fibrillation. In general, however, VF does not have to consist of closed circuits such as that diagrammed in Figure 6. Reset in this setting therefore does not have to occur with respect to any particular wave front head or tail. The concept of reset was introduced to describe how a shock can terminate all preshock VF wave fronts without interrupting VF itself. By "resetting" VF, the shock instantaneously replaces one set of wave fronts with another. Thus, the global pattern of activation can be altered with a discrete defibrillation-pause-refibrillation scenario as envisioned by the upper limit of vulnerability hypothesis.[50] This simple concept is also applicable to explaining the ability of shocks to initiate VF when applied during the vulnerable period of a regular rhythm. Clearly, a sufficiently strong shock will not be able to evoke the propagating wave fronts that induce VF if the areas of shock-induced depolarization border effectively refractory myocardium. Less strong shocks carry the possibility of evoking propagating wave fronts, which, for a variety of reasons including the critical point reentry mechanism,[51] may break down into disorganized conduction and fibrillation. Thus, a single electrophysiological mechanism, the ability of a shock to depolarize all of the non effectively refractory myocardium in the ventricle, may explain the numeric correlation[18,52] between shock strengths that are not able to initiate VF, i.e., the upper limit of vulnerability, and those that are able to defibrillate. In both cases the shock is too strong to evoke propagating wave fronts to either initiate VF or continue it. We are encouraged to take this viewpoint by the results of another of our optical mapping studies which showed that the lower defibrillation threshold of a biphasic shock waveform relative to a comparable monophasic waveform was consistent with a greater ability of the biphasic waveform to prevent postshock wave fronts.[53] This was shown to be a result of the biphasic waveform being able to depolarize, on a volt-per-volt basis, myocardium that was more refractory than that which the monophasic shock could.

The preceding does not explain all of the important phenomena related to defibrillation. A crucial question that remains to be addressed is why, when there is propagating activity after the shock, wave fronts either continue fibrillation or spontaneously die out. Another important issue is the mechanism coupling the electrical field established by the shock to the membrane voltage change it evokes. It is likely that, given the ability of optical mapping to obtain high-resolution, shock-proof recordings of membrane potential in the heart, this method will continue to be applied to the study of defibrillation.

References

1. Prevost J-L, Battelli F. La mort par les courants electriques. (Courants alternatifs et courants continus.). *Rev Med d l Suisse Rom* 1899;19:545–574.
2. Colavita PG, Wolf P, Smith WM, et al. Determination of effects of internal countershock by direct cardiac recordings during normal rhythm. *Am J Physiol* 1986;250:H736-H740.
3. Witkowski FX, Penkoske PA, Plonsey R. Mechanism of cardiac defibrillation in open-chest dogs with unipolar DC-coupled simultaneous activation and shock potential recordings. *Circulation* 1990;82:244–260.
4. Dillon SM, Wit AL. Use of voltage sensitive dyes to investigate electrical defibrillation. *Proc IEEE Eng Med Biol* 1988;10(Pt. 1):215–216.
5. Dillon SM. Optical recordings in the rabbit heart show that defibrillation strength shocks prolong the duration of depolarization and the refractory period. *Circ Res* 1991;69:842–856.
6. Kwaku KF, Dillon SM. Shock-induced depolarization of refractory myocardium prevents wave-front propagation in defibrillation. *Circ Res* 1996;79:957–973.
7. Knisley SB, Blitchington TF, Hill BC, et al. Optical measurements of transmembrane potential changes during electrical field stimulation of ventricular cells. *Circ Res* 1993;72:255–270.
8. Knisley SB, Hill BC. Optical recordings of the effect of electrical stimulation on action potential repolarization and the induction of reentry in two-dimensional perfused rabbit epicardium. *Circulation* 1993;88(Pt. 1):2402–2414.
9. Knisley SB, Hill BC, Ideker RE. Virtual electrode effects in myocardial fibers. *Biophys J* 1994;66:719–728.
10. Dillon SM, Kwaku KF. The electrophysiological effects of defibrillation shocks. In Kroll MW, Lehmann MH (eds): *Implantable Cardioverter-Defibrillator Therapy: The Engineering-Clinical Interface.* Norwell, MA: Kluwer Academic Publishers; 1996:31–61.

11. Walcott GP, Knisley SB, Zhou X, et al. On the mechanisms of ventricular defibrillation. *Pacing Clin Electrophysiol* 1997;20:422–431.
12. Mower MM, Mirowski M, Spear JF, et al. Patterns of ventricular activity during catheter defibrillation. *Circulation* 1974;69:858–861.
13. Zipes DP, Fischer J, King RM, et al. Termination of ventricular fibrillation in dogs by depolarizing a critical amount of myocardium. *Am J Cardiol* 1975;36:37–44.
14. Dillon SM, Kwaku KF. Progressive depolarization: A unified hypothesis for defibrillation and fibrillation induction by shocks. *J Cardiovasc Electrophysiol* 1998;9:529–552.
15. Swartz JF, Jones JL, Fletcher RD. Symmetrical biphasic defibrillator waveforms enhance refractory period stimulation in the human heart. *J Am Coll Cardiol* 1991;17:335.
16. Sweeney RJ, Gill RM, Steinberg MI, et al. Ventricular refractory period extension caused by defibrillation shocks. *Circulation* 1990;82:965–972.
17. Dillon SM. Synchronized repolarization after defibrillation shocks. A possible component of the defibrillation process demonstrated by optical recordings in rabbit heart. *Circulation* 1992;85:1865–1878.
18. Chen PS, Shibata N, Dixon EG, et al. Comparison of the defibrillation threshold and the upper limit of ventricular vulnerability. *Circulation* 1986;73:1022–1028.
19. Pogwizd SM, Corr PB. Reentrant and non-reentrant mechanisms contribute to arrhythmogenesis during early myocardial ischemia: Results using three-dimensional mapping. *Circ Res* 1987;61:352–371.
20. Hill BC, Courtney KR. Design of a multi-point laser scanned optical monitor of cardiac action potential propagation: Application to microreentry in guinea pig atrium. *Ann Biomed Eng* 1987;15:567–577.
21. Salama G, Lombardi R, Elson J. Maps of optical action potentials and NADH fluorescence in intact working hearts. *Am J Physiol* 1987;252:H384-H394.
22. Rosenbaum DS, Kaplan DT, Kanai A, et al. Repolarization inhomogeneities in ventricular myocardium change dynamically with abrupt cycle length shortening. *Circulation* 1991;84:1333–1345.
23. Efimov IR, Huang DT, Rendt JM, et al. Optical mapping of repolarization and refractoriness from intact hearts. *Circulation* 1994;90:1469–1480.
24. Rohr S, Salzberg BM. Multiple site optical recording of transmembrane voltage (MSORTV) in patterned growth heart cell cultures: Assessing electrical behavior, with microsecond resolution, on a cellular and subcellular scale. *Biophys J* 1994;67:1301–1315.
25. Fast VG, Kleber AG. Microscopic conduction in cultured strands of neonatal rat heart cells measured with voltage-sensitive dyes. *Circ Res* 1993; 73:914–925.
26. Muller W, Windisch H, Tritthart HA. Fast optical monitoring of microscopic excitation patterns in cardiac muscle. *Biophys J* 1989;56:623–629.
27. Nassif GN, Dillon SM, Wit AL. Video mapping of cardiac activation. *J Mol Cell Cardiol* 1990;22(Suppl IV):S44.
28. Davidenko JM, Pertsov AM, Salomonz R, et al. Stationary and drifting spiral waves of excitation in isolated cardiac muscle. *Nature* 1992;355:349–351.
29. Wikswo JP Jr, Lin S, Abbas RA. Virtual electrodes in cardiac tissue: A common mechanism for anodal and cathodal stimulation. *Biophys J* 1995;69:2195–2210.
30. Witkowski FX, Leon LJ, Penkoske PA, et al. A method for visualization of ventricular fibrillation. *Chaos* 1998;8:942–1002.
31. Dillon S, Morad M. A new laser scanning system for measuring action potential propagation in the heart. *Science* 1981;214(4519):453–456.
32. Gupta RK, Salzberg BM, Grinvald A, et al. Improvements in optical methods for measuring rapid changes in membrane potential. *J Membr Biol* 1981; 58:123–137.

33. Bove R, Dillon SM. A new high performance system for imaging cardiac electrical activity. *Circulation* 1996;98(Suppl):I714.

34. Dillon SM, Mehra R. Prolongation of ventricular refractoriness by defibrillation shocks may be due additional depolarization of the action potential. *J Cardiovasc Electrophysiol* 1992;3:442–456.

35. Korpel A, Adler R, Desmarnes P, et al. A television display using acoustic deflection and modulation of coherent light. *IEEE Proc* 1966;54:1429–1437.

36. Dillon S, Morad M. A new optical technique for scanning action potential in the heart. *Circulation* 1981;64:IV171.

37. Girouard SD, Laurita KR, Rosenbaum DS. Unique properties of cardiac action potentials recorded with voltage-sensitive dyes. *J Cardiovasc Electrophysiol* 1996;7:1024–1038.

38. Jones JL, Swartz JF, Jones RE, et al. Increasing fibrillation duration enhances relative asymmetrical biphasic versus monophasic defibrillator waveform efficacy. *Circ Res* 1990;67:376–384.

39. Surawicz B, Gettes LS, Ponce-Zumino A. Relation of vulnerability to ECG and action potential characteristics of premature beats. *Am J Physiol* 1967; 212:1519–1528.

40. Efimov IR, Cheung Y, Van Wagoner DR, et al. Virtual electrode-induced phase singularity. A basic mechanism for defibrillation failure. *Circ Res* 1998; 82:918–925.

41. Girouard SD, Pastore JM, Laurita KR, et al. Optical mapping in a new guinea pig model of ventricular tachycardia reveals mechanisms for multiple wavelengths in a single reentrant circuit. *Circulation* 1996;93:603–613.

42. Kirchhof C, Chorro F, Scheffer GJ, et al. Regional entrainment of atrial fibrillation studied by high-resolution mapping in open-chest dogs. *Circulation* 1993;88:736–749.

43. Kenknight BH, Bayly PV, Gerstle RJ, et al. Regional capture of fibrillating ventricular myocardium. Evidence of an excitable gap. *Circ Res* 1995;77:849–855.

44. Pertsov AM, Davidenko JM, Salomonsz R, et al. Spiral waves of excitation underlie reentrant activity in isolated cardiac muscle. *Circ Res* 1993;72:631–650.

45. Pruente HM, Bove R, Kwaku KF, et al. Animated images of cardiac membrane voltage during defibrillation. *J Electrocardiol* 1995;28(Suppl):7–15.

46. Gillis AM, Fast VG, Rohr S, et al. Spatial changes in transmembrane potential during extracellular electrical shocks in cultured monolayers of neonatal rat ventricular myocytes. *Circ Res* 1996;79:676–690.

47. White JB, Walcott GP, Pollard AE, et al. Myocardial discontinuities. A substrate for producing virtual electrodes that directly excite the myocardium by shocks. *Circulation* 1998;97:1738–1745.

48. Gray RA, Jalife J, Panfilov AV, et al. Mechanisms of cardiac fibrillation. *Science* 1995;270:1222–1223.

49. Janse MJ, Wilms-Schopman FJ, Coronel R. Ventricular fibrillation is not always due to multiple wavelet reentry. *J Cardiovasc Electrophysiol* 1995;6:512–521.

50. Chen PS, Shibata N, Dixon EG, et al. Activation during ventricular defibrillation in open-chest dogs. Evidence of complete cessation and regeneration of ventricular fibrillation after unsuccessful shocks. *J Clin Invest* 1986;77:810–823.

51. Frazier DW, Wolf PD, Wharton JM, et al. Stimulus-induced critical point. Mechanism for electrical initiation of reentry in normal canine myocardium. *J Clin Invest* 1989;83:1039–1052.

52. Fabiato A, Coumel P, Gourgon R, et al. Le seuil de reponse synchrone des fibres myocardiques. Application a la comparison experimentale de l'efficacite des differentes formes de chocs electriques de defibrillation. *Arch Mal Coeur* 1967;60:527–544.

53. Kwaku KF. *On The Mechanism of Cardiac Defibrillation: Optical Mapping of*

Chapter 22

Mechanisms of Defibrillation:

3. Virtual Electrode-Induced Wave Fronts and Phase Singularities; Mechanisms of Success and Failure of Internal Defibrillation

Igor R. Efimov and Yuanna Cheng

Introduction

Delivery of a strong electrical shock to the heart remains the only effective therapy against ventricular fibrillation (VF). It has been more than a century since the first evidence was presented that a strong electrical shock can stop VF in dogs.[1] Fifty years after this was demonstrated in animals, the same effect was observed in humans in an open-chest[2] and transthoracic[3] defibrillation. In 1970, the idea of an automatic implantable cardioverter-defibrillator (ICD) was proposed.[4,5] The recent clinical success of the ICD has been driven primarily by purely empirical studies. Despite significant research efforts, the basic mechanisms of defibrillation are not fully understood. Systematic investigation of the effects of strong electrical shocks on the heart has been difficult, mostly due to the presence of shock-induced artifacts in any recordings obtained with conventional (electrical) electrophysiological recording techniques. These artifacts make it impossible to record during defibrillation shocks and for periods of up to tens of milliseconds after the shock. Therefore, most of our knowledge of events occurring during and immediately after defibrillation shocks has been based on indirect evidence. The recent application of fluorescent methods using voltage-sensitive dyes in the area of cardiac electrophysiology has finally delivered a technique capable of recording transmembrane voltage changes during shocks that are free of electrical artifacts. These recordings can be obtained from a single site,[6] from several sites,[7] and from several hundred recording sites simultaneously with nearly microelectrode quality.[8,9]

Application of the voltage-sensitive dye techniques has permitted us to map, for the first time, transmembrane polarization during and immediately after defibrillation shocks with a high temporal (350 to 1000 μs)

From Rosenbaum DS, Jalife J (eds): *Optical Mapping of Cardiac Excitation and Arrhythmias.* ©Futura Publishing Co., Inc., Armonk, NY, 2001.

and spatial (275 to 1000 μm) resolution, and also to directly relate the electrical activity produced by the shocks with mechanisms of defibrillation.

In this chapter we present experimental evidence, obtained using voltage-sensitive dye techniques, of the following:

1. Monophasic shocks produce complex spatiotemporal transmembrane polarization responses with large areas of positive and negative polarization present simultaneously, which are referred to as virtual electrode polarization (VEP).
2. A second phase of biphasic shocks nonlinearly reverses VEP produced by the first phase, with less energy required to reverse negative polarization compared with positive polarization.
3. Optimal biphasic defibrillation waveforms produce most homogeneous polarization with no VEP.
4. VEPs are strongly influenced by electrical and structural characteristics of myocardium and interface between heart and elements of the tissue bath.
5. A sharp VEP gradient between positively and negatively polarized areas may result in new propagated activation wave fronts regardless of preshock electrical activity.
6. VEP may produce virtual electrode-induced phase singularities (VEIPS; i.e., points of intersection of areas of positive, negative, and no polarization), which may result in induction of reentrant arrhythmias and in failure to defibrillate.

Methods

Experimental Model of Defibrillation

Langendorff-perfused rabbit hearts are one of the most popular in vitro models of defibrillation. This model was used in this study. Detailed protocols have been previously published[8–10] and are only briefly described in this chapter. The intact heart stained with di-4-ANEPPS (Molecular Probes Inc., Eugene, OR) was perfused via the aorta and kept in a temperature-controlled bath containing 15 mmol/L 2,3-butanedione monoxime, diacetyl monoxime (BDM; Fisher Scientific Co., Pittsburgh, PA) to remove motion artifacts. We have recently demonstrated that, unlike in canine, guinea pig, or sheep heart, in rabbit BDM does not significantly affect action potential duration (APD) and conducting properties at this concentration.[11] While we recognize that BDM interacts with a number of ionic channels and may influence the electrophysiological response to electrical shocks, there are few alternatives with their own even more significant side effects in this model. We have therefore concluded that the benefits associated with the judicious use of BDM greatly exceed the drawbacks.

Numerous theoretical studies have predicted that geometry is one of the most important factors modulating shock-induced electrical fields. We have taken great care in trying to reproduce the geometry of the human thorax and the position of the defibrillation electrodes in it. Figure 1 shows the front and top views of the experimental chamber and two positions of a pair of

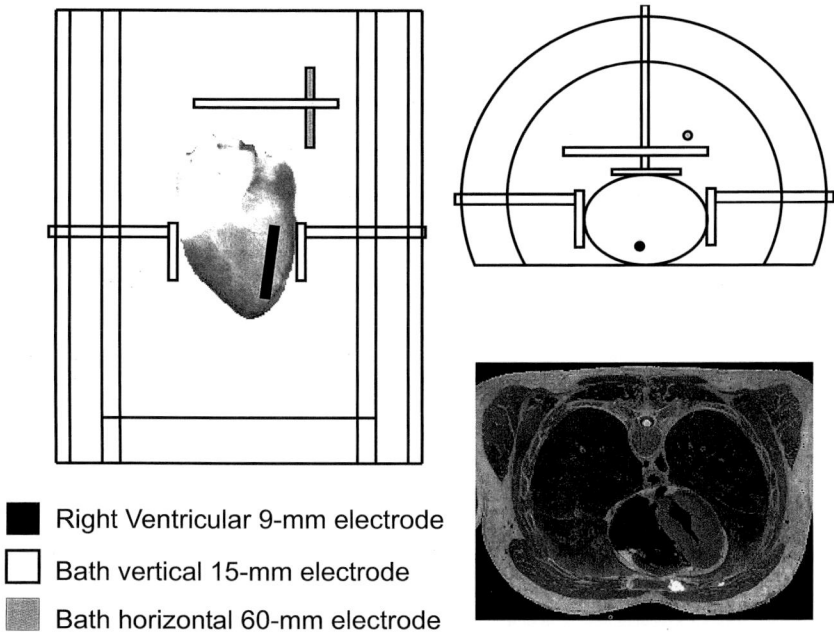

Figure 1. Experimental chamber design and its relation to the anatomy of the human thorax. Experiments were conducted using a Langendorff-perfused rabbit heart. The heart, tissue chamber, and defibrillation electrodes reproduced major geometrical characteristics of the human thorax. At left is the anterior view of the heart and the chamber, as it is viewed by the photodiode array. At the top right is the top superior view. At the bottom right is a cryosection of the human thorax. Reproduced with permission from the Visible Human Project, Multimedia Medical Systems. See text for details.

defibrillation electrodes. The chamber had a water jacket to maintain constant temperature ($36\pm1°C$). The water jacket surrounded the bath everywhere except in the front. This was done in order to simplify access of the optical apparatus to the anterior aspect of the heart. The heart was then confined between the glass wall and the three plastic pads. Isolating electrical properties of these materials simulated high impedance of the interface between the heart muscle and such elements of thorax as fat, lungs, and bones.

Stimulation Protocol

The heart was stimulated by a bipolar electrode, sutured to the apex of the left ventricle, with a basic cycle length of 300 ms. Shocks were delivered during different phases of the ventricular action potential by a clinical defibrillator (HVS-02, Ventritex, Sunnyvale, CA) between the two coil electrodes. Two sets of electrodes were used in this study (see in Fig. 1 for positions): 1) a set made from a clinical dual-coil lead (4007L, Angeion, Minneapolis, MN): one 9-mm coil inside of the right ventricle and another 6-cm coil floating horizontally above the heart in the perfusate; and 2) custom-made 15-mm platinum electrodes (Guidant, St. Paul, MN). Different shock waveforms were used (see Fig. 2): in each, the first phase (truncated

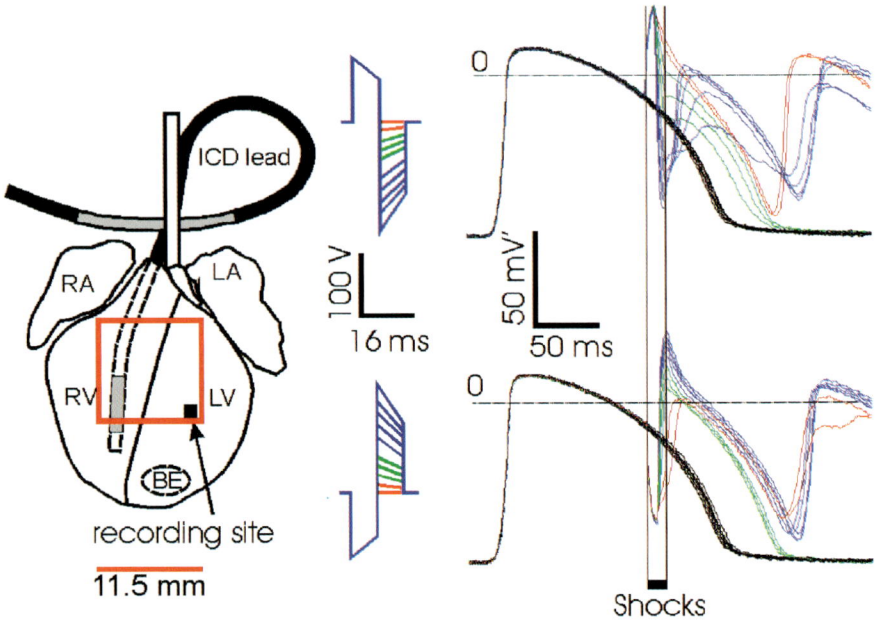

Figure 2. Superimposed optical recordings from a single site during basic beats and 20 different biphasic and monophasic shocks. Langendorff-perfused rabbit hearts were paced at a basic cycle length of 300 ms with a bipolar electrode (BE) sutured to the apex of the left ventricle (LV). Biphasic shocks of different polarity were applied during the plateau phase of an action potential. Shock waveforms are shown in the middle upper (anodal) and lower (cathodal) panels. The first phase of each shock was 100 V in amplitude, while the second phase was varied in the range from 0 V to 200 V. At top right and bottom right are 10 superimposed recordings during the last basic beat, and 10 recordings during the application of shocks. The timing of the 16-ms shock application is shown with a black bar and two vertical lines. Transmembrane voltage was calibrated based on the assumption of a 100-mV control action potential amplitude and a -85-mV resting potential. A single recording site out of 256 (red square) is shown by the solid black square. Reproduced, with permission, from refer-

exponential waveform) had a leading edge voltage of 100 V, while the leading edge voltage of the second phase was always of the opposite polarity and varied from 0 to 200 V. The duration of each phase was 8 ms. Just more than half of the shocks (55.4%, 112/202) resulted in extra beats, ventricular tachycardias, and/or VF. Sustained episodes of VF were defibrillated with either monophasic or biphasic shocks. Both successful (n = 12) and failed (n = 19) defibrillation shocks were analyzed. The timing of shock delivery was set as previously described[8]: a mean activation time was defined in the field of view during basic cycle length activation, then the S1-S2 coupling interval for the shock application was set to occur at a required time delay from the mean activation time.

Data Acquisition, Processing, and Visualization

The field of view of the imaging system could be easily readjusted from 3×3 to 25×25 mm. Fluorescence was excited by a semi-monochromatic light source (520±45 nm) and collected above 610 nm by a 16×16 photo-diode array (C4675, Hamamatsu Photonics Corp., Bridgewater, NJ). Optical signals were amplified, filtered at 1 kHz, and sampled at a rate of 2 kHz with 12-bit resolution. Figure 3 shows an example of 256 basic beat recordings superimposed with 256 optical recordings obtained during a biphasic shock applied at a 100-ms coupling interval after the onset of the action potential. Near-microelectrode quality optical recordings (peak-to-peak signal-to-noise [S/N] ratio 49±13, mean±SD; n = 25 hearts ×256 recordings) were accompanied by conventional electrocardiograms and aortic pressure recordings, and the pacing and shock hardware triggers. These signals were acquired for documentation and off-line signal analysis. S/N ratios decreased during the experiment because of dye washout and/or internalization. The kinetics of the decay of the S/N ratios were measured using a single exponential fit. The time constant of this decay was 76±16 minutes (n = 5 hearts), as summarized in Figure 4.

Data processing included several previously described computer algorithms implemented in the software, developed by Igor Efimov, based on the LabVIEW environment (National Instruments, Austin, TX). These algorithms automatically calculated activation,[12] repolarization,[13] and shock-induced polarization[8] maps which were displayed as grayscale

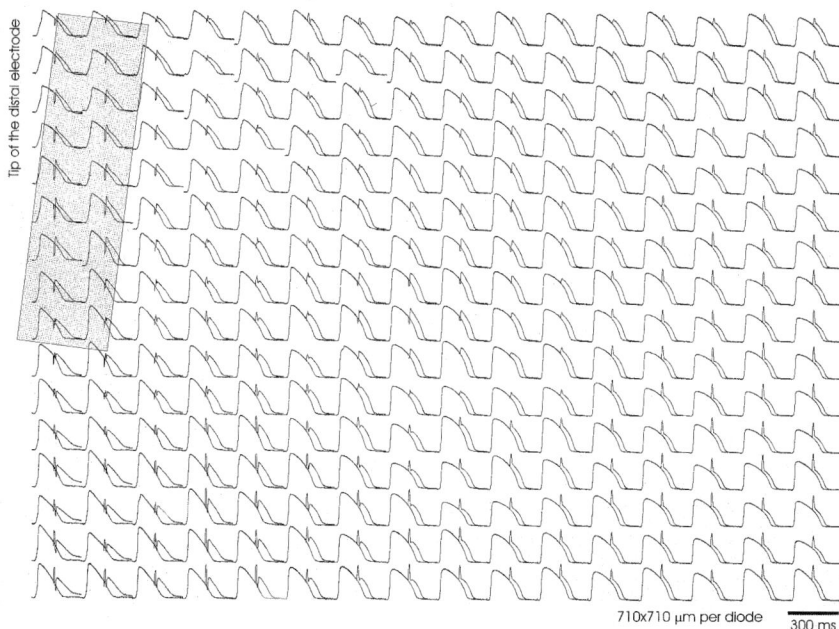

710x710 μm per diode   300 ms

Figure 3. Maps of optical recordings. Two superimposed maps of 256 optical action potentials recorded from the anterior ventricular epicardium during normal rhythm and during application of a truncated exponential biphasic shock (+100/−50 V, 8/8 ms, 200-μs delay between phases, 150-μF capacitor). The average signal-to-noise ratio of this recording was 47±15 (mean±SD; n = 256). Optical recordings were obtained from the 11.5×11.5-mm area of epicardium. Each signal was recorded from an area of 710×710 μm. The shaded box indicates the position of the distal defibrillation electrode. Reproduced, with permission, from reference 9.

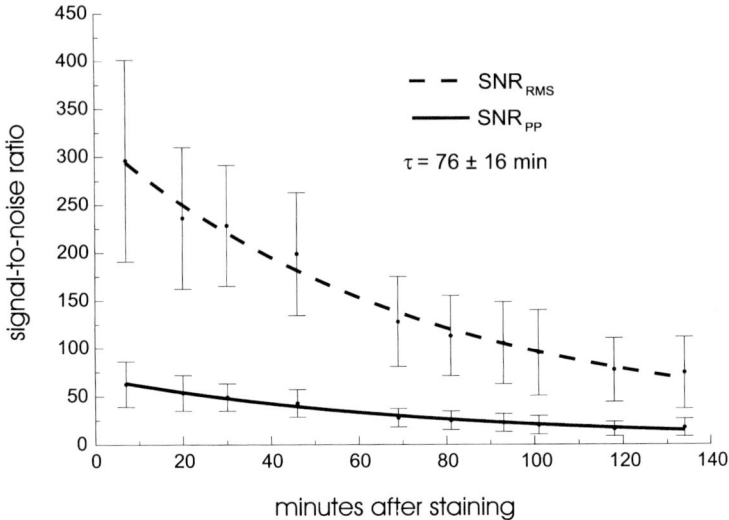

Figure 4. Decay of the signal-to-noise ratio (SNR) during experiment.

plots. Final publication-quality color contour plots were produced using Origin 5.0 graphing software (Microcal Software, Northampton, MA) and LabVIEW-generated data.

Activation maps were reconstructed using a $-(dF/dt)_{max}$ algorithm.[12] This algorithm finds the maximum of the first derivative of the inverted fluorescence intensity ($-dF/dt$). The time of the maximum $-(dF/dt)_{max}$ was considered as the activation time point at the recording site from which the signal was acquired. Repolarization was calculated from the second derivative of the inverted fluorescent signal intensity, and locating the local maximum peak $-(d^2F/dt^2)_{max}$, which corresponds to the repolarization time point at the recording site.[13] Shock-induced polarization was calculated by subtracting signals recorded during the last basic beat action potentials from the signals acquired during the shock application.[8] Since the fluorescent signal cannot be absolutely calibrated with respect to the mV value of transmembrane voltage, we used a pseudo-mV calibration (mV'), based on the assumption that the normal action potential recorded from every site has a 100-mV amplitude and a -85-mV resting potential.

Results

Real and Virtual Electrodes Produce Heterogeneous Polarization Pattern during Defibrillation Shock

Epicardial polarization patterns were first investigated in the simplest model of internal defibrillation. In this model monophasic shocks were delivered at the right ventricular free wall endocardium during the plateau phase of an action potential produced by pacing. Figure 5 demonstrates snapshots of the polarization pattern produced by an anodal 10-ms/+100-V truncated exponential shock. Polarization was recorded from an 11×11-mm

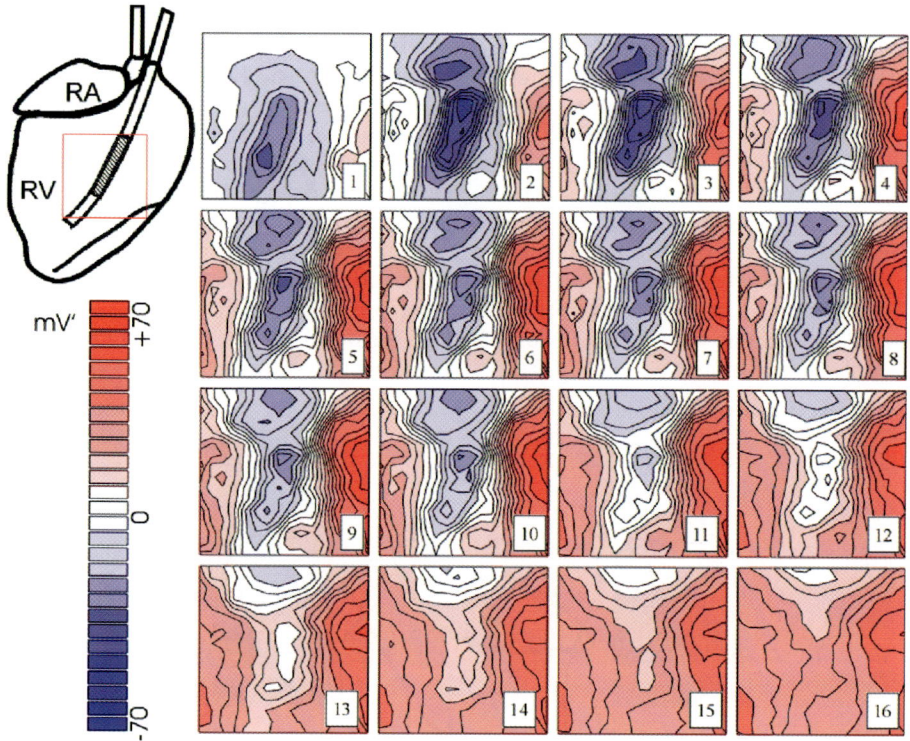

Figure 5. Dynamics of polarization produced by real and virtual electrodes during anodal monophasic shock. The location of the electrode is shown at the top left of the figure. Sixteen successive frames are shown. The time between frames is 1.056 ms. Contour maps represent the distribution of transmembrane voltage changes with respect to the value of the normal action potential at the same phase in the response induced by the electrical shock. Lines are drawn with 10-mV' steps, where 100 mV' is the assumed amplitude of the normal action potential preceding the action potential interrupted by the shock. Blue areas represent negative polarization produced by the real electrode (anode in this example), red areas represent positive polarization produced by the virtual electrodes (virtual cathodes in this example). Each frame was recorded from an 11×11-mm area of right ventricular epicardium. The first 10 frames were recorded during a 10-ms shock, the remaining six maps were recorded after the shock withdrawal. Reproduced, with permission, from reference 8.

area of the right ventricular epicardium. Polarization maps are shown starting from the onset of the shock. The last six maps show polarization after the shock withdrawal. The field of view was chosen immediately against defibrillation electrode (see red box in the upper left diagram). As seen from the picture, the first-millisecond frame shows the formation of a relatively large central area of negative polarization, occupying almost the entire field of view. During the second millisecond, this negative polarization reaches its maximum in amplitude but decreases slightly in area. At the same time the formation of virtual cathodes was observed: areas to the right and to the left of the area of real electrode-induced negative polarization were positively polarized such that two cathodes were present next to these areas. Since these cathodes were not real, we called these areas of polarizations areas of virtual electrodes, or cathodes in this case. In contrast, the central area of negative polarization was called the area of real electrode (anode in this case). In frames 3 to 10, the spatial pattern does not show any significant changes except a slight further reduction in the amplitude of negative polarization, which appeared to follow the exponential discharge of the capacitor in the defibrillator. Following the completion of an electrical shock at the 11th millisecond, the area of negative polarization rapidly decreased in size and amplitude, while areas of virtual cathodes expanded, bringing depolarization to almost the entire area by the 16th millisecond. Depolarization of the entire field of view was observed at the 18th millisecond (not shown).

Differences between the responses produced by anodal and cathodal shocks are illustrated in Figure 6. Shocks of both polarities produced a

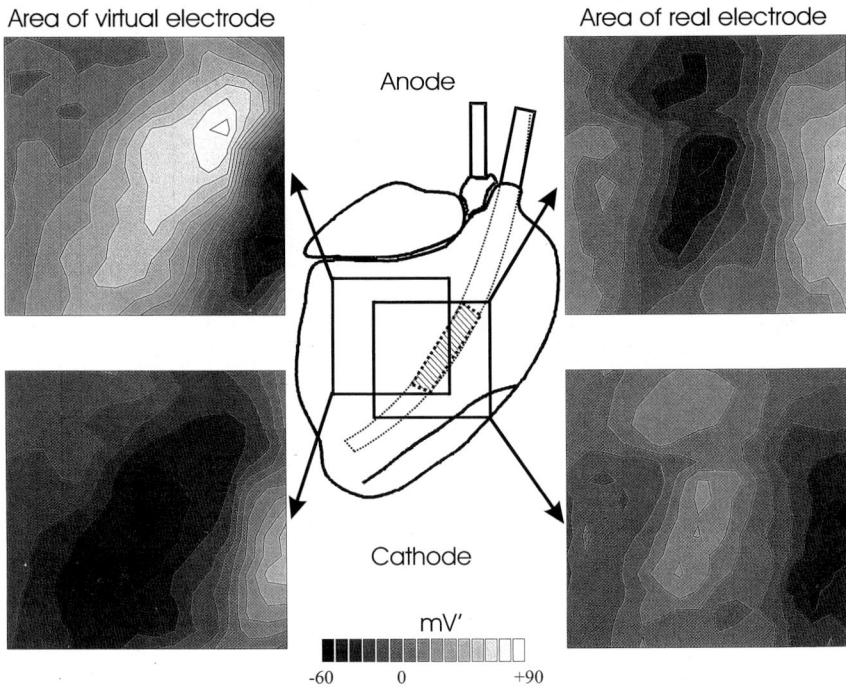

Figure 6. Areas of real and virtual electrodes. Spatial distributions of amplitudes of responses at the third millisecond of anodal and cathodal 10-ms shocks are shown. The changes in the amplitudes were measured as a signal change in each recording site relative to the action potentials recorded before the shocks, and are expressed in percentages relative to the action potential amplitudes (see text for details). Using these values, contour maps were built with 10-mV' steps between the isolevel lines. Dark areas represent negative polarization, light areas represent positive polarization. Areas of recordings are shown on the middle diagram. At the top and bottom right are areas of the real electrode produced by 100-V anodal and cathodal shocks, respectively. At the top and bottom left are areas of virtual electrodes induced by 50-V anodal and cathodal shocks, respectively. The upper left panel represents a virtual cathode, while the lower left panel shows polarization in an area of virtual anode. Reproduced, with permission, from reference 8.

real-electrode polarization area immediately against the electrode (right top and bottom panels). The anodal shock (right top panel) resulted in negative polarization of this real electrode area, while the cathodal shock produced a positive polarization (right bottom panel) in the real electrode area. In addition to the differences in polarity, the responses were different in amplitude. The maximum amplitude of depolarization during cathodal shock was smaller than the maximum hyperpolarization during anodal shocks in the same area. The cathodal response amplitude was 68±12% of the anodal shock amplitude (mean±SD; n = 14 pairs of shocks from 12 hearts). However, no difference in the size of these two areas was observed.

The areas on either side of the electrode placed in the center of the right ventricular free wall had responses of opposite polarity to the area near the electrode. Anodal shocks created two "virtual cathodes," which produced two areas of depolarization (the left one is shown in the upper left panel of Fig. 6). Conversely, cathodal stimulation produced two areas of "virtual anodes" located by both sides adjacent to the shock electrode (the left area of virtual electrode is shown in lower left panel of Fig. 6).

The area of measurement in these experiments was limited to 11×11 mm. Therefore, the position of the photodiode array versus the heart was adjusted in order to better measure the optical action potentials in the area of the virtual electrodes. The left upper and lower panels of Figure 6 illustrate typical patterns of changes in transmembrane voltage during anodal (upper left panel) and cathodal (lower left panel) shocks of 50 V in amplitude. Virtual electrode polarization areas had an elliptical shape, with the long axis oriented along the electrode. The size of the areas of virtual electrodes depended on both the applied voltage and the time from the onset of the monophasic shock. We estimated the size of the virtual cathode area (anodal shock) as an area of depolarization by 30 mV' or more. The virtual anode (cathodal shock) was estimated by the area negatively polarized by −30% mV' or more. For a 50-V shock, the length of the virtual electrode ellipse was estimated to be 11.4±1.2 mm for anodal shocks and 10.9±1.6 mm for cathodal shocks (mean±SD; n = 15 from 12 hearts). One virtual electrode area of both polarities was measured from nine hearts, and two areas of both polarities were measured from three hearts. No statistically significant difference was observed between anodal and cathodal virtual electrode areas ($P = 0.21$).

Modulation of the Virtual Electrode Pattern by Defibrillation Waveform: Asymmetric Response to the Second Phase of Biphasic Shock

The success of defibrillation is known to strongly depend on the shock waveform used. It has been shown that some biphasic waveforms require significantly lower energy to successfully defibrillate, compared with monophasic or other biphasic waveforms.[14] The mechanisms of these differences are not fully understood. During the second stage of our project, we tried to delineate the VEP produced by different biphasic waveforms with their defibrillation efficacy.

Figure 2 shows representative superimposed recordings from 1 of 256 recording sites (black square in left panel). Figure 3 shows a representative map of action potentials recorded from all 256 recording sites during a basic beat, superimposed with a recording during a shock of +100/-50 V applied at the plateau phase of the ventricular action potential. This shock waveform corresponds to a clinically optimal defibrillation waveform.[14]

The right upper and lower panels of Figure 2 show superimposed optical recordings performed during 10 basic beats (control action potentials) and 10 applications of different waveforms for anodal (upper panel) and cathodal (lower panel) shocks, respectively. These recordings demonstrate that the recording site underwent either positive (upper) or negative (lower) polarization during the first phase of the shock relative to the preshock transmembrane potential. The magnitude of the polarization depended upon both the polarity of the shock and the location of the recording site (see Figs. 3, 5, 6, 7, and 8). Spatially, the polarization produced by the first phase was arranged in the virtual electrode pattern qualitatively similar to our data reported for monophasic waveforms.[8] There are quantitative differences related to the different position of the electrode with respect to interventricular septum, which is discussed later in this chapter.

The second phase of the shock is partially or fully reversed in the polarization produced by the first phase in every recording site, in an amplitude-dependent fashion, for either shock polarity. However, there was a striking difference in the reversal of the polarization, depending on the sign of the polarization produced by the first phase. In this example, more than 70 V was required to fully reverse the positive polarization (Fig. 2, blue traces in upper panel), while only 20 V or more was required to reverse the negative polarization (Fig. 2, green and blue traces in lower panel). Therefore,

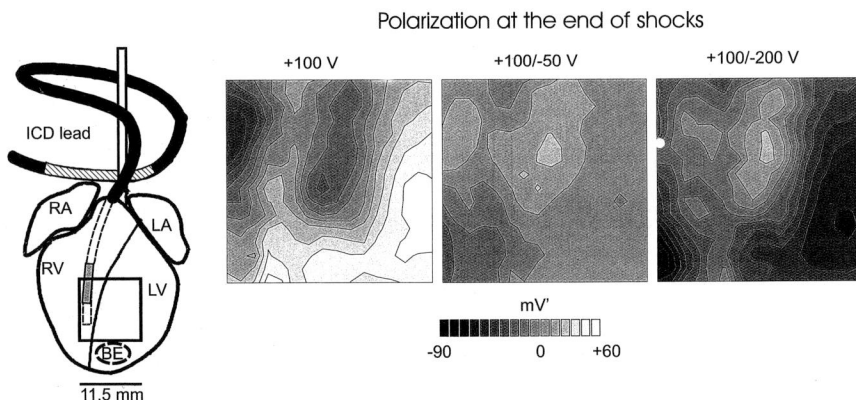

Polarization at the end of shocks

Figure 7. Modulation of virtual electrode pattern by the amplitude of the second phase. The spatial patterns of polarization are shown at the end of shocks produced by a monophasic (+100 V, seventh ms of 8-ms shock), optimal biphasic (+100/−50 V, 15th ms of 16-ms shock), and nonoptimal biphasic (+100/−200 V, 15th ms of 16-ms shock) shocks. Fig. 3 shows raw data used for calculating the middle map in this figure. The area of recording (11.5×11.5 mm) is represented by the black box. Values of polarization are shown relative to the preshock transmembrane voltage, with light color assigned to positive polarization and dark color to negative polarization. Reproduced, with permission, from reference 9.

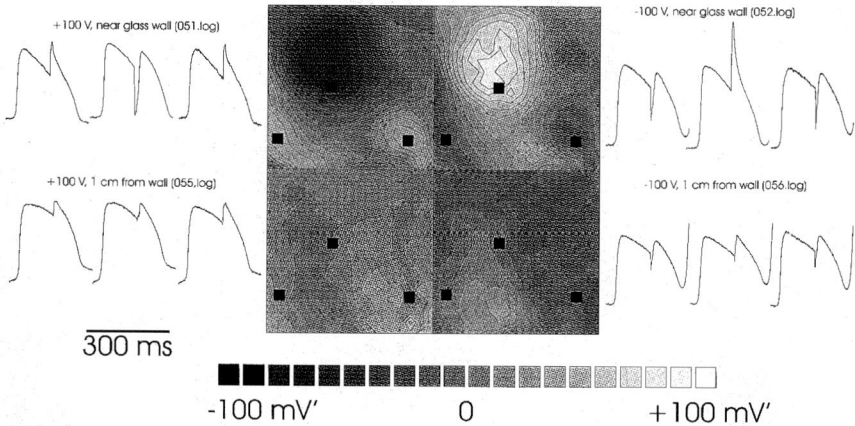

Figure 8. Modulation of virtual electrode-induced phase singularity by tissue-bath interface. Epicardial transmembrane polarization during anodal (left maps and corresponding optical traces, +100 V, 8 ms) and cathodal shocks (right maps and corresponding traces, −100 V, 8 ms), applied during plateau phase of an action potential. The upper maps and traces show data recorded from the left ventricular epicardium, pressed against the glass wall (see Fig. 1). The lower maps and traces show data recorded in heart 1 cm from the glass wall. Representative traces were recorded in sites shown by solid black boxes. Equipotential contours are drawn every 10 mV′. Redrawn from reference 18, with permission.

waveforms with a second phase leading edge voltage between 20 V and 70 V (Fig. 2, green traces in both upper and lower panels) produced a positive polarization nearly everywhere throughout the field of view (Fig. 7, middle panel). Waveforms with a second phase leading edge voltage either weaker than 20 V or stronger than 70 V created a highly heterogeneous polarization pattern, with the simultaneous occurrence of positive (light area) and negative (dark area) polarizations (Fig. 7, left and right maps). Furthermore, as seen in Figure 2, shocks with a second phase leading edge voltage between 20 V and 70 V resulted in no postshock evoked responses, while every other shock initiated postshock extra beats or sustained VF (see examples in Figs. 9 and 10, respectively).

Based on these data, we concluded that work on defibrillation waveform optimization might be guided by measurements of homogeneity of the VEP rather than on the degree of action potential prolongation. Action potential prolongation is commonly used as a predictor for defibrillation waveform efficacy. In the example shown in Figure 2, optimal waveforms produced the least action potential prolongation compared with recording from the same site, but in response to less efficient waveforms.

Virtual Electrode Pattern Modulation by the Myocardial Structure and Tissue-Bath Interface

Bidomain mathematical models predicted that structural characteristics of the myocardium may be responsible for exact shape of the virtual electrode pattern in the myocardium. Anisotropic fiber orientation[15] and

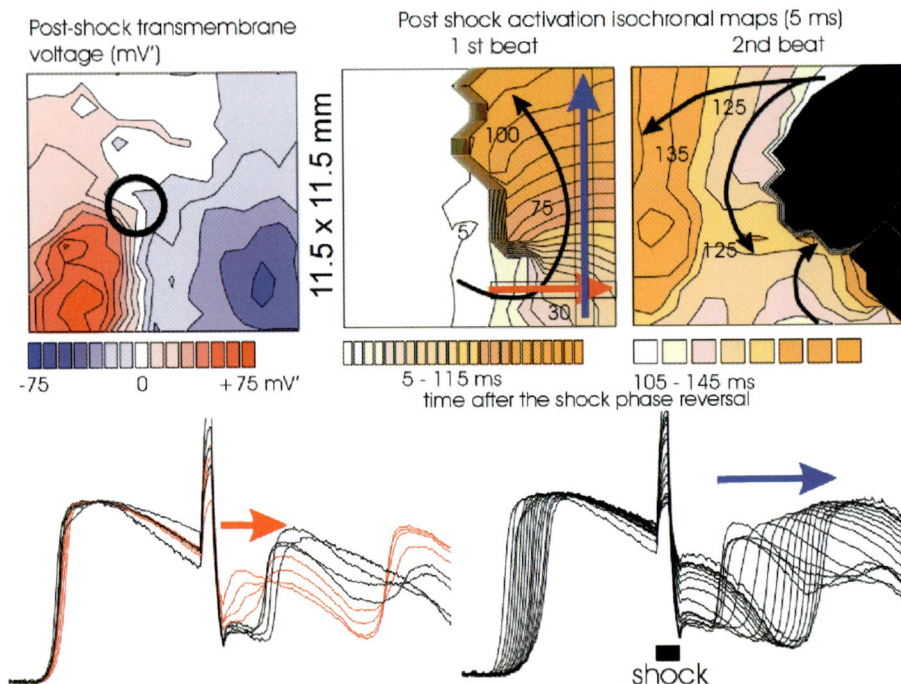

Figure 9. Virtual electrode-induced phase singularity. Electrical activity was recorded from the area shown by the red box in Fig. 2. The upper left map shows the polarization pattern at the end of a +100/−200 V biphasic shock (15th millisecond of 16-ms shock) that resulted in a single extra beat. The scale is shown in mV, calibrated in the same manner described in Fig. 2. The point of phase singularity is shown with the black circle. The upper middle map is a 5-ms isochronal map depicting the initiation of postshock spread of activation. The map starts at the onset of the 8-ms second phase of the shock (phase reversal). Shown at the bottom left and bottom right are optical recordings from several recording sites used to reconstruct the activation maps: the eight sites in the middle top map marked with a red arrow correspond to the left-lower panel, and the 16 sites marked with a blue arrow correspond to the lower-right panel. The upper right map shows a continuation of the reentrant activation that follows the middle map. Reentrant activity then self-terminated, after encountering refractory tissue in the lower-right corner of the field of view (see lower-right traces). Reproduced, with permission, from reference 9.

syncytial heterogeneities[16,17] have been directly implicated in the formation of VEPs. Another possible factor that may modulate exact 3-dimensional organization of VEPs is the passive electrical properties of tissues surrounding the heart. We conducted a series of experiments (n = 4) to explore the effects of the tissue-bath interface on epicardial VEPs.

Figure 8 shows left ventricular patterns of polarization produced by anodal shocks (right panels) and cathodal shocks (left panels) with leading edge voltage of 100 V. The shock electrode was positioned in the left ventricular cavity. Data in the upper panels were recorded while the heart was in direct contact with the glass wall. Both anodal and cathodal shocks produced sharp VEP gradients. Data shown in the lower panels were

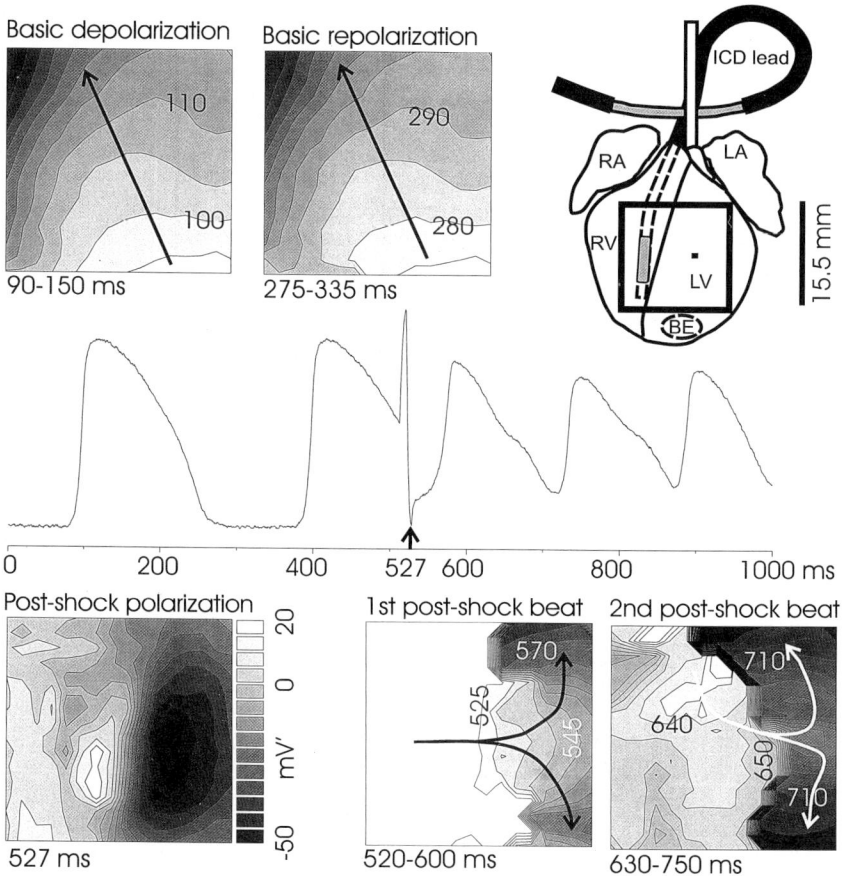

Figure 10. Evidence of difference between virtual electrode-induced phase singularity and Frazier's critical point mechanism: implications to near-field versus far-field differences. A pair of phase singularity points was produced by a +100/−170-V shock. The upper left and middle maps show activation and repolarization patterns of the basic beat, respectively. Time in all maps is given with respect to the beginning of the recording. The trace in the middle represents one recording from a left ventricular site shown with a black box at the top right of the figure. The left lower map shows transmembrane polarization at the end of the shock (15th millisecond of 16-ms biphasic shock). Lower middle and right maps are 5-ms isochronal maps for the first and second reentrant beats, respectively. The time starts at the phase reversal (520 ms). Reproduced, with permission, from reference 9.

recorded while the heart was 1 cm from the glass wall. No sharp gradients were observed: VEPs were not present (left lower panel) or were greatly reduced in amplitude (right lower panel), yielding to a single polarity polarization. Bidomain simulations were conducted by Entcheva et al.,[18] who predicted qualitatively similar patterns of polarization at the epicardium. However, unlike with optical mapping, these simulations could demonstrate the entire 3-dimensional structure of VEP. Figure 11 shows VEP calculated in a model of free right and left ventricular walls that in-

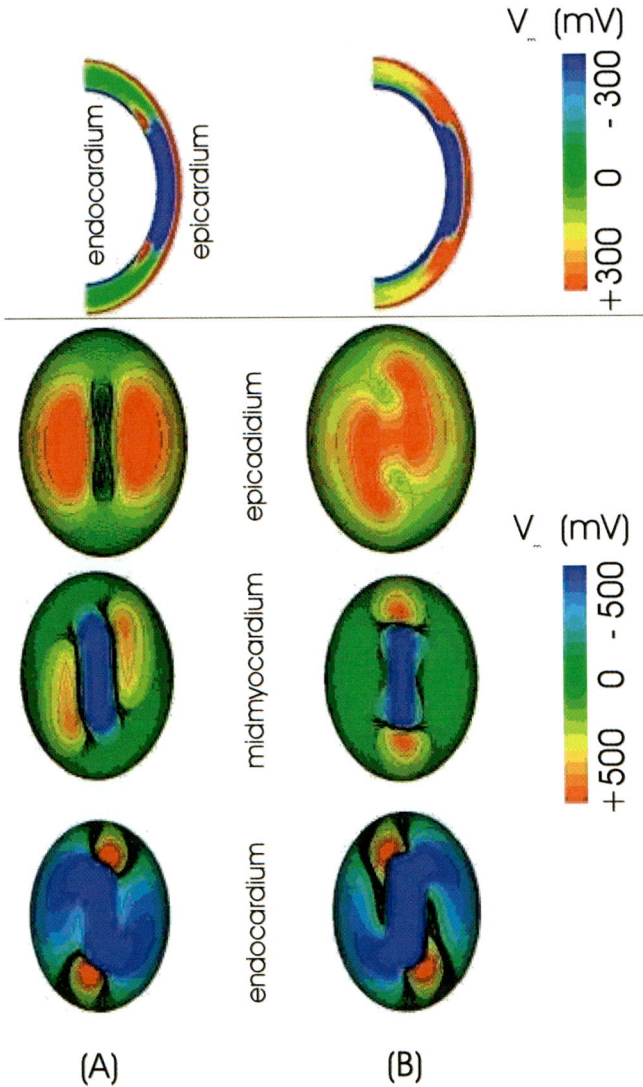

(A)   **(B)**

Figure 11. Bidomain simulations of the effects of fiber rotation and tissue-bath interface on the 3-dimensional structure of virtual electrode polarization. *Left:* Transmembrane potential distribution for linear counterclockwise rotation (from −30° to +90°). *Right:* Linear counterclockwise rotation (+30° to +150°). The first row shows V_m on transmural slices. The second, third, and fourth rows show V_m distribution at the subepicardial layer (1 mm from epicardium), midmyocardium, and subendocardium (1-mm from endocardium). The heart is positioned 1 cm from the insulating boundary, the bath conductivity is nominal, and the internal lead is in longitudinal position. For the transmural slices, the range of values is from −300 mV′ to +300 mV′. For other surfaces, the range of values is from −500 mV′ to +500 mV′. The equipotential contours are given for every 100 mV above 100 mV and for every 10 mV below 100 mV. Redrawn from reference 18, with permission.

cludes different rotations of myocardial fiber orientation from the epicardium to the endocardium. As in the lower panels of experimental Figure 8, the heart was 1 cm from the glass wall. VEPs were not present at the epicardium in both cases, while spanning the entire midmyocardial and endocardial layers. The exact arrangement of the fibers has a dramatic impact on the 3-dimensional structures of VEPs (compare left and right panels of Fig. 11).

Another important determinant of the exact 3-dimensional structure of VEP is the gross structure of the heart. For example, the interventricular septum may play an important role in forming VEP. Comparisons of the epicardial VEP obtained during shocks from electrodes positioned in the middle of the right ventricular free wall and those near the septum show that the presence of the septum dramatically altered the polarization pattern. A single virtual electrode area was present on either side of the real electrode area when the shock electrode was placed in the middle of the right ventricular free wall (see Figs. 5 and 6). It appears that the interventricular septum caused fractionation of the area of the virtual electrode such that anodal monophasic shocks produced a virtual cathode that was split in the middle by another virtual anode, which then caused negative polarization in the middle of positive polarization (see gray area in the middle of the left polarization map in Fig. 7). The exact mechanism of this modulation of VEP by the septum remains unknown, but one might suggest that the septum is another myocardial structure, which may support VEP. Septal VEP may interact with VEP on the ventricular walls, altering their epicardial appearance.

Phase Resetting by Virtual Electrodes: Prolongation and Shortening of APD

Since the first introduction of optical recordings to the field of defibrillation research, it has been assumed that strong electrical shock prolongs APD and refractory period.[6] This prolongation causes termination of preshock fibrillatory dispersion of refractoriness and therefore terminates fibrillation.[19] We investigated the role of virtual electrodes in the prolongation of APDs, and measured high-resolution patterns of APD changes caused by the shock.

The first striking finding was the observation that APD may be prolonged and shortened at the same time in different areas of the epicardium due to the virtual electrode effect. Figure 12 shows a part of 16×16 optical recordings from the left ventricular epicardium. These data illustrate that action potentials were prolonged in the area of positive polarization (lower traces), while in the area of negative polarization they were shortened (upper traces). Typically, shortening is not readily observed after shocks of defibrillation strength. Strong negative polarization and, therefore, shortening is likely to lead to the reopening of sodium channels and restoration of excitability. In the majority of cases, the presence of an area of strong negative polarization shortening will necessitate the presence of neighboring areas with strong positive polarization and APD prolongation (see Figs. 5, 6, and 7). Electrotonic interaction between these two neigh-

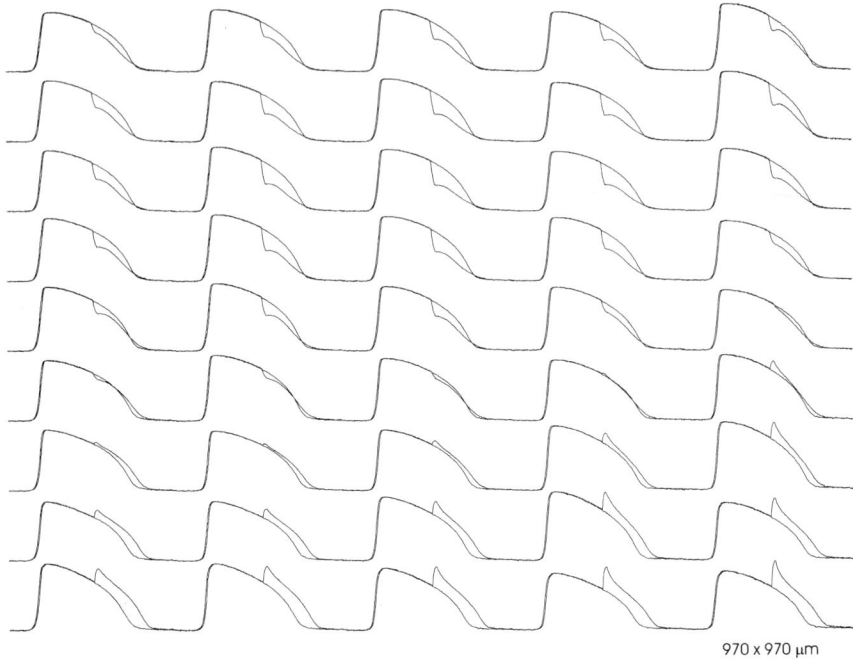

970 x 970 μm

Figure 12. Virtual electrode polarization is responsible for prolongation and shortening of the action potential duration and the dispersion of repolarization. Superimposed traces were recorded from the left ventricular epicardium during basic beat, and an anodal shock was applied at the left ventricular endocardium. The upper traces with shock-induced shortening were recorded from the area of the real electrode. The lower prolonged traces were recorded from an area of virtual cathode.

boring areas will produce rapid reactivation of negatively polarized areas with restored excitability. Therefore, action potential shortening caused by negative polarization will be hidden by subsequent relatively rapid reactivation spread from the positively polarized area, and can only be seen if sufficient temporal and spatial resolution is provided.

These data demonstrate that VEP produced dispersion of APD and/or refractoriness, which provided a substrate for postshock arrhythmias. Therefore, the presence of VEP may be linked to postshock arrhythmias during failed defibrillation shocks.

Mechanism of Shock-Induced Activation Wave Fronts

Presence of dispersion of repolarization is a necessary condition for arrhythmogenesis. However, in order for arrhythmias to develop, another condition must be met: an ectopic beat must arrive to the area with dispersion of repolarization and produce a unidirectional block and reentry. During this stage of our study, we investigated mechanisms of inducing new wave fronts by strong electrical shocks.

As shown in the previous section of this chapter, strong negative polarization produced action potential shortening with possible reactivation of sodium channels. Therefore, it may be subsequently reexcited and support an active propagated response. Figure 13 demonstrates one such example. The upper panel shows nine optical recordings from a line of photodiodes 710 μm apart. Recording sites were chosen based on increasing distance from the shock electrode. All of these sites were negatively polarized at the end of a +100/−170-V biphasic shock (upper panel). As seen in the lower right panel of this figure, all nine recording sites were reexcited, starting from sites near the electrode. Then, excitation was spread from the electrode. The sequence of reexcitation may not be explained by the passive discharge of the membrane. A purely electrotonic response also fails to explain this sequential depolarization, because distant recordings sites are located farther than several space constants and a delay is clearly seen between the first electrotonic foot and subsequent depolarization, especially in the most remote sites. In this example, the conduc-

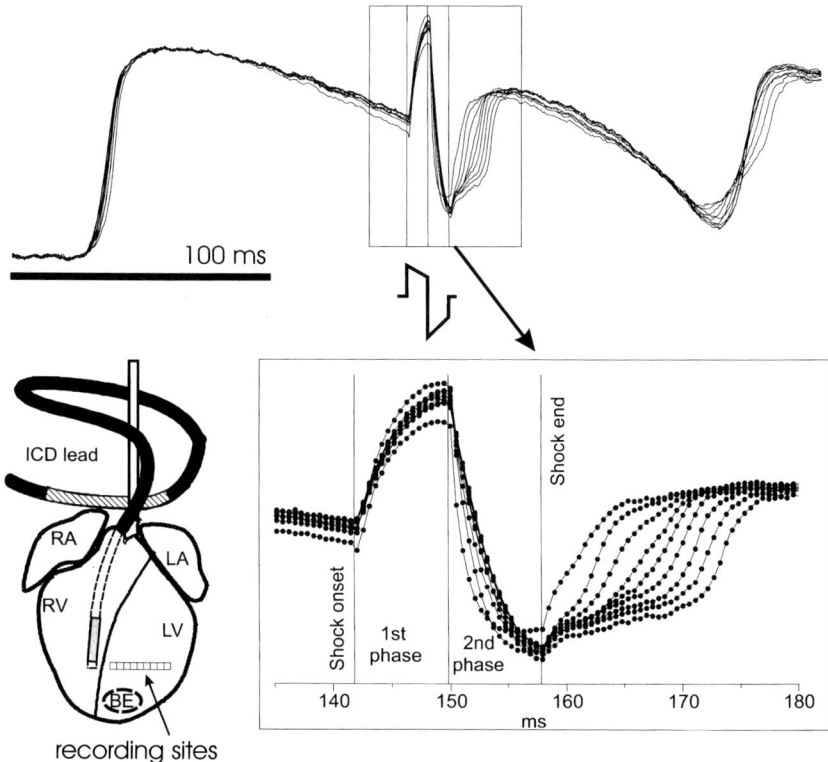

Figure 13. Mechanism of generation of active propagated responses by virtual electrode polarization gradients. At top are nine representative traces recorded at the anterior epicardium during the application of a biphasic shock (+100/−170 V, 8/8 ms). The shock produced negative polarization in all nine sites (710 μm apart). The location of the recording sites is shown in the lower left panel. The lower right panel shows expanded traces from these recordings during and immediately after the shock (sampled at 2 kHz). As evident from the traces, recording sites were progressively activated after the shock withdrawal with a conduction velocity of 35 cm/s (65% of normal conduction velocity in this area during basic beat produced by epicardial pacing).

tion velocity was 65% of the normal conduction velocity recorded at the same site during paced rhythm. As seen in Figure 2 (upper right panel), progressively stronger negative polarization resulted in a progressively sharper onset of the postshock depolarization. Conduction velocity of postshock active response also was faster in more negatively polarized areas. This was consistently observed in all 24 hearts studied.

As seen from these data, there is a presence of strongly negatively polarized areas next to positively polarized areas providing two of the conditions for reentry: dispersion of repolarization and new wave fronts of activation, generated at the boundary between real and virtual electrode areas of the VEP.

Mechanism of Virtual Electrode-Induced Phase Singularities Leading to Reentry and Failure to Defibrillate

Unidirectional blocks and slow conduction are present during arrhythmogenesis via a reentrant mechanism. We have investigated the possible role of VEP in providing these two conditions for arrhythmogenesis. We have carefully analyzed shock-induced arrhythmias, paying special attention to shock-induced polarization maps and postshock propagation.

We reconstructed isochronal activation maps of postshock beats resulting from VEP using the $-(dF/dt)_{max}$ technique.[13] Figure 9 shows a typical pattern of activation produced by a shock resulting in arrhythmia. This pattern of activation was reproduced in all 12 hearts after shocks resulting in a strongly polarized VEP. The upper left panel shows the transmembrane voltage distribution at the end of a $+100/-200$-V biphasic shock, which was applied during the plateau phase of an action potential. The area of the recordings and the location of the electrodes were the same as in Figure 2 (red box). Tissue located close to the electrode underwent a strong depolarization, which decreased with the distance from the electrode in the superior direction (red), while the lateral area underwent negative polarization (blue), which also decreased in the superior direction. The black circle indicates a point of shock-induced phase singularity (see Discussion).

Tissue in the lower left quadrant of the field of view was strongly depolarized, while the tissue in the lower right quadrant was negatively polarized, restoring excitability in that area. As shown in the eight superimposed optical recordings in the lower left corner of Figure 9, the depolarized area excited the negatively polarized areas (see red arrows and corresponding traces in the left lower panel). First, this excitation was transmitted electrotonically, via a mechanism similar to the "break" excitation described by Roth,[20] through a narrow isthmus between the areas that were strongly negatively polarized and those that were strongly depolarized (slow-rising, low-amplitude decaying responses in first four red traces in postshock time window). This functional isthmus was formed by cells that were put into different phases of refractoriness by the shock. Thus, the electrotonus first activated the excitable negatively polarized area (presumably containing reactivated sodium channels), resulting in fast propagation with full-amplitude action potentials (last four black recordings).

At the same time, the upper half of the field of view demonstrated unidirectional conduction block in the left-to-right direction (Fig. 9, thick black line in the middle upper panel). The lower driving force provided by the upper left depolarized area was unable to activate the less negatively polarized area in the upper right panel. Activation in this area followed the restoration of the resting potential from the lower right area (see blue arrow in traces in lower right panel and the middle upper panel). The right upper panel demonstrates the continuation of the reentrant activity, from right to left, in the upper half of the field of view. In addition, as seen in the lower right corner of this panel, an additional activation wave front spread from an area below the field of view. This indicates that additional phase singularities may have been induced by the shock in areas beyond our field of view.

Figure 10 presents postshock maps of activation recorded from a larger field of view (15.5×15.5 mm) than that in Figure 9. The lower middle and right maps demonstrate that, indeed, there are two reentrant circuits formed at one side from the electrode. This finding was observed in both of two different experiments performed with a larger field of view (15.5×15.5 mm), after a total of five shocks.

The results shown in Figures 9 and 10 were confirmed in all 12 hearts. A total of 38 of 112 shocks resulted in extra beats and/or arrhythmias. Of these, 31 shocks were applied at 102 ± 12 ms from the upstroke and seven shocks were applied at 50 ± 7 ms from the upstroke.

The above data were obtained with shocks applied during the plateau phase of a normally propagating action potential. In order to demonstrate that the same underlying mechanism is involved in defibrillation, we analyzed 19 unsuccessful defibrillation shocks (6 hearts). Fibrillation was induced by shocks applied as previously described, during the plateau phase of the action potential. Figure 14 shows the activation pattern recorded during one of these shocks. The lower left map shows the spread of activation during the last beat of VF, before the defibrillation attempt. Conduction was slow and emerged from several foci at the same time (white areas). Trace F (fluorescence) shows that during fibrillatory electrical activity the transmembrane potential did not reach either full depolarization or resting potential, and therefore there was no excitable gap. Recordings in none of the 256 channels demonstrated the presence of an excitable gap. A cathodal monophasic shock (−150 V) produced a VEP pattern similar to the one shown in Figure 9, with positive polarization near the electrode and negative polarization on both sides (not shown). The middle activation map (isochrones 1 ms apart) shows that activation rapidly spread in the right half of the field of view, near the electrode. Then it spread to the left in the upper half, while it was blocked in the lower half. Activation then spread downward, completing the reentrant cycle. The point of phase singularity is shown with a white circle. Similar results, with clear evidence of the occurrence of a phase singularity followed by reentry, were observed in 14 of 19 unsuccessful defibrillation shocks. A phase singularity was also created in 2 of 12 successful defibrillation shocks. However, in these cases, reentry persisted for only 1 and 3 beats, respectively. If the postshock arrhythmias lasted more than 3 beats, the shock was considered unsuccessful.

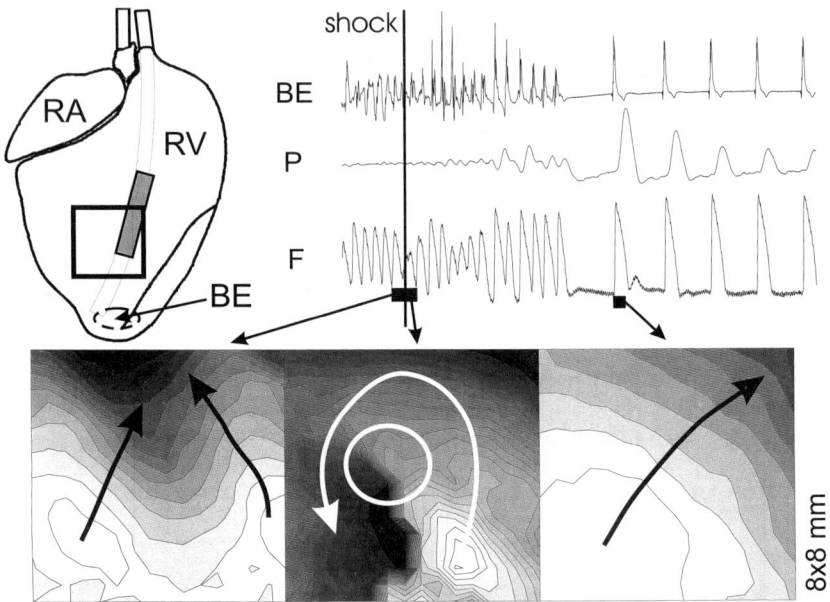

Figure 14. Virtual electrode-induced phase singularity is responsible for failure to defibrillate. A phase singularity is produced during a failed defibrillation shock. The top left panel shows the location of the field of view with respect to the defibrillation electrode. The top right panel shows a bipolar electrogram (BE), aortic pressure (P), and a fluorescent signal (F) from one of the optical recording sites. Timing of the shock application is shown with the vertical line labeled "shock." The lower maps show activation sequences (1-ms isochrones) just before (left) and immediately after (middle) the shock, and after restoration of sinus rhythm (right). Redrawn from reference 9, with permission.

Discussion

Theories of Fibrillation and Defibrillation

Lewis[21] suggested in 1925 that fibrillation has a reentrant nature and that the difference between fibrillation and tachycardia is that the reentrant pattern in tachycardia is repeated accurately while in fibrillation it is not. Our findings demonstrate that in the rabbit heart VF may be initiated via the mechanism of VEIPS. This leads to the creation of multiple reentrant circuits that comprise the fibrillatory substrate. The failure to defibrillate in our experiments also occurred via the VEIPS mechanism.

Two main hypotheses have previously been proposed to explain the mechanisms of defibrillation: the critical mass hypothesis[22–24] and the upper limit of vulnerability hypothesis.[25] The first hypothesis suggests that a critical amount of tissue is required to sustain fibrillation. Two underlying mechanisms have been proposed to support the critical mass hypothesis: statistical and dynamical. Both postulate that *VF must be extinguished in a significant portion of the myocardium, while the remaining fibrillatory activity will self-terminate.* The statistical critical mass hypothesis[26] postulates that a critical number of wavelets is required to sustain fibrillation, because of the statistical nature of their birth and death.[23] The dynamical critical mass hypothesis is based on the observation that some critical amount of tissue is required to support even a single reentry, which may evolve indefinitely in a nonstationary fashion if provided with sufficient space.[27,28] In contrast to these, the upper limit of vulnerability hypothesis postulates that for successful defibrillation VF must be extinguished *everywhere throughout the heart.* To succeed, a critical voltage gradient (called the upper limit of vulnerability) must be reached everywhere in order to fully extinguish VF and not reinduce a new one via a critical point mechanism.[29] The primary area of disagreement between the two theories is not in the mechanism of defibrillation, but rather in the understanding of the mechanisms of the failure to defibrillate.

The upper limit of vulnerability hypothesis insists that VF will be reinduced unless critical voltage is reached everywhere. The suggested mechanism responsible for the reinduction of VF was named the critical point mechanism.[29] The idea of this mechanism can be traced back more than half a century. In 1946, Wiener and Rosenblueth[30] proposed a mechanism by which reentry can be induced. They predicted "*the initiation of a one-way wave by successive stimulation of two overlapping small regions of two dimensional system*" (see p. 219 and Fig. 5 of reference 30), which may lead to a pattern of electrical activity similar to what is known now as a figure-of-8 reentry. This mechanism has been carefully explored, both theoretically and in the chemical Belousov-Zhabotinsky reaction, by Winfree,[31] who recognized in this electrophysiological mechanism the abstract concept of a *point of singularity,* which has long been known in physics and mathematics. An experimental protocol of inducing the point of singularity qualitatively similar to that of Wiener and Rosenblueth[30] was first successfully applied in the heart by Frazier et al.,[29] who named this protocol cross-field stimulation, and named the point of singularity the critical point. We refer to the cross-filed stimulation for inducing critical points[29] as the critical point mechanism.

As pointed out by Winfree,[31] a functional reentrant circuit presents an example of an abstract concept known in mathematics as a point of singularity. In fact, this is the only known example of this concept in electrophysiology. Term singularity refers to the impossibility of defining a value of a function at some unique point. The electrical activity of cardiac muscle can be described in terms of phase, with phase $\varphi = 0$ being assigned to onset of an action potential and $\varphi = 2\pi$ assigned to the fully repolarized state. In two dimensions, a point of phase singularity is defined as a point in which the following is true, $\lim_{L\to 0} \oint \vec{\nabla}\phi \bullet \vec{dl} \neq 0$, where $L = \oint |\vec{dl}|$. The virtual electrode pattern may contain a point that is surrounded by depolarized (excited), nonpolarized (refractory), and polarized (excitable) areas. Therefore, the phase in such a point will yield the above equation, and this point of phase singularity may be responsible for the initiation of reentrant activity.

The concept of VEIPS was clearly visualized in our experiments. The map of transmembrane potential shown in the upper left of Figure 9 can be interpreted in terms of the phase of the electrical activity. The transmembrane voltage shown in the right panel can then be translated into a phase value by using additional information about dV/dt. The sign of dV/dt is needed to distinguish phases corresponding to the activation (dV/dt>0) from phases corresponding to the repolarization (dV/dt<0). The area marked with a black circle contains a point that yields the mathematical definition of a phase singularity, known also as a critical point, which has been previously demonstrated to result in reentrant activity.[29]

However, the mechanism of creating phase singularities and reentry in this study is significantly different from that in the critical point concept as described by Frazier et al.[29] Indeed, the repolarization map of the last basic beat, shown in the upper middle row in Figure 10, shows that repolarization gradient is directed from apex to the base, while the polarization gradient is pointed from left to right. According to the critical point mechanism, one would expect only the upper phase singularity to be formed by the shock, because this is the only site at which an appropriate cross-field pattern between repolarization and electrical field gradients is formed. The lower phase singularity cannot be explained by the critical point mechanism and therefore provides compelling evidence of the novelty of our finding.

Our data indicate that the phase singularity mechanism is indeed involved in electrical activity resulting from proarrhythmic ICD shocks. However, point singularities resulted in self-sustained arrhythmias (>3 min) in only 10.7 % of cases (12 of 112), while the remaining reentries self-terminated. In 24 cases we could clearly identify that the reentrant wave front propagated along a line of a conduction block, turned around a pivoting point, and then self-terminated by encountering refractory tissue (see the example in Fig. 9). Therefore, the arrhythmia may halt spontaneously, as according to the critical mass hypothesis. However, it is important to note that our data cannot clearly identify which is the correct theory, because we did not look at the nonextinguished preshock fibrillatory electrical activity and we could not map the electrical activity of the entire heart.

The critical mass theory and the upper limit of vulnerability theory both have limitations. Critical mass does not specify exactly how the remaining VF will self-terminate. Upper limit of vulnerability fails to recognize the vector nature of voltage gradients, for example the difference between positively and negatively polarizing voltage gradients, referring to only absolute amplitude of voltage gradients. It also fails to consider boundaries between the two areas that are associated with the creation of new wave fronts and phase singularities. The upper limit of vulnerability hypothesis states that new wave fronts and new reentrant circuits (critical points) may only occur in areas of low voltage gradient, typically far from electrodes. Our finding indicates that VEP may be responsible for phase singularities and reentry near the electrode. We believe that both mechanisms may participate in failure to defibrillate: the critical point and the VEIPS. The critical point may induce reentry in the far-field low voltage gradients, while VEIPS is responsible for reentry in the near-field strong voltage gradients. In the case of optimal biphasic defibrillation waveforms, when virtual electrodes are canceled by the second phase and therefore VEIPS are less likely to occur, the critical point may be the only participant in failure to defibrillate. This, however, remains to be investigated, because structural heterogeneities of heart with coronary artery disease may induce new virtual electrode polarizations, also known as secondary sources,[16] and, therefore, new VEIPS.

Further, neither the critical mass hypothesis nor the upper limit of vulnerability hypothesis specifies exactly how fibrillatory electrical activity is extinguished at the cellular level. Several basic mechanisms have been proposed to explain defibrillation at the cellular level, including 1) prolongation of APD[6] and refractoriness,[32,33] known also as graded responses,[34] and 2) reactivation of sodium channels[35] with possible subsequent break excitation.[20]

Our optical data indicate that *nearly all* of these effects may be involved in defibrillation, at the same time, in different parts of the heart, in which extracellular field gradients of opposite polarity produce either inward or outward current sources. However, our data demonstrate that the success of the shock is not related solely to the degree of action potential prolongation, but rather to the homogeneity of postshock transmembrane polarization. Indeed, Figure 2 indicates that shocks which resulted in no postshock extra beats or arrhythmias prolonged the action potential least of all (see green traces). Thus, their defibrillation efficacy is more likely related to the homogenization of the postshock phase distribution, because strong phase gradients may produce propagated responses via the break excitation mechanism.[20] The latter can form a reentrant circuit if a phase singularity is created in addition to the phase gradient.

Numerous basic and clinical studies have empirically identified certain monophasic and biphasic defibrillation waveforms that are relatively more efficient than others.[36–38] Our data support a logical explanation for why a specific waveform may be better than others. We have shown that if the ratio between the leading edge voltage of the second phase and that of the first phase is in the range of 0.2 to 0.7, then the shock creates a relatively homogeneous postshock transmembrane polarization and phase pattern with no substrate for creating points of phase singularity. Therefore, we suggest that these waveforms will be the least likely to induce postshock arrhythmias via the VEIPS mechanism. Our results are consistent with defibrillation threshold measurements in humans.[14]

Limitations of the Study

This study has several limitations. Mapping of electrical activity was confined to only a limited epicardial area. Therefore, we may have missed the induction of some other phase singularities that may have occurred beyond our field of view, and at the endocardium and midmyocardium. Asynchronous measurements indicated that phase singularities are likely to occur at four sites around the right ventricular electrode in areas where negative, positive, and no polarization meet. This is qualitatively similar to the theoretical prediction of Roth and Saypol,[39] who proposed the involvement of a virtual electrode pattern in the proarrhythmic response to a premature pacing stimulus applied at the vulnerable period of an action potential. Their hypothesis was based on the interaction of stimulus-induced VEP and the preshock phase pattern. Our data indicate that a strong shock may overcome the preshock electrical activity and create phase singularities, regardless of the preshock phase distribution (see Fig. 9). Furthermore, unlike low-energy pacing, defibrillation shocks create virtual electrode patterns comparable to the size of the heart. Therefore, additional areas of opposite polarization may be present, for example at the septum. Thus, additional phase singularities may be generated.

Our study does not address the issue of a 3-dimensional pattern of polarization. We can only record the average electrical activity from a 500-μm superficial layer of the epicardium.[40] However, our findings can be easily extended to a 3-dimensional case. Reversal of negatively polarized areas should be easier than the reversal of positively polarized patterns, presumably because of the involvement of different ionic currents at different levels of transmembrane polarization and, therefore, different transmembrane impedance to the polarizing effects of the shock. Postshock propagation from depolarized to negatively polarized areas must occur in the 3-dimensional case as well. The exact 3-dimensional organization of the propagation pattern remains to be elucidated, perhaps by use of a bidomain simulation approach. Our new data[18] indicate that 2-dimensional phase singularities and vortices in three dimensions may correspond to filaments of phase singularity and twisted and curved scrolls, respectively. The twisted shape of the filament is a result of the rotation of the fiber orientation within the ventricular wall. Detection of the virtual electrode pattern on the epicardium suggests that these scrolls are likely to be transmural and therefore may evolve into stable 3-dimensional sources of reentrant activity. Alternatively, in hearts with a low-impedance tissue-bath interface, one might expect no virtual electrodes protruding at the epicardium, but spanning the endocardium and midmyocardium. Therefore, U-shaped scroll waves will be formed. Questions on their relative stability remains unanswered experimentally and theoretically.

Another limitation of this study is a common limitation of nearly all animal models of defibrillation, which, however, becomes most compelling in view of the data presented. Internal defibrillation therapy is primarily applied in hearts with structural heart disease. Presence of scars may alter VEP dramatically, causing new sources of VEIPS. Most of animal models are based on structurally normal hearts, which is clearly a limiting factor.

References

1. Prevost JL, Battelli F. Sur quel ques effets des dechanges electriques sur le coer mammifres. *Comptes Rendus Seances Acad Sci* 1899;129:1267.
2. Beck CS, Pritchard WH, Feil HS. Ventricular fibrillation of long duration abolished by electric shock. *JAMA* 1947;135:985.
3. Zoll PM, Linethal AJ, Gibson W, et al. Termination of ventricular fibrillation in man by externally applied electric shock. *N Engl J Med* 1956;254:727.
4. Mirowski M, Mower MM, Staewen WS, et al. Standby automatic defibrillator: An approach to prevention of sudden coronary death. *Arch Intern Med* 1970;126:158–161.
5. Schuder JC, Stoeckle H, Golg JH, et al. Experimental ventricular defibrillation with an automatic and completely implanted system. *Trans Am Soc Artif Organs* 1970;16:207–212.

6. Dillon SM. Optical recordings in the rabbit heart show that defibrillation strength shocks prolong the duration of depolarization and the refractory period. *Circ Res* 1991;69:842–856.
7. Zhou X, Ideker RE, Blitchington TF, et al. Optical transmembrane potential measurements during defibrillation-strength shocks in perfused rabbit hearts. *Circ Res* 1995;77:593–602.
8. Efimov IR, Cheng YN, Biermann M, et al. Transmembrane voltage changes produced by real and virtual electrodes during monophasic defibrillation shock delivered by an implantable electrode. *J Cardiovasc Electrophysiol* 1997; 8:1031–1045.
9. Efimov IR, Cheng Y, Van Wagoner DR, et al. Virtual electrode-induced phase singularity: A basic mechanism of failure to defibrillate. *Circ Res* 1998;82:918–925.
10. Efimov IR, Fahy GJ, Cheng YN, et al. High resolution fluorescent imaging of rabbit heart does not reveal a distinct atrioventricular nodal anterior input channel (fast pathway) during sinus rhythm. *J Cardiovasc Electrophysiol* 1997;8:295–306.
11. Cheng Y, Mowrey KA, Efimov IR, et al. Effects of 2,3-butanedione monoxime on the atrial-atrioventricular nodal conduction in isolated rabbit heart. *J Cardiovasc Electrophysiol* 1997;8:790–802.
12. Salama G, Kanai A, Efimov IR. Subthreshold stimulation of Purkinje fibers interrupts ventricular tachycardia in intact hearts. Experimental study with voltage-sensitive dyes and imaging techniques. *Circ Res* 1994;74:604–619.
13. Efimov IR, Huang DT, Rendt JM, Salama G. Optical mapping of repolarization and refractoriness from intact hearts. *Circulation* 1994;90:1469–1480.
14. Feeser SA, Tang AS, Kavanagh KM, et al. Strength-duration and probability of success curves for defibrillation with biphasic waveforms. *Circulation* 1990;82:2128–2411.
15. Roth BJ, Wikswo JP. Electrical stimulation of cardiac tissue: A bidomain model with active membrane properties. *IEEE Trans Biomed Eng* 1994;41:232–240.
16. Fast VG, Rohr S, Gillis AM, Kléber AG. Activation of cardiac tissue by extracellular electrical shocks: Formation of 'secondary sources' at intercellular clefts in monolayers of cultured myocytes. *Circ Res* 1998;82:375–385.
17. Fishler MG. Syncytial heterogeneity as a mechanism underlying cardiac far-field stimulation during defibrillation-level shocks [In Process Citation]. *J Cardiovasc Electrophysiol* 1998;9:384–394.
18. Entcheva E, Eason J, Efimov IR, et al. Virtual electrode effects in transvenous defibrillation-modulation by structure and interface: Evidence from bidomain simulations and optical mapping. *J Cardiovasc Electrophysiol* 1998;9:949–961.
19. Dillon SM. Synchronized repolarization after defibrillation shocks. A possible component of the defibrillation process demonstrated by optical recordings in rabbit heart. *Circulation* 1992;85:1865–1878.
20. Roth BJ. A mathematical model of make and break electrical stimulation of cardiac tissue by a unipolar anode or cathode. *IEEE Trans Biomed Eng* 1995;42:1174–1184.
21. Lewis T. *The Mechanism and Graphic Registration of the Heart Beat.* 3rd ed. London: Shaw & Sons; 1925.
22. Garrey WE. The nature of fibrillary contraction of the heart. Its relations to tissue mass and form. *Am J Physiol* 1914;33:397–414.
23. Krinskii VI, Fomin SV, Kholopov AV. [Critical mass during fibrillation]. *Biofizika* 1967;12:908–914.
24. Zipes DP, Fischer J, King RM, et al. Termination of ventricular fibrillation in dogs by depolarizing a critical amount of myocardium. *Am J Cardiol* 1975;36:37–44.
25. Chen PS, Shibata N, Dixon EG, et al. Comparison of the defibrillation threshold and the upper limit of ventricular vulnerability. *Circulation* 1986;73:1022–1028.

26. Moe GK. A conceptual model of atrial fibrillation. *J Electrocardiol* 1968; 1:145–146.
27. Zykov VS. Cycloidal circulation of spiral waves in excitable medium. *Biofizika* 1986;31:862–865.
28. Efimov IR, Krinsky VI, Jalife J. Dynamics of rotating vortices in the Beeler-Reuter model of cardiac tissue. *Chaos Solitons Fractals* 1995;5:513–526.
29. Frazier DW, Wolf PD, Wharton JM, et al. Stimulus-induced critical point. Mechanism for electrical initiation of reentry in normal canine myocardium. *J Clin Invest* 1989;83:1039–1052.
30. Wiener N, Rosenblueth A. The mathematical formulation of the problem of conduction of impulses in a network of connected excitable elements, specifically in cardiac muscle. *Arch Inst Cardiologia de Mexico* 1946;16:205–265.
31. Winfree AT. *When Time Breaks Down: The Three-Dimensional Dynamics of Electrochemical Waves and Cardiac Arrhythmias.* Princeton, NJ: Princeton University Press; 1987:125–153.
32. Swartz JF, Jones JL, Jones RE, Fletcher R. Conditioning prepulse of biphasic defibrillator waveforms enhances refractoriness to fibrillation wavefronts. *Circ Res* 1991;68:438–449.
33. Sweeney RJ, Gill RM, Reid PR. Characterization of refractory period extension by transcardiac shock. *Circulation* 1991;83:2057–2066.
34. Kao CY, Hoffman BF. Graded and decremental responses in heart muscle fibers. *Am J Physiol* 1958;194:187–196.
35. Jones JL, Jones RE, Milne KB. Refractory period prolongation by biphasic defibrillator waveforms is associated with enhanced sodium current in a computer model of the ventricular action potential. *IEEE Trans Biomed Eng* 1994;41:60–68.
36. Walcott GP, Walcott KT, Knisley SB, et al. Mechanisms of defibrillation for monophasic and biphasic waveforms. [Review]. *Pacing Clin Electrophysiol* 1994;17:478–498.
37. Shorofsky SR, Foster AH, Gold MR. Effect of waveform tilt on defibrillation thresholds in humans. *J Cardiovasc Electrophysiol* 1997;8:496–501.
38. Huang J, KenKnight BH, Walcott GP, et al. Effect of electrode polarity on internal defibrillation with monophasic and biphasic waveforms using an endocardial lead system. *J Cardiovasc Electrophysiol* 1997;8:161–171.
39. Roth BJ, Saypol JM. The formation of a re-entrant action potential wave front in tissue with unequal anisotropy ratios. *Int J Bifurc Chaos* 1991;4:927–928.
40. Girouard SD, Laurita KR, Rosenbaum DS. Unique properties of cardiac action potentials recorded with voltage-sensitive dyes. *J Cardiovasc Electrophysiol* 1996;7:1024–1038.

Chapter 23

Optical Mapping of Cardiac Defibrillation:
Clinical Insights and Applications

Douglas P. Zipes

Introduction

Wearing my clinician's hat, as I have been requested to do while writing this chapter, I will start by asking the question, why apply electricity to the heart? This fundamental query underlies the important research presented in this section, in which scientists have explored various ways to deliver electricity to the heart and determine the cardiac response. For the clinician, the answer to this somewhat rhetorical question is obvious: to achieve radiofrequency catheter ablation, pacing, and defibrillation. Pacing and defibrillation are "old hat," while the newest application, of course, has been radiofrequency catheter ablation.[1] This technique has literally revolutionized the treatment of patients with a variety of tachyarrhythmias. We now have the ability to routinely cure patients with several types of supraventricular tachyarrhythmias, with the exception, perhaps, of atrial fibrillation[2]; and that old citadel will fall to the ablationist's catheter soon also. Ventricular tachyarrhythmias in patients with normal hearts are eminently erasable, but patients with ventricular tachycardias resulting from coronary disease still offer a challenge. While the full potential of radiofrequency ablation has scarcely been realized, it has profoundly impacted clinical care by permitting *cures* of disease—the only cardiovascular modality to do so. However, it is not a subject covered in this section, and I will not discuss it further.

The second reason to apply electricity to the heart is to achieve cardiac pacing to treat patients with symptomatic bradyarrhythmias. Recently, this application celebrated 50 years of successful clinical use. No one would argue that there have been very important improvements in cardiac pacing over these past 50 years. However, to play the devil's advocate, one could point out that the major advance from cardiac pacing in terms of *lives saved* came with the formulation of the very first pacemaker,

Supported in part by the Herman C. Krannert Fund, Indianapolis, and Grant HL-52323 from the National Heart, Lung, and Blood Institute, National Institutes of Health, Bethesda, MD.

From Rosenbaum DS, Jalife J (eds): *Optical Mapping of Cardiac Excitation and Arrhythmias.* ©Futura Publishing Co., Inc., Armonk, NY, 2001.

the ponderous, asynchronous ventricular pacemaker (VOO). The very first VOO units, once lead and pulse generator reliability were established, restored the complete heart block patient to a normal life span. All the following iterations, one could argue, were mere "bells and whistles" that reduced pacemaker size, increased longevity, eliminated competition with spontaneous rhythms (VVI), and provided more physiological responses (DDD, DDDR). Subsequent models have incremented the quality of life, clearly an important factor, but have probably not added many years to that life.

The third reason to apply electricity to the heart, and the subject of this chapter, is to achieve defibrillation. This application, too, has a long history, and recently celebrated its centennial; Prevost and Batelli[3] used a strong electrical shock to terminate ventricular fibrillation (VF) in dogs in 1899. The clinical application of *external* cardioversion and defibrillation pioneered by Zoll, Lown, Schuder, and others, achieved an apogee of clinical success 25 or more years ago and subsequent improvements, as with pacing, have improved quality of use but have not represented major breakthroughs.

In contrast, the type of defibrillation application that *has* proved revolutionary and *has* had an enormous impact on patient survival and how we practice medicine has been the implantable defibrillator, beginning with its first report more than 20 years ago[4] (the initial implantable system did not cardiovert, i.e., use a synchronous shock to terminate an organized rhythm; that came 4 years later[5]). It has been this device more than any other that, in my view, has spurred the work presented in this section. To create implantable cardioverter-defibrillator (ICD) *systems* (we must include the leads as well) that are smaller, more reliable, longer lasting, and less painful, it now becomes imperative to learn about mechanisms responsible for defibrillation. And to do that, we must also learn about the mechanisms responsible for fibrillation. But, as with pacing, one can ask the question, have we achieved the pinnacle of patient survival with the present ICD, and are we now just adorning it with more bells and whistles to improve quality of life, since sudden cardiac death mortality in patients with an ICD is less than 1% per year?[6,7] This topic is further discussed later in the chapter.

Ventricular Defibrillation Hypotheses

At least three hypotheses have been proffered to explain defibrillation, including the critical mass hypothesis,[8] the upper limit of vulnerability hypothesis,[9] and the progressive depolarization hypothesis.[10] Additional hypotheses have been suggested but are not considered in this chapter. In each hypothesis, defibrillation must terminate propagating electrical activity so that fibrillation ceases; in addition, the shock cannot initiate new propagating wave fronts that restart fibrillation. One must ask how these concepts differ and whether it matters to the clinician. Will it alter the way we use ICDs or the way they are built?

Garrey[8] first suggested the critical mass hypothesis, and early work from our laboratory supported his conclusions.[11] The critical mass hypothesis is predicated on the concept that a minimum amount of myocardium is required to sustain a critical number of reentrant wavelets necessary to perpetuate fibrillation. Naturally, a basic assumption here is that fibrillation is maintained by multiple reentrant wavelets. When fibrillation is extinguished in a critical amount of myocardium, the remaining myocardium has insufficient mass to maintain the reentrant activity and fibrillation terminates. In contrast, the upper limit of vulnerability hypothesis proposes that for successful ventricular defibrillation to occur, VF must be extinguished everywhere in the heart and not be restarted by the shock. For this to happen, a critical voltage gradient, i.e., the upper limit of vulnerability, must be achieved everywhere in the ventricle in order to fully extinguish VF[12] and not induce new fibrillation via such responses as the critical point mechanism.[13]

Recently, a third defibrillation hypothesis has been suggested, the progressive depolarization hypothesis, which attempts to unite the critical mass and the upper limit of vulnerability hypotheses.[10] The major point of the progressive depolarization hypothesis is that progressively stronger shocks depolarize progressively more refractory myocardium. This, then, progressively prevents shock wave fronts and prolongs and synchronizes postshock repolarization in a progressively larger volume of the ventricle. In turn, these changes progressively decrease the probability of fibrillation after the shock.

Mechanisms of Defibrillation

We do not fully understand at a cellular level the mechanism by which VF terminates after an electrical shock. Importantly, neither the critical mass nor the upper limit of vulnerability hypotheses specify *how* fibrillatory activity is extinguished at the cellular level, and they do not consider mechanisms such as prolongation of action potential duration and refractoriness[14] or the homogeneity of postshock transmembrane polarization.[15] These responses may explain why certain waveforms, such as biphasic defibrillation waveforms, are more efficient than are others. It is also clear that ventricular defibrillation is not an all-or-none phenomenon, but rather a probabilistic function.[12]

The cable model, resulting from early work of Hodgkin, Rushton, and Huxley on the squid axon, and from subsequent studies on Purkinje fibers by Weidmann, has recently been expanded to include the bidomain model.[16,17] The bidomain model assumes that conductivities for the intracellular, interstitial, and extracellular spaces remain independent from each other but are interconnected so that the intracellular space forms one domain separated by a highly resistive membrane from the interstitial space which connects to the extracellular space to form the second domain. This model most accurately describes the electrical response of cardiac tissue to strong electrical shocks and, particularly when tempered by unequal anisotropy, the model helps explain how cathodal and anodal make and break stimuli induce propagating activation. Modification by the secondary source model incorporates the influence of interruptions in intracellular coupling caused by nonpropagating segments of the myocardium such as blood vessels, collagen, or scar.[18] The concept of an activating function has been used to reproduce the response of all mathematical models to date.[19]

Understanding the response of the myocardium to electrical stimulation using the bidomain model has enhanced our understanding of how the heart responds to electrical activity. Important to this concept is the idea of a virtual electrode, which represents a reversal of polarity several millimeters from a stimulated site[18,20] that influences alterations in membrane potential produced by the primary stimulation site. In addition, understanding propagation of electrical activity through ventricular myocardium requires knowledge of the response of the electrical behavior of individual cardiac cells as well as the cardiac syncytium that binds them together. Therefore, the response of cardiac myocytes to electrical fields is important and may be complex. For example, the transmembrane potential beneath the electrode can respond in a manner that reflects the nonlinear impedance properties of the cell membrane while virtual electrode effects may be prominent near the electrode and cause regions of oppositely polarized responses. Virtual sources may form far from the electrode at the border of strands or bundles of cardiac cells.[21]

Let us briefly consider the insight offered by the hypotheses above about how the heart defibrillates. The critical mass hypothesis[8,10,11] states that a shock delivered during fibrillation cannot depolarize all of the myocardium because some cells will be in an absolutely refractory period and thus resistant to the effects of the shock. We now know that that is not entirely true since these cells can still be affected to some degree and can undergo prolongation of their action potential, which can influence termination of fibrillation.[22] But, still, the basic tenet holds that when fibrillation is eliminated in a critical mass of myocardium, fibrillation in the remaining myocardium ceases. Justification for this concept is founded in the unequivocal observations—from multiple sources and studies—that very small hearts and pieces of myocardium cannot maintain fibrillation. What can be argued is whether an electrical shock leaves refractory myocardium entirely unaffected, and the latter just spontaneously defibrillates, or whether the shock impacts it in some way, such as prolonging action potential duration, that facilitates termination.

The upper limit of vulnerability[9] is defined as the current strength of a shock at or above which VF cannot be induced. Important in understanding the upper limit of vulnerability concept is the observation that, after unsuccessful defibrillation, all wave fronts in the ventricle are terminated but new wave fronts arise from low voltage gradient field area and it is these new wave fronts that reinitiate VF. Thus, VF is stopped and reinitiated. How can this happen? It is proposed that during fibrillation, an electrical shock likely induces graded responses in some cells that contribute to prolonging the action potential duration and effective refractory period but do not result in an all-or-none excitation because the neighboring cells have not recovered excitability. However, when the strength of the stimulus is large, a graded response can propagate into sufficiently recovered tissue to produce an all-or-none response in that tissue. This generally occurs more than a few millimeters away from the site of stimulation, a virtual electrode effect, and may be responsible for reinitiating fibrillation. The appropriately timed shock excites the myocardium, evokes a graded response, or has no effect. The propagating wave front leaves the area of direct excitation but can undergo unidirectional block in the graded response zone due to spatial gradients in myocardial refractoriness and shock voltage gradient. Reentry arises when the intersection of the gradient in refractoriness with the gradient in shock strength occurs at a point on the ventricle experiencing a critical degree of refractoriness and the critical shock voltage gradient. A point cathodal electrode can modify the refractory period differently in directions perpendicular and parallel to the fibers,[23] and quatrefoil reentry may be induced by a related mechanism.[24] Thus, the nonuniformity of voltage change produced by point stimulation, in which the voltage change has opposite signs on different axes, may be disadvantageous and reinitiate VF.[25] A stronger stimulus may induce excessive prolongation of refractoriness at the site of stimulation and the long refractory period caused by the graded response can cause bidirectional block and prevent reentrant excitation. Line stimulation may produce a more uniform response.[25]

Thus, the major aspect of the upper limit of vulnerability hypothesis that disagrees with the critical mass hypothesis is the concept that a defibrillation shock could be unsuccessful even if it has terminated all fibrillation wave fronts. Defibrillation could occur transiently but the shock would simultaneously reinitiate VF. According to the critical mass hypothesis, defibrillation would be guaranteed if all fibrillation wave fronts were terminated.

The basis for the upper limit of vulnerability hypothesis lies in studies showing cessation of all recorded electrical activity following an unsuccessful defibrillation shock. This observation was interpreted to indicate termination and then reinitiation of fibrillation.[9] Critics point out that electrical activation could have continued without interruption within the ventricle in unmapped areas even when the electrical mapping system indicated that all wave fronts were apparently eliminated on the epicardium.[10] Therefore, the alleged spontaneous regeneration of fibrillation after the shock, explained by the graded response reinitiation of fibrillation, could be a result of epicardial breakthrough of fibrillation wave fronts from within the ventricle that had continued unmapped. Consistent with this view is the fact that not all studies have found abolition of all electrical activity in failed defibrillation shocks.[10] In these latter studies, the shock was able to modify the temporal and spatial patterns of activation and permit the process of fibrillation to continue.

An advantage of the upper limit of vulnerability hypothesis is that it apparently unifies shock-induced fibrillation and defibrillation because the upper limit of vulnerability correlates with the defibrillation threshold in animals and humans. However, if it can be demonstrated that there is no obligate initial defibrillation event in failed defibrillation, the upper limit of vulnerability hypothesis loses its strongest distinction from the critical mass hypothesis.[10] None of the other known factors in defibrillation are different between the two hypotheses even though the critical mass hypothesis does not account for the linkage between VF induction and defibrillation. One could argue, however, that this linkage is not necessarily important. Fibrillation is different from defibrillation and the correlation achieved by the upper limit of vulnerability hypothesis could be just happenstance or at least not related to similar mechanisms.

Clinically Relevant Issues

The study of defibrillation mechanisms briefly outlined above is of unquestioned importance. However, in my view, even more important is the study of fibrillation—not what causes it to perpetuate, but what causes it to *start*. The main clinical issue confronting us today is the 300,000 to 400,000 sudden cardiac deaths annually in the US, and the problem of identifying the at-risk patient before the sudden death event, so as to prevent it. Our problems include the fact that known risk factors are nonspecific, nonsensitive, and nonmechanistic, i.e., they do not provide an understanding of the *mechanism* causing the sudden cardiac death. For example, heart rate variability, or even the presence of premature ventricular complexes, fails to offer clues about the initiation and maintenance of the ventricular arrhythmia, thus precluding interventions based on their presence. Even when the spontaneous onset of ventricular tachycardia/fibrillation is recorded, distinguishing features about mechanistic causality are usually absent.[26] More importantly, modification of some risk factors, when used as a surrogate for sudden cardiac death, can actually worsen the clinical outcome, as was found in the Cardiac Arrhythmia Suspension Trial II.[27] These facts make it difficult, in most instances, to identify the person at risk prior to an arrhythmic event in a cost-effective manner and with a degree of sensitivity, specificity, and predictive accuracy that justifies a therapeutic intervention, such as implanting an ICD.

While we understand the basis for many arrhythmic mechanisms, e.g., reentry, triggered activity, and automaticity, we do not understand very well the interactions between the anatomical/functional cardiac substrate of a patient and the *transient* risk factors that may finally precipitate sudden cardiac death in a particular individual (Fig. 1). Further, our testing paradigms are limited because initiation of arrhythmias in most, but not all,[28] animal models does not occur spontaneously but is investigator-controlled, using artificial methods such as coronary occlusion/release, prolonged rapid pacing, drug administration, or autonomic manipulation. Most of these experimental manipulations do not accurately replicate the clinical onset of arrhythmias in patients with coronary disease and dilated cardiomyopathy, the two largest groups of patients with sudden cardiac death. These factors, plus the varied routes leading to the final common pathway of ventricular tachycardia/fibrillation or to a bradyarrhythmia, make testing interventions difficult and hinder the arrhythmologist's ultimate quest, that of matching the precise arrhythmia mechanism with a specific therapeutic intervention. We may be close to achieving this goal in some disease states, such as the long QT syndrome,[29] but the latter is rare and represents the exception rather than the rule. While we do have acceptable therapy to terminate the ventricular arrhythmia after its onset, i.e., the ICD, the biggest challenge is to identify the at-risk patient before the event and then to be able to prevent the ventricular arrhythmia from occurring at all. Those two steps, *identification* and *prevention,* are very difficult to achieve given the present state of the art, but, in addition to prevention of the primary disease state, which is a *very* long-term goal, are the most important long-term goals that we have.

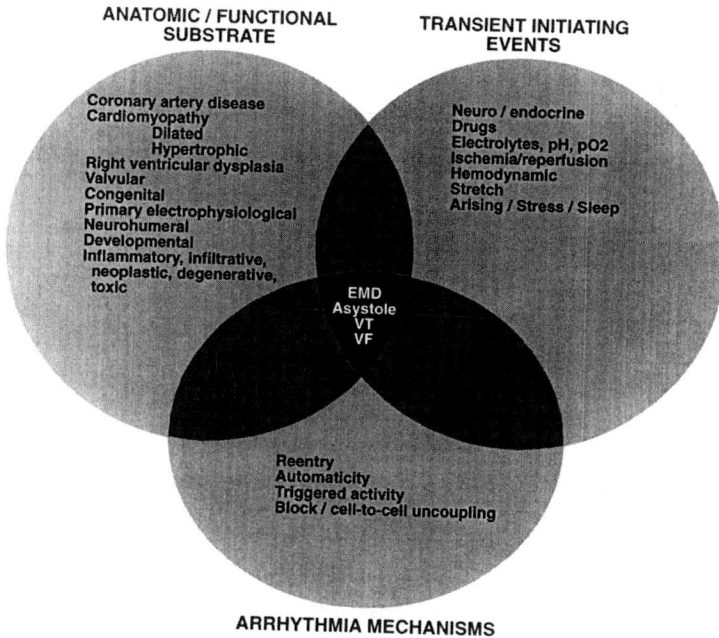

Figure 1. Interaction between cardiac substrate and transient events that can precipitate sudden cardiac death. Reproduced, with permission, from reference 31.

Mechanisms of Sudden Cardiac Death

It is likely that structural abnormalities of the myocardium and its innervation lead to electrophysiological disturbances responsible for cardiac arrhythmias. Some of these abnormalities, once identified, can be corrected or modified, resulting in the elimination of the propensity of arrhythmia development. It is also likely that characterization of these abnormalities in animal models will lead to identification of mechanistically based risk factors that will increase the specificity and sensitivity in identifying patients at risk of sudden cardiac death. Inevitably, these observations will lead to new therapeutic interventions.

The exploration of mechanisms responsible for sudden cardiac death, in my view, must be divided into three parts that include a search for the trigger precipitating the lethal cardiac arrhythmia, a study of the underlying substrate upon which the trigger acts, and investigation of the interaction(s) between the two that caused the event to generate the arrhythmia (Fig. 1). Triggers are very difficult to evaluate because they are evanescent and variable, and there exist few models other than humans of truly spontaneous sudden cardiac death. Substrates are much easier to control and characterize, and therefore represent the bulk of most research efforts to date. One of the generally accepted triggers is the autonomic nervous system via its influence on cardiac excitable properties. Thus, while studies must be directed on the receptive substrate necessary to create an arrhythmia, investigation of myocardial structure-function patterns, particularly when modulated by the autonomic nervous system, is mandatory.

While the responses to autonomic stimulation have been well studied, the arrhythmogenic/antiarrhythmic influences of the autonomic nervous system are still not well understood. For example, it is generally accepted that increasing sympathetic or decreasing vagal activity most often is arrhythmogenic, while the reverse usually protects against the development of a wide variety of ventricular arrhythmias.[30] However, the mechanism(s) that actually mediates autonomic impact on arrhythmogenesis is not known and could include direct electrophysiological impact on impulse formation, excitability, refractoriness and conduction, as well as indirect actions on infarct size or ischemic metabolism, coronary/myocardial blood flow, platelet clumping, free radical formation, and other actions. It is very likely that autonomic modulation can induce competing antiarrhythmic and arrhythmogenic effects. For example, sympathetic stimulation might be antiarrhythmic by improving contractility and coronary blood flow in a failing heart, but the increased myocardial oxygen demand or promotion of abnormal automaticity or reentry could cause arrhythmias.[31]

The complexity of these systems is apparent from a review of the literature. Until the 1970s, an increase in vagal activity was thought to be proarrhythmic. More recent studies have reversed that concept.[30] Yet, on close inspection, the putative protective effects of vagal stimulation against ventricular tachyarrhythmias are predicated on surprisingly incomplete data. Such data include the observations that vagal stimulation opposes sympathetic actions at pre- and postjunctional sites,[32] minimally prolongs ventricular refractoriness,[33] has modest effects on raising VF thresholds,[34] and prevents VF in an occlusion/reperfusion ischemic canine model, mostly, though not entirely, through rate reduction.[30] Two recent studies using scopolamine patches to increase vagal tone failed to demonstrate antiarrhythmic effects.[35,36]

Abnormalities in central neural regulation of sympathetic-parasympathetic interactions have been implicated in precipitating or facilitating sudden cardiac death for many years. For example, frontocortical brain stimulation in pigs was shown to prevent VF during acute coronary artery ligation.[37,38] Clinically, we know that emotional stress can cause arrhythmias, and recent experiments show that such stress can induce expression of immediate early genes/proto-oncogenes in the rat brain and heart via activation of alpha- and beta-adrenoreceptors.[39] Until now, it has been difficult to study potential central neural mechanisms in humans. However, recent advances in positron-emission tomography technology[40] now make it possible to image various centers in the human brain that could serve as transient precipitators or preventors of ventricular arrhythmias. Central sympathetic stimulation, for example, could help explain the relatively small number of individuals who have sudden cardiac death during exercise, compared with those who have sudden cardiac death while engaged in normal physical activities or during sleep.[30,41] Interestingly, paroxetine (Paxil®, GlaxoSmithKline, Research Triangle Park, NC), a selective serotonin reuptake inhibitor used as an antidepressant, has recently been shown to restore heart rate variability and baroreflexes in patients with panic disorders who had blunted vagal responses due to excessive sympathetic activity.[42] These autonomic changes have been linked to reduced risk of having a life-threatening arrhythmia. Paroxetine potentiates serotoninergic activity in the brain, with only weak effects on norepinephrine and dopamine reuptake.

It is obvious that the normal heart, despite its cellular complexity and heterogeneity, rarely, if ever, develops VF. However, when it becomes injured from a variety of processes such as rate, ischemia/infarction, or dilation/stretch,[43] the normal electrophysiological processes can become sufficiently modified to now make the patient a sudden cardiac death candidate. In recent years, we have become aware that the heart can undergo progressive changes in structure and function, including electrophysiological characteristics, due to a variety of stimuli, such as rate,[44-46] ischemia, dilation,[43] genetic predisposition, and others. Remodeling, as this process is often called, likely plays a critical role in the pathogenesis of many arrhythmias, particularly as it influences and potentially remodels the autonomic nervous system and its interaction with altered cardiac excitable properties. Remodeling has different causes, depending on the initiating event and its duration. Remodeling can range from short-term alterations of ion concentration and channel function, perhaps due to metabolic influences, to longer term changes due to altered gene expression in regulating protein synthesis and assembly, to very long-term structural revisions from damage caused by fibrosis, fatty infiltration, and similar processes.[47-50] Remodeling-induced alternations can significantly impact cardiac structure and function in the atrium[44-47,51,52] and ventricle.[43,53-55]

It is clear that study of the causes of the *initiation* of fibrillation, the mechanisms responsible for its perpetuation, and how it can be terminated are all important. It is our hypothesis that sudden cardiac death results from an interaction between a transient trigger, which very often is provided by the autonomic nervous system, and a remodeled, receptive myocardial substrate in which basic electrophysiological characteristics such as cell-to-cell communication and/or repolarization have been modified by ischemia/infarction, scar, dilation, rate, etc. This interaction between a transient trigger and a remodeled substrate in turn activates one of several fundamental arrhythmia mechanisms, including reentry, abnormal automaticity, and triggered activity, which provokes a ventricular tachyarrhythmia, causing sudden cardiac death. Some of these abnormalities of trigger, substrate, or interaction, once identified, can be corrected or modified, with a concomitant reduction/elimination of the risk for sudden cardiac death. It is toward this end that we must direct major research initiatives. Accurate identification of the patient at risk, with an acceptable degree of specificity, sensitivity, and predictive accuracy, as well as the development of acceptable, cost-effective treatments that can be applied to large numbers of patients at risk to prevent the (tachyarrhythmic, in most instances) episode responsible for sudden cardiac death, is a major goal. While this emphasis in no way minimizes the importance of the work highlighted in this section, I have tried to stress that we have extremely effective electrical therapies that have already achieved a high degree of clinical success, even if they have not reached their utopian applicability or mechanistic understanding. Yet, we are still in the relatively dark ages when it comes to identifying the fairly asymptomatic patient at risk for a cardiac catastrophe and, once the patient has been identified, to preventing the catastrophe. It is toward understanding *how* and *why* fibrillation *starts* that we have to concentrate our research efforts in the next decade.

References

1. Morady F. Radio-frequency ablation as treatment for cardiac arrhythmias. *N Engl J Med* 1999;340:532–544.
2. Zipes DP. Atrial fibrillation: From cell to bedside. *J Cardiovasc Electrophysiol* 1997;8:927–938.
3. Prevost JL, Batelli F. Sur qul ques effets des dechanges electriques sur le coer mammifres. *Comptes Rendus Seances Acad Sci* 1899;129:1267.
4. Mirowski M, Reid PR, Mower MM, et al. Termination of malignant ventricular arrhythmias with an implanted automatic defibrillator in human beings. *N Engl J Med* 1980;303:322–324.
5. Zipes DP, Heger JJ, Miles WM, et al. Early experience with an implantable cardioverter. *N Engl J Med* 1984;311:485–490.
6. Zipes DP, Roberts D. Results of the international study of the implantable pacemaker cardioverter-defibrillator. A comparison of epicardial and endocardial lead systems. The Pacemaker-Cardioverter-Defibrillator Investigators. *Circulation* 1995;92:59–65.
7. A comparison of antiarrhythmic-drug therapy with implantable defibrillators in patients resuscitated from near-fatal ventricular arrhythmias. The Antiarrhythmics versus Implantable Defibrillators (AVID) Investigators [see comments]. *N Engl J Med* 1997;337:1576–1583.
8. Garrey WE. The nature of fibrillatory contraction of the heart. Its relation to tissue mass and form. *Am J Physiol* 1914;33:397–414.
9. Chen PS, Shibata N, Dixon EG, et al. Comparison of the defibrillation threshold and the upper limit of ventricular vulnerability. *Circulation* 1986;73:1022–1028.
10. Dillon SM, Kwaku KF. Progressive depolarization: A unified hypothesis for defibrillation and fibrillation induction by shocks. *J Cardiovasc Electrophysiol* 1998;9:529–552.
11. Zipes DP, Fischer J, King RM, et al. Termination of ventricular fibrillation in dogs by depolarizing a critical amount of myocardium. *Am J Cardiol* 1975;36:37–44.
12. Chen PS, Swerdlow CD, Hwang C, Karagueuzian HS. Current concepts of ventricular defibrillation. *J Cardiovasc Electrophysiol* 1998;9:553–562.
13. Frazier DW, Wolf PD, Wharton JM, et al. Stimulus-induced critical point. Mechanism for electrical initiation of reentry in normal canine myocardium. *J Clin Invest* 1989;83:1039–1052.
14. Dillon SM. Optical recordings in the rabbit heart show that defibrillation strength shocks prolong the duration of depolarization and the refractory period. *Circ Res* 1991;69:842–856.
15. Efimov IR, Cheng Y. Mechanisms of defibrillation: 3. Virtual electrode-induced wavefronts and phase singularities; Mechanisms of success and failure of defibrillation. In Rosenbaum DS, Jalife J (eds): *Optical Mapping of Cardiac Excitation and Arrhythmias*. Armonk, NY: Futura Publishing Co., Inc.; 2001: 407–432.
16. Newton JC, Knisley SB, Zhou X, et al. Review of mechanisms by which electrical stimulation alters the transmembrane potential. *J Cardiovasc Electrophysiol* 1999;10:234–243.

17. Lin S-F, Wikswo JP Jr. New perspectives in electrophysiology from the cardiac bidomain. In Rosenbaum DS, Jalife J (eds): *Optical Mapping of Cardiac Excitation and Arrhythmias*. Armonk, NY: Futura Publishing Co., Inc.; 2001:335–359.

18. Fast VG, Rohr S, Gillis AM, Kléber AG. Activation of cardiac tissue by extracellular electrical shocks: Formation of 'secondary sources' at intercellular clefts in monolayers of cultured myocytes. *Circ Res* 1998;82:375–385.

19. Sobie EA, Susil RC, Tung L. A generalized activating function for predicting virtual electrodes in cardiac tissue. *Biophys J* 1997;73:1410–1423.

20. Sepulveda NG, Roth BJ, Wikswo JP Jr. Current injection into a two-dimensional anisotropic bidomain. *Biophys J* 1989;55:987–999.

21. Tung L. Response of cardiac myocytes to electrical fields. In Rosenbaum DS, Jalife J (eds): *Optical Mapping of Cardiac Excitation and Arrhythmias*. Armonk, NY: Futura Publishing Co., Inc.; 2001:313–333.

22. Dillon S. Mechanisms of defibrillation: 2. Application of laser scanning technology. In Rosenbaum DS, Jalife J (eds): *Optical Mapping of Cardiac Excitation and Arrhythmias*. Armonk, NY: Futura Publishing Co., Inc.; 2001:381–405.

23. Saypol JM, Roth BJ. A mechanism for isotropic reentry in electrically active tissue. *J Cardiovasc Electrophysiol* 1992;3:558–566.

24. Lin S-F, Roth BJ, Wikswo JP. Quatrefoil reentry in myocardium: An optical imaging study of the induction mechanism. *J Cardiovasc Electrophysiol* 1999;10:574–586.

25. Knisley SB. Mechanisms of defibrillation: 1. Influence of fiber structure on tissue response to electrical stimulation. In Rosenbaum DS, Jalife J (eds): *Optical Mapping of Cardiac Excitation and Arrhythmias*. Armonk, NY: Futura Publishing Co., Inc.; 2001:361–380.

26. Bardy GH, Olson WH. Clinical characteristics of spontaneous-onset sustained ventricular tachycardia and ventricular fibrillation in survivors of cardiac arrest. In Zipes DP, Jalife J (eds): *Cardiac Electrophysiology. From Cell to Bedside*. 2nd ed. Philadelphia: W.B. Saunders Co.; 1990:778–790.

27. Effect of the antiarrhythmic agent moricizine on survival after myocardial infarction. The Cardiac Arrhythmia Suppression Trial II Investigators. *N Engl J Med* 1992;327:227–233.

28. Dae MW, Lee RJ, Ursell PC, et al. Heterogeneous sympathetic innervation in German shepherd dogs with inherited ventricular arrhythmia and sudden cardiac death. *Circulation* 1997;96:1337–1342.

29. Moss AJ. Management of patients with the hereditary long QT syndrome. *J Cardiovasc Electrophysiol* 1998;9:668–674.

30. Schwartz PJ, Zipes DP. Autonomic modulation of cardiac arrhythmias. In Zipes DP, Jalife J (eds): *Cardiac Electrophysiology. From Cell to Bedside*. 3rd ed. Orlando: W.B. Saunders Co.; 2000:300–314.

31. Zipes DP, Wellens HJ. Sudden cardiac death. *Circulation* 1998;98:2334–2351.

32. Takahashi N, Zipes DP. Vagal modulation of adrenergic effects on canine sinus and atrioventricular nodes. *Am J Physiol* 1983;244:H775–H781.

33. Martins JB, Zipes DP. Effects of sympathetic and vagal nerves on recovery properties of the endocardium and epicardium of the canine left ventricle. *Circ Res* 1980;46:100–110.

34. Mitrani RD, Miles WM, Klein LS, et al. Phenylephrine increases T wave shock energy required to induce ventricular fibrillation. *J Cardiovasc Electrophysiol* 1998;9:34–40.

35. Hull SS Jr, Vanoli E, Adamson PB, et al. Do increases in markers of vagal activity imply protection from sudden death? The case of scopolamine. *Circulation* 1995;91:2516–2519.

36. Casadei B, Pipilis A, Sessa F, et al. Low doses of scopolamine increase cardiac vagal tone in the acute phase of myocardial infarction. *Circulation* 1993;88:353–357.

37. Skinner JE, Reed JC. Blockade of frontocortical-brain stem pathway prevents ventricular fibrillation of ischemic heart. *Am J Physiol* 1981;240:H156–H163.
38. Oppenheimer SM, Cechetto DF, Hachinski VC. Cerebrogenic cardiac arrhythmias. Cerebral electrocardiographic influences and their role in sudden death. *Arch Neurol* 1990;47:513–519.
39. Senba E, Ueyama T. Stress-induced expression of immediate early genes in the brain and peripheral organs of the rat. *Neurosci Res* 1997;29:183–207.
40. Drevets WC, Videen TQ, MacLeod AK, et al. PET images of blood flow changes during anxiety: Correction. *Science* 1992;256:1696.
41. Lavery CE, Mittleman MA, Cohen MC, et al. Nonuniform nighttime distribution of acute cardiac events: A possible effect of sleep states. *Circulation* 1997;96:3321–3327.
42. Tucker P, Adamson P, Miranda R Jr, et al. Paroxetine increases heart rate variability in panic disorder. *J Clin Psychopharmacol* 1997;17:370–376.
43. Satoh T, Zipes DP. Unequal atrial stretch in dogs increases dispersion of refractoriness conducive to developing atrial fibrillation. *J Cardiovasc Electrophysiol* 1996;7:833–842.
44. Wijffels MC, Kirchhof CJ, Dorland R, Allessie MA. Atrial fibrillation begets atrial fibrillation. A study in awake chronically instrumented goats. *Circulation* 1995;92:1954–1968.
45. Morillo CA, Klein GJ, Jones DL, Guiraudon CM. Chronic rapid atrial pacing. Structural, functional, and electrophysiological characteristics of a new model of sustained atrial fibrillation. *Circulation* 1995;91:1588–1595.
46. Elvan A, Wylie K, Zipes DP. Pacing-induced chronic atrial fibrillation impairs sinus node function in dogs. Electrophysiological remodeling. *Circulation* 1996;94:2953–2960.
47. Elvan A, Huang XD, Pressler ML, Zipes DP. Radiofrequency catheter ablation of the atria eliminates pacing-induced sustained atrial fibrillation and reduces connexin 43 in dogs. *Circulation* 1997;96:1675–1685.
48. Katz AM. T wave "memory": Possible causal relationship to stress-induced changes in cardiac ion channels. *J Cardiovasc Electrophysiol* 1992;3:150–159.
49. Zipes DP. Electrophysiological remodeling of the heart owing to rate. *Circulation* 1997;95:1745–1748.
50. Allessie MA. Atrial electrophysiological remodeling: Another vicious circle? *J Cardiovasc Electrophysiol* 1998;9:1378–1393.
51. Jayachandran JV, Zipes DP, Weksler J, Olgin JE, Role of the Na^+/H^+ exchanger in short-term atrial electrophysiological remodeling. *Circulation* 2000; 101:1861–1866.
52. Sih HJ, Zipes DP, Berbari EJ, et al. Differences in organization between acute and chronic atrial fibrillation in dogs. *J Am Coll Cardiol* 2000;36:924–931.
53. Satoh T, Zipes DP. Rapid rates during bradycardia prolong ventricular refractoriness and facilitate ventricular tachycardia induction with cesium in dogs. *Circulation* 1996;94:217–227.
54. Krebs ME, Szwed JM, Shinn T, et al. Short-term rapid ventricular pacing prolongs ventricular refractoriness in patients. *J Cardiovasc Electrophysiol* 1998;9:1036–1042.
55. Rubart M, Fineberg N, Zipes DP. Ionic remodeling following one hour of ventricular tachycardia superimposed on bradycardia in the adult dog heart. *J Cardiovasc Electrophysiol* 2000;11:652–664.

Index

Page numbers in italics indicate a table or figure; terms followed by [**glossary**] indicate glossary terms.